White Coat Companion

Michael Lorinsky, MD
Sana Majid, MD
and
Jason Ryan, MD
Creator of Boards & Beyond

2019 Edition

Disclaimer:
The topics discussed in this book are not intended as a substitute for the medical advice of physicians, and should not be used to diagnose or treat patients. Application of any of this information for the care of patients is the sole responsibility of the physician or practitioner.

Considerable effort has been taken to confirm the accuracy of the information in this book and the content reflects generally accepted best medical practices. However, medical practice is constantly evolving and practice may change after the printing of this text.

This book is produced independently from the institutions in which the authors of the book are affiliated. This book is not produced by or affiliated with the National Board of Medical Examiners or the USMLE.

Copyright © 2019 by Lorinsky Clinician Education LLC

All rights reserved. This book is protected by copyright. No part of this book may be reproduced or used in any manner without written permission of the copyright owner, including photocopying or reproduction in electronic forms.

First edition: 2019

ISBN-13: 978-0-578-50605-0
ISBN-10: 0-578-50605-X

Introduction

While studying during my clinical years of medical school, I found there was a dearth of succinct, well-structured, and current resources. During my preclinical years, I found tremendous value in First Aid for Step 1, largely because it was one consolidated resource to use as a reference throughout studying for medical school exams as well as the Step 1 exam. I sought a resource similar to that for Step 2, but instead found current textbooks out of date, poorly organized, and too verbose to serve as my singular primary resource.

Ultimately, that led me to the creation of this review text. The information provided here is synthesized from a variety of textbooks, online videos, and formal teaching that I received as a medical student. It then was refined using primary resources to ensure that everything contained is as updated and evidence-based as possible. It is designed to be a singular comprehensive resource that can serve as your foundation while going through core clerkships, and later can be used as a review for Step 2CK and Step 3.

I hope you find this book fills the void for which it was created.

Michael Lorinsky, MD

About the Authors

Dr. Michael Lorinsky is an Internal Medicine resident and clinical fellow at Harvard Medical School's Beth Israel Deaconess Medical Center in Boston, MA, where he is a member of the Clinician-Educator Track. He received his undergraduate degree in biophysics from Brown University and his MD from the University of Connecticut School of Medicine, where he graduated with the Dean's Award for most outstanding academic achievement. Michael's academic interests include medical education, diagnostic reasoning, and outcomes research. He has also been extremely successful on the USMLE exams, scoring 275 on Step 1 and 283 on Step 2 CK.

Dr. Sana Majid is a future Radiology resident at Brigham and Women's Hospital in Boston, MA. She is currently completing an internship in Internal Medicine at Beth Israel Deaconess Medical Center. She received her undergraduate degree in Biochemistry and Molecular Biology from Brown University and her MD from the University of Massachusetts Medical School, where she was elected to the Alpha Omega Alpha Medical Honor Society. She is a passionate medical educator, and tutors for both the USMLE Step 1 and 2 exams.

Dr. Jason Ryan is the creator of the website Boards and Beyond. Thousands of students from around the globe use his online videos and practice questions to prepare for the USMLE Step 1 exam. Dr. Ryan trained in Internal Medicine and cardiology at Harvard's Beth Israel Deaconess Medical Center, where he also served as a chief resident. In addition to his MD, he holds a Master of Public Health degree and a Bachelor of Science degree in Chemical Engineering. He has been a faculty member at the University of Connecticut School of Medicine in Farmington, Connecticut for over 10 years.

Topic	Page(s)	Topic	Page(s)	Topic	Page(s)
Cardiovascular		**Pulmonary/Critical Care**		**Renal**	
Coronary Artery Disease	Cards 1	Physical Exam	Pulm 1	Volume	Renal 1
Acute Coronary Syndrome	Cards 2	COPD	Pulm 2	Sodium/Potassium	Renal 2
Heart Failure	Cards 4	Asthma/Bronchiectasis	Pulm 4	Calcium/Magnesium/Phosphate	Renal 8
Cardiomyopathy	Cards 6	Restrictive Lung Disease	Pulm 6	Acid Base	Renal 12
Malignancy	Cards 7	Pulmonary Hypertension	Pulm 11	Acute Renal Failure	Renal 14
Pericardial Disease	Cards 8	DVT/PE	Pulm 12	Chronic Kidney Disease	Renal 15
Inflammatory Cardiac Disease	Cards 10	Pleural Effusion	Pulm 15	Glomerular Pathology	Renal 17
Valvular Heart Disease	Cards 13	Pneumothorax	Pulm 16	Tubulointerstitial Disease	Renal 20
Electrophysiology	Cards 15	Hemoptysis	Pulm 17	Renal Vascular Disease	Renal 22
Hyperlipidemia	Cards 20	Respiratory Failure	Pulm 18	Cystic Kidney Disease	Renal 23
Hypertension	Cards 21	Shock	Pulm 20	Nephrolithiasis	Renal 24
Congenital Defects	Cards 22	Sepsis	Pulm 21	Incontinence	Renal 25
Pediatric Murmurs	Cards 25	Malignancy	Pulm 22	Urinary Tract Infections	Renal 26
Pediatric Arrhythmia	Cards 26	Allergy	Pulm 24	Malignancy: Renal, Bladder, Prostate	Renal 28
Atherosclerotic Disease	Cards 27	Respiratory Tract Infections	Pulm 25	Pediatric Renal Neoplasia	Renal 31
Aortic Disease	Cards 29	Acute Pediatric Lung Disease	Pulm 35	Congenital Renal/Urologic Disease	Renal 32
Aneurysms	Cards 31	Chronic Pediatric Lung Disease	Pulm 36	Testicular Cancer	Renal 38
Vascular Emergencies	Cards 32	Congenital ENT Lesions	Pulm 38	BPH/Prostate Cancer	Renal 39
CV Pharmacology	Cards 33	Adult ENT	Pulm 39	Penile/Testicular/Scrotal Pathology	Renal 40
		Pulm Pharmacology	Pulm 46	Hematuria	Renal 43
				Renal/Urology Pharmacology	Renal 44

vii

Topic	Page(s)	Topic	Page(s)	Topic	Page(s)
Endocrine		**Gastrointestinal Medicine**		**Hematology/Oncology**	
Hypothalamic Pituitary Axis	Endo 1	Esophageal Disease	GI 1	Anemia	Heme 1
Thyroid (Hypo/Hyper)	Endo 2	Gastric Disease	GI 7	Microcytic Anemia	Heme 2
Thyroid Nodules	Endo 6	Small Bowel Pathology	GI 12	Macrocytic Anemia	Heme 4
Diabetes Insipidus	Endo 7	Functional Bowel Disorders	GI 19	Normocytic Anemia	Heme 5
Hyperaldosteronism	Endo 8	Inflammatory Bowel Disease	GI 20	Disorders of Heme Synthesis	Heme 10
Hyper and Hypocortisolism	Endo 9	Colorectal Pathology	GI 21	Thrombocytopenia	Heme 11
Hypopituitarism	Endo 11	Approach to GI Bleeds	GI 25	Coagulopathy/Thrombophilia	Heme 14
Pituitary Adenoma	Endo 12	Anal/Rectal Pathology	GI 26	Oncology Overview/Emergencies	Heme 17
Growth Hormone	Endo 13	Biliary Pathology	GI 28	Plasma Cell Dyscrasias	Heme 20
Calcium Homeostasis	Endo 14	Pancreatic Pathology	GI 33	Myeloproliferative Disease	Heme 21
Hypo and Hyperparathyroidism	Endo 15	Cirrhosis	GI 36	Leukemia	Heme 23
Male Reproductive Endocrinology	Endo 17	Acute Liver Failure	GI 39	Lymphoma	Heme 26
Adrenal Neoplasia	Endo 19	Etiologies of Liver Disease	GI 40	Misc Malignancies	Heme 28
Pancreatic Neuroendocrine Tumor	Endo 21	Viral Hepatitis	GI 42	Amyloidosis	Heme 29
Hypoglycemia	Endo 23	Liver Malignancy and Masses	GI 44	Blood Product Transfusions	Heme 30
Diabetes Mellitus	Endo 24	Diarrhea	GI 46	Transplant	Heme 32
Pediatric Thyroid Disease	Endo 28	Constipation	GI 49	Immunologic Reactions	Heme 33
Pediatric Reproductive Disease	Endo 29	Neonatal/Congenital GI	GI 50	Immunodeficiencies	Heme 34
Pediatric Adrenal Disease	Endo 31	GI Pharmacology	GI 58	Cryoglobulinemia	Heme 37
Growth	Endo 33			Heme/Onc Pharmacology	Heme 38
Endocrine Pharmacology	Endo 34				

viii

Topic	Page(s)	Topic	Page(s)	Topic	Page(s)
Rheumatology/MSK		**Dermatology**		**Infectious Disease**	
Arthritis	Rheum 1	Dermatology Basics	Derm 1	Fevers	ID 1
Crystal Arthropathy	Rheum 4	Pigmented Disorders	Derm 2	Gram Positive	ID 2
Reynaud	Rheum 5	Benign/Miscellaneous Disorders	Derm 4	Gram Negative	ID 5
Connective Tissue Disease	Rheum 6	Inflammatory Disorders	Derm 7	Atypical Bacteria	ID 9
Seronegative Spondyloarthropathy	Rheum 9	Blistering Disorders	Derm 13	Fungal Organisms	ID 12
Sarcoidosis	Rheum 10	Sun-Related Skin Disorders	Derm 14	Protozoal Organisms	ID 14
Myopathy	Rheum 11	Microbial Skin Reactions	Derm 15	Helminth Infections	ID 17
Vasculitis	Rheum 14	Fungal Skin Disorders	Derm 16	DNA Virus	ID 20
Bones	Rheum 18	Parasitic Skin Disorders	Derm 17	DNA Virus (Herpes)	ID 21
Bone and Joint Infections	Rheum 20	Bacterial Skin Disorders	Derm 18	RNA Virus	ID 23
Bone and Soft Tissue Malignancy	Rheum 22	Soft Tissue Ulcers	Derm 21	HIV/AIDS	ID 27
MSK: Back	Rheum 23	Hair Disorders	Derm 22	STIs	ID 35
MSK: Upper Extremity	Rheum 28	Vascular Skin Tumors	Derm 23	Infection Prophylaxis	ID 38
MSK: Lower Extremity	Rheum 33	Dermatologic Malignancy	Derm 24	Antibiotics	ID 39
MSK: Neurovascular	Rheum 36			Antifungals	ID 43
Rheumatology Pharmacology	Rheum 38			Antivirals	ID 44

Topic	Page(s)	Topic	Page(s)	Topic	Page(s)
Neurology		**Neurology**		**Primary Care/Emergency Medicine**	
Neurologic Examination	Neuro 1	Vertigo	Neuro 36	Adult Preventative Care	PC/EM 1
Stroke	Neuro 2	Seizure	Neuro 37	Smoking	PC/EM 3
Subdural/Epidural Bleeds	Neuro 8	Neuropathy/Neuropathic Pain	Neuro 40	Obesity	PC/EM 4
Intracranial Hypertension	Neuro 9	CNS Infection	Neuro 42	Geriatrics	PC/EM 5
Traumatic Brain Injury	Neuro 10	CNS Malignancy	Neuro 46	Vitamins/Minerals	PC/EM 6
Complications of Head Trauma	Neuro 11	Hearing Loss	Neuro 49	Toxicology	PC/EM 9
Hypokinetic Movement Disorders	Neuro 12	Auditory Pathology	Neuro 50	Ingestions	PC/EM 12
Hyperkinetic Movement Disorders	Neuro 14	Ophthalmology	Neuro 51	Heat Illness	PC/EM 13
Gait/Cerebellar Dysfunction	Neuro 17	Congenital Neurological Defects	Neuro 62	Cold	PC/EM 14
Cerebellar Disorders	Neuro 18	Neurocutaneous Disorders	Neuro 63	Drowning/Lightning	PC/EM 15
Central Demyelinating Disease	Neuro 19	Cerebral Palsy	Neuro 64	Bites	PC/EM 16
Peripheral Demyelinating Disease	Neuro 21	Neurology Pharmacology	Neuro 65		
Spinal Cord Lesions	Neuro 22				
Neuromuscular Disease	Neuro 23				
Ventricular Pathology	Neuro 26				
Dementia	Neuro 27				
Prion Disease	Neuro 29				
Altered Mental Status	Neuro 30				
Headache	Neuro 32				
Syncope	Neuro 34				

Topic	Page(s)	Topic	Page(s)	Topic	Page(s)
Psychiatry		**Pediatrics**		**Surgery**	
Mental Status Examination	Psych 1	Neonatology	Peds 1	Pre-Operative Evaluation	Surg 1
Psychiatry Basics	Psych 2	Pediatric Vaccinations	Peds 11	Post-Operative Fever	Surg 2
Psychotic/Delusional Disorders	Psych 3	Developmental Milestone	Peds 12	Post-Operative Complications	Surg 3
Mood Disorders	Psych 5	Screening	Peds 14	Emergencies	Surg 4
Anxiety Disorders	Psych 9	Anticipatory Guidance	Peds 15	Fractures	Surg 4
Personality Disorders	Psych 13	Growth Disturbances	Peds 19	Pediatric Orthopedics	Surg 9
Dissociative Disorders	Psych 16	SIDS/Child Abuse	Peds 21	Trauma	Surg 11
Somatic and Factitious	Psych 17	Colic/Pediatric Constipation	Peds 22	Burns	Surg 19
Impulse Control Disorders	Psych 19	Chromosomal Abnormalities	Peds 23	Anesthesia	Surg 21
Eating Disorders	Psych 20	Genetic Diseases	Peds 25		
Sexual/Sexuality Disorders	Psych 21	Approach to Fevers	Peds 36		
Sleep Disorders	Psych 23				
Child Psychiatry	Psych 27				
Substance Abuse	Psych 32				
Psychotherapy	Psych 37				
Psychopharmacotherapy	Psych 38				

Topic	Page(s)	Topic	Page(s)
Obstetrics and Gynecology		**Obstetrics and Gynecology**	
Normal Pregnancy	OBGYN 1	Amenorrhea	OBGYN 57
Routine Prenatal Care	OBGYN 3	Hyperandrogenism	OBGYN 60
Prenatal Testing	OBGYN 4	Dysmenorrhea	OBGYN 62
Teratogenesis (Drugs)	OBGYN 6	Menorrhagia	OBGYN 64
Teratogenesis (TORCH Infections)	OBGYN 8	Vaginitis	OBGYN 65
Other Perinatal Infections	OBGYN 9	Upper Gynecologic Infections	OBGYN 66
Abortion	OBGYN 11	Congenital Gynecologic Disorders	OBGYN 67
Ectopic Pregnancy	OBGYN 15	Miscellaneous Vaginal Lesions	OBGYN 68
Gestational Trophoblastic Disease	OBGYN 16	Miscellaneous Cervical Lesions	OBGYN 69
Placental Pathology	OBGYN 18	Pelvic Organ Prolapse	OBGYN 70
Multiple Gestation	OBGYN 20	Cervical Neoplasia	OBGYN 71
Normal Labor and Delivery	OBGYN 22	Endometrial Neoplasia	OBGYN 74
Operative Labor and Delivery	OBGYN 25	Ovarian Neoplasia	OBGYN 76
Complications of Labor and Delivery	OBGYN 27	Vulvar/Vaginal Neoplasia	OBGYN 79
Fetal Complications	OBGYN 34	Breast	OBGYN 80
Maternal Pregnancy Complications	OBGYN 37	OB-GYN Pharmacology	OBGYN 86
Postpartum Complications	OBGYN 44		
Postpartum Management	OBGYN 47		
Menstrual Cycle	OBGYN 49		
Contraception	OBGYN 52		
Infertility	OBGYN 55		

CORONARY ARTERY DISEASE
Cardiovascular Medicine

Asymptomatic Coronary Artery Disease

General: Gradual narrowing of arteries by lipid plaques. Generally asymptomatic until > 70% stenosis.

Risk: Atherosclerotic risk factors include diabetes, hypertension, hyperlipidemia, smoking, ↑ age (> 45 M/ 55 F), family history (> 55 M/ 65 F)

Management: Aspirin + Statin. Lifestyle modifications.

Stable Angina

General: Fixed atherosclerotic lesions → Inadequate perfusion (O_2 demand > supply)

Clinical: Chest pain occurring with exertion, relieved with rest or nitroglycerin.

Typical Angina: (3/3)	1) Substernal (diffuse, pressure/squeeze)
Atypical Angina: (2/3)	2) Brought on by exertion/emotion
Non Cardiac: (0-1/3)	3) Relieved with rest or nitro

Note: ECG (perform on all with symptoms, but generally nonspecific or normal)

Diagnosis: Clinical (classic symptoms + risk factors)
 - Stress test (to help confirm disease and evaluate severity)

Management:
 - Angina: Beta-blockers (alternatives: CCB, nitrates, Ranolazine)
 - Disease Progression: ASA, statin, smoking cessation, HTN/DM control
 - Revascularization (PCI or CABG) only indicated if:
   (1) Functional impairment despite medical therapy
   (2) High risk lesions (such as left-main, 3-vessel, proximal LAD)

| PCI | Single vessel circumflex, right main, some LAD |
| CABG | Multivessel, some LAD |

Stress Tests

Type	Features
Exercise Stress	- First line, but must be able to achieve target HR/interpret ECG - ECG always used (look for ST changes) - Can add imaging modality (ECHO/MPI) to increase sensitivity

Pharm Stress	- Use if unable to exercise
	- Must have imaging (ECHO or MPI)
	- Drug Choice:
	  - Adenosine/Dipyridamole/Regadenoson (contraindicated with reactive airway disease)
	  - Dobutamine (risk for ventricular arrhythmias)

Myocardial Perfusion Imaging (MPI): Tc-99/SPECT or Rb-82/PET
 - Visualize myocardial perfusion before/during/after stress
 - Defects that occur with stress but improve with rest → Likely ischemia
 - Stable defects (poor perfusion throughout study) → Likely old scar tissue

ACUTE CORONARY SYNDROME (ACS)
Cardiovascular Medicine

Unstable Angina/NSTEMI

General:
- Unstable Angina: Ischemic symptoms without elevation in biomarkers
- NSTEMI: Ischemic symptoms with elevated cardiac biomarkers
  - Type I NSTEMI: Acute plaque rupture
  - Type II NSTEMI: Imbalance of oxygen supply/demand

Clinical:
- Chest pain (at rest, new onset with physical limitation, or angina that is increasing in frequency or duration)
- Other symptoms: Dyspnea, nausea/vomiting (especially in elderly/women)

Diagnosis: Clinical features, plus ECG and Biomarkers (TnI or CKMB)

Management:

Initial (Acute)	- ASA 325 mg chewed - Statin (as early as possible) - O_2 (to maintain O_2 saturation > 90 %) - Nitroglycerin (persistent pain, HTN, or HF) - Morphine (if unacceptable, persistent pain) - Beta-Blocker (contraindicated with HF, bradycardia) - 2nd ("Dual") Antiplatelet Agent (either Ticagrelor or Clopidogrel) - Anticoagulation (Heparin or LMWH)
Reperfusion	- Immediate PCI: Indicated if shock, severe CHF, ventricular arrhythmias, structural complications (ie papillary muscle rupture) - Reperfuse others within 24-48 hours depending on risk (ie TIMI risk score)

STEMI

General: Defined as chest pain + ECG Δ + Cardiac Enzyme ↑ (TnI/CKMB)

Clinical:
- Persistent substernal chest pain > 20 min
- Radiation of pain (jaw, arm, or neck), diaphoresis, dyspnea

Location	Artery	ECG
Anteroseptal	LAD	V1-V2
Anteroapical	LAD	V3-V4
Anteriorlateral	LCX	I, V5-V6
Inferior	RCA	II, III, aVF
Posterior	PDA	V1-V3 ST Dep.

Diagnosis:
- Cardiac biomarkers (TnI appears within 2-3 hours, CK-MB within ~6 hours)
- ECG: ST elevation in ≥ 2 contiguous leads, > 0.1 mV (> 0.2 mV in V2/V3)

Treatment: Initial management similar to UA/NSTEMI above

Reperfusion (PCI)	- Ideally door-to-balloon of 90 min or 120 min if transferred - Benefits all within 12 hours of symptom onset - If at 12-24 hours: Reperfuse if ongoing ischemia, HF, or hypotension
Fibrinolysis (Tenecteplase, Alteplase)	- Used if PCI not available in timely manner - Contraindications similar to those in stroke [See: Neuro]

Note: Drug eluting/bare metal stents require 6-12 months of dual antiplatelet therapy.

ACUTE CORONARY SYNDROME (ACS)

Cardiovascular Medicine

Myocardial Infarction Complications

Disorder [Timing]	Clinical Features
Arrhythmia [any time]	- Commonly ventricular arrhythmias - Most common cause of death within 24 hours - [See: Arrhythmia] for management of VTach/VFib
RV Failure [any time]	- Seen with inferior MI (typically RCA) - Presents with hypotension, elevated JVP, peripheral edema - Tx: Avoid beta-blockers, nitro (preload dependent), watch for AV block or bradycardia
LV Failure [any time]	- Tx: Diuresis (Furosemide), avoid beta-blockers, inotropic or mechanical support if severe
Fibrinous Pericarditis [< 1 week]	- Tx: ASA plus Colchicine
Papillary Muscle Rupture [< 1 week]	- Presents with acute onset HF due to mitral regurgitation - Dx: ECHO - Tx: Stabilize with nitrates, diuresis, followed by surgical repair
Interventricular Septal Rupture [< 1 week]	- Presents with VSD formation (holosystolic murmur at LLSB), biventricular CHF, hemodynamic instability - Dx: ECHO - Tx: Stabilize with afterload reduction (nitrates), followed by surgical repair
Ventricular Free Wall Rupture [1-2 weeks]	- Complete rupture presents with hemopericardium and cardiac tamponade, while incomplete rupture presents with recurrent chest pain - Dx: ECHO, +/- pericardiocentesis - Tx: Surgical
Ventricular Pseudoaneurysm [1-2 weeks]	- Free wall rupture contained by scar/pericardium - Dx: ECHO, angiography - Tx: Surgical (high risk of rupture)
True Ventricular Aneurysm [weeks to months]	- Dyskinetic, scarred LV wall that balloons during systole - Tx: Medical (ACEi +/- anticoagulation) Surgery: Indicated if frequent arrhythmia or CHF
Dressler Syndrome [weeks to months]	- Post MI autoimmune pericardial inflammation - Tx: NSAIDs or ASA, +/- Colchicine

HEART FAILURE — Cardiovascular Medicine

HF: Overview, Chronic Management

General: Clinical syndrome of dyspnea and fatigue resulting from cardiac disorder that impairs ventricular filling or ejection

Subtype	Definition	Causes
HFpEF	Ejection Fraction > 50%	- Diastolic dysfunction (associated w/ obesity, HTN, DM) - Hypertrophic/restrictive cardiomyopathy - Pericardial disease
HFrEF	Ejection Fraction < 40%	- Ischemic heart disease (can also cause HFpEF) - Other cardiomyopathies or myocarditis - Infiltrative disease

Clinical:
- Right Sided: Peripheral edema, JVD elevation, hepatomegaly
- Left Sided: Pulmonary edema, orthopnea, paroxysmal nocturnal dyspnea
- Exam: S3, displaced PMI, bibasilar rales, jugular venous distension
- CXR: Interstitial edema, Kerley B lines, pleural effusion, alveolar edema
- BNP: > 500 pg/mL has high PPV

Diagnosis: Clinical as above, but initial workup should include:
- ECHO: Evaluates systolic ejection fraction and diastolic function
- Coronary angiogram to assess for underlying CAD in new HF presentation

Management:

Reduced EF	Symptomatic Interventions:
	- Salt/Water Restriction (< 2g / < 2L)
	- Diuretic (Furosemide, Torsemide)
	- Digoxin (if symptomatic despite above measures)
	
	Mortality Improving ("Guideline Directed") Interventions:
	- ACEi, ARB, or angiotensin receptor-neprilysin inhibitor
	- Beta-blocker (Carvedilol, Metoprolol, Bisoprolol)
	- K-sparing diuretic (Spironolactone)
	- Hydralazine + nitrate (black patients)
	
	Other Interventions:
	- ICD (Implantable Cardiac Defibrillator), indicated if:
	    > 1 month post MI, class II/III symptoms on therapy, EF < 35%
	- BiV-Pacer (Biventricular Pacer), indicated if:
	    Same criteria as ICD, plus wide QRS (> 120 ms)

Preserved EF	- Treat underlying disease - Diuretics (if volume overloaded) - Spironolactone (controversial, modest mortality improvement)

New York Heart Classification

Stage	Symptoms	Management
I	Asymptomatic	ACEi + Beta Blocker
II	Symptoms with moderate exertion	Spironolactone, Hydralazine + Nitrate ICD/BiVD if indicated
III	Symptoms with activities of daily living	
IV	Symptoms at rest	Transplant, LVAD, end-of-life discussion

HEART FAILURE — Cardiovascular Medicine

Acute HF Exacerbation

General: Acute worsening of new or underlying heart failure

Risk: Precipitated by dietary/medication noncompliance, ischemia, arrhythmia (ie AFib), severe HTN, renal failure, pulmonary emboli, sepsis

Clinical: Dyspnea, peripheral edema, exercise intolerance, weight gain
- Exam demonstrated rales, jugular venous distension

Diagnosis: Clinical

Management:
- Respiratory support: Supplemental O_2, with NIV/intubation if required
- Diuretics: Furosemide (2.5x home oral dose, generally as IV)
- Vasodilators (Nitroprusside, Nitroglycerin) in some cases
- Inotropic agents (Dobutamine, Milrinone) if refractory to above

High Output Heart Failure

General: Elevated cardiac output, usually secondary to chronically increased volume status OR decreased peripheral vascular resistance

Risk: Arteriovenous shunting (Congenital [PDA, AVF], trauma, malignancy), anemia, sepsis, hyperthyroidism, pregnancy, erythroblastosis fetalis

Clinical: Presents similar to heart failure (both pulmonary edema, peripheral edema, elevated JVP, bounding pulses, warm, flow murmur, venous hum)

Management:
- Volume overload → Diuresis, salt/water restriction
- Decreased SVR → Manage underlying condition

Cor Pulmonale

General: Right ventricular hypertrophy with eventual RV failure. A complication of advanced pulmonary hypertension (due to mechanism other than left heart failure).

Risk: COPD, interstitial lung disease, OSA, idiopathic pulmonary hypertension

Clinical:
- Exertional dyspnea, angina, and syncope
- Right heart failure (JVD, edema), prominent S2, RV heave
- ECG: RBBB, RVH, right axis
- ECHO: Right ventricular dilatation, possible tricuspid regurgitation

Diagnosis: Right heart catheterization

Management:
- Treat underlying pulmonary disorder. Supplemental O_2 if hypoxemic.
- May be preload dependent, must be careful with diuretics

CARDIOMYOPATHY
Cardiovascular Medicine

Type	Definition/Etiology	Clinical/Diagnosis	Management
Dilated	- Dilation and impaired contraction of one or both ventricles (EF < 40%) with diffuse dilation and decreased wall thickness Causes - Idiopathic (50%, many genetic), Myocarditis (Viral [ie coxsackie], chagas, lyme), ischemia, infiltrative (sarcoid), peripartum, toxin (alcohol, Doxorubicin), collagen vascular disease (SLE, scleroderma)	- Presents with HF - Diagnosis: ECHO Note: Dilated CM has diffuse "global" hypokinesis, while ischemic CM appears with focal areas of hypokinesis	- Standard HF management
Restrictive	- Process infiltrates myocardium, resulting in impaired ventricular diastolic relaxation Causes - Amyloid, Sarcoid, Hemochromatosis - Young Children: Endocardial fibroelastosis, Loeffler's syndrome (endomyocardial fibrosis with prominent eosinophilic infiltrate)	- Presents with HF - Diagnosis: ECHO (diastolic dysfunction with restrictive filling pattern)	- Treat underlying cause - Standard HF management
Hypertrophic	- Genetic disorder of sarcomere proteins resulting in disorganized/hypertrophied myocytes - Most commonly AD b-myosin heavy chain or myosin binding protein C mutations	- Presents with dyspnea, chest pain, syncope, or sudden cardiac death. Exam reveals harsh systolic murmur (LLSB). - Diagnosis: ECHO (asymmetric septal hypertrophy, LVH, systolic anterior motion of the mitral valve)	- Beta or Ca Channel Blocker - Diuretics (if fluid retention) Note: Avoid preload or afterload reducers (ie nitrates or ACEi) - Myectomy or alcohol ablation for persistent symptoms despite therapy

Cards6

CARDIOMYOPATHY/MALIGNANCY — Cardiovascular Medicine

Other Cardiomyopathy

Takotsubo ("Stress Cardiomyopathy")
- Non-ischemic temporary hypokinesis of myocardium. Patients can develop chest pain and symptoms of acute HF. ECHO shows apical ballooning (typically diagnostic). Treatment is supportive, as cardiac function can often return.

RV Arrhythmogenic Cardiomyopathy
- Genetic non-ischemic RV cardiomyopathy associated with ventricular arrhythmias. Can present as cardiogenic syncope or sudden cardiac death in young adults.

Cardiac/Vascular Malignancy

Cardiac Malignancies	
Metastases	- 75% of cardiac neoplasm - Primary most commonly melanoma. Others include lung, breast, soft tissue, liquid tumors.
Atrial Myxoma	***General***: Benign mesenchymal growth, often pedunculated and located in the left atrium. Most common primary cardiac malignancy. ***Clinical:*** Cardiovascular symptoms (ie chest pain, dyspnea, palpitations), embolization (stroke, arterial occlusion), constitutional (fever, weight loss). Low pitched diastolic murmur (diastolic plop). ***Diagnosis:*** ECHO ***Management***: Surgery
Rhabdomyomas	- Almost entirely in children - Associated with tuberous sclerosis
Vascular Malignancies	
Angiosarcoma	- Rare blood vessel malignancy typically occurring in the head, neck, and breast areas (sun exposed areas). Usually in elderly. - Associated with radiation therapy, chronic postmastectomy lymphedema - Hepatic angiosarcoma associated vinyl chloride and arsenic exposures

PERICARDIAL DISEASE — Cardiovascular Medicine

Acute Pericarditis

General: Inflammation of the pericardial sac

Etiology:
- Viral (Coxsackie, echovirus, adenovirus)
- Bacterial (TB), fungal, parasitic
- Acute MI, Dressler
- Uremia
- Autoimmune (ie collagen vascular diseases)
- Surgery/Trauma/Radiation

Clinical:
- Severe, pleuritic chest pain (improves leaning forward)
- Pericardial friction rub (specific)
- ECG (PR depressions, diffuse ST changes)
- ECHO (~50% have pericardial effusion)

Diagnosis: Clinical Criteria (≥ 2/4 of the following)
1) Classic positional chest pain   2) Friction rub
3) Typical ECG changes   4) Pericardial effusion

Management: Generally self-limited (1-3 week resolution)
- Idiopathic → NSAIDs (Ibuprofen or Indomethacin) PLUS Colchicine
- Post MI → ASA PLUS Colchicine
- Uremic → Dialysis

Note: Glucocorticoids reserved for those with contraindication for NSAIDs

Constrictive Pericarditis

General: Fibrous scarring of pericardium resulting in rigid and thick pericardium. Restricts diastolic filling of the heart. Increased ventricular interdependence.

Etiology: Idiopathic, bacterial (ie TB), connective tissue disease, surgery, radiation

Clinical:
- Presents with signs of low cardiac output, signs of heart failure
- Elevated JVP, Kussmaul sign (JVP up with deep breath), pulsus paradoxus, pericardial knock

Diagnosis:
- Initial Workup: ECHO
- Surgical Planning or Uncertain Diagnosis: CT/MRI
    (See pericardial thickening +/- calcification)

Treatment: Pericardiectomy

PERICARDIAL DISEASE — Cardiovascular Medicine

Pericardial Effusion

General: Fluid between the visceral and parietal layers of the pericardial sac

Risk:
- Pericarditis (of any cause)
- Hypervolemia (as seen with CHF, cirrhosis, nephrotic syndrome)

Clinical:
- Often asymptomatic, but can develop signs of impaired cardiac function
- Muffled heart sounds, soft PMI, dullness at left lung base (compressed by pericardial fluid), friction rub
- CXR (water bottle appearance)
- ECG (low voltage, electrical alternans)

Diagnosis:
- ECHO (best at establishing effusion and assess hemodynamic compromise)
- Pericardial fluid analysis (if etiology is unknown)

Treatment:
- Stable: Treat underlying disease. Can sample fluid if etiology unclear. Avoid diuretics. Follow with ECHO.
- Unstable: Urgent pericardiocentesis (alternative: Surgical drainage)

Cardiac Tamponade

General: Impaired diastolic function of heart due to pericardial effusion that is under pressure. Results from either a large effusion (> 2L) OR rapid accumulation of smaller effusion.
- Equalization of cardiac pressures and decreased cardiac output/stroke volume (ventricular interdependence)

Clinical:
- Presents with signs of hemodynamic compromise, chest pain, dyspnea
- Cardiogenic shock without pulmonary edema
- Tachycardia, elevated JVP, hypotension, pulsus paradoxus, narrowed pulse pressure, distant heart sounds
- Beck's Triad: (1) Hypotension (2) JVD (3) Muffled heart sounds
- ECG with decreased voltage, electrical alternans

Diagnosis: ECHO, plus clinical syndrome as above

Management:
- Nonhemorrhagic → Urgent pericardiocentesis or surgical drainage
- Hemorrhagic (traumatic) → Surgical drainage and repair

INFLAMMATORY CARDIAC DISEASE
Cardiovascular Medicine, Pediatrics

Myocarditis

General: Myocardial inflammation, that may be accompanied by cardiac dysfunction

Etiology:
- Infectious (viral [Coxsackie B, parvo, adeno, etc], bacterial, Chagas)
- Rheumatism, Cardiotoxicity

Clinical:
- Variable presentation. Ranges from subclinical to highly symptomatic (chest pain, heart failure, shock)
- Can see nonspecific ECG changes, ECHO with wall motion abnormalities

Diagnosis:
Criteria:
(1) Elevated cardiac biomarkers
(2) ECG changes (myocardial injury)
(3) Abnormal cardiac function (on ECHO/MRI)
PLUS
Low suspicion for CAD (based on clean cardiac catheterization or age)

*Cardiac MRI and/or myocardial biopsy can further characterize

Management: Supportive (ICU monitoring, heart failure/arrhythmia management)

Rheumatic Heart Disease

General: Sequella (~2-4 weeks) of group A *Streptococcus* pharyngitis, from M protein cross reactivity (molecular mimicry)

Clinical/Diagnostic Criteria: Either 2 major OR 1 major + 2 minor

Major (JONES)	Minor
1) Joints (migratory polyarthritis)	1) Fever
2) Pancarditis (endocarditis, pericarditis, myocarditis)	2) Elevated ESR
3) Nodules (subcutaneous)	3) Polyarthralgias
4) Erythema marginatum	4) Prolonged PR
5) Sydenham's chorea	

*Evidence of previous *Streptococcus* infection (helpful, but not necessary) with either (+) throat *Streptococcus* test or ASO titer

Management:
- *Streptococcus* Eradication: Penicillin G
- Joint pain: NSAIDs
- Heart failure management (if necessary)

Prophylaxis:
Penicillin G (IM q4 weeks), Penicillin V (daily), or Azithromycin (daily)

Rheumatic fever w/ carditis + valve disease	Until 40 y/o OR 10 years
Rheumatic fever w/ carditis	Until 21 y/o OR 10 years
Rheumatic fever w/o carditis	Until 21 y/o OR 5 years

INFLAMMATORY CARDIAC DISEASE

Cardiovascular Medicine

Endocarditis

General: Infection of the endocardial surface of the heart, generally of a valve
- Location (in order of frequency): (1) Mitral (2) Aortic (3) Tricuspid (IVDU)
- Can be acute (rapidly progressive symptoms) or subacute

Risk: Prosthetic valve, cardiac devices, valvular disease, congenital heart disease, IV drug use

Organism	Presentation
Staphylococcus aureus	- IV drug use, prosthetic valve, cardiac device
Streptococci viridans	- Gingival manipulation or poor dentition - Subacute presentation
Enterococcus	- Genitourinary problems - Subacute presentation
Streptococcus bovis	- Association with colon cancer
Coagulase negative *Staph*	- Prosthetic devices, valves
HACEK *Haemophilus aphrophilus* *Aggregatibacter aphrophilus* *Actinobacillus actinomyc.* *Cardiobacterium hominis* *Eikenella corrodens* *Kingella kingae*	- *Eikenella*: Found in human mouths
Fungi (*Candida*)	- IV drug use, immunocompromised status
Brucella, Coxiella	- Animal exposures

Clinical:
- Constitutional: Fever, weight loss, night sweats, etc
- New murmur, petechiae, splinter hemorrhage (nails)
- Janeway's lesions (nontender macules on extremities), Osler nodes (tender nodules fingers/toes), Roth spots (exudative lesions of retina). All highly specific but rare findings.

Diagnosis: Modified Duke Criteria

Definite IE: 2 Major OR 1 Major + 3 Minor OR 5 Minor	Major Criteria 1) Positive blood culture of typical organism 2) Evidence of endocardial lesion (ie + ECHO for vegetation, abscess, or new regurgitation)
Possible IE: 1 Major + 1 Minor OR 3 Minor	Minor Criteria 1) Risk factor (IV drug, prosthetic valve) 2) Fever > 38°C 3) Vascular event (arterial emboli, septic infarcts, etc) 4) Immunologic (glomerulonephritis, Osler, Roth, RF+) 5) Atypical blood cultures or serologic evidence of infection

INFLAMMATORY CARDIAC DISEASE — Cardiovascular Medicine

Endocarditis (cont)

Management:
- Workup → 3x Blood cultures, prior to empiric therapy
- Antibiotics: Empiric (acutely ill patients) → Vancomycin
- Transition to specific drug once blood cultures result
- Generally 4-6 weeks total therapy

Complications:
- Heart Failure
- Perivalvular abscess (suspect in patients developing conduction defects or persistent bacteremia)
- Septic embolization (strokes, pulmonary infarcts, metastatic abscesses)
- Mycotic aneurysms
- Glomerulonephritis

Endocarditis Prophylaxis Guidelines

Drug Choice (Single dose pre-procedure)
- Amoxicillin (alt: Cephalexin, Clindamycin, Azithromycin)
- If IV required: Ampicillin/Cefazolin/Vancomycin

Indicated Conditions
1) Prosthetic valves/cardiac material
2) History of endocarditis
3) Unrepaired cyanotic congenital heart disease

Indicated Procedures
1) Dental (with gingival manipulation: extraction, implants, periodontal, cleaning with bleeding)
2) Respiratory biopsy
3) Procedure on infected GI, GU, skin
4) Heart surgery involving prosthetic valves or intracardiac materials

Nonbacterial Thrombotic Endocarditis

General: Non-infectious endocarditis characterized by thrombi deposition on valves

Risk: Associated with advanced malignancy ("Marantic") and SLE ("Libman-Sacks"), other inflammatory conditions

Clinical: Typically asymptomatic until embolization

Diagnosis: ECHO

Management: Anticoagulation (Heparin). Surgery.

VALVULAR HEART DISEASE
Cardiovascular Medicine

Aortic Stenosis

General: Left ventricular outflow obstruction at the aortic valve

Risk: Idiopathic "wear & tear" (age > 65), bicuspid valve (~50 y/o), rheumatic valve

Clinical:
- Asymptomatic or nonspecific findings early in disease
- Severe disease → Classic triad (Heart failure, angina, syncope)
- Systolic ejection (crescendo-decrescendo) murmur at second right intercostal, radiates to carotids, soft S2. Carotid pulse ("parvus et tardus" or weak and delayed), sustained PMI.

Diagnosis: ECHO

Management: Aortic valve replacement if severe grade stenosis/highly symptomatic

Aortic Insufficiency

General: Inadequate closure of aortic valve leaflets with regurgitation that increases LV diastolic pressure/volume, resulting in dilatation and hypertrophy of the LV to maintain cardiac output, but eventually leading to heart failure

Risk:
- Acute: Endocarditis, aortic dissection
- Chronic: Valve issues (bicuspid valve, rheumatic disease, autoimmune and congenital connective tissue disorders), root issues (syphilis aortitis)

Clinical:
- Presents with heart failure symptoms (more severe with acute AI)
- Diastolic decrescendo murmur at lower left sternal border, wide pulse pressure, water hammer pulse, head/uvula bobbing, Austin Flint murmur

Diagnosis: ECHO

Management:
- Acute: Emergent aortic valve replacement/repair
- Chronic: Manage heart failure medically
  - Severe/highly symptomatic disease → Aortic valve replacement

Tricuspid Regurgitation

Risk: Functional (ie from dilation of right atrium/ventricle), valve damage (from endocarditis, rheumatic fever, injury from invasive cardiac device), congenital (Ebstein's anomaly)

Clinical:
- Right sided CHF signs (JVD, RV heave, hepatomegaly, peripheral edema)
- Holosystolic murmur heard best at the left mid sternal border

Diagnosis: ECHO

Management:
- Functional regurgitation: Treat underlying disorder
- Primary valve disease: If severe → Tricuspid valve repair or replacement

VALVULAR HEART DISEASE
Cardiovascular Medicine

Mitral Regurgitation

Risk:
- Acute: Endocarditis, papillary muscle/chordae rupture
- Chronic: MVP, rheumatic valve, functional (cardiomyopathy or HF)

Clinical:
- Ranges from asymptomatic to left sided heart failure (dyspnea, fatigue)
- Holosystolic murmur at apex, radiates to axilla

Diagnosis: ECHO (regurgitation, LA dilatation)

Management:
- Acute: Emergent valve repair or replacement
- Chronic: Medical therapy (for heart failure), surgery if severe

Mitral Valve Prolapse

General: Myxomatous degeneration of mitral valve leaflets, with excessive or redundant tissue, leading to prolapse into LA. Can develop mitral regurgitation.

Risk: Primary (idiopathic/familial), Secondary (CT disorders like Marfans, Ehlers-Danlos, etc)

Clinical:
- "MVP Syndrome": Nonspecific symptoms (ie chest pain, palpitations, dyspnea) that are controversial regarding true causality/existence
- Midsystolic click and murmur (standing/valsalva increases the murmur, make click earlier; squatting decreases click/murmur)

Diagnosis: ECHO

Management: Reassurance

Mitral Stenosis

General: Obstruction of blood flow from left atrium to the ventricle, with resulting ↑ pressure in the pulmonary circulation and right heart

Risk: Rheumatic heart disease

Clinical:
- Exertional dyspnea, decreased exercise tolerance, hemoptysis, AF
- Opening snap followed by mid diastolic rumble (Loud S1, P2)
- ECG: Can show RVH, supraventricular tachyarrhythmias, atrial enlargement

Diagnosis: ECHO (MV thickening/calcification, decreased valve mobility, +/- regurg)

Management:
- Medical: Anticoagulation (for AFib or hx of embolism), manage CHF/AF
- Severe symptoms or severe grade disease: Mitral valvotomy

ELECTROPHYSIOLOGY (BRADY)

Cardiovascular Medicine

Sinus Bradycardia

General: Sinus rhythm with rate < 60 bpm

Etiology:
- Benign (sleep, well-conditioned athletes)
- Drugs (beta-blockers, CCBs)
- Pathologic (SA node disease, increased ICP, OSA, hypothyroidism, medications)

Clinical: Generally asymptomatic until < 45 bpm, then syncope/dizziness

Diagnosis: ECG (sinus origin of p waves, HR < 60 bpm)

Management:
Hemodynamically Stable: Work-up for underlying cause (infection, hypothyroidism, medication, sick sinus)
Hemodynamically Unstable: Defined as bradycardia causing CHF, altered mentation, shock, hypotension, or chest pain. Follow algorithm on right.

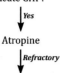

Identify/Treat Underlying
Start Supportive Care
(airway, O_2, cardiac monitoring)
↓
Persistent Bradyarrhythmia Causing:
Shock?
Altered Mentation?
Ischemic chest pain?
Acute CHF?
↓ Yes
Atropine
↓ *Refractory*
Transcutaneous Pacing OR
Dopamine Drip OR
Epinephrine Drip

Atrioventricular Block

General: Abnormal conduction through the AV/His system

Etiology: Idiopathic, ischemia, drugs, congenital abnormalities

Degree	ECG Findings	Management
1°	PR > 0.2 sec (AV Nodal delay)	Reassurance
2° Mobitz I (Wenckebach)	Progressive PR lengthening into dropped beat	Reassurance (generally benign)
2° Mobitz II	Consistent PR interval with dropped beats	Pacemaker (risk to progress to complete block)
3° (Complete)	Complete P/QRS disassociation	Pacemaker

Note: If reversible cause is identified, pacemaker not indicated. Ischemia, drugs, and excessive vagal tone states may be reversible, so temporarily pace first.

Sick Sinus Syndrome

General: SA nodal dysfunction, diagnosed by the combination of ECG abnormalities plus clinical symptoms

Clinical: Fatigue, presyncope, palpitations, dizziness, dyspnea, angina

Diagnosis:
- ECG (sinus brady, sinus pauses, SA exit block, or alternating tachy/brady)
- If diagnosis unclear, ambulatory cardiac monitor

Management: Permanent pacemaker (for symptomatic patients)

ELECTROPHYSIOLOGY (TACHY) — Cardiovascular Medicine

Atrial Fibrillation

General: Ectopic atrial rhythm most commonly originating from abnormal foci near pulmonary veins. Atrial HR ~400, but AV nodal conduction is variable, so ventricular rate is ~75-125. Can be paroxysmal or permanent.

Risks: HTN, CHF, diabetes mellitus, older age, alcohol, MR/MS

Clinical: Can be asymptomatic or symptomatic (palpitations, syncope, dyspnea)

Diagnosis: ECG (irregularly irregular rhythm without distinct P waves)

Management:
New Onset
Step 1: Rate control (if necessary: Beta-blocker or Ca-Channel blocker)
Step 2: Cardioversion (if still in AF after trial of rate control)
Note: Patient must be anticoagulated for at least 3 weeks OR have developed AF within last 48 hr
Step 3: Chronic therapy (as below)

Cardioversion: DC electrical cardioversion preferred to pharmacologic (drug options include flecainide, propafenone, or ibutilide)

Chronic Therapy:
Rate Control (Rate Control = Rhythm Control)
  - Goal HR: < 85 (symptomatic) and < 110 (asymptomatic)
  - Drug Choice: Beta-Blocker (ie Metoprolol) (alt: Diltiazem/Verapamil)
    * Combine both if necessary for proper control of rate
Rhythm Control
  - Used for: < 65 y/o, symptomatic patients for whom restoration of sinus rhythm is desired.
  - Flecainide or Propafenone. If CAD → Sotalol. If CHF → Amiodarone.
Anticoagulation

Indications [CHA2DS2-VASc]	Score: ≥ 2 → Anticoagulate = 1 → Clinical Judgement = 0 → No anticoagulation indicated
CHF (1 point) HTN (1 point)	
Age (≥ 75 2 points) DM (1 point) Stroke/TIA/Thromboembolism (2 point) Vascular disease (1 point) Age 64-75 (1 point) Sex female (1 point)	**Drug Choice** 1) DOAC (Dabigatran, Rivaroxaban, Apixaban) Note: Contraindicated in renal insufficiency 2) Warfarin (INR 2-3)

Rapid Ventricular Response:
  - Hemodynamic Instability: Emergent DC Cardioversion (or rate control trial)
  - No CHF/Hypotension: IV Diltiazem or Metoprolol
  - If CHF/Hypotension OR If additional rate control required: Digoxin
  - If intolerant to all of the above: Amiodarone

Complications:
  - Tachyarrhythmia induced cardiomyopathy: Dilated cardiomyopathy from prolong tachyarrhythmias
  - Embolic events (stroke, mesenteric ischemia, limb ischemia, etc)

ELECTROPHYSIOLOGY (TACHY) — Cardiovascular Medicine

Atrial Flutter

General: Rapid, regular atrial depolarizations with an atrial rate ~300 bpm and ventricular rate of 150 bpm. Thought to be on a spectrum between sinus rhythm and atrial fibrillation. Typically generates from reentrant circuit that revolves around the tricuspid annulus or atrial scar tissue.

Risk: Cardiovascular risk factors (CHF, MI, HTN, etc), AF risk conditions (Thyrotoxicosis, obesity, OSA), cardiac surgery, atrial ablation procedures.

Clinical: Palpitations, dyspnea, fatigue, dizziness, presyncope. Risk for atrial thrombus.

Diagnosis: ECG (atrial rate 300 bpm [saw-tooth shaped waves], with variable levels of conduction across the AV node [most commonly 2:1], resulting in a ventricular rate around 150 bpm)

Management:
Medical
- Rate control with beta-blocker or non-dihydropyridine Ca-channel blocker
- Anticoagulate as in atrial fibrillation

Definitive
- DC Cardioversion (if ablation is delayed/not planned)
- Radiofrequency catheter ablation (definitive therapy)

Multifocal Atrial Tachycardia

General: Arrhythmia with HR > 100 bpm PLUS variable P-wave morphology
Note: Variable P-wave morphology w/ normal rate is called wandering pacemaker.

Risk: Most commonly associated with pulmonary disease, but other cardiovascular conditions also associated (HF)

Clinical: Generally asymptomatic

Diagnosis: ECG (rate > 100 bpm with P waves of at least 3 different morphologies)

Management: Only indicated if the elevated rate is worsening underlying disease (ie heart failure), in which case rate control with beta-blockers

AV Nodal Reentry Tachycardia

General: Most common paroxysmal SVT, caused by a reentry circuit in the AV node

Risk: Idiopathic, generally with onset in young adulthood

Clinical: Acute onset palpitations, dizziness, dyspnea

Diagnosis: ECG (regular narrow complex tachycardia without P waves, +/- retrograde P waves)

Management:
- Unstable: DC Cardioversion
- Stable: Valsalva maneuvers. IV Adenosine if the rhythm persists. Beta-blockade if all else fails.

ELECTROPHYSIOLOGY (TACHY)

Cardiovascular Medicine

Ventricular Tachycardia

General: Rapid firing of > 3 PVCs (originating below the bundle of his), with HR of 120-250 bpm. Subtypes:
- Non-sustained (< 30 sec, but > 3 beats. Generally asymptomatic)
- Sustained (> 30 sec, generally symptomatic)
- Can also be categorized as monomorphic or polymorphic

Risk: Typically related to ischemic heart disease, cardiomyopathy, structural abnormalities, or prolonged QT

Management:
Non-sustained VT: Search for underlying etiology and treat
Sustained VT:
- No pulse → ACLS
- Pulse found: Stable → IV Amiodarone (alt: Lidocaine, Procainamide)
                Unstable → Synchronized cardioversion

Long-term
- ICD Placement
- Meds: Beta-blocker or Amiodarone may be indicated in certain patients

Torsades de Pointes

General: Polymorphic VT with cyclic, sinusoidal changes in the QRS

Risk: Long QT (Congenital, Drugs [macrolides/fluoroquinolones, antipsychotics/TCA, Methadone, antiemetics, anti-arrhythmics], electrolytes [hypocalcemia, hypokalemia, hypomagnesemia])

Management: Stable → IV Magnesium. Unstable → Electric defibrillation.

Ventricular Fibrillation/ACLS

General: Arrest of systolic cardiac function from disorganized electrical activity in the ventricles. Often preceded by runs of ventricular tachycardia.

Management: See ACLS algorithm below
- ICD indicated for patients that survive

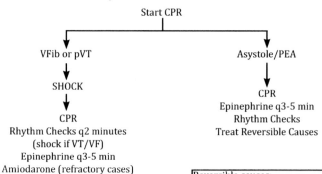

Reversible causes:
Hypovolemia, hypoxia, acidosis, electrolyte abnormalities, hypothermia, tension pneumothorax, tamponade, toxin, PE

ELECTROPHYSIOLOGY (MISC) — Cardiovascular Medicine

PAC/PVC

Premature Atrial Complex: Generally benign and asymptomatic ectopic (non-sinus) atrial beats. No treatment necessary. Symptomatic patients can try beta-blocker.

Premature Ventricular Complex: Ectopic ventricular beats. Generally asymptomatic, but can experience palpitations. Workup patients with unexplained PVCs with 24-hour ambulatory monitoring/ECHO/exercise stress test. Symptomatic patients can try beta-blocker.

Pacemaker Basics

Types:
- Single-chamber pacemaker – 1 pacing lead is implanted in the RA or RV
- Dual-chamber pacemaker – 2 pacing leads are implanted (1 in RV, 1 in RA)
- Biventricular pacing (cardiac resynchronization therapy [CRT])
    - Single or dual-chamber leads, PLUS coronary sinus lead

Indications:

ICD

1) Anyone who suffers a cardiac arrest or sustained ventricular tachycardia (unless reversible cause was identified). This includes structural causes, such as ischemic cardiomyopathy/HCM.
2) EF < 35% in NYHA Class II/III CHF
3) Channelopathies, including long QT and Brugada

Resynchronization Therapy
1) LVEF ≤ 0.35, a QRS > 0.12 seconds, sinus rhythm and NYHA Functional Classes III–IV while on optimal medical therapy

Permanent Pacemaker
1) Symptomatic bradycardia (for any reason)
2) < 40 HR and asymptomatic
3) Any irreversible Mobitz type II heart block OR Complete heart block

Cardiac Event Monitors

Types:
1) Holter (1-2 day continuous ECG monitor)
2) Loop event monitor (weeks long, patient activated when symptomatic)
3) Implantable loop recorder (months of monitoring, subcutaneous recorder)

Indications:
1) Unexplained syncope, near syncope
2) Recurrent unexplained palpitations
3) Monitor atrial fibrillation (monitor rate control, determine possible occult AF in cryptogenic stroke)
4) Screen for ventricular arrhythmia in structural heart disease

HYPERLIPIDEMIA
Cardiovascular Medicine

General: Elevated levels of LDL are known to be atherogenic, while HDL is anti-atherogenic. Triglycerides do not have clear association with atherosclerosis, but at very high levels are associated with pancreatitis.

Clinical: Generally asymptomatic. If very high, can develop deposition:
- Xanthoma (lipid deposit, commonly of tendon and eyelid ["xanthelasma"])
- Corneal arcus (lipid deposit in cornea)

Management:
- Lifestyle modification for all (healthy diet, weight loss, quit smoking)
- Indications for Statin therapy
- If patient extremely high risk and LDL remains > 70-100, can consider ezetimibe or PCSK-9 inhibitor

Indication	Statin
ASCVD	High Intensity
LDL > 190	High Intensity
40-75 y/o Diabetics	Moderate to High Intensity
ASCVD risk > 7.5%	Moderate to High Intensity

Notes on Statins:
- If patient develops myalgias or transaminitis on statins, stop drug, retry at lower dose
- Obtain baseline LFTs and CK, but no need to screen for LFTs/CK unless symptomatic

Drug	LDL	HDL	Trig	Mechanism	Adverse Reaction
Statin Atorva, Rosuva Simva, Prava	↓↓	↑	↓	HMG-CoA inhibitor	Hepatotoxicity Myopathy
Bile Resin Cholestyramine, Colestipol	↓	↑	↔	Inhibit bile resorp	GI Disturbance Drug malabsorption
Ezetimibe	↓	↔	↔	Inhibit cholesterol absorp (NPC1L1)	Diarrhea
Fibrate Gemfibrozil Fenofibrate	↔	↑	↓↓	Upregulate LPL Activate PPAR-a	Cholesterol stone
Niacin	↓	↑	↓	Inhibit lipolysis	Flushing (use ASA) Hyperglycemia, uricemia
Omega-3	↔	↔	↓	Decrease hepatic fat secretion	
PCSK-9 Inhibitor Evolocumab Alirocumab	↓↓↓	↑	↓	Prevent LDL-R uptake/breakdown	Reaction at injection site

Genetic Dyslipidemia:

Class	Name	Mxn	Clinical
I (AR)	Hyperchylomicronemia	LPL Deficiency	Trigs up → Pancreatitis
IIa (AD)	Hypercholesterolemia	LDL-R Def.	Elevated cholesterol (LDL)
III (AR)	Dysbetalipoproteinemia	APO-E Def.	Atherosclerosis
IV (AD)	Hypertriglyceridemia	VLDL Overpdx	Trigs up → Pancreatitis

HYPERTENSION — Cardiovascular Medicine

Stage	SBP mmHg	DBP mmHg	Management
Normotensive	< 120	< 80	
Prehypertensive	120-129	< 80	- Lifestyle modification, routine follow-up
Stage 1	130-139 or	80-89	- Lifestyle (all) - Pharm (for high risk individuals§)
Stage 2	> 140 or	> 90	- Lifestyle + Pharm (for all)
Severe	> 180	> 110	- Management below

§High Risk: CAD, HF, Diabetes, CKD, Age > 65 (controversial), ASCVD 10 year risk > 10%

Hypertensive Urgency	- Severe grade hypertension with possible mild headache, but no end organ damage

Hypertensive Emergency	- Severe grade hypertension with evidence of end organ damage, including:
	  - CNS: Encephalopathy, stroke, elevated ICP
	  - Renal: AKI
	  - Cardiovascular: ACS, angina, worsening CHF, dissection

White Coat Hypertension	- Elevated blood pressure in doctor's office - Diagnose with either 24 hour ambulatory or home BP monitoring
Secondary Hypertension	- Etiologies: CKD, renal arterial stenosis, hyperaldosteronism, pheochromocytoma, Cushing's, aortic coarctation, meds (OCP), OSA - Workup for secondary hypertension indicated if: Young (age < 35), severely elevated BP, refractory BP, or sign specific to certain pathologies (ie bruit, hypokalemia, etc)

Diagnosis: Two seperate clinic readings over 4 weeks
- Ambulatory or home blood pressure monitoring preferred to confirm diagnosis, but not widely available

Management:

Essential	Lifestyle Modification (in order of efficacy) - Weight Loss > DASH Diet > Exercise > Salt Restriction > Alcohol Limitation - Pharm indicated if > 140/90 in average risk adult, or > 130/80 in high risk adult - First Line Meds: Include ACEi/ARB, thiazides, or Ca-Channel Blockers - Med choice should be tailored based on patient's comorbid conditions
Severe	Overall goal for either is either 25% reduction from baseline or < 160/100 mmHg Emergency - Drop MAP by ~20% in first hour, with total of no more than 25% in 24 hrs - Overly aggressive reduction can lead to ischemic end organ damage (unable to autoregulate in time), but lack of control risks hypertensive related complications (stroke, ACS, etc) - Drug Choice: IV Hydralazine, Esmolol, Nitroprusside, Labetalol, Clevidipine, Nicardipine, etc Urgency (Asymptomatic Severe HTN) - Lower within 24 hours using oral meds (Captopril, Clonidine, Labetalol, etc)

CONGENITAL DEFECTS (ACYANOTIC) — Cardiovascular Pediatrics

Ventricular Septal Defect

General: Most common congenital heart defect, typically located in the membranous septum

Risk: Often idiopathic, associated with Down's and fetal alcohol syndrome

Clinical:
- Small defects often asymptomatic, while larger defects can lead to tachypnea, failure to thrive, within 1-2 months of birth
- Harsh holosystolic murmur at left sternal border, which can often be louder with smaller defects. Severe defects cause diastolic rumble (high mitral flow), sternal lift (RV enlargement).

Diagnosis: ECHO

Management:
- Small Defects / Asymptomatic → ECHO surveillance, monitoring
- Small Defects / Symptomatic → Medical therapy (Furosemide). Surgery if refractory.

- Moderate/Large Defects // Asymptomatic → Close monitoring, with surgery if PAH/LV Dilatation or symptoms develop
- Moderate/Large Defects // Symptomatic → Surgical Closure

Atrial Septal Defect

General: Congenital defect of the atrial septum, occurring in the following locations:
- Secundum: Arrested growth of the septum secundum or excessive septum primum absorption
- Primum: Septum primum does not fuse with the endocardial cushions, associated with AV canal defects

Note: Patent foramen ovale not considered an atrial septal defect

Risk: Down's (primum)

Clinical:
- Asymptomatic until middle age, then can develop dyspnea, fatigue, exercise intolerance
- Systolic ejection murmur at pulmonary area (due to increased pulmonary blood flow), fixed split S2, diastolic flow rumble murmur across tricuspid area (due to increased blood flow)

Diagnosis: ECHO

Management:
Children
- Small / Asymptomatic: Monitor, as spontaneous closure is likely
- Large / Symptomatic: Surgical or percutaneous closure

Adults
- Symptomatic / RV overload / Embolic stroke: Surgical or percutaneous closure
- Severe PAH → No surgical closure

CONGENITAL DEFECTS (ACYANOTIC) — Cardiovascular Pediatrics

Patent Ductus Arteriosus

General: Communicating vessel from aorta to pulmonary artery, which typically remains open in the fetus due to low O_2 and elevated PGE2 levels, but closes shortly after birth. If it remains patent, a left-to-right shunt occurs.

Risk: Prematurity, Rubella infection

Clinical:
- Asymptomatic to heart failure. Persistent large shunts can lead to shunt reversal and Eisenmenger.
- Continuous "machinery murmur," wide pulse pressure/bounding pulse, differential cyanosis

Diagnosis: ECHO

Management:
- Preterm infants: Indomethacin/Ibuprofen. Surgery if ineffective.
- Term infants and older: Surgical closure

Note: If patient has significant shunt reversal +/- severe pulmonary hypertension, it is too late, and surgical closure is likely harmful

Coarctation of the Aorta

General: Narrowing of the descending aorta, typically just distal to the left subclavian artery origin

Risk: Generally an idiopathic, congenital structural abnormality. Associated with Turner syndrome. Can be acquired with Takayasu arteritis.

Clinical:
- Upper-lower body blood pressure differential, brachial-femoral pulse delay, upper body hypertension (headaches, epistaxis)
- Interscapular murmur (from collateral circulation)
- CXR can show rib notching (arterial collaterals). ECG can show LVH.

Diagnosis: ECHO

Management: In patients with significant stenosis (causing elevated pressure gradient), correction via surgery or balloon angioplasty is indicated

Vascular Rings

General: Congenital anomalies of the aortic arch that result in compression of the trachea or esophagus

Risk: Idiopathic. Can be associated with Down's or DiGeorge.

Clinical: Can present with respiratory distress, tachypnea, cyanosis (arching back and extending head relieves obstruction)

Diagnosis: ECHO plus MRI angiography

Management: Surgical correction

CONGENITAL DEFECTS (CYANOTIC)

Cardiovascular Pediatrics

	Definition/Risk	Clinical	Management
Truncus Arteriosus	- Common truncal artery that gives rise to aorta and pulmonary arteries - Often have VSD - Risk: DiGeorge	- Presents within first weeks of life with cyanosis, heart failure, respiratory distress - Dx: ECHO	- Medical stabilization followed by surgical repair during the neonatal period
D-Transposition of the Great Vessels	- Aorta arises from RV, pulmonary artery from the LV - Utilizes some combination of VSD, ASD, PFO, PDA to survive - Risk: Pre-existing maternal diabetes	- Presents within hours of birth with cyanosis and respiratory distress - Dx: ECHO. CXR ("eggs on a string" narrowed mediastinum).	- Alprostadil (PGE1), which maintains patent ductus - Balloon atrial septostomy (allow for interarterial blood mixing) - Surgical correction (arterial switch)
Tricuspid Atresia	- Absence of the tricuspid valve, with no direct connection between RA/RV - All have ASD, RV hypoplasia, and most VSD. Many also have PDA.	- Presents within days of birth with cyanosis +/- a murmur - Dx: ECHO. CXR (minimal pulmonary markings). ECG (left axis).	- Alprostadil (PGE1), which maintains patent ductus - Surgical correction
Tetralogy of Fallot	- Syndrome of: (1) RVH (2) VSD (3) Overriding aorta (4) Obstructed RV outflow	- Clinical severity varies with degree of out flow obstruction. Can be immediately to within weeks of birth with cyanosis, distress. - "Tet Spell" or Hypercyanotic spells with periods of agitation. Squatting relieves symptoms. - Harsh systolic murmur from RV outflow - Dx: ECHO, CXR (boot-shaped heart).	- Medical Stabilization: Alprostadil - Tet spell: Knee-chest position, O$_2$, pain control - Surgical closure (3-6 months of life)
Total Anomalous Pulmonary Venous Return	- Four pulmonary veins fail to make connection to LA, drain to systemic system, mixing oxygenated blood with deoxygenated from venous return	- Can have acute or subacute presentation of cyanosis and heart failure - Dx: ECHO, CXR ("snowman" sign from enlarge vein)	- Surgical Repair

Cards24

CONGENITAL DEFECTS/PEDS MURMURS
Cardiovascular Pediatrics

Hypoplastic Left Heart Syndrome

General: Hypoplasia of the LV and abnormal development of mitral/aortic valves. Requires RV to help deliver both pulmonary and systemic circulation.

Clinical: Presents with cyanosis, respiratory distress, decreased peripheral pulses

Diagnosis: ECHO

Management: Alprostadil and transcatheter septoplasty to maintain shunting, followed by three-staged surgical repair

Ebstein's Anomaly

General: Malformed and displaced tricuspid valve displaced through the valve annulus and attached to the RV endocardium

Clinical: Severe disease presents with cyanosis and heart failure in infants

Diagnosis: ECHO (Tricuspid regurgitation and RV dilatation occur)

Management: Medically stabilize (Alprostadil, HF and arrhythmia management), followed by surgical repair

Supravalvular Aortic Stenosis

General: A rare cause of aortic stenosis, due to thickening of the ascending aorta

Risk: Characteristic of William's syndrome, but can be idiopathic

Clinical: Features are variable depending on the degree of obstruction, but causes a systolic ejection murmur

Management: Surgical correction for high grade stenosis

Approach to Pediatric Murmurs

Innocent Murmurs
1) Vibratory Still's (Most common innocent murmur)
   - Low pitched vibratory crescendo-decrescendo systolic murmur at left lower sternal border

2) Cervical Venous Hum
   - Low pitched crescendo-plateau-decrescendo, continuous, below clavicle
   - Begins in mid systole, crosses S2, and is loudest in diastole

3) Pulmonary or Aortic Flow
   - Systolic ejection murmurs

"Red Flags" (that workup is indicated)
   - If > 3/6 in intensity and harsh in quality
   - Diastolic or continuous
   - Holosystolic murmurs
   - S3 or S4 gallop

PEDIATRIC ARRHYTHMIA

Wolff Parkinson White

General: Accessory electrical pathway ("Bundle of Kent") that can lead to premature ventricular excitement. Tachycardia can be caused by either AFib/Flutter OR re-entry of normal conduction (Atrioventricular reentrant tachycardia or AVRT).

Clinical: Asymptomatic unless arrhythmia develops

Diagnosis: ECG shows shortening PR interval and presence of delta wave

Treatment:
- Unstable arrhythmia → Cardioversion
- Antidromic or Orthodromic AVRT → Vagal maneuvers, Adenosine
- Atrial Fibrillation → Ibutilide or Procainamide
- Definitive therapy → Catheter ablation of accessory pathway

Brugada Syndrome

General: AD genetic condition with increased risk of ventricular arrhythmias and sudden cardiac death

Diagnosis: ECG typically shows pseudo-right bundle branch block with ST elevations in V1-V3

Management: ICD placement

Congenital Long QT

General: Congenital defect in sodium or potassium channels resulting in delayed cardiac repolarization. High risk for ventricular tachycardia (Torsades). (Refer to Torsades in arrhythmia section for discussion on acquired causes of long-QT and management of Torsades)

Etiology: Many mutations in Na/K channels have been implicated
- Romano-Ward: AD LQTS without deafness
- Jervell and Lange Nielsen: AR LQTS with sensorineural deafness

Management: Exercise avoidance, beta-blocker, with ICD or pacemaker in certain situations

ATHEROSCLEROTIC DISEASE (NON-CAD) — Cardiovascular Surgery

Carotid Artery Disease

General: Atherosclerotic stenosis of the carotid artery. Plaques develop just inside the internal carotid at the bifurcation. Considered "symptomatic" if the patient has stroke like symptoms (ie stroke, TIA, amaurosis fugax) in the previous 6 months. Events occur due to thrombus formation, which either causes low flow state or embolizes.

Clinical:
- Stroke (Anterior circulation TIA/stroke features [ie MCA, ACA, retinal])
- Amaurosis fugax
- Hollenhorst plaques in retina. Rare, but specific.
- Carotid bruit

Diagnosis: Imaging (the following modalities have similar efficacies)
- Carotid Duplex US
- MRA
- CTA

Treatment:

Symptomatic	Intervention
100% Stenosis	- Medical management
70-99% Stenosis	- Carotid endarterectomy (ideally performed between 3-14 days after stroke symptoms) - Carotid artery stenting (if high risk for surgery or lesion is not surgically accessible)
Men 50-69% Stenosis	- Carotid endarterectomy
Women 50-69% Stenosis	- Medical management (statins, antiplatelets, antihypertensives)
< 50% Stenosis	- Medical management
Asymptomatic	**Intervention**
≥ 80 % Stenosis	- Carotid endarterectomy
< 80 %	- Medical management (statin, antiplatelet, BP control, etc)

Subclavian Steal

General: Flow reversal in vertebral artery ipsilateral to significant stenosis of subclavian artery

Clinical: Asymptomatic, or causes arm ischemia and/or vertebrobasilar ischemia
- BP on affected side > 15 mmHg less than normal arm, pulse differential

Diagnosis: Clinical (ie pulse exam, BP) plus Duplex US Scan

Treatment: Bypass surgery or stenting

ATHEROSCLEROTIC DISEASE (NON-CAD) — Cardiovascular Surgery

Peripheral Artery Disease

General: Atherosclerosis of vessels most commonly in the lower extremities

Risk: Smoking, hypertension, hyperlipidemia, diabetes mellitus

Clinical:
- Initial symptom is claudication, induced by walking, relieved with rest
- Quads, calves, and gluteal muscles most commonly involved
- Severe symptoms: Rest pain, purple/blue, hairless legs, ulcers, shiny skin, atrophy of muscles
- Buerger's Sign (elevation turns foot pale, then dangling turns in bright red)
- Rutherford Symptom Scale (see right)

Diagnosis:
- ABI (arterial-brachial index): ≤ 0.9 is abnormal
- Can add exercise to test if equivocal
- Elevated values can be seen with calcified vessels
- US/Doppler
- CT/MRI Angiography: Reserved for uncertain cases

Category	Symptoms
0	Asymptomatic
1	Mild claudication
2	Moderate claudication
3	Severe Claudication
4	Rest pain
5	Minor tissue loss
6	Major tissue loss

Management:
- Medical Therapy:
    - Antiplatelets (ASA/Clopidogrel)
    - Smoking cessation
    - Anti-lipid therapy
    - Cilostazol (for claudication symptoms)
- Exercise Therapy
- Revascularization (either surgical bypass or endovascular stenting)
    - Indications: Disabling symptoms refractory to medical therapy OR limb-threatening ischemia (ie rest pain, skin ulcerations)

Leriche Syndrome

General: Obstruction of aortoiliac vessels

Clinical: Presents as bilateral thigh/quad claudication, erectile dysfunction, and absent/diminished femoral pulse

AORTIC DISEASE
Cardiovascular Surgery

Aortic Dissection

General: Separation of the layers of the aortic wall, due to an intimal tear. Stanford subtypes:
- A (ascending): Involves ascending aorta
- B (arch/descending): Distal to the subclavian artery

Risk:
- Spontaneous (long standing HTN, Marfan's/Ehlers-Danlos, bicuspid aortic valve)
- Iatrogenic (instrumentation)
- Traumatic

Clinical:
- Severe chest pain, radiating to back, "tearing" quality
- Asymmetric BP (> 20 mmHg)
- CXR showing widened mediastinum
- Type A: Risk for MI, stroke, aortic regurgitation, or tamponade
- Type B: Risk for limb, renal, mesenteric ischemia

Diagnosis:
- CTA (test of choice in hemodynamically stable patients)
- TEE (test of choice in hemodynamically unstable or CKD patients)

Management:

Both Subtypes	- Maintain HR < 60 and BP between 100-120 mmHg systolic (IV beta blockers: Esmolol or Labetalol. Add Nitroprusside if BP still elevated) - IV opioid analgesia
Type A	- Surgical emergency
Type B	- Medically managed, unless any complication below - Surgery indicated if evidence for ischemic complication or disease propagation/progression (Note: Intervention can be either endovascular or open surgery)

AORTIC DISEASE — Cardiovascular Surgery

Abdominal Aortic Aneurysm

General: Focal aortic dilatation, generally > 3 cm in size

Risk: ↑ Age, males, smoking, HTN, atherosclerotic disease

Clinical:
- Usually asymptomatic if AAA is stable
- Symptomatic, but not ruptured: Can cause pressure/pain in back/flank area

Diagnosis: Abdominal US (initial modality of choice)

Management:
- Symptomatic: Elective repair
- Asymptomatic:
    - Surgery (EVAR or TAVR): If ≥ 5.5 cm, or rapidly expanding (> 1cm/yr), coexisting peripheral artery aneurysms
    - Observation: In anyone not meeting surgical criteria
        - q6-12 month screening ultrasounds
        - Treat modifiable risk factors (ie smoking cessation)

Ruptured Abdominal Aortic Aneurysm

Clinical: Classic triad: Abdominal pain, shock, pulsatile abdominal mass

Diagnosis:
- Stable: Abdominal CT
- Unstable: Bedside US

Management:
- Endovascular or open surgical repair

Complications:
- Aortoenteric fistula (causes large GI bleed)

Thoracic Aortic Aneurysm

General: Localized dilatation of thoracic aorta, > 50% larger in diameter than normal

Risk: Most commonly due to HTN/HLD/smoking, but can be associated with vasculitis (ie Takayasu's, Giant cell) or genetic syndromes (Marfan, Loeys-Dietz, or vascular ED)

Clinical: Most commonly asymptomatic
- Rupture, or imminent rupture: Can cause chest/back pain, nerve compression, thromboembolism, aortic dissection, hypotension, shock
- XR: Can show widened mediastinum

Diagnosis: CTA or MRA

Management:
- Surgery (open or endovascular): > 5.5 cm or rapid expansion (> 1cm/yr)
- Observation/serial monitoring if does not meet surgical criteria

ANEURYSMS — Cardiovascular Surgery

General:
- Definition: Aneurysms are focal dilatations that are > 50% larger than the normal calibre of a vessel

Risk:
- Similar to aortic aneurysms (atherosclerotic risk factors)

Management: Surgical intervention is either endovascular stenting or surgical bypass

	General/Clinical	Management
Popliteal	- Most common peripheral aneurysm - Can cause arterial obstruction due to thrombosis or distal embolization of the thrombus	Dx: US (alt: CTA/MRA) Tx: Surgery if: Ischemic symptoms or > 2 cm
Femoral	- Usually asymptomatic, but can cause leg claudication or localized groin pain/pulsatile mass	Dx: US (alt: CTA/MRA) Tx: Surgery if: Ischemic symptoms or > 3 cm
Visceral	- Can affect splenic artery, hepatic artery, or SMA - Most often picked up incidentally on abdominal imaging	Tx: Surgery if: Ischemic symptoms or > 2 cm
Pseudoaneurysm	- False aneurysm, occurring with injured blood vessel wall, with contained bleeding into surrounding tissues - Common complication of femoral access site for coronary catheterization	Tx: Ultrasound guided thrombin injection, stenting, or surgical ligation

VASCULAR EMERGENCIES — Cardiovascular Surgery

Acute Limb Ischemia

General: Sudden decrease in limb perfusion

Etiology:
- Thrombosis (at site of atherosclerosis, aneurysm)
- Embolism
- Phlegmasia (extensive venous backup, very rare)
- Iatrogenic Injury
- Trauma [See: Trauma]

Clinical:
- Six P's (pain, pallor, pulselessness, poikilothermia, paresthesia, paralysis)
- Sensory symptoms are early symptoms, while motor loss is severe

Diagnosis: CTA

Management: Fluids, Heparin, place limb in dependent position

Class	Definition	Intervention
Viable (I)	- Mild pain, but intact capillary refill, peripheral pulses	None
Marginally threatened (IIa)	- Moderate pain, diminished pulses, possible sensory deficit	Urgent revascularization
Immediately threatened (IIb)	- Severe pain, sensory/motor deficits, no pulses	Emergent revascularization
Irreversible ischemia (III)	- Complete paralysis/no sensation - Signs of dead tissue	Amputation

*Depending on type of obstruction, procedure could be open embolectomy, endovascular thrombectomy, medical thrombolysis, etc.

CARDIOVASCULAR PHARM
Cardiovascular Medicine

	Mechanism	Indication	Side Effects/Management
Antiarrhythmics			
Class Ia Quinidine Procainamide Disopyramide	- Na⁺ Channel Inhibitor - ↑ QRS Duration, ↑ QT Duration	- Ventricular arrhythmias - Atrial arrhythmias - WPW (procainamide)	- ↑ QT → Torsades, ventricular arrhythmias (all) - Quinidine: Cinchonism (tinnitus, confusion, psychosis) - Procainamide: Drug-induced SLE - Disopyramide: Anticholinergic, myocardial depression
Class Ib Lidocaine Mexiletine	- Na⁺ Channel Inhibitor - ↑ QRS Duration, ↓ QT Duration	- Ventricular arrhythmias	- Ventricular arrhythmias - Cardiovascular depression (hypotension, sinus slowing) - CNS (drowsiness, agitation, etc)
Class Ic Flecainide Propafenone	- Na⁺ Channel Inhibitor - ↑ QRS Duration	- Atrial arrhythmias	- Ventricular arrhythmias *Not used if structural heart disease
Class II **Beta-Blockers** Atenolol Bisoprolol Carvedilol Esmolol Labetalol Metoprolol Propranolol	- β-adrenergic antagonist β1- Selective: "A-M" Nonselective: "N-Z" Exceptions: Carvedilol/Labetalol: α/β block	- Atrial fibrillation/flutter - AVNRT - Angina/ACS - Hypertension - Heart Failure - Migraine PPX (propranolol) - Thyrotoxicosis (propranolol) - Variceal PPX (nadolol) - Glaucoma (timolol)	- Exacerbation of HF - Bradyarrhythmias - Increased airway resistance (if underlying lung disease) - Fatigue - Sexual dysfunction Beta Blocker Overdose: Fluids, Atropine, Glucagon
Class III Amiodarone Ibutilide Dofetilide Sotalol	- K⁺ Channel Blocker	- Ventricular arrhythmias - Atrial arrhythmias	- ↑ QT → Torsades, ventricular arrhythmias (all) Amiodarone: - Pulmonary fibrosis/pneumonitis, hepatotoxicity - Hypo or hyperthyroidism. Bradyarrhythmias. - Corneal deposits, blue/gray skin
Class IV Diltiazem Verapamil	- Ca²⁺ Channel Blocker (Non-Dihydropyridine)	- Atrial fibrillation/flutter - AVNRT - Angina - Hypertension	- Constipation - Edema - Heart block or heart failure

CARDIOVASCULAR PHARM

Cardiovascular Medicine

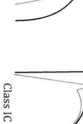

| | Class IA | Class IB | Class IC |

- Class IA-IC antiarrhythmics exhibit "use dependency." They bind more regularly to on/off Na+ channels, rather than resting channels.
- Class C > A > B in terms of strength of effect.

Antihypertensives

	Mechanism	Indication	Side Effects/Management
Ca²⁺ Channel Blocker Amlodipine Nicardipine Nifedipine Nimodipine	- Ca²⁺ Channel Blocker (Dihydropyridine)	- Hypertension - Angina - Raynaud's	- Peripheral Edema - Flushing - Dizziness
Hydralazine	- Direct arteriolar vasodilation	- Hypertension	- Reflex tachycardia - Headache, Edema - Angina - Drug-induced SLE
Fenoldopam	- D1 receptor partial agonist (maintains renal perfusion)	- Hypertension (emergency, post-op)	- Reflex tachycardia
Nitroprusside	- Arterial/venous dilator (NO release → ↑ cGMP)	- Hypertension (emergency)	- Cyanide toxicity - Methemoglobinemia
Nitrovasodilators Nitroglycerin Isosorbide mono or dinitrate	- Vasodilatation (veins > arterial) - NO release → ↑ cGMP	- Angina - HF (Isosorbide dinitrate + Hydralazine)	- Reflex tachycardia - Flushing, Headache

Cards34

CARDIOVASCULAR PHARM

Cardiovascular Medicine

	Mechanism	Indication	Side Effects/Management
Glycosides Digoxin	- Direct inhibition of Na/K ATPase - Results in increased cardiac calcium and contractility - Increased vagal tone	- HF - Atrial fibrillation	- GI (nausea, vomiting, abdominal pain) - Neurologic (confusion and weakness) - Visual disturbances (scotomas, change in color vision) - Arrhythmias: Ventricular arrhythmias, heart block, bradycardia - Hyperkalemia Toxicity: - ↑ Risk for toxicity with renal failure, hypokalemia - Reverse severe toxicity with digoxin Fab
Ranolazine	- Inhibits late Na current, reducing diastolic wall tension and O_2 consumption	- Angina	- QT prolongation
Adenosine	- Transient induction of heart block by decreasing AV nodal cAMP, increasing K^+ efflux, and hyperpolarization of cells	- Supraventricular tachycardia	- Effects blunted by caffeine and theophylline - Flushing, chest pain, sense of impending doom - Bronchospasm
Nesiritide	- Recombinant BNP	- HF	- Controversial in terms of efficacy and indication
Sacubitril	- Neprilysin inhibitor, increasing levels of ANP/BNP	- HF	- Hypotension - Hyperkalemia, AKI - Hypersensitivity
Ivabradine	- Inhibits funny channel, slowing heart rate	- HF requiring rate control	- Bradycardia - Visual changes

Cards35

PHYSICAL EXAM/PFTs

Pulmonary/Critical Care Medicine

Pulmonary Physical Exam

	Sounds	Percussion	Fremitus	Trachea
Pleural Effusion	Decreased	Dull	Decreased	Midline (away from large effusions)
Consolidation	Increased (Rales)	Dull	Increased	Midline
Pneumothorax	Decreased	Hyperresonant	Decreased	Away from tension pneumothorax
Atelectasis	Decreased	Dull	Decreased	Towards large atelectasis
COPD (emphysema)	Decreased	Hyperresonant	Decreased	Midline

Clubbing

General: Associated with pulmonary or cardiovascular diseases, including lung cancer, interstitial pulmonary fibrosis, pulmonary tuberculosis, pulmonary lymphoma, HF, infective endocarditis, and cyanotic congenital heart disease. Unknown pathophysiology, thought to involve excess growth factor production in the lungs (ie PDGF).

Clinical: Increased convexity of the nail bed. Can progress to hypertrophic osteoarthropathy, which presents with focal distal extremity bone and joint pain.

Pulmonary Function Tests

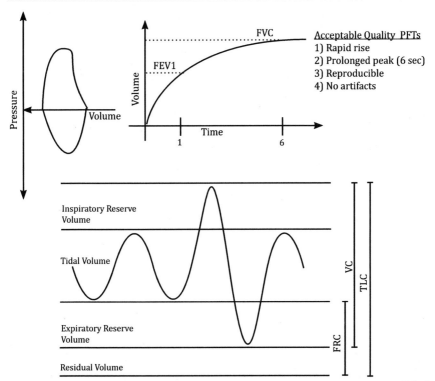

Acceptable Quality PFTs
1) Rapid rise
2) Prolonged peak (6 sec)
3) Reproducible
4) No artifacts

Pulm1

COPD
Pulmonary/Critical Care Medicine

Overview of COPD

General: Chronic lung disease, with multiple subtypes:

Chronic Bronchitis	- Cough > 3 months for at least 2 years - Caused by excessive mucus production
Emphysema	- Enlarged air spaces with alveolar destruction, secondary to excess protease activity from chronic bronchoalveolar inflammation - Centrilobular (smokers) vs Panlobular (α1-antitrypsin)
Asthma-COPD overlap	- Asthma with persistent airflow obstruction

Risk: Smoking, genetic (α1-antitrypsin), environmental (occupational exposure, air pollution, second-hand smoke), chronic poorly controlled asthma

Clinical: Dyspnea, cough, sputum, wheezing, or chest tightness
- Chronic bronchitis (prolonged expiration, rhonchi, wheeze)
- Emphysema (decreased breath sounds, hyperinflation, barrel chest, pursed lip breathing)
- X-ray: Can show hyperinflation, increased lung translucency, flat diaphragm, enlarged retrosternal air space, subpleural blebs

Diagnosis: Pulmonary Function Testing (Original Gold Classification, see right)

Note: FEV1/FVC ratio < 70%. Increased TLC, FRC, RV. DLCO decreased in emphysema.

Class	Severity	FEV1
1	Mild	≥ 80%
2	Moderate	50-79%
3	Severe	30-49%
4	Very Severe	< 30%

Management: Revised GOLD Classification (used to determine management)

	mmRC 0-1	mmRC ≥ 2	mmRC Dyspnea Scale
0 or 1 Exacerbation	Class A	Class B	0: Dyspnea w/ strenuous exercise 1: Dyspnea w/ hills 2: Walks slower than others 3: Takes break after 100 yard walk 4: Dyspneic w/ dressing
≥ 2 Exacerbation or > 1 Hospitalization	Class C	Class D	

- Class A: Short acting agent (beta-agonist Albuterol or anticholinergic Ipratropium)
- Class B: Short acting PLUS LAMA or LABA
- Class C: Short acting PLUS LAMA or LABA +/- inhaled corticosteroid
- Class D: Short acting PLUS LAMA, LABA, inhaled corticosteroid

LAMA options: Aclidinium, Tiotropium
LABA options: Formoterol, Salmeterol

Other measures:
- Group B and above: Pulmonary rehab
- PDE4 inhibitor (in severe chronic bronchitis)
- Supplemental oxygen, if O_2 saturation < 55 mmHg or 88%

COPD — Pulmonary/Critical Care Medicine

Acute Exacerbation of COPD

General: Worsening of respiratory symptoms, characterized by one or more of the following:
- (1) Increased cough/cough severity
- (2) Increased sputum production
- (3) Increased dyspnea

Risk: High severity COPD at higher risk. Trigger most commonly bacterial or viral infection.

Diagnosis: Clinical diagnosis (worsening respiratory status, exam, and vitals)

Management:
- Short acting β-agonists (albuterol) +/- anticholinergic (ipratropium)
- Systemic glucocorticoids
- Oxygen titrated to 88-92% (to avoid CO_2 retention from loss of hypoxemic respiratory drive, Haldane effect)
- If necessary, NIV preferred to invasive mechanical ventilation
- No evidence for mucoactive agents or mucus clearance techniques

Antibiotics
- Indicated if ≥ 2/3 cardinal symptoms
- Uncomplicated COPD (age < 65, FEV1 > 50%, < 2 exacerbations a year)
    - Azithromycin, Doxycycline, TMP-SMX, 2nd/3rd Gen Cephalosporin
- Complicated COPD (age > 65, FEV1 < 50%, > 2 exacerbations a year)
    - Cover *Pseudomonas* if patient has risk factors
    - Fluoroquinolone, Amoxicillin-Clavulanate if outpatient
    - IV fluoroquinolone, Cefepime, Piperacillin-Tazobactam if inpatient

Alpha-1 Antitrypsin Deficiency

General: Deficiency in antiprotease protein, which results in abnormal excess elastase activity
- M allele (normal protein levels), Z allele (deficient alpha-1 antitrypsin)
- MM (normal), MZ (normal or mild increase in COPD risk), ZZ (high-risk)

Clinical:
- (1) Early onset panacinar COPD (Age~40's)
- (2) Liver disease (on a spectrum from mild transaminitis to cirrhosis)
- (3) Panniculitis (rare complication)

Diagnosis:
- AAT Levels
- Genotype (PCR)

Management:
- Avoid cigarette smoke and occupational exposures
- Normal COPD Management
- IV Human AAT

ASTHMA — Pulmonary/Critical Care Medicine

Asthma Overview

General: Condition of bronchial hyperresponsiveness, in which inflammation results in episodes of reversible airflow obstruction

Risk:
- History of atopy (most commonly IgE against environmental allergens)
- Triggers include allergens, tobacco smoke, air pollution, respiratory infections, and exercise

Clinical:
- Intermittent dyspnea, wheezing, chest tightness, and cough
- Wheezing may or may not be present

Diagnosis:
- Most often a clinical diagnosis (confirmed by improvement with albuterol)
- Spirometry: Demonstrates reversible airflow obstruction (> 12%/200cc improvement in FEV1 after bronchodilator administration)
    - If inconclusive: Methacholine or exercise challenge testing
- Peak Flow Testing: Can help to monitor symptoms
    - > 10% worsening from baseline suggests asthma exacerbation

Management: Note: For >12 y/o

	Intermittent	Mild Persistent	Moderate Persistent	Severe Persistent
Symptoms	≤ 2 days/week	> 2 days/week	Daily	Constant
Short Acting Agent Use	≤ 2 days/week	> 2 days/week	Daily	Multiple times per day
Nighttime Awakenings	≤ 2 times/month	3-4 times/month	Multiple nights weekly	Most nights
Lung Function	FEV1 Normal (outside of episodes)	FEV1 > 80%	FEV1 60-80%	FEV1 < 60%
Exacerbations	0-1 per year	≥ 2 per year	≥ 2 per year	≥ 2 per year
Management Step	Step 1	Step 2	Step 3	Step 4 or 5

Step 1: SABA prn (Note: Used in all asthma patients, in addition to the steps below)
Step 2: Low dose inhaled glucocorticoids
Step 3: Low dose inhaled glucocorticoids + LABA or Med dose inhaled glucocorticoids
Step 4: Med dose inhaled glucocorticoids + LABA
Step 5: High dose inhaled glucocorticoids, LABA, consider Omalizumab
Step 6: High dose inhaled glucocorticoids, oral glucocorticoids, + LABA and consider omalizumab

Evaluate at each visit for symptoms control:
- If uncontrolled, step up
- If under good control, consider step down in therapy (if stable > 3 months)

ASTHMA/BRONCHIECTASIS
Pulmonary/Critical Care Medicine

Acute Asthma Exacerbation

Clinical:
- Breathlessness, wheezing, coughing, chest tightness
- Decreased I:E ratio, accessory muscle use, tachypnea

Diagnosis: Primarily clinical
- Peak flow testing (worsened from baseline)

Management:
- Beta agonists +/- Ipratropium
- Supplemental oxygen (> 92%). NIV/Mechanical ventilation if this goal cannot be achieved.
- Early steroids (Oral Prednisone or IV Methylprednisolone for ICU)
- Severe exacerbations: Intravenous Mg

Note: Patients with normal/increasing CO_2 may have impending respiratory failure.

Aspirin-exacerbated Respiratory Disease

General: Imbalance in which leukotrienes > prostaglandins, due to NSAIDs or ASA use, leading to respiratory symptoms and airway hyperreactivity

Clinical: (1) Rhinosinusitis (2) Nasal polyposis (3) Asthma

Management: NSAID/ASA avoidance, normal asthma management, plus addition of leukotriene antagonists (Montelukast, Zileuton)

Bronchiectasis

General: Permanent, abnormal dilation and destruction of bronchial walls with inflammation and airway collapse. Due to chronic inflammation with impaired mucous clearance.

Risk:
- Recurrent infections (ie airway obstruction, immunodeficiency, allergic bronchopulmonary aspergillosis)
- Cystic fibrosis, primary ciliary dyskinesia, or autoimmune (RA/SLE)

Clinical: Chronic cough (with lots of mucopurulent sputum), dyspnea, hemoptysis

Diagnosis:
- High Res CT (Study of choice) → Bronchial dilatation/wall thickening
- PFTs (show obstructive disease)
- Workup for underlying etiology (CF test, sputum culture, Ig quantification)

Management:
<u>Acute Exacerbations</u>
- Antibiotics (tailored to previous infectious agents; normally Amoxicillin-Clavulanate or fluoroquinolone, but *Pseudomonas*/MRSA coverage if hx)
- If history of asthma → May require oral glucocorticoids/bronchodilators

<u>Chronic</u>
- Chest physiotherapy/mucus clearance techniques
- Azithromycin if ≥ 2 exacerbations per year

RESTRICTIVE LUNG DISEASE

Pulmonary/Critical Care Medicare

Overview (Pulmonary Processes)

General: Heterogenous group of processes that distort the pulmonary interstitium and alveolar walls, resulting in fibrosis, distortion of the lung structure, and impaired gas exchange

Etiologies:
- Environmental (pneumoconiosis)
- Granulomatous (sarcoid, vasculitis, histiocytosis X)
- Alveolar filling disease (goodpasture, alveolar proteinosis)
- Hypersensitivity (pneumonitis, eosinophilic pneumonia)
- Drug induced (Amiodarone, Nitrofurantoin, Bleomycin, Methotrexate)
- Autoimmune CT disorders (RA, SLE, scleroderma)
- Others (idiopathic pulmonary fibrosis, cryptogenic organizing pneumonia)

Clinical:
- Dyspnea, nonproductive cough, +/- symptoms of a specific above etiology
- Rales, clubbing

Workup:
- High Resolution CT
- Pulmonary Function Testing
    - Decreased lung volumes, FEV1/FVC ≥ 85%, decreased DLCO
- Bronchiolar Lavage (if hemoptysis)
- ECHO (to evaluate for pulmonary HTN)
- Lung Biopsy (if workup is inconclusive of etiology)

Classifying Interstitial Lung Disease

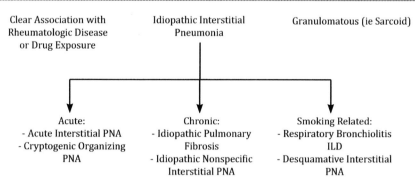

Overview (Extrinsic Processes)

General: Restrictive disease due to abnormalities in chest wall structure or respiratory musculature

Etiologies:
- Neuromuscular (myasthenia gravis, ALS, multiple sclerosis)
- Chest wall (obesity, kyphoscoliosis)

RESTRICTIVE LUNG DISEASE — Pulmonary/Critical Care Medicine

	Definition/Risk	Clinical/Diagnosis	Management
Idiopathic Interstitial PNA			
Acute Interstitial Pneumonia	- Rare, fulminant form of diffuse lung injury without clear cause	- Presents with acute respiratory failure (very similar to ARDS), but without catastrophic event - Dx: Clinical presentation above, plus biopsy showing diffuse alveolar damage	- High dose corticosteroids
Cryptogenic Organizing Pneumonia	- Idiopathic, noninfectious inflammatory pneumonia of the distal bronchioles and alveolar walls	- Two month onset of cough, dyspnea, fever, malaise (often starts with flu-like illness) - Dx: CT (patchy interstitial opacities, ground glass, nodular opacities). Biopsy for definitive diagnosis.	- Corticosteroids +/- an additional immunosuppressive agent
Idiopathic Pulmonary Fibrosis ("Usual Interstitial Pneumonia")	- Chronic fibrosing interstitial pneumonia - Can be idiopathic (6th/7th decade) or genetically based (earlier onset)	- Gradual onset dyspnea, cough, rales - Dx: CT (classic honeycombing and reticular opacities). Biopsy for definitive diagnosis.	- Supportive (supplemental O_2, vaccines, pulmonary rehab) - Pirfenidone or Nintedanib (growth factor inhibitors) - Lung transplant

RESTRICTIVE LUNG DISEASE — Pulmonary/Critical Care Medicine

		Definition/Risk	Clinical/Diagnosis	Management
Granulomatous	Sarcoid	- Idiopathic disorder characterized by noncaseating granuloma formation in multiple systems, especially lung - Most commonly in 20-60 y/o, black females	- Often presents with dyspnea, cough - [See: Rheum] for full discussion - CXR (bilateral hilar LA, +/- infiltrates) - Dx: CT (further characterizes disease) - Biopsy to confirm (can biopsy most accessible lesion, such as peripheral skin lesion/lymph node if possible)	- Asymptomatic/limited disease → Monitor, high rate of self-resolution - Symptomatic/progressive → Glucocorticoids
	Histiocytosis X	[See: Heme-Onc]		
	Vasculitis	[See: Rheum]		
Alveolar Filling Disorders	Goodpasture's	- Circulating antibodies against alpha-3 chain of type IV collagen (expressed in GBM and alveoli)	- Typically presents with rapidly progressive glomerulonephritis and alveolar hemorrhage - Dx: Kidney biopsy (linear IgG deposits), serology (for anti-GBM)	- Plasmapheresis - Prednisone + Cyclophosphamide
	Alveolar Proteinosis	- Intraalveolar accumulation of phospholipids and apoproteins. There is no disturbance of lung architecture.	- Progressive dyspnea, cough, sputum production, fatigue, weight loss. Exam with crackles, clubbing, cyanosis. - Dx: CT, Bronchiolar lavage	- Supportive Care - Whole lung lavage (if severe)
Other	Radiation Induced Lung Disease	- Acute: Pneumonitis occurring immediately secondary to radiation of the chest wall - Permanent fibrosis can occur over time	- 1-3 months following radiation, develop cough, dyspnea, chest pain, fever - Dx: CT (patchy ground glass/opacities)	- Supportive care - If severe, prednisone therapy

Pulm8

RESTRICTIVE LUNG DISEASE — Pulmonary/Critical Care Medicine

Pneumoconiosis	General/Risk	Clinical/Diagnosis	Management
Coal Miner's Lung	- Inhalation of coal dust, resulting in formation of nodular opacities, fibrosis, and areas of necrosis, most commonly in upper lung lobes	- Simple Disease: Most commonly asymptomatic - Can develop fibrosis, restrictive lung disease	- Supportive care, avoid exposure
Silicosis	- Inhalation of silica particles that results in pulmonary fibrosis - Sandblasting, mining, masonry - Increased risk for TB, lung malignancy	- Can present acutely (months to years after exposure) or chronically (> 10 years after exposure). Dyspnea and chronic cough most common. - Dx: CT (upper lobe opacities, possible "eggshell" calcifications of lymph nodes)	- Supportive care, avoid exposure
Asbestosis	- Inhalation of asbestos fibers, resulting in progressive pulmonary fibrosis - Typically occurs in individuals in construction exposed to older asbestos containing buildings - Elevated risk of bronchogenic carcinoma and mesothelioma	- Presents 20-30 years after exposure with exertional dyspnea, dry cough - Dx: CT (subpleural linear opacities, diffuse fibrosis, pleural plaques)	- Supportive care, avoid exposure
Berylliosis	- Beryllium exposure → Noncaseating lung granulomas (looks like sarcoid) - Seen in aerospace, computers, automotive industries	- Presents with progressive dyspnea, cough	- Supportive care, avoid exposure

RESTRICTIVE LUNG DISEASE — Pulmonary/Critical Care Medicine

Hypersensitivity Pneumonitis

General: Alveolar inflammation due to type III/IV hypersensitivity against inhaled organic dusts

Etiologies:
- Farmer's Lung (moldy hay, or thermophilic actinomycetes)
- Silo filler's
- Bird breeder's lung (avian droppings)
- Bagassosis (moldy sugar cane)
- Byssinosis (textiles)

Clinical: Can present acutely (within hours) or chronically with cough, dyspnea, fatigue, weight loss

Diagnosis:
- Inhalation challenge (reexposure)
- CT (ground glass/nodular opacities)
- BAL (marked lymphocytosis with decreased CD4/CD8 ratio)
- Biopsy (poorly formed granulomas)

Management:
- Avoid exposure
- If severely symptomatic → Steroids
- If severe, irreversible fibrosis develops → Transplant

Eosinophilic Pneumonia

General: Eosinophilic infiltration of the pulmonary parenchyma, thought to be hypersensitivity against inhaled antigen

Clinical:
- Acute (< 4 week) illness with cough, dyspnea, fever, and systemic symptoms
- Hypoxemic respiratory failure

Diagnosis: CT (diffuse pulmonary opacities), BAL with > 25% eosinophilia

Management:
- Supportive care
- Glucocorticoids

PULMONARY HYPERTENSION
Pulmonary/Critical Care Medicine

Pulmonary Hypertension (Overview)

General: Mean pulmonary arterial pressure ≥ 25 mmHg

Etiology	Name	Description
Class 1	Pulmonary Arterial HTN	*Below
Class 2	Left Heart Disease	- Elevated LAP (PCWP)
Class 3	Chronic Lung Disease	- COPD, ILD, OSA, etc
Class 4	Chronic Thromboembolism (CTEPH)	- Occurs after PE/multiple PE's - V/Q scan can aid in diagnosis
Class 5	Multifactorial/Unclear Mechanism	- Variety of causes (sickle cell, systemic disorders, metabolic disorders)

Clinical:
- Progressive exertional dyspnea, presyncope/syncope, exertional angina
- Signs of right heart failure (peripheral edema, elevated JVP, increased pulmonary component of S2)

Diagnosis: Right Heart Cath
- Note: ECHO can be used for noninvasive evaluation of pressures

Management:
- Treat underlying (ie treat heart failure for Class 2, manage lung disease for Class 3, etc)
- Class 4: Warfarin and surgical thromboendarterectomy

Pulmonary Arterial Hypertension (PAH)

General: Pulmonary hypertension from proliferation of smooth muscle in pulmonary arterioles

Etiology:
- Idiopathic
- Familial: BMPR-2 mutation (commonly young adult females)
- Drugs, toxins, connective tissue disease, HIV, schistosomiasis

Clinical/Diagnosis: Overview above

Management:
- CCB (Diltiazem)
- Oral endothelin antagonists (Bosentan)
- Oral phosphodiesterase inhibitors (Sildenafil, Tadalafil)
- Oral prostacyclin agonists (Selexipag)
- For severe: IV prostacyclin agonists (Epoprostenol or Treprostinil)

Note: Transplantation is last line for severe refractory cases

DVT/PE — Pulmonary/Critical Care Medicine

DVT

General: Formation of blood clot within a deep vein of the legs. 90% are proximal (most commonly femoral, iliac), 10% distal (posterior tibial).

Risk: Virchow Triad (endothelial injury, stasis, and hypercoagulability)
- Hypercoagulability risks include cancer, surgery, obesity, smoking, birth control, pregnancy, any genetic or autoimmune thrombophilia

Clinical:
- ~50% have calf pain, tenderness, erythema, and superficial vein dilatation
- Homan Sign: Calf pain on ankle dorsiflexion

Diagnosis: Lower Extremity US. Risk stratify utilizing modified Wells score below.

Simplified Wells Score (Pretest Probability of DVT)	
- Previous DVT - Active cancer diagnosis - Recent immobilization or bedridden - Localized tenderness along venous distribution - Leg swelling - Asymmetric calf swelling - Pitting edema - Collateral superficial nonvaricose veins *Alternative diagnosis more likely (-2 points)	< 1: Low probability (DVT unlikely) 1-2: Moderate probability 3-8: High probability (DVT likely) - **Low/Moderate PTP** → D-Dimer: If elevated, then US. - **High PTP** → US

Old methods: CTV, MRV, contrast venography, impedance plethysmography rarely used

Management:

Proximal DVT	- Anticoagulate (Heparin, Warfarin, LMWH, or DOAC) - Contraindication to Anticoagulation → IVC Filter
Massive Proximal DVT	- Defined by severe swelling, soft tissue ischemia, etc - Thrombolytic or surgical thrombectomy
Distal DVT	- Anticoagulate (if contraindication, then observe closely with LE US)

- Follow-up:
  - Work up for underlying cause if unknown (ie age appropriate cancer screening, if young then hereditary thrombophilia panel)
  - 3 months of anticoagulation required, continue indefinitely if cause is unknown or irreversible

Complications:
Phlegmasia cerulea dolens: Severe pain/edema/blue discoloration due to ischemia from extensive proximal DVT. Indication for thrombolytic/surgical thrombectomy.

Post-thrombotic syndrome: Chronic venous insufficiency that can occur after DVT. Presents as chronic extremity pain, edema, and venous changes. Manage with symptomatic therapy, such as limb elevation, compression therapy, exercise.

DVT/PE — Pulmonary/Critical Care Medicine

Pulmonary Embolism

General: Embolization of a thrombus into the pulmonary vasculature. Subtypes:
- Massive (high-risk): Hemodynamically unstable
- Submassive (intermediate-risk): Hemodynamically stable with RV strain
- Low risk: Hemodynamically stable, no RV dysfunction

Can also be characterized by anatomic location: Saddle, lobar, segmental, subsegmental

Clinical:
- Dyspnea, pleuritic chest pain, hemoptysis. Syncope possible.
- Tachypnea, tachycardia. Small pleural effusions possible.

Wells Criteria [Pretest Probability of PE]	
Clinical symptoms of DVT	3 points
Other diagnoses less likely	3 points
HR > 100 bpm	1.5 points
Immobilization or recent surgery	1.5 points
Hx of DVT/PE	1.5 points
Hemoptysis	1 point
Malignancy	1 point
High Probability: ≥ 6 points Medium Probability: 2-6 points Low Probability: < 2 points	

Diagnosis:
- Spiral CT Angiography (first line)
- V/Q Scan (for those who cannot tolerate contrast)
- If patient is unstable despite resuscitation → Bedside ECHO (Right heart hypokinesis/dilatation, called McConnell's sign)

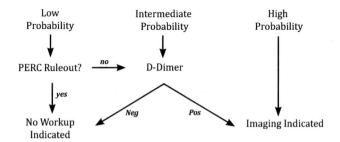

PERC (Ruleout criteria):

Age < 50	No prior PE/DVT
BPM < 100	No leg swelling
O_2 Sat > 95%	No recent surgery/trauma
No hemoptysis	No estrogen use

| DVT/PE | Pulmonary/Critical Care Medicine |

Pulmonary Embolism (Management)

Management:
- Initial:
    - Suspected PE: Supplemental O_2, ventilation, hemodynamic support
    - If high probability for PE and low bleeding risk, empiric anticoagulation

- Unstable:
    - Thrombolytic therapy, followed by anticoagulation
    - Alternative is catheter or surgical embolectomy

- Stable: Anticoagulation
    - Initial: Heparin, LMWH, Fondaparinux, Apixaban/Rivaroxaban
        - UFH if renal failure, as LMWH and DOAC contraindicated
    - Long term: DOAC (Factor Xa or thrombin inhibitor), Warfarin, LMWH

Note: Anticoagulation contraindicated → IVC filter

If any evidence of worsening hemodynamics, thrombolytic therapy can be considered on case-to-case basis

DVT/PE Prophylaxis

Indications:
- Hospitalized patients with ≥ 1 following risk factor deserve prophylaxis
    - Risks: ICU, cancer, stroke, CHF, MI, age > 75, hx of VTE, renal failure, obesity, prolonged immobility
- Essentially all acutely ill hospitalized patients will get pharm DVT ppx unless young/healthy/short hospitalization

Pharm	- LMWH, subcutaneous unfractionated Heparin - Contraindicated with bleeding risk/current active bleeding
Non-pharm	- Mechanical compression devices (intermittent pneumatic compression or graduated compression stockings) - Early ambulation

PLEURAL EFFUSION
Pulmonary/Critical Care Medicine

Pleural Effusion (Overview)

General: Excess fluid in pleural cavity, from either increased fluid production or impaired drainage

Etiology:
- Transudative (HF, hypoalbuminemia, cirrhosis)
- Exudative (parapneumonic, malignancy, TB, autoimmune [RA, SLE], trauma)
- Chylothorax (rupture of thoracic ducts)

Clinical:
- Often asymptomatic, but can cause dyspnea
- Decreased breath sounds, dullness to percussion, decreased fremitus

Diagnosis:
- CXR (blunting of costophrenic angle)
- CT (can confirm/reveal small effusions)
- Thoracentesis (can be diagnostic/therapeutic, obtain on all large effusions unless clear cut HF)
- Light's Criteria:
    (1) Pleural protein/Serum protein ratio > 0.5
    (2) Pleural LDH/Serum LDH > 0.6
    (3) Pleural LDH > $2/3$ upper limit of normal serum LDH
- Other pleural fluid findings:
    - Glucose low in infection, malignancy
    - pH (7.6 normal, 7.4-7.55 transudative, 7.3-7.45 exudative)
    - Cytology
    - Amylase (esophageal rupture)

Management:

Transudative	- Treat underlying condition - Therapeutic thoracentesis may be useful in large effusions
Exudative	- Depends on underlying etiology, but in general thoracentesis, +/- chest tube - Surgical intervention for those that are loculated/difficult to drain

Parapneumonic Effusions

	Uncomplicated	Complicated	Empyema
General	Sterile exudate	Bacterial invasion	Frank pus
Pleural Fluid	WBC < 50k pH > 7.2	WBC > 50k pH < 7.2	
Gram Stain/Culture	Negative	Usually negative	Positive
Management	Antibiotics	Antibiotics +/- Drainage	Antibiotic + Drainage

Pulm15

PNEUMOTHORAX
Pulmonary/Critical Care Medicine, Surgery

Pneumothorax (Overview)

General: Accumulation of air in the pleural space

Etiology:
- Spontaneous
    - Primary (due to subpleural bleb rupture, young tall male)
    - Secondary (due to underlying lung disease, like COPD)
- Traumatic
- Iatrogenic (mechanical ventilation, thoracentesis, central lines, CPR)

Clinical:
- Acute onset ipsilateral chest pain, dyspnea, cough
- Decreased breath sounds, hyperresonance

Diagnosis: CXR (absent lung markings, with pleural line)

Management:
- Small (< 2 cm): Observation and supplemental oxygen +/- drainage of air
- Large (> 2 cm) or Clinically Unstable: Chest tube placement

Tension Pneumothorax

General: Subtype of pneumothorax characterized by accumulation of subpleural air resulting in increased pressure and collapse of lung tissues. Elevated thoracic pressures result in hemodynamic compromise.

Etiology: Trauma or mechanical ventilation

Clinical:
- Hemodynamic collapse, hypotension (impaired venous return)
- Decreased breath sounds, hyperresonance, plus possible tracheal deviation, and distended neck veins

Diagnosis: CXR will confirm, but treat if high clinical suspicion

Management:
- Immediate needle thoracostomy
- Followed by chest tube placement

HEMOPTYSIS
Pulmonary/Critical Care Medicine, Surgery

Hemoptysis (Overview)

General: Expectoration of blood, most commonly from bronchial arteries. Classified based on amount of blood.
- < 500 mL: Mild to moderate
- > 500 mL or 100 mL/hr: Massive

Etiology:
- Airway disease (bronchitis, bronchiectasis, neoplasm, trauma, iatrogenic)
- Parenchymal disease (infection, autoimmune/genetic CT disorders)
- Vascular (PE, AV malformation)

Management:

Mild/Moderate	- Workup/treat underlying cause - CT scan or flexible bronchoscopy reserved for cases of active bleeding
Massive	- Establish airway, maintain hemodynamics (ie ABC's) - Flexible bronchoscopy (electrical cautery or balloon tamponade) - Arteriographic embolization (if bronchoscopy fails to identify and reverse bleed)

RESPIRATORY FAILURE
Pulmonary/Critical Care Medicine

Acute Respiratory Failure

General: Inadequate ventilation leading to hypoxemia. Subtypes:
- Hypoxemic (V/Q mismatch, shunting, or decreased diffusion)
   - Associated with high A-a gradient
- Hypercapnic (decreased alveolar ventilation from decreased respiratory rate, minute ventilation, or increased dead space)

Clinical: Dyspnea, accessory muscle use, inability to complete sentences, hypoxemia

Diagnosis: ↓ O_2 saturation and ABG

Management:

	Method	Oxygen Delivery
Floors	Nasal Cannula	- 2-6 L/min (FiO_2: 24-40%)
	Face Mask	- 5-8 L/min (FiO_2: 30-50%)
	Venti Mask	- 6-10 L/min (FiO_2: 24-50%)
	Non-rebreather	- 8-10 L/min (FiO_2: 60-80%)
ICU	High-dose Nasal Cannula	- 10-60 L/min (FiO_2: up to 100%)
	CPAP	- Provides positive end-expiratory pressure
	BIPAP (NIPPV)	- Provides positive end-expiratory pressure AND additional pressure support with breaths
	Mechanical Ventilation	

Mechanical Ventilation

Indications: Apnea, acute respiratory failure, impending respiratory failure, or need for airway protection

Note: Typically start in volume-control, with V(t) of 6-8 ml/kg, RR 12-16, FiO_2 100%, PEEP 5cm H_2O

Mode	Description	Trigger	Cycle
Assist Control (Volume Control)	Set tidal volume delivered at set rate, fully machine supported. Pressure varies with compliance.	Time/pt	Volume
Pressure Control (PCV)	Set inspiratory positive pressure administered over a set time. Tidal volume varies with compliance.	Time	Time
Pressure Support	No set tidal volume or rate, but set inspiratory pressure to reduce work of breathing.	Pt	Flow

Sedation: Utilize medication pairings with analgesic and amnesic effects:
- Opiates (Fentanyl or Hydromorphone)
- Propofol
- Midazolam
- Dexmedetomidine

RESPIRATORY FAILURE
Pulmonary/Critical Care Medicine

Mechanical Ventilation (Management Basics)

After intubation, check for proper placement (2-5 cm above carina) and ABG

Situation	Adjustment
$paCO_2$ is high + respiratory acidosis	Increase RR/ VT to increase ventilation
$paCO_2$ is low + respiratory alkalosis	Decrease RR/ VT to decrease ventilation
paO_2 is low	FIO_2 and PEEP in steps to achieve $paO_2 > 60$ mmHg
paO_2 is high	Decrease FIO_2 in steps to 50% and then slowly reduce PEEP in 3-5mmHg increments, maintaining $paO_2 > 60$
Refractory Hypoxemia	Pressure control mode, prone ventilation, or ECMO
↑ Peak Pressure	Can be elevated with low lung compliance, but also ↑ airway resistance (mucus plugging, obstructed ET tube)
↑ Plateau Pressure	Elevated with low lung compliance

Weaning (patient must have $FIO_2 < 50\%$ and PEEP < 5 mmHg)
- Spontaneous Breathing Trial: Most commonly trial of pressure support
- RSBI < 105 (RR/Vt)

Complications:
- Barotrauma (can lead to pneumothorax)
- Oxygen Toxicity
    - Absorptive atelectasis
    - Parenchymal injury (worsening lung disease due to high O_2 sats)

Acute Respiratory Distress Syndrome (ARDS)

General: Hypoxemic respiratory failure secondary to alveolar injury, which results in accumulation of proteinaceous fluid in the alveoli, impairing gas exchange and decreasing compliance. Results in massive pulmonary shunt physiology.

Etiology: Sepsis, aspiration, pneumonia, trauma, transfusions (TRALI), pancreatitis

Clinical: Respiratory distress, dyspnea, hypoxemia, cyanosis, tachypnea, rales

Diagnosis: Berlin Definition
   (1) Acute onset < 1 week
   (2) Bilateral infiltrates on chest imaging
   (3) Pulmonary edema not explained by fluid overload or CHF
       (no CHF and PCWP is < 18 mmHg)
   (4) Abnormal PaO_2/FiO_2 ratio < 300
       (Mild: 200-300, Moderate: 100-200, Severe: 100)

Management:
- Mechanical Ventilation (high PEEP, low tidal volume ventilation)
    - Neuromuscular blockade (helps ventilator synchrony)
    - Conservative fluid strategy (to avoid worsened pulmonary edema)
- Treat underlying condition

SHOCK
Pulmonary/Critical Care Medicine

Shock Overview

General: Low tissue perfusion, resulting in cellular injury and tissue hypoxia

Subtypes	Cause	Clinical	PCWP	CO	SVR
Hypovolemic	Hemorrhage, Dehydration, Burn	Cold, clammy	↓	↓	↑
Cardiogenic	MI, CHF, Valvular, Arrhythmia	Cold, clammy	↑	↓	↑
Obstructive	Cardiac Tamponade, PTX, PE Pulmonary Embolism	Cold, clammy	↑/↓	↓	↑
Distributive	Sepsis, Anaphylaxis	Warm, dry	↓	↑	↓

Clinical: Hypotension (MAP < 70 mmHg), clinical signs of hypoperfusion (cool skin, altered mental status, low urine output), increased serum lactate

Management: Treat underlying etiology. To improve hypotension:
- Fluids (generally LR or NS, but not in cardiogenic shock)
- Vasopressors if BP remains critically low

Drug	Activity	Effect	Indications
Norepinephrine	α1>α2>β1	↑ SVR, CO	- Initial vasopressor of choice in septic, cardiogenic and hypovolemic shock
Phenylephrine	α1>α2	↑ SVR	- Alternative or add on to norepinephrine - Indicated if norepi induces tachyarrhythmia
Vasopressin	V_1, V_2	↑ SVR	- Used as adjunctive agent to reduce primary agent dosage
Epinephrine	β>α	↑ SVR, HR, CO	- Agent of choice in anaphylaxis, cardiac arrest - High doses → α effects predominate - Low doses → Decreases peripheral tone
Dopamine	D1>β1>α1	↑ SVR, CO	- Second line agent - Low Dose: Dilates renal veins (D1) - Medium Dose: Increase heart contractility (β) - High Dose: Vasoconstriction (α)
Midodrine (PO)	α1	↑ SVR	- Mild vasoconstrictor, only oral agent
Inotropic Agents			
Dobutamine	β1>β2>α	↑ CO	- Initial agent of choice in cardiogenic shock with low cardiac output and normal blood pressure - Also used in stress tests - Inotropic > chronotropic. Also causes mild peripheral vasodilation (so can ↓ BP).
Milrinone	PDE3 Inhibitor	↑ CO	- Alternative for short-term cardiac output augmentation in refractory cardiogenic shock

SEPSIS

Pulmonary/Critical Care Medicine

Sepsis Overview

Definitions: (Note: SIRS and severe sepsis no longer used)
- Infection: Invasion of sterile tissue by organisms
- Bacteremia: Bacteria in blood
- Sepsis: Organ dysfunction from infection (≥ 2 SOFA score from baseline)
- Septic shock: Sepsis plus hemodynamic compromise. Despite resuscitation, requires pressors to maintain MAP and have elevated lactate (> 2 mmol/L)

Diagnosis:

SIRS Criteria (Old)	qSOFA (New)
≥ 2/4 of the following:	≥ 2 of the following:
(1) Temperature > 38°C or < 36°C (2) HR > 90 bpm (3) RR > 20 or paCO$_2$ < 32 mmHg (4) WBC > 12k, < 4k, or > 10% bands	(1) RR > 22 (2) Altered mentation (3) SBP < 100 mmHg Note: Applies to patients outside the ICU

SOFA Score (ICU mortality increases with increased score)

Variable	0	1	2	3	4
Respiratory - PaO$_2$/FiO$_2$	> 400	≤ 400	≤ 300	≤ 200	≤ 100
Coagulation - Platelets x 10^3	> 150	≤ 150	≤ 100	≤ 50	≤ 20
Liver - Bilirubin	< 1.2	1.2-1.9	2.0-5.9	6.0-11.9	> 12.0
CV - Hypotension	None	MAP < 70	Dop < 5 Dob (any)	Dop > 5 Epi ≤ 0.1 Norepi ≤ 0.1	Dop > 15 Epi > 0.1 Norepi > 0.1
CNS - Glasgow Coma	15	13-14	10-12	6-9	< 6
Renal - Creatinine/UO	< 1.2	1.2-1.9	2.0-3.4	Cr 3.5-4.9 UO < 500mL/d	Cr > 5.0 UO < 200mL/d

*Dop=Dopamine, Dob=Dobutamine, Epi=Epinephrine, Norepi=Norepinephrine. All rates in ug/kg/min

Management:
- Early antibiotic therapy
    - Broad spectrum with gram positive and negative coverage
- Vascular access and IV fluids (bolus 30mL/kg or NS or LR)
    - Give fluids to maintain > 65 mmHg MAP and urine > 0.5 ml/kg/hr
    - RBC transfusion if Hgb < 7 g/dL
- Vasopressors if MAP goal (> 65 mmHg) not achieved

LUNG MALIGNANCY

Pulmonary/Critical Care Medicine

Lung Cancer (Overview)

Subtype	Location	Characteristics
Small Cell Carcinoma	Central	- Undifferentiated → Very aggressive - Associated w/ paraneoplastic syndromes
Non-Small Cell Lung Cancer (NSCLC)		
Squamous Cell Carcinoma	Central	- Arises from bronchus - Associated with cavitation, hypercalcemia
Adenocarcinoma	Peripheral	- Most common lung cancer (and most common in non-smokers) - Bronchioloalveolar (low-grade subtype with improved prognosis)
Large Cell Carcinoma	Peripheral	- Highly anaplastic, undifferentiated tumor
Bronchial Carcinoid	Either	- Excellent prognosis with rare metastasis - Symptoms due to mass effect or carcinoid syndrome - Flushing, diarrhea, wheezing

Risk: Smoking (~90% of cases), second hand smoke, radon (basements), asbestos

Clinical: Variable presentation. Can present as cough, hemoptysis, wheezing, dyspnea, recurrent pneumonia, weight loss, fever. Or with complication/paraneoplastic syndrome.

Diagnosis:
- CT Chest
- Confirm diagnosis with biopsy or cytology
    - Bronchoscopy, CT-guided biopsy or VATS for tissue sample

Management:
- NSCLC: Surgery +/- Chemo and/or Radiation
- SCLC: Chemotherapy, +/- prophylactic cranial irradiation

Complications:
- Paraneoplastic
    - Small Cell (SIADH, lambert-eaton, ectopic ACTH production)
    - SCC (PTHrP → Hypercalcemia)
- Pleural Effusions
- Horner Syndrome (ptosis, miosis, anhidrosis from cervical chain invasion)
- Pancoast (Superior Sulcus) Tumors
    - Upper lobe tumors that can invade cervical chain (Horner's) and Brachial Plexus (Shoulder pain, C8-T1 weakness/atrophy/paresthesias)
- Superior Vena Cava Syndrome [See: Heme-Onc]

LUNG MALIGNANCY

Pulmonary/Critical Care Medicine

Lung Nodules

Note: Any nodule found on CXR should be evaluated with CT

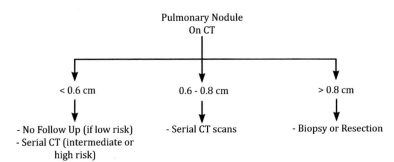

Risk	Age	Smoking	Size (cm)	Characteristics
Low	< 40	Never	< 0.8	Smooth, fat inside (hamartoma), or calcifications (granuloma)
Intermediate	40-60	Current or quit 5-15 yr	0.8-2.0	Scalloped
High	> 60	Current or quit < 5 yr	≥ 2.0	Spiculated

- Benign nodules most commonly hamartomas, granulomas, or focal PNA
- Any growing nodule should undergo biopsy or resection

Mediastinal Mass

Anterior Mediastinum	Teratoma, thyroid mass, thymoma, lymphoma
Middle Mediastinum	Bronchogenic cyst, lymph nodes, pericardial or enteric cyst
Posterior Mediastinum	Neurogenic tumors

Mesothelioma

General: Rare neoplasm arising from mesothelial surface of pleural cavity. Associated with asbestos exposure.

Clinical: Generally insidious, with symptoms including dyspnea, chest pain, cough

Diagnosis:
- CT (unilateral pleural thickening, calcification, pleural effusion)
- Cytology (thoracentesis, closed biopsy, or VATS)

Management:
- Surgery (pleurectomy or radical pneumonectomy) + Chemotherapy

| ALLERGY | | Pulmonary/Critical Care Medicine |

Chronic Rhinitis

General: Rhinorrhea, sneezing, congestion. Can be allergic, nonallergic, or mixed.

	Allergic	Nonallergic (Vasomotor)
Gen	- Associated with atopic disorders (eczema, asthma, conjunctivitis)	- Excess fluid leakage from nasal vasculature - Can be triggered by odors, fragrance, smoke, etc
Clin	- Prominent nasal itching - Sneezing, rhinorrhea, congestion - Can be seasonal/related to allergens - Commonly presents in childhood - Possible IgE sensitivity	- Prominent congestion - Sneezing, rhinorrhea - Commonly presents in adulthood
Dx	- Clinical - Allergy testing if severe/refractory	- Clinical (diagnosis of exclusion)
Tx	- Intranasal glucocorticoid (first line) - Intranasal antihistamine or oral antihistamine (second generation) are adjuncts	- Intranasal glucocorticoids and/or intranasal antihistamines (Azelastine) - Intranasal Ipratropium (for pure watery rhinitis)

Anaphylaxis

General: Sudden systemic syndrome caused by massive mast cell release into the bloodstream

Etiology: Common triggers include food reaction, drug, insect sting, or any other allergen

Clinical: Rapid onset (minutes to hours) of;
- Generalized hives, pruritus
- Swollen lips/tongue/oropharynx
- Respiratory failure (hypoxemia, dyspnea, bronchospasm, stridor)
- Shock (hypotension, signs of end-organ malperfusion)

Management:
- Epinephrine (used in all cases, from mild hives, to life-threatening shock)
  - IM Epi for most, IV if patient is severely ill
  - No absolute contraindications to Epinephrine
- Fluids (for those in shock)
- Symptomatic: Albuterol, antihistamines

LOWER RESPIRATORY INFECTIONS
Pulmonary/Critical Care Medicine

Pneumonia

	Definition	Organisms
Community-Acquired	Within 72 hours of hospitalization	- *S. pneumoniae* - *H. Influenzae* - *Moraxella* - Atypicals (see below)
Hospital-Acquired	> 72 hours after hospitalization	- MSSA/MRSA/*Strep* - *Pseudomonas* - *E. Coli, Klebsiella, Enterobacter*
Ventilator-Acquired	> 48 hours after ventilation	

Etiology:

Group	Organism	Group	Organism
< 4 weeks old	*E. Coli* Group B *Strep*	*IV Drug Use*	MSSA/MRSA *Pseudomonas*
4 weeks-18 y/o	*Mycoplasma* *Chlamydia* Virus (RSV) Pneumococcus	*Alcoholic*	*Klebsiella* Anaerobes
Postviral	MSSA/MRSA Pneumococcus	*Cystic Fibrosis*	MRSA/MSSA *Pseudomonas*

Clinical:
- Acute onset fever/chills, productive cough, dyspnea, pleuritic chest pain
- Hypoxemia, rales, dullness to percussion, increased tactile fremitus

Diagnosis:
- Chest X-ray (Gold standard, infiltrates are classic)
- Sputum Culture, Blood Culture, Pneumococcal/*Legionella* urine antigen test
  - These are indicated in certain circumstances (ICU admissions, certain underlying comorbidities/past medical history)

Atypical Pneumonia

Etiology:
- *Mycoplasma pneumoniae, Chlamydia pneumoniae, Chlamydia psittaci, Coxiella burnetii* (Q fever), *Legionella*
- Viruses: Influenza, adenoviruses, RSV

Clinical:
- Insidious onset (headache, sore throat, fatigue), dry cough, fever
- Diffuse wheezing, rhonchi, or rales
- CXR (Diffuse reticulonodular infiltrates)

LOWER RESPIRATORY INFECTIONS
Pulmonary/Critical Care Medicine

Pneumonia Management

Curb-65 (aid for disposition)

- Confusion - Urea (BUN) > 19 mg/dL - RR > 30 - BP < 90/60 mmHg - Age > 65	0-1 → Outpatient 2 → Inpatient ≥ 3 → ICU

Subgroup	Intervention
Outpatient	- <u>Empiric Antibiotic</u>: Macrolide or Doxycycline. - If high rate of resistance to above, or antibiotic use within the last 3 months → β-lactam (ie Amox) PLUS Azithromycin or Levofloxacin - 5 day course. Must be afebrile for > 48 hours upon termination of antibiotics.
Inpatient CAP	<u>Empiric Antibiotics</u>: - Beta-lactam (Ceftriaxone, Ampicillin-Sulbactam) PLUS macrolide (Azithromycin) - OR respiratory fluoroquinolone (Levo/Moxifloxacin)

ICU CAP	- Empiric Antibiotics: Beta-lactam (Ceftriaxone, Ampicillin-Sulbactam) PLUS Macrolide (Azithromycin) or respiratory fluoroquinolone (Levo/Moxifloxacin)
	
	- MRSA Coverage (Vancomycin or Linezolid) IF:
	    Septic shock/mechanically ventilated, known MRSA colonization or risk factors for colonization
	
	- *Pseudomonas* coverage (Piperacillin-Tazobactam, Cefepime, Meropenem) IF:
	    Structural lung disease (bronchiectasis), gram negative rods on gram stain, frequent COPD exacerbations
	
	- Adjunctive glucocorticoids (in certain severe situations)

HAP or VAP	- MRSA Coverage (Vancomycin or Linezolid) PLUS - *Pseudomonas* coverage: Pip-Tazo, Cefepime, Gentamicin Note: Very sick patients (septic shock, ARDS) can get 2x anti-pseudomonal agents

CAP: Other General Rules
- Narrow therapy based on culture results, change to oral meds when stable
- X-ray will not improve for 4-6 weeks after treatment
- High risk individuals should receive follow up X-ray in ~ 7 weeks
- For example, male smokers, age > 50 y/o

LOWER RESPIRATORY INFECTIONS
Pulmonary/Critical Care Medicine

Recurrent Pneumonia

Recurrent PNA in same location:
- Most likely anatomical abnormality
    - Obstructive lesions like neoplasms
    - Bronchial abnormalities (bronchiectasis)
- If right lower or middle lobe: Consider recurrent aspiration

Recurrent PNA in different location:
- Primary or secondary immunodeficiency

Lung Abscess

General: Local area of necrotic pulmonary parenchyma

Risk: Most commonly secondary to aspiration with anaerobes (*Bacteroides, Peptostreptococcus, Prevotella*). Others: MRSA, *Klebsiella*.

Clinical: Presents with subacute onset of fever and productive cough, with systemic symptoms such as night sweats/weight loss. Can also present as a secondary complication of pneumonia in hospitalized patients.

Diagnosis: CXR or CT: Pulmonary infiltrate with cavitary area

Management: Antibiotics (anaerobic coverage)
- Ampicillin-Sulbactam, Piperacillin-Tazobactam, or a carbapenem

Aspiration Pneumonitis/Pneumonia

General: Pulmonary consequences resulting from the entry of exogenous fluid or particles into the lower airway. Syndromes attributed to aspiration include chemical pneumonitis, bacterial pneumonia, and simple mechanical obstruction.

Risk: Reduced consciousness, dysphagia, esophageal disorders, vomiting, large volume tube feedings, disruption of glottic closure mechanism

	Pneumonitis	Pneumonia
Gen	- "Flash burn" from aspiration of gastric acid	- Aspiration of oropharyngeal or upper airway contents (anaerobes, but also common upper airway bacteria)
Clin	- Acute onset of dyspnea, often after witnessed aspiration event - Hypoxemia, respiratory distress	- Insidious onset of classic pneumonia symptoms, in someone with the above risk factors
Dx	- Clinical diagnosis, based on the presentation above, presence of risk factors, and XR demonstrating infiltrates	
Tx	- Tracheal suctioning - Supplemental O$_2$ - Antibiotics are controversial	- Antibiotics (Amp-Sulbactam, Pip-Tazo)

Pulm27

LOWER RESPIRATORY INFECTIONS
Pulmonary/Critical Care Medicine

Tuberculosis

General: Infection due to *Mycobacterium tuberculosis*. The organism can be immediately cleared, or result in primary infection, latent infection, or reactivation disease.

Risk: Prisoners, healthcare workers, recent immigrants (within 5 years), close contact with someone with TB, IV drug use, immunodeficiency (HIV, glucocorticoid use, hematologic malignancy)

	Primary	Reactivation
Definition	- New TB infection in naive host	- Reactivation of previous TB infection
Clinical	- Often asymptomatic - Acute pneumonia is also possible (middle/lower lobe)	- Fever, night sweats, weight loss, dyspnea, cough
Diagnosis	- Positive PPD or IFN-γ assay	- Positive CXR (pulmonary infiltrate, most commonly upper lobe) PLUS sputum culture

Diagnosis:
Screening:
  - Positive PPD (or IFN-γ assay), with normal X-ray → Latent TB
  - Positive PPD with abnormal x-ray → Active TB or Reactivation

Suspicion for active disease:
  - CXR (Looking for: Focal infiltrates most commonly in apex, +/- cavitation)
  - Cultures (Three sputum cultures, taken at various times)
    - Test with AFB smear, mycobacterial culture, and NAA test

PPD Interpretation	
Induration	Group
≥ 5 mm	- HIV, Recent TB contact, Immunosuppressed, Evidence of prior TB infection
≥ 10 mm	- Recent (< 5 year) immigrant from endemic country, IV drug use, high-risk exposure (prison, healthcare, TB lab) - High risk for reactivation (DM, CKD, leukemia, glucocorticoid use)
≥ 15 mm	- Everyone else

Management:
Latent
  - Isoniazid + Pyridoxine (6-9 months) or
  - Isoniazid + Rifapentine (3 months) or
  - Rifampin (4 months)

Active
  - 2 months of RIPE (Rifampin, Isoniazid, Pyrazinamide, Ethambutol) PLUS 4 months of Isoniazid+Rifampin

LOWER RESPIRATORY INFECTIONS
Pulmonary/Critical Care Medicine

Tuberculosis Complications

Complications:
- Hemoptysis, bronchiectasis, pneumothorax
- Bone involvement ("Pott's")
- Pleural, pericardial, or peritoneal disease

<u>Miliary TB</u>
- Hematogenous dissemination of TB, resulting in multiorgan failure and septic shock
- Pulmonary disease with small "millet seed-like" lesions
- Can involve bones, adrenal, CNS, GU (sterile pyuria)
- Diagnosis: Acid-fast blood cultures, tissue biopsy (culture/NAA testing)
- Treat similarly to pulmonary tuberculosis

Acute Bronchitis

General: Large airway inflammation resulting in a clinical syndrome defined by a cough > 5 days that can last up to 3 weeks

Risk: Typically follows viral URI, with < 10% of cases bacterial

Clinical:
- Cough +/- sputum production. URI symptoms can overlap early on.
- Cough can be subacute (ie multiple weeks)
- Physical exam typically unremarkable. Wheezing/rhonchi/rales possible.

Diagnosis: Clinical diagnosis. CXR in those with suspicion for PNA.

Management:
- Reassurance/Education (antibiotics not indicated)
- Cough
    - Nonpharm options preferred (tea, lozenges)
    - Dextromethorphan or Guaifenesin if refractory
    - Albuterol if wheezing component

UPPER RESPIRATORY INFECTION
Pulmonary/Critical Care Medicine

Upper Respiratory Infection (Common Cold)

General: Common, self-limited syndrome from upper respiratory virus infection. Term URI includes viral rhinosinusitis, pharyngitis.

Etiology: Rhinovirus, coronavirus, influenza, parainfluenza, RSV

Clinical:
- Rhinitis, nasal congestion
- Sore throat, cough
- Malaise
- Can be complicated by bacterial sinusitis/otitis, bronchitis

Diagnosis: Clinical

Management:
- Self-limited (1-1.5 weeks)
- Symptomatic care
    - NSAIDs for pain
    - If severe cough: Dextromethorphan
    - Congestion: Antihistamine/decongestant combination

Influenza

General: Acute respiratory illness due to influenza A or B virus infection. Transmitted via respiratory droplets/aerosols.

Clinical:
- Sudden onset of malaise, fever, headache, myalgia
- URI symptoms possible (cough/sore throat/rhinitis)
- Complications
    - PNA (can be primary viral or secondary bacterial)
        - Pneumococcus, *S. aureus*

Diagnosis:
- Molecular Tests: RT-PCR (alt. rapid molecular assay)
    - Both are sensitive, can reveal subtype of flu
- Antigen tests (ie rapid antigen assay) less sensitive (possible false negative)

Management:
- Antiviral therapy (Oseltamivir, Zanamivir, Peramivir [IM]). Indicated if:
    - < 48 hours of symptoms
    - > 48 hours of symptoms, if high risk for complications
- Consider prophylactic antivirals if close contact AND high risk for influenza complication or are members of long-term care facility

UPPER RESPIRATORY INFECTION
Pulmonary/Critical Care Medicine

Rhinosinusitis

General: Inflammation in the nasal cavity and paranasal sinuses. Sinusitis most commonly viral/associated with common cold, but can be bacterial (most common organisms pneumococcus, *H. influenzae, and Moraxella*).

Risk: Often associated with polyps, deviated septum, foreign body

Clinical:
Acute (< 4 weeks):
- Facial pain/pressure
- Nasal congestion with purulent nasal discharge
- Maxillary tooth discomfort
- Other symptoms (fever, malaise, headache, ear pain/pressure)

Key Bacterial Features:
(1) > 10 days without improvement
(2) "Double Worsening" (gets worse after seems to improve)
(3) Severe symptoms for ≥ 3 days (T > 102°F, heavy purulent drainage)

Chronic (> 12 weeks):
- Purulent drainage, nasal obstruction, facial pain, decreased olfaction

Diagnosis: Clinical (see key bacterial features above to differentiate from viral)
- Imaging (ie head CT) only indicated if concerned about complication
- Chronic disease: Require clinical symptoms plus imaging or endoscopic evidence of inflammation

Management:

Viral	- Self-limited - Symptomatic (analgesia, saline irrigation, intranasal steroids)
Bacterial	- Symptomatic therapy (as above) - Antibiotics (Amoxicillin-Clavulanate; alt: Doxycycline) - Note: Many with bacterial sinusitis improve without antibiotics, so it is clinical decision to give antibiotics
Chronic	- Extended antibiotic therapy (Amoxicillin-Clavulanate; alt: Clindamycin) - Oral glucocorticoids, plus long term intranasal glucocorticoids - Surgery for refractory/severe cases

Complications:
- Orbital/periorbital cellulitis
- CNS (abscess, meningitis, cavernous sinus thrombosis)

UPPER RESPIRATORY INFECTION
Pulmonary/Critical Care Medicine, Pediatrics

Pharyngitis

General: Acute inflammation of the oropharynx. Most commonly due to respiratory viruses (self-limited). Bacterial cases usually due to Group A *Streptococcus*. Differential also includes:
- Bacterial: *Mycoplasma*, diphtheria, *Gonorrhea*, *Chlamydia*
- Viral: EBV, HSV, acute HIV

Clinical:
- Viral: Sore throat. Associated with cold symptoms (nasal congestion, cough, rhinorrhea, etc)
- Bacterial: Sore throat, associated with fever, tonsillar exudates, tender anterior cervical lymphadenopathy. Cold symptoms missing (vs viral).

Diagnosis:
Adults
- Rapid antigen test preferred (culture only required in rare, high-risk cases)
- Centor Criteria (below) can be used to help determine who needs testing

(1) Fever
(2) Tonsillar Exudates
(3) Tender Cervical LA
(4) No Cough

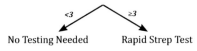

Children
- Rapid antigen test (alt: culture)
- Test those with signs of bacterial pharyngitis that lack any other viral URI symptoms

Management:

Viral	- Self-limited
GAS	- Penicillin V or Amoxicillin (alt: Macrolides, Clindamycin, cephalosporin)

Complications:
- Rheumatic fever, poststreptococcal glomerulonephritis (GAS)
- Abscess, recurrent infection

PEDIATRIC RESPIRATORY INFECTIONS
Pulmonary/Critical Care
Pediatrics

Croup

General: Laryngotracheobronchitis, which produces characteristic barking cough

Etiology: Most commonly parainfluenza virus (others include RSV, adeno, influenza)

Clinical:
- Starts with congestion/coryza, fever
- Followed by hoarseness, barking cough, +/- stridor
- Spasmodic Subtype (Recurring Croup)
    - Recurrent nighttime episodes of barking cough
    - Self-limited, short episodes

Diagnosis:
- Clinical Diagnosis
- XR (may show steeple sign, referring to tapering of upper trachea)

Management:
- Corticosteroids
- PLUS Nebulized Epinephrine (if severe)

Bronchiolitis

General: Lower respiratory tract infection of the bronchioles. Most common in children < 2 years old.

Etiology: RSV is most common (others: rhino, parainfluenza, metapneumo, influenza)

Clinical:
- URI prodrome (mild fever, rhinorrhea, etc)
- Followed by respiratory distress (tachypnea, labored breathing, nasal flaring, retractions)
    - Exam may reveal wheezing, crackles, hypoxemia

Diagnosis: Clinical diagnosis

Management:
- Supportive care
- Supplemental oxygen (may require non-invasive PAP or mechanical vent)
- No evidence for bronchodilators, corticosteroids, or other medical interventions

Prophylaxis: Palivizumab
- Indicated in premature infants (< 29-32 weeks), some bronchopulmonary dysplasia patients, congenital heart disease, immunocompromised

PEDIATRIC RESPIRATORY INFECTIONS
Pulmonary/Critical Care — Pediatrics

Epiglottitis

General: Acute inflammation and edema of the epiglottis and surrounding area

Etiology: *H. Influenzae* type B (rare now due to immunizations), group A *Streptococcus*, *Staphylococcus aureus*, pneumococcus

Clinical:
- Rapidly progressive high fever/toxic appearance, drooling, dysphagia
- Respiratory distress (tripod or sniffing posture, stridor)

Diagnosis: Enlarged epiglottis on imaging or direct visualization

Management:
- Airway management
- Antibiotics: Amox-Clav or cephalosporin usually sufficient for *H. Influenzae*, but broad spectrum Vanc/Ceftriaxone usually started prior to determining cause
- PPX: Rifampin (young, at risk household contacts of HiB epiglottitis)

Pertussis

General: *Bordetella pertussis* infection, which causes "whooping cough"

Clinical:
- Catarrhal (1-2 weeks): Flu like prodrome (cough/rhinitis)
- Paroxysmal (2-6 weeks): Severe cough with inspiratory whoop, post-tussive emesis
- Convalescent stage: Eventual resolution of symptoms

Diagnosis: Culture or PCR for < 4 weeks of symptoms. Serology for > 4 weeks.

Management: Macrolides. Update Tdap.
- Post-exposure PPX: Macrolide for close contacts

Pediatric Pneumonia (Management)

Situation	Regimen
CAP (outpatient)	- Amoxicillin (typical) or macrolide (if suspected atypical)
CAP (inpatient)	- Ampicillin or cephalosporin (suspected typical) - Macrolide (suspected atypical) - Combination therapy if severe or requires ICU admission

ACUTE PEDIATRIC LUNG DISEASE — Pulmonary/Critical Care — Pediatrics

Foreign Body Aspiration

General: Most commonly occurs in children between 1-3 y/o

Clinical:
- Partial Obstruction: Cough, stridor, tachypnea/respiratory distress
    - Extremely acute in onset, often while child playing alone or witnessed choking event
    - Trachea: Stridor
    - Bronchi: Can cause unilateral ↓ breath sounds, focal wheeze
- Complete Obstruction: Respiratory distress, cyanosis, altered mental status

Diagnosis:
- CXR: Inspiratory/expiratory films can reveal air trapping
- Can consider CT if XR equivocal

Management:
- Partial: Bronchoscopy
- Complete:
    - Emergency care (back blows in infants, Heimlich in older children)
    - Emergent rigid bronchoscopy

CHRONIC PEDS LUNG DISEASE
Pulmonary/Critical Care — Pediatrics

Bronchopulmonary Dysplasia

General: Immature pulmonary system, resulting in long term oxygen requirement and respiratory support at birth

Risk: Prematurity, low birth weight, mechanical ventilation/oxygen toxicity

Clinical:
- Infant, with the above risk factors, presenting with respiratory distress (tachypnea, retractions, possible rales)

Management:
- Mechanical ventilation (utilizing as low of oxygen and as little pressure as possible)
- No evidence for steroids, bronchodilators, etc
- In general, lung function should recover months to a few years after birth

Pediatric Asthma Management

Note: [See: Asthma] for remainder of asthma discussion

Management:
Acute Exacerbation
- Inhaled SABA
- Systemic corticosteroids
- Supplemental oxygen (> 92%)
- Magnesium sulfate
    - Use acutely in ED in severe cases

Chronic
- Stepwise pharm therapy
    - SABA prn
    - Inhaled glucocorticoids (start low, increase if necessary)
    - Add LABA if medium glucocorticoids not sufficient
    - Add systemic corticosteroids if above not sufficient
- Other general counseling advice
    - Monitor peak flow/symptoms
    - If worsening, initiate an asthma control plan (emergency plan to help prevent serious exacerbations)
- Physicians should review asthma control test results at each visit (a simple symptoms scale to assess success of treatment)

CHRONIC PEDS LUNG DISEASE
Pulmonary/Critical Care — Pediatrics

Cystic Fibrosis

General: Chronic multi-system disorder from AR inherited mutations of the CFTR gene on chromosome 7. Most commonly due to F508del. Results in abnormal chloride channel, abnormally thickened secretions in the lungs, GI tract, and elsewhere.

Clinical:
- Pulmonary (Productive cough, hyperinflation, signs of airway obstruction)
    - Increase risk for bacterial infections (ie PNA)
        - *Staph* (kids)/*Pseudomonas* (adults)
    - Risk for bronchiectasis long term
- Chronic rhinosinusitis/Nasal polyps
- Gastrointestinal
    - Pancreatic insufficiency/malabsorption
        - Fecal elastase for screening
    - Meconium ileus (at birth)
    - Hepatobiliary disease
- Infertility
    - Men: Defective sperm transport
    - Women: Abnormal cervical mucus (but still can get pregnant)

Diagnosis: Criteria require:
- Symptoms consistent with CF PLUS
- Lab evidence of CFTR dysfunction
    - Elevated sweat chloride
        - Preferred first line. Confirm indeterminate or (+) results with follow up genetic testing.
    - Genetic testing (confirming two disease causing mutations)
    - Abnormal nasal potential difference
- Newborn Screening (Immunoreactive trypsinogen) in all 50 states

Management:
Pulmonary
- Chronic
    - Hypertonic saline, DNase
    - Chest physiotherapy
    - If reversible airflow obstruction: Inhaled beta agonists
    - CFTR modulators (Ivacaftor, Lumacaftor, Tezacaftor)
        - Used in patients with certain mutations, including F508
    - Chronic Azithromycin or Ibuprofen (anti-inflammatory)
- Acute exacerbations: Antibiotics (need to cover for *Staph/Pseudomonas*)

Gastrointestinal
- Pancreatic enzyme replacement therapy
- Nutritional/vitamin supplementation as necessary

CONGENITAL ENT LESIONS
Otorhinolaryngology, Pediatrics, Surgery

	General/Clinical	Management
Choanal Atresia	- Blockage of the posterior nasal passage, by bony or membranous abnormality - Associated with CHARGE, Treacher-Collins - Bilateral: Presents in infancy, with cyclic cyanosis, worse with activities not allowing for mouth breathing (ie feeding) and better with crying, noisy breathing, failure in ability to pass catheter through nares - Unilateral: Presents later in life with unilateral nasal discharge, obstruction	Dx: CT scan (confirms narrowing of pterygoid plate in posterior nasal cavity) Tx: - Initial: Establish oral airway and feeding tube - Definitive: Endoscopic or surgical correction
Laryngomalacia	- Increased laxity of supraglottic structures (worse with inspiration) - Infants (~3-9M): Inspiratory stridor, noisy respiration, possible poor feeding/respiratory distress if severe - Worse supine, improves when prone	Dx: Flexible fiberoptic laryngoscope Tx: Reassurance for most cases (resolves by 1.5 years). Supraglottoplasty for severe cases.
Cystic Hygroma	- Congenital obstruction of the lymphatic system in neck, resulting in lymph accumulation in jugular lymphatic sacs - ↑ risk for fetal aneuploidy	Dx: Prenatal US (fetus) or clinical exam (after birth)
Torus Palatinus	- Bony exostosis of the hard palate - Presents as a hard nodule on palate with normal overlying mucosa	Dx: Clinical Tx: Reassurance. Can surgically remove if symptomatic.

EYE — Otorhinolaryngology Surgery

Preseptal (Periorbital) and Orbital Cellulitis

	Preseptal	Orbital
Gen	- Infection of anterior portion of eyelid - Risk: Sinusitis, contiguous SST infection (ie post bug bite, trauma)	- Infection of orbit (fat and ocular muscles) - Risk: Sinusitis, orbital trauma, eye surgery
Clin	- Eyelid erythema, edema, pain - Possible fever, leukocytosis	- Eyelid erythema, edema, tenderness - Possible fever, leukocytosis - Ophthalmoplegia, painful EOM - Possible proptosis/visual blurring High risk for complications: - Subperiosteal/orbital abscess - Intracranial extension (Cavernous sinus thrombosis, meningitis, abscess) - Blindness
Dx	- CT scan of orbit/sinuses	
Tx	- Oral ABX (Clindamycin or TMP-SMX)	- IV ABX (Vancomycin + 3rd gen cephalosporin or Amp-Sulbactam) - Surgery for severe/refractory cases

	EAR	Otorhinolaryngology Medicine, Pediatrics, Surg
	Otitis Media	
	Otitis with Effusion (Serous)	**Acute Otitis Media**
Gen	- Middle ear effusion without signs of active infection	- Acute infection of the middle ear - Bulging of the TM (distinguishes AOM from OME) - Organisms: Pneumococcus, *H. influenzae*
Risk	- Post AOM - Eustachian tube dysfunction (kids) - Barotrauma, allergy (adults)	- Viral URI
Clin	- Generally asymptomatic - Can cause ↓ hearing, pain, tinnitus, "full" feeling	- Ear pain, otorrhea - Nonspecific symptoms in young kids (fever, fussiness, ear tugging)
Dx	- Pneumatic otoscopy (immobile TM, air-fluid levels, opacification)	- Pneumatic otoscopy (middle ear effusion PLUS bulging TM)
Tx	- Observation for 3 months (most resolve) - No use for nose sprays/decongestants Kids: - Tympanostomy: If > 3 months, recurrent disease, high risk for developmental delay, or hearing loss	- Antibiotics (Amoxicillin, or Amox-Clav for severe/refractory cases) Indications for abx: - All adults receive abx - Kids < 2 y/o, or kids > 2 y/o that appear toxic, have Temp > 102.2°F, or > 48 hrs of ear pain
Cp	No significant acute complications If Chronic (> 3 months): - Conductive hearing loss - Tympanosclerosis - Cholesteatoma	Acute Complications: - TM perforation - Mastoiditis - Labyrinthitis - Intracranial infection spread (rare) If Chronic (> 6 weeks): - Conductive hearing loss - TM perforation

EAR

Otorhinolaryngology
Medicine, Pediatrics, Surg

	General/Clinical	Management
Bullous Myringitis	- AOM, complicated by bullae on the tympanic membrane - Causes ↑ pain compared to AOM	- Dx/Tx same as AOM
Hemotympanum	- Blood in middle ear, causing dark opacification of TM - Usually associated with trauma (ie basilar skull fracture)	
Mastoiditis	- Complication of AOM, with purulent material in mastoid cavity - Presents with postauricular erythema, tenderness, swelling - Normally also have the fever/ear pain associated with AOM - Complications: Osteomyelitis, CNS spread (meningitis or abscess), facial nerve palsy	Dx: Clinical plus radiographic (CT w/ contrast is best initial imaging test) Tx: - IV Antibiotics (Vanco + Pip-Tazo or Cefepime) - Myringotomy +/- tympanostomy tube
Otitis Externa (Swimmer's Ear)	- Inflammation of the external auditory canal - Risk: Swimming (gram negative like *Pseudomonas*), ear canal trauma, intra-ear devices - Ear pain, itching, and otorrhea	Dx: Clinical (otoscopy shows edematous and erythematous external ear canal) Tx: Clean out ear canal, topical ear drops (antibiotics, steroids, and antiseptic)
Malignant Otitis Externa	- Invasive, necrotizing infection of the ear canal and skull base - Almost always *Pseudomonas* - Risk: Diabetes, immunocompromised - Can spread to bone and cause osteomyelitis, cranial nerve lesions - Ear pain, otorrhea, facial nerve palsy - Otoscopy shows granulation tissue, erythema	Dx: CT/MRI Tx: IV Fluoroquinolone

< OROPHARYNGEAL | Otorhinolaryngology Medicine >

Salivary Glands

Disorder	Features
Sialolithiasis	- Parotid, submandibular, and sublingual stone formation - Occurs with dehydration, anticholinergic drugs - Presents as pain/swelling with salivation (ie while eating) - Tx: Hydration, compression/massage
Sialadenitis	- Infection of salivary gland. Associated with stones or poor hygiene. - Can be bacterial (ie *S. aureus*) or viral (ie Mumps) - Presents with painful swelling, erythema, edema - Tx: Antibiotics, hydration, compression/massage
Sialadenosis	- Benign noninflammatory, bilateral swelling of salivary glands (abnormal autonomic innervation) - Associated with liver disease (both alcoholic and nonalcoholic cirrhosis), diabetes, bulimia - Presents as bilateral nontender enlargement of the salivary glands
Malignancy	Subtypes: - Pleomorphic Adenoma (benign mixed tumor) - Mucoepidermoid Carcinoma (most common malignant tumor, has mucinous and squamous components) - Warthin's Tumor (papillary cystadenoma lymphomatosum): Benign cystic tumor with germinal centers Tx: Superficial or deep parotidectomy

Temporomandibular Joint Disorders

General: Jaw joint pain. Common complaint, but often difficult to determine exact etiology or pathophysiology.

Clinical: Limited jaw mobility, pain, cracking/popping upon opening mouth

Diagnosis: Clinical

Management:
- Patient education, physical therapy
- NSAIDs, muscle relaxants
- Surgery if refractory

OROPHARYNGEAL — Otorhinolaryngology Medicine

Peritonsillar Cellulitis/Abscess

General: Infectious inflammation in the soft tissues surrounding the palatine tonsil. Can cause distinct pus pocket (abscess) or just soft tissue infection (cellulitis). Often a complication of usual tonsillitis/pharyngitis.

Clinical:
- Severe throat pain, fever
- Muffled voice, trismus (spasming of the jaw muscles), pooling of saliva
- Swelling of soft tissues, deviation of the uvula, unilateral lymphadenopathy

Diagnosis: Clinical (uvula deviation is classic)

Management:
- Antibiotics (Amp-Sulbactam or Clindamycin)
- Needle aspiration or I&D
- Severe, recurrent disease → Tonsillectomy

Retropharyngeal Abscess

General: Infection in the retropharynx, with high risk for spread into the danger space that leads into the mediastinum. Occurs after trauma to retropharynx (ie fish bone injury), or from spread from local pharyngitis or dental infection.

Clinical: Neck pain, fever, odynophagia, drooling, muffled voice

Diagnosis: Neck CT or XR (widened prevertebral space)

Management:
- Antibiotics (ie Amp-Sulbactam or Clindamycin)
- Surgical drainage (if abscess is present)

Ludwig's Angina

General: Bilateral cellulitis of the submandibular space. Polymicrobial infection, most often an extension of molar dental infections.

Clinical:
- Mouth pain, stiff neck, drooling, dysphagia
- Submandibular swelling
- Fever/chills
- Possible airway compromise (ie hoarse voice, stridor, respiratory distress)

Diagnosis: Clinical plus CT scan

Management:
- Antibiotics (ie Amp-Sulbactam or Clindamycin; Vancomycin if MRSA)
- Airway management (if necessary)
- Surgical drainage if not improving

OROPHARYNGEAL — Otorhinolaryngology Medicine, Surgery

Oral Lesion DDx

Candida	- Candidal infection of mucosa, associated with immunocompromised states and inhaled corticosteroids - Scrapable white plaques
Leukoplakia	- Premalignant hyperplasia of the squamous epithelium, associated with classic head/neck cancer risk factors - White patches or plaques of the oral mucosa
Oral Hairy Leukoplakia	- EBV infection, associated with immunocompromised states - White plaque most commonly covering lateral tongue, not easily scraped off
Aphthous Stomatitis	- "Canker sores" - Painful, shallow, round ulcers with gray base - Tx: Self-limited. Symptomatic control with topical steroid gel.

Head/Neck Cancer

Head/Neck Cancer	- General term for squamous cell carcinoma, originating from oropharynx - Associated with smoking, EtOH use, HPV - Presentation varies by site: Otalgia, oral lesions, dysphagia/odynophagia, neck lymphadenopathy are all possible - Dx: CT Head/Neck, with biopsy for definitive diagnosis *Note: If presented with SCC of neck node → Panendoscopy to find primary source in head/neck - Tx: Surgery/radiation, plus chemotherapy for higher stages
Nasopharyngeal Carcinoma	- Epithelial malignancy of the nasopharynx (usually SCC) - Associated with EBV infection, HPV, southeast Asia - Headache, diplopia, facial numbness, cervical LA - Dx: Endoscopic biopsy + MRI - Tx: Radiation +/- chemotherapy

Nasal Pathology

Epistaxis	- Anterior (Kiesselbach's plexus). Posterior bleeds (rare, cause significant hemorrhage). - Risk: Trauma, coagulopathy/platelet disorder, vascular lesions, tumor - Tx: Tamponade maneuvers, topical α_1 adrenergic agonists - Cautery or nasal packing for refractory cases
Septal Perforation	- Risk: Trauma, cocaine, post rhinoplasty, autoimmune disorder - Presents with whistling noise when breathing, bleeding
Septal Deviation	- Congenital or acquired displacement of nasal septum, causing obstruction (difficulty breathing, congestion, snoring, etc) - Tx: Septoplasty
Nasal Fracture	- Tx: Ice, head elevation, with reduction of displaced fractures
Septal Hematoma	- Traumatic complication, high risk for necrosis of septum if not drained

LARYNGEAL DISEASE
Otorhinolaryngology
Medicine, Surgery

Hoarseness DDx

Etiology:
- Acute laryngitis (associated w/ URI, lasts < 3 weeks, self-limited)
- Laryngeal cancer (anyone w/ > 3 weeks of hoarseness needs laryngoscopy)
- Benign polyps/nodules
- Neurologic (recurrent laryngeal nerve injury, diseases like Parkinson's)
- Spasmodic dysphonia

Clinical:
- Breathy voice: Incomplete adduction of cords
- Aphonia (lack of voice): Completely abducted cords
- Strained: Large mass on cords

Laryngeal Mass

Nodules	- Benign masses that arise from chronic irritation of vocal cord - Risk: Smoking, GERD, vocal overuse/abuse
Papilloma	- Benign papillary vocal cord tumor, associated with HPV 6, 11 - Can present with hoarseness/upper airway obstruction - Juvenile: Rape/abuse can get multiple papillomas - Dx: Laryngoscopy with biopsy
Squamous Cell Carcinoma	- Risk: Tobacco, alcohol - Presents with hoarseness - Dx: Laryngoscopy with biopsy (appears as white plaques) - Tx: Surgery or radiation. Chemotherapy for advanced disease.

PULMONARY PHARM

Pulmonary Medicine

Decongestants and Antihistamines

	Mechanism	Indication	Side Effects/Management
1st Gen Antihist Diphenhydramine Dimenhydrinate Chlorpheniramine Meclizine Promethazine Hydroxyzine	- H1 Antagonist - Anti M1, 5-HT, α-adrenergic effects as well	- Allergy - Motion Sickness - Insomnia	- Sedation - Antimuscarinic (Urinary retention, dry mouth, constipation, confusion in elderly) - Anti-α (Postural hypotension) - Anti-serotonergic (Increase appetite, weight gain)
2nd Gen Antihist Loratadine Fexofenadine Desloratadine Cetirizine	- H1 Antagonist (more selective than 1st gen)	- Allergy	- All of the above, but much less frequent
Guaifenesin	- Increases volume, decreases viscosity of sputum	- Expectorant	- N/A
Pseudoephedrine Phenylephrine	- α1 agonists	- Decongestant	- Hypertension, tachycardia - Tachyphylaxis; Rebound rhinorrhea if overuse

Pulmonary Hypertension

	Mechanism	Indication	Side Effects/Management
Ambrisentan Bosentan	- Endothelin receptor antagonist	- Pulmonary hypertension	- Hepatotoxicity
Sildenafil Tadalafil	- PDE-5 inhibitors	- Pulmonary hypertension	- Headache, flushing, blurry/blue vision - Avoid with nitric oxide donating drugs
Epoprostenol (IV) Iloprost (inhaled)	- Prostacyclin agonist	- Pulmonary hypertension	- Jaw pain, flushing - High output cardiac states (at high doses)

Pulmonary Fibrosis

	Mechanism	Indication	Side Effects/Management
Nintedanib	- TK inhibitor	- Idiopathic pulmonary fibrosis	- GI Disturbances
Pirfenidone	- Anti-inflammatory/fibrotic		- Hepatotoxicity

PULMONARY PHARM

Pulmonary Medicine

	Mechanism	Indication	Side Effects/Management
Asthma/COPD			
Albuterol	- β2 receptor agonists - Relaxation of smooth muscle in large airways	- Asthma - COPD	- Tachycardia - Tremor, anxiety/agitation, insomnia
Salmeterol Formoterol Vilanterol			
Fluticasone Budesonide Mometasone	- Inhaled corticosteroids	- Asthma - COPD	- Oral/Esophageal Thrush (rinse to avoid)
Ipratropium Tiotropium Glycopyrronium Aclidinium	- Muscarinic antagonist	- Asthma - COPD	- Dry mouth
Montelukast Zafirlukast Zileuton	- Leukotriene receptor antagonists (-ukast) - Lipoxygenase inhibitor (Zileuton)	- Asthma - COPD	- GI Disturbances, hypersensitivity (anaphylaxis) - Hepatotoxicity (Zileuton)
Omalizumab	- Monoclonal antibody against free IgE	- Asthma - Urticaria	- Hypersensitivity (anaphylaxis)
Methylxanthine Theophylline	- Induces bronchodilation via PDE inhibition	- Asthma - COPD	*Narrow therapeutic window - Cardiotoxic (tachyarrhythmias) - Neurotoxic (seizures)
Roflumilast	- PDE-4 Inhibitor	- COPD	- Weight loss
Methacholine	- M3 agonist	- Induces bronchospasm (for PFTs)	
Cromolyn	- Mast cell stabilizer	- Asthma	

Pulm48

VOLUME

Renal Medicine

Volume Basics

Fluid Balance:
- TBW is estimated at 60% of weight
  - $2/3$ of this is ICF, $1/3$ ECF
- Normal Intake: ~2L / day (fluids + solids)
- Normal Output: 0.75-1.5 L Urine, 0.25 L stool, 0.5-1 L insensible losses

Note: Insensible losses ↑ in patients with sepsis, fever, burns

Intracellular Fluid (67%)	Extracellular Fluid (33%)
	Plasma (25% ECF)

Fluid Options:

	Indications	Notes
Normal Saline	Volume Replacement	Strong anion gradient → Acidosis
Lactated Ringers	Volume Replacement	Contains small amounts of K^+
D5 1/2 NS	Maintenance Fluid	20 mEq KCl often added
D5W	Hypernatremia (Free water replacement)	
Hypertonic Saline	Severe Hyponatremia Elevated ICP	
Mannitol	Elevated ICP	

Maintenance Fluid Calculations:

100/50/20 Rule (Daily Rate)	4/2/1 Rule (Hourly Rate)
- 100 mL/kg for first 10 kg - 50 mL/kg for next 10 kg - 20 mL/kg for remainder	- 4 mL/kg for first 10 kg - 2 mL/kg for next 10 kg - 1 mL/kg for remainder

Hypovolemia

Etiology: GI Loss (vomit/diarrhea/NG suction), renal loss (DKA, diuretic abuse), poor intake, third spacing (ascites, effusions, burns, pancreatitis), sepsis, trauma

Clinical: Poor skin turgor, dry mucous membranes, oliguria, decreased CVP, low BP

Management:
- For mild cases: Oral replacement generally sufficient
- For severe cases:
  - Initial bolus of 1-2 L of isotonic crystalloid (NS or LR)
  - Further fluid to maintain MAP > 65 mmHg, urine output > 0.5 ml/kg/hr

Hypervolemia

Etiology: (1) Iatrogenic (2) Volume Retaining States (CHF, CKD, Cirrhosis)

Clinical: Weight gain, edema, elevated JVP or CVP

Management: Salt/Water restriction, diuretics

SODIUM — Renal Medicine

Hyponatremia

General: Sodium < 135 meq/L
- Mild (130-135 meq/L)
- Moderate (120-130 meq/L)
- Severe (< 120 meq/L)

Etiology		Specific Findings
True Hyponatremia (Serum Osm: < 275 mOsm/kg)		
Hypovolemic	Renal Salt Loss (U_{Na} > 40 meq/L)	- Causes: Diuretics, post ATN, low aldosterone (ie primary adrenal insufficiency)
	Extrarenal Salt Loss (U_{Na} < 40 meq/L)	- Causes: GI loss (diarrhea, vomit), sweat, dehydration ("non-osmotic ADH release")
Normovolemic	SIADH	[See: SIADH]
	Primary Polydipsia	- Abnormal thirst response resulting in excess water intake/abnormal ADH levels - Associated with psychiatric illness
	Beer Potomania	- Excess intake of solute-poor beer
	Other: Postoperative Hypothyroid	
Hypervolemic	CHF Cirrhosis Nephrotic Syndrome Renal Failure	
Isotonic (Serum Osm: 275-295 mOsm/kg)		
	"Pseudo"-Hyponatremia	- Elevated levels of lipids or proteins in serum, which results in abnormal lab calculation of serum sodium - Causes include hyperlipidemia, monoclonal gammopathy, iatrogenic administration of certain substances
Hypertonic Hyponatremia (Serum Osm > 295 mOsm/kg)		
	Hyperglycemia	
	Exogenous Substance	- Mannitol, Sorbitol

Clinical:
- Mild Symptoms: Nausea, vomiting, headache, lethargy, confusion
- Severe Symptoms: Lethargy, coma, seizure, respiratory arrest

SODIUM — Renal Medicine

Hyponatremia (Management)

Acute (< 48 hours)	
Mild (> 130 mEq/L)	- Identify and treat underlying cause
Moderate-Severe (ie < 130 mEq/L)	- Can consider small hypertonic saline bolus (to prevent lowering further, but only use if convinced of acute ↓) - Identify and treat underlying cause
Symptomatic	- Hypertonic Saline
Chronic (> 48 hours)	
Asymptomatic or Mild symptoms	- Continue to treat underlying cause - Fluid restriction
Severe (< 120 mEq/L) and/or Symptomatic	- Hypertonic saline
Treatment Based on Volume Status	
Hypovolemic	- Restore volume (ie isotonic fluids)
Isovolemic	- Fluid restriction - Consider salt tabs, urea, or vaptans
Hypervolemic	- Fluid restriction

- Sodium should not be corrected faster than 8 mEq/L in 24 hour period

Osmotic Demyelination Syndrome

General: Rapid correction of hyponatremia can lead to irreversible demyelination. More likely to occur with severe and chronic hyponatremia (< 120 mEq/L).

Clinical: Delayed (2-5 day) onset of neurologic symptoms, including dysphagia, dysarthria, paralysis, mental status changes, and other focal neurologic deficits

Diagnosis: MRI

Management: Supportive. Can attempt to re-lower sodium.

SODIUM — Renal Medicine

SIADH

General: Inappropriately elevated ADH levels, leading to hyponatremia from impaired clearance of free water

Etiology:
- CNS (traumatic, stroke, infection)
- Paraneoplastic (lung cancer)
- Drugs (cyclophosphamide, chlorpropamide, carbamazepine, SSRI)
- Pulmonary disease

Clinical: [See: Hyponatremia] Note that patients are euvolemic.

Diagnosis: Hypotonic hyponatremia, plus $U_{osm} > 100$ mOsm/kg H_2O, $U_{Na} > 40$ meq/L

Management:
- [See: Hyponatremia] for acute management
- For chronic
    - Fluid restriction
    - Consider salt tabs, urea, or vaptans

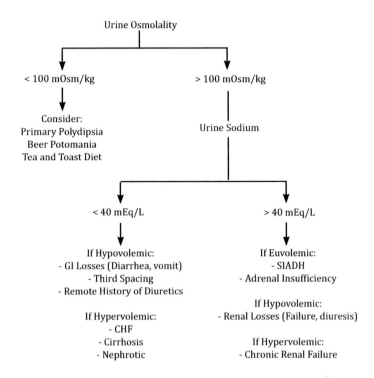

SODIUM

Renal Medicine

Hypernatremia

General: Sodium > 145 mEq/L

Etiology:

Etiology	Specific Findings
Hypovolemic Hypernatremia	
Renal Loss	- Osmotic diuresis (hyperglycemia), diuretics, renal failure
Extrarenal Loss	- GI losses, insensible (skin/respiratory fluid loss), poor free water intake
Isovolemic Hypernatremia	
Diabetes Insipidus	
Hypervolemic Hypernatremia	
Iatrogenic	- TPN, hypertonic fluids
Hyperaldosteronism	
Excess corticosteroids	- Cushing's or exogenous

Clinical: Altered mental status, weakness, neurologic deficits, seizures, coma

Management:
- Isovolemic/Hypervolemic: D5W
- Hypovolemic
    - Patients will require both D5W/Normal Saline
    - Can either accomplish with separate drips or D5-1/4NS
- Note: Maximum correction is 12 mEq/L/day (0.5 mEq/L/hr)

Complications:
- Cerebral edema (can result in encephalopathy and seizures if severe)
- Generally occurs with too rapid sodium correction

◁ **POTASSIUM** | **Renal Medicine** ▷

Hypokalemia

General: Potassium < 3.5 mEq/L

Etiology:

	Etiology	Specific Findings
Potassium Depletion		
Extrarenal	Diarrhea Fistula Laxative abuse	Urine K < 20 mEq/L
Renal	Renal Tubular Acidosis DKA Diuretics Hyperaldosteronism	Urine K > 20 mEq/L Note: Hypovolemia can activate RAAS, with aldosterone promoting K secretion
	Hypomagnesemia	Mg normally inhibits ROMK in distal tubule. Replace Mg before K can be corrected.
	Bartter ≈ loops	AR defect in Na-K-Cl symporter in thick ascending limb
	Gitelman ≈ thiazides	AR defect in NaCl absorption in distal tubule
Redistribution		
	- Increased insulin - Increased beta-adrenergic activity - Metabolic or respiratory alkalosis	

Clinical: Generally asymptomatic until well below 3 mEq/L
- Muscle weakness
- Arrhythmias (PAC, PVC, bradycardia, AV block, and ventricular tachycardia)
- ECG changes: Depressed ST, flattened T, U-waves

Management:
- K > 3.0: Oral K replacement
- K < 3.0 or symptomatic: High dose oral replacement or IV
*Note: IV K can cause phlebitis at rates > 10 mEq/hr in peripheral veins

- Hyperaldosteronism: Spironolactone/Eplerenone
- Chronic renal potassium wasting: K-Sparing Diuretic

POTASSIUM

Renal Medicine

Hyperkalemia

General: Potassium > 5.0 mEq/L

Etiology:

Etiology		Specific Findings
Potassium Excess		
Renal (↓ urine K)	Acute/Chronic kidney disease	
	Decreased ECV	- Low distal solute delivery
	Decreased aldosterone	- Hyporeninemic-Hypoaldosteronism (type 4 RTA) - Addison's - ACEi use
	Resistance to aldosterone	- Potassium sparing diuretics
Extrarenal	Tissue catabolism	
Redistribution		
	- Insulin deficiency - Beta-adrenergic blockade - Metabolic or respiratory acidosis	
Laboratory Error		
	- Hemolysis - Prolonged tourniquet use (can cause movement of K out of cells after venipuncture)	

Clinical: Generally asymptomatic, but > 7 mEq/L can result in below symptoms
- Weakness/paralysis
- Cardiac arrhythmias (including VT/VF)
- ECG: Peaked T-waves, lengthened PR/QRS duration

Management:
    K > 6.0-6.5 mEq/L or Symptomatic
        - IV Ca Gluconate
        - IV Insulin/D5W (2nd line: Sodium bicarbonate or beta-agonists)
        - Remove K from body
            - Diuretic (if renal status is good)
            - K-Binding Resin (sodium polystyrene or patiromer)
            - Hemodialysis (if severe renal compromise)

    All Others:
        - Find and reverse underlying cause

CALCIUM — Renal Medicine

Hypocalcemia

General: Calcium < 8.5 mg/dL
- Note: For every 1 g/dL below 4 in albumin, correct Ca by adding 0.8 mg/dL

Etiology	Specific Findings
Low PTH Levels	
Parathyroidectomy	
Hypoparathyroidism	- Autoimmune
Infiltrative Parathyroid Disease	
Elevated PTH Levels	
Vitamin D Deficiency	
Chronic Kidney Disease	- ↓ Vitamin D production
Pancreatitis	
Tumor Lysis Syndrome	- Hyperphosphatemia, AKI
Pseudohypoparathyroidism	- [See: Endocrine]
Other	
Hypomagnesemia	
Transfusion	- Citrate binds Ca

Clinical:
- Neuromuscular: Irritability/tetany, paresthesias
    - Chvostek sign (Tap on facial nerve → Contraction of facial muscle)
    - Trousseau sign (Carpal spasm with inflated blood pressure cuff)
    - Hyperactive DTR
- Cardiac:
    - Prolonged QT, possible cardiac arrhythmias (ie Torsades)

Management:
- Severely Symptomatic or < 7.5 mg/dL: IV Calcium
- Symptomatic or > 7.5 mg/dL: Oral calcium
- Hypomagnesemia: Correct Mg first

CALCIUM

Renal Medicine

Hypercalcemia

General: Calcium > 10.0 mg/dL

	Etiology	Specific Findings
Endocrine	Primary Hyperparathyroid	- [See: Endocrine]
	Tertiary Hyperparathyroid	
Malignancy	Bone Metastasis	
	Paraneoplastic	- PTHrP production
	Multiple Myeloma	
Pharm	Vitamin A/D Toxicity	
	Thiazides, Lithium	
	Milk-Alkali Syndrome	- Excessive intake of absorbable alkali (ie antacids) → Renal vasoconstriction, decreased GFR - Nausea, vomit, constipation, polyuria - Dx: Triad of hypercalcemia, alkalosis, AKI
Other	Granulomatous	- Excess vitamin D production
	Immobilization	
	Genetic	- Familial Hypocalciuric Hypercalcemia

Clinical:
Note: Generally asymptomatic < 12
- Stones (nephrolithiasis, other urinary including polydipsia)
- Bones (bone pain)
- Groans (muscle weakness, nausea, vomit, constipation, pancreatitis)
- Psychiatric overtones (confusion, fatigue, poor concentration)
- Cardiac: Shortened QT

Management:

Severe (> 14 mg/dL) Symptomatic	- IV Normal Saline and calcitonin (acutely) - Bisphosphonate (chronic). Denosumab is 2nd line.
Moderate (12-14 mg/dL)	- Treat if patient is symptomatic
Mild (< 12 mg/dL)	- Treat underlying condition - Avoid exacerbating agents
Other	- Glucocorticoid in lymphoma, MM, or granulomatous disease - Dialysis in renal failure

MAGNESIUM
Renal Medicine

Hypomagnesemia

General: < 1.8 mEq/L   [handwritten: Mg 1.8-2.5]

Etiology:
- GI Losses (diarrhea, malabsorption, PPI use, pancreatitis)
- Renal Loss (diuretic use, ATN recovery)
- Malnutrition (alcoholism)
- Genetic Disorders (such as Gitelman's)

Clinical:
- Neuromuscular/CNS irritability
- Hypocalcemia, hypokalemia
- Cardiac: Prolonged QT, t-wave flattening, Torsades

Management:
- Mild/Asymptomatic: Oral Mg replacement
- Severe/Symptomatic: IV Mg replacement

Hypermagnesemia

General: > 2.5 mEq/L

Etiology:
- Renal insufficiency
- Iatrogenic (Mg infusions, enemas)
- Laxative or antacid abuse

Clinical:
- Neuromuscular Effects (starts around 4-6 mEq/L)
    - Loss of DTR, somnolence, muscle weakness/paralysis
- Cardiac Effects (starts around 4-5 mEq/L)
    - Prolonged PR, QRS, and QT
    - Complete heart block/cardiac arrest at very high levels
- Transient hypocalcemia from PTH receptor blockade

Management:
- For all: Stop any Mg medications

- Normal Renal Function: Correcting underlying etiology generally sufficient
- Moderate Renal Insufficiency: Normal Saline + Loop Diuretics
- Severe Renal Failure: Dialysis

PHOSPHATE
Renal Medicine

Hypophosphatemia

General: < 2.5 mg/dL

Etiology:
- Decreased intestinal absorption (chronic diarrhea, PPI use, low intake)
- Extracellular shift (↑ insulin, refeeding syndrome, glucose/glucagon)
- Renal excretion (hyperparathyroid, vitamin D deficiency)
- Removal in dialysis
- Hungry bone syndrome

Clinical:
- Increased bone turnover
    - Chronic deficiencies can lead to rickets and osteomalacia
    - Decreased distal tubule calcium resorption
- ATP Depletion
    - Metabolic encephalopathy
    - Impaired myocardial contractility
    - Muscular weakness

Management:
- If < 2.0 mg/dL or symptomatic, provide oral phosphate replacement
- Severely low phosphate can receive IV phosphate replacement

Hyperphosphatemia

General: > 4.5 mg/dL

Etiology:
- Phosphate load (tumor lysis, rhabdo, phosphate laxatives)
- Acute/Chronic kidney disease
- Increased renal phosphate absorption (hypoparathyroidism)

Clinical:
- Ectopic calcification if extremely high
    - Risk is high if Ca x Phos > 70

Management:
<u>If Severe, Symptomatic</u>
- Normal saline (↑ renal phosphate clearance if normal renal function)
- Hemodialysis (severe renal failure)

<u>Kidney Disease</u>
- Low phosphate diet, +/- phosphate binders (ie sevelamer)

ACID-BASE — Renal Medicine

Respiratory Acidosis
Alveolar Hypoventilation:
- COPD
- CNS depression
- Neuromuscular weakness
- Respiratory muscle fatigue

Metabolic Alkalosis
Saline Responsive ($U_{Cl} < 20$)
- Vomit
- Laxative/Diuretic abuse
- GI suctioning
- Dehydration

Saline Unresponsive ($U_{Cl} > 20$)
- 1°/2° Hyperaldosteronism
- Cushing's
- Severe hypokalemia

Metabolic Acidosis
Elevated Anion Gap (GOLD MARK)
- Glycols
- Oxoproline
- L-Lactate
- D-Lactate
- Methanol
- Aspirin
- Renal failure (late)
- Ketones

Normal Anion Gap
- Renal tubular acidosis
- GI Loss of HCO_3 (diarrhea, fistula)
- Infusion of HCO_3-free Fluids
- Acetazolamide
- Post-hypocapnia
- Renal failure (early)

Respiratory Alkalosis
- Alveolar hyperventilation (anxiety, PE, hypoxemia)
- Salicylate toxicity (early)
- Pregnancy
- Sepsis

Y-axis: HCO_3 (10 to 40)
X-axis: pH (7.2 to 7.6)

Renal12

ACID-BASE

Renal Medicine

Compensation

Disorder	Primary	Comp	Compensation Calculation
Metabolic Acidosis	↓ HCO_3	↓ CO_2	$PCO_2 = 1.5 [HCO_3] + 8 \pm 2$
Metabolic Alkalosis	↑ HCO_3	↑ CO_2	↑ $PCO_2 = 0.7 [\Delta HCO_3]$
Respiratory Acidosis	↑ CO_2	↑ HCO_3	Acute: ↑ HCO_3 1.0 mEq/L for each 10 mmHg CO_2 Chronic: ↑ HCO_3 3.5 mEq/L for each 10 mmHg CO_2
Respiratory Alkalosis	↓ CO_2	↓ HCO_3	Acute: ↓ HCO_3 2.0 mEq/L for each 10 mmHg CO_2 Chronic: ↓ HCO_3 4.0 mEq/L for each 10 mmHg CO_2

Other Formulas

Anion Gap
   $AG = Na - Cl - HCO_3$
   Expected gap: 2.5 x [Albumin]

Urine Anion Gap
   $UAG = [Na^+] + [K^+] - [Cl^-]$
   Should be negative with acidosis, but is positive with Type I/IV RTAs

Osmolar Gap
   Osmolar Gap = Measured P_{osm} – Calculated P_{osm}
   P_{osm} (calculated) = $2[Na]$ + glucose/18 + BUN/2.8

   Common substances that increase the osmolar gap are ethanol, ethylene glycol, methanol, acetone, isopropyl ethanol and propylene glycol

Delta/Delta
   Delta ratio = Δ Anion Gap/Δ [HCO_3]
   Interpretation
      < 0.4: Normal Anion-Gap Acidosis (non-gap)
      < 1: Mixed normal and elevated anion-gap acidosis
      1-2: Pure anion-gap acidosis
      > 2: Elevated AG acidosis, plus concurrent metabolic alkalosis + compensation

Alkalosis/Acidosis Systemic Effects

	Acidosis	Alkalosis
Resp	Hyperventilation	Hypoventilation
CV	Myocardial depression	Myocardial depression
CNS	Increased cerebral blood flow/ICP	Decreased cerebral blood flow/ICP
Hgb	Right-shifts oxyhemoglobin curve	Left-shifts oxyhemoglobin curve
Other		Increased neuromuscular excitability (albumin binds ↑ Ca)

ACUTE RENAL FAILURE
Renal Medicine

General: A rapid decline in renal function, reflected in decreased glomerular filtration

RIFLE	Creatinine	GFR	Urine Output
Risk	1.5 fold ↑	↓ 25%	< 0.5 mL/kg/hr for 6 hours
Injury	2.0 fold ↑	↓ 50%	< 0.5 mL/kg/hr for 12 hours
Failure	3.0 fold ↑	↓ 75%	< 0.3 mL/kg/hr for 24 hours or Anuria
Loss	- Complete loss of kidney function for > 4 weeks		
ESRD	- Complete loss of kidney function for > 3 months (requiring dialysis)		

KDIGO Guideline Definition
(1) Abrupt (< 48 hr) increase in Cr by > 0.3 mg/dL
(2) Increase in creatinine 50% from baseline in last week
(3) Reduction in urine output to < 0.5 mL/kg/hr for > 6 hr

Etiology:

	Prerenal	Renal	Post-renal
Etiology	- Hypovolemia - Hypoperfusion (↓ECV) - Hepatorenal - Cardiorenal - Renal arterial stenosis	- Glomerular disease - ATN - AIN - Vascular (PAN, TTP, DIC, etc)	- Obstruction (BPH, nephrolithiasis, neoplasm, bladder dysfunction)
BUN/Cr	> 20	< 15	Varies
FE_{Na}	< 1%	> 2%	> 2%
U_{Osm} (mOsm/kg)	> 500	< 350	< 350
U_{Na} (mEq/L)	< 40	> 40	> 40

Clinical: Often asymptomatic, can cause edema, hypertension, decreased urine output

Diagnosis: Renal function (as above). Other useful tests include urinalysis, urine sodium excretion, urine volume monitoring. Renal US to rule out post-renal etiology.

Management:
- Correct volume status, underlying disorder
- Monitor for below complications, which (if severe) are dialysis indications
- Acute renal failure (requiring hemodialysis) can be treated with CVVH, which is continuous veno-venous hemodialysis

Dialysis Indications: (AEIOU)
- Acidosis
- Electrolyte abnormalities (hyperkalemia)
- Intoxication (ethylene glycol, lithium, etc)
- Overload (volume)
- Uremia (pericarditis, encephalopathy, platelet dysfunction)

CHRONIC KIDNEY DISEASE

Renal Medicine

General: Decreased kidney function for > 3 months, with GFR < 60 mL/min
- Stage III (Moderate): GFR < 60 mL/min
- Stage IV (Severe): GFR < 30 mL/min
- Stage V (ESRD): GFR < 15 mL/min

Etiology: Most commonly due to diabetes mellitus or hypertension, followed by all other causes of renal disease (ie PCKD, glomerulonephritis, etc)

Clinical: CKD is associated with increased risk for cardiovascular disease, end-stage renal disease, infection, malignancy, and mortality

System	Findings
Fluids/Lytes	- Volume overload - Hyperkalemia - Metabolic acidosis

Endocrine	- Vitamin D Deficiency/Hyperparathyroidism
	   - Leads to hypocalcemia, hyperphosphatemia
	   - Bone disease (osteomalacia/osteodystrophy)

Cardiovascular	- Hypertension - Dyslipidemia - Accelerated atherosclerosis - Uremic pericarditis
Hematologic	- Normocytic anemia (low EPO) - Uremic platelet dysfunction
Reproductive	- Erectile dysfunction, decreased libido
Neurologic	- Uremic encephalopathy

Workup:
- Urinalysis, urine microscopy (for casts or dysmorphic RBCs)
- Protein-to-creatinine ratio, albumin-to-creatinine ratio
- Renal US
- Consider SPEP/UPEP

Management: Treat underlying condition

Complication	Intervention
Hypertension	- ACEi or ARB preferred
Anemia	- EPO if Hgb < 10 g/dL
Electrolyte Issues	- Low phosphate, potassium diets (for hyperkalemia/phosphatemia)
Acidosis	- PO NaHCO$_3$
Hyperparathyroidism	- Calcitriol, vitamin D, or calcimimetics - Phosphate binders (if phosphatemia refractory to dietary control)

Renal Replacement Therapy:
- Indicated once GFR falls < 5 OR GFR 5-15 with AEIOU symptoms

CHRONIC KIDNEY DISEASE — Renal Medicine

Renal Replacement

	Hemodialysis	Peritoneal Dialysis
Process	- Blood pumped out of body to artificial semipermeable membrane, with dialysate on other side	- Dialysate is infused into peritoneal space, which acts as membrane for exchange
Access	- Catheter, AV Graft, AV Fistula	- Implanted peritoneal catheter
Timing	~ 3 days/week	~ 4-6 hours/day
Pro	- Efficient and emergent	- Convenience, more physiologic
Con	- Less physiologic, so elevated risk of hypotension - Requires access	- Peritonitis

Transplantation
- More natural renal replacement
- Requires immunosuppressive therapy, risk for acute or chronic rejection

Continuous Veno-Venous Hemofiltration (CVVH)
- Filters blood along highly permeable membrane, removing water and solute
- Short term, continuous form of renal replacement used if critically ill

NEPHRITIC/NEPHROTIC SYNDROME — Renal Medicine

Nephritic Syndrome

General: Glomerular inflammation resulting in the clinical syndrome of hematuria, proteinuria, and renal failure

Etiology:
- Post Streptococcal Glomerulonephritis
- Crescentic Glomerulonephritis
    - ANCA + Vasculitis
    - Goodpasture's and Anti-GBM disease
- Lupus Nephritis
- IgA Nephropathy

Clinical:
- Hematuria
- Proteinuria (< 3.5 g/day)
- Hypertension
- Azotemia

Management: Depends on underlying etiology

Nephrotic Syndrome

General: Nephrotic syndrome is defined by protein excretion > 3.5 g/day, due to a variety of glomerular processes that allow for leakage of protein through glomerular basement membrane and into urine

Etiology:
- Minimal Change Disease
- Focal Segmental Glomerulosclerosis (FSGS)
- Membranous Nephropathy
- Amyloidosis
- Diabetic Nephropathy

Clinical:
- Proteinuria (>3.5 g/day), hypoalbuminemia (<3.5 mg/dL), and edema
- Hyperlipidemia (increased liver protein synthesis)
- Hypercoagulability (loss of anti-plasmin III)
- Increased infection risk (IgG loss in urine)

Management:
- Treat underlying disease
- Proteinuria: ACEi/ARB
- Edema: Loop diuretics
- Hyperlipidemia: Statin

GLOMERULONEPHRITIS
Renal — Medicine, Pediatrics

	General/Pathophysiology	Findings	Management
Post-Strep GN	- Occurs ~2 weeks after group A *Strep* infection of skin or respiratory tract - Much more common in children	- Antistreptolysin O ↑, Complement ↓ - LM: Glomeruli enlarged/hypercellular - IF: Granular appearance - EM: Subepithelial humps (IgG/C3)	- Generally self-limited
Rapidly Progressive GN	Type I: Goodpasture's or anti-GBM Type II: Progressed lupus/post-strep GN Type III: "pauci-immune" - Granulomatosis with polyangiitis - Microscopic polyangiitis - Eosinophilic granulomatosis with polyangiitis	- LM/IF: Crescent moon shapes of fibrin - Linear immunofluorescence (for anti-GBM), granular pattern immunofluorescence (for type II), and no immunofluorescence (for type III)	- Methylprednisolone, Cyclophosphamide - +/- Plasmapheresis (for IgG antibodies)
Diffuse Proliferative GN	- Common subtype of lupus nephritis (type IV)	- LM: Wire-looping of capillaries - EM: Subendothelial immune complex deposition	- Immunosuppressive therapy (steroids plus cyclophosphamide or mycophenolate)
IgA Nephropathy	- Gross hematuria days after a URT infection, with preserved renal function - Often chronic, recurrent process. Some will progress to ESRD.	- IM: Globular IgA deposits in the mesangium	- ACEi/ARB - Steroids (if disease is severe/progressing)
Membrano-proliferative GN (can cause nephritic, nephrotic, or mixed picture)	Type I: Immune-Complex Mediated: Occurs with viral infection (hepatitis) and autoimmune disease Type II: Complement Mediated: Occurs with genetic or acquired overactivation of complement (ie C3 Nephritic Factor)	- LM: "Tram-track" GBM splitting - IF: Continuous, dense ribbon-like deposits along the glomeruli	- Work up for infections if immune-complex mediated
Alport's	- X-linked inherited nephritis due to abnormal type IV collagen	- ESRD, ocular abnormalities, sensorineural hearing loss - EM: "Split" basement membrane	- Early: Supportive (ACEi) - Late: Transplant/Dialysis

NEPHROPATHY
Renal Medicine

	General/Pathophysiology	Findings	Management
Minimal Change Disease	- Most common cause of childhood nephrotic syndrome - Primary: Idiopathic, or associated with recent infection or immunization - Secondary (lymphoma)	LM: Normal glomeruli EM: Effacement of foot processes - Selective Proteinuria (albumin)	- Prednisone
Focal Segmental Glomerulosclerosis	- Most common cause of nephrotic syndrome in black patients - Primary [Idiopathic] - Secondary (HIV ["collapsing subtype"], sickle cell, IFN, heroin, congenital abnormalities, severe obesity)	LM: Segmental sclerosis and hyalinosis IF: Generally negative EM: Effacement of foot process similar to MCD	- Primary: Give steroids/immunosuppressive agents - Secondary: Treat underlying
Membranous Nephropathy	Primary (idiopathic): Ig against phospholipase A2 receptor Secondary: - Infections (Hep B/C, syphilis) - Drugs (gold, Captopril, penicillamine, NSAIDS) - Autoimmune (SLE) - Solid Malignancy	LM: Diffuse capillary and GBM thickening IF: Granular (IC deposition) EM: Spike and dome appearance with subepithelial deposits	- Treat underlying - ACEi for proteinuria control - Immunosuppressive therapy for idiopathic MN
Amyloid	- Complication of systemic amyloidosis	LM: Congo red stain shows apple-green birefringence	- Treat underlying
Diabetic	- Possible complication of diabetic nephropathy	LM: Mesangial expansion, GBM thickening, "Kimmelstiel-Wilson" nodules	- Treat underlying

TUBULOINTERSTITIAL DISEASE
Renal Medicine

Acute Tubular Necrosis

General: Necrosis of tubular epithelium, resulting in renal dysfunction

Etiology:
- Renal Ischemia (sepsis, hypotension, surgery)
- Toxins: Radiocontrast, heme pigments, Ig light chains, crystals
    - Aminoglycosides, cisplatin, other nephrotoxic drugs

Clinical:
- Oliguric phase (1-2 weeks): Uremia, azotemia, hyperkalemia, acidosis
- Diuretic phase: High urine output, with risk for electrolyte depletion

Diagnosis:
- Azotemia, plus FeNa > 2% (to differentiate from pure prerenal azotemia)
- Urinalysis (muddy brown granular/epithelial cell casts)
- Limited improvement in kidney function with fluids (versus prerenal)

Management:
- Supportive
- Prophylaxis: Patients at high risk (ie CKD, other comorbid conditions) should be volume optimized and avoid nephrotoxic agents

Acute Interstitial Nephritis

General: Inflammatory renal interstitial disease

Etiology:
- Drugs (NSAIDs, Penicillin/cephalosporin, PPI, loop diuretics, other abx)
- Infection (pyelonephritis, systemic legionella or TB)
- AI (Sjogren's, SLE, sarcoid)

Clinical: 1-3 weeks post insult, patients develop AKI plus the triad of fever, rash, and eosinophilia (serum and/or urinary)

Diagnosis: Clinical. AKI + urinalysis showing WBC, WBC casts, or (rarely) eosinophils.

Management:
- Remove offending agent
- Glucocorticoids

Renal Papillary Necrosis

General: Necrosis of the renal papilla from ischemia

Etiology: Analgesic abuse (ie NSAIDs), sickle cell, pyelonephritis

Clinical: Variable time course and degree of symptoms. Symptoms include hematuria, colicky flank pain, passage of sloughed papilla in urine.

Diagnosis: Urinalysis, urine cytology. CT can show small, irregular kidneys.

Management: Supportive. Treat underlying condition.

TUBULOINTERSTITIAL DISEASE — Renal Medicine

Renal Tubular Acidosis

General: Disorder of abnormal renal tubular acid secretion

Type	1	2	4
Location	Distal	Proximal	Hypoaldosteronism
Abnormality	Secretion	Absorption	Generation
K+	Low	Low	High
Urine pH	> 5.5	< 5.5	< 5.5
Causes	- AI Disease (Sjogrens/ RA) - Drugs (Amp B, Ifosfamide, Lithium) - Hypercalciuric conditions - Genetic	- M-protein disorders (MM, amyloid) - Drugs (Acetazolamide, Ifosfamide) - Heavy metals - Fanconi syndrome	- Hyporenin/Hypoaldo (seen in a variety of renal disease) - ACEi/ARB use - Aldo resistance (ie K sparing diuretics, or Trimethoprim)
Tx	- NaHCO$_3$	- Potassium Citrate - Thiazide	- Fludrocortisone
Other	- Nephrolithiasis (Ca phosphate)		

can't secrete H+   *can't reabs. bicarb*

Other Tubular Abnormalities

Disease	Findings
Hartnup	- AR abnormality in amino acid transport, with decreased resorption of neutral amino acids like tryptophan
Fanconi's	- Hereditary or acquired proximal tubule dysfunction, leading to defective transport of glucose, amino acids, sodium, potassium, phosphate, uric acid, bicarbonate - Treat with phosphate, potassium, alkali and salt supplements
Bartter	- Resorptive defect in thick ascending loop of Henle NaKCl transporter - Appears like chronic loop diuretic use
Gitelman	- Resorptive defect in DCT NaCl transporter
Liddle	- Gain of function to increase Na reabsorption in collecting tubules - Presents like hyperaldosteronism, but low aldosterone levels in serum - Tx: Amiloride
Syndrome of Apparent Mineralocorticoid Excess	- Hereditary deficiency of 11b-hydroxysteroid dehydrogenase (inability to convert cortisol to cortisone) - Can acquire from glycyrrhetinic acid (in licorice) - Presents as hypertension, hypokalemia, metabolic alkalosis - Treatment: Corticosteroids (down-regulate own cortisol production)

RENAL VASCULAR DISEASE
Renal Medicine

Renal Artery Stenosis

General: Decreased renal perfusion, leading to elevated RAAS activity and secondary hypertension

	Atherosclerotic Disease	Fibromuscular Dysplasia
Gen	- Most common, seen in those with usual atherosclerotic risk factors	- Angiopathy of medium sized vessels, resulting in areas of stenosis and aneurysm - Commonly seen in women of child bearing age
Clin	- Secondary hypertension in someone with high likelihood for vascular disease - Abdominal bruit	- Renal Stenosis (secondary hypertension, flank pain) - Carotid Stenosis (headache, TIA/stroke, carotid bruit, tinnitus) - Vertebral Stenosis
Dx	- CTA, MRA, or Duplex US	- CTA, MRA, or Duplex US ("String of Beads")
Tx	- Pharm: ACEi/ARB - Percutaneous transluminal angioplasty - Surgical bypass if all else fails	

Renal Vein Thrombosis

General: Renal venous thrombus, highly associated with nephrotic syndrome (especially membranous nephropathy)

Clinical: Generally asymptomatic, but can result in pulmonary embolism or worsening renal failure

Diagnosis: CT, MRI, or Duplex US

Treatment:
- Acute: Local thrombolytic therapy plus anticoagulation
- PPX: Individuals with low risk of bleeding can receive anticoagulation

Renal Infarction

General: Arterial infarction from cardioembolism, dissection, or hypercoagulability

Clinical: Acute onset flank/abdominal pain, nausea/vomiting

Diagnosis: CT/CTA

Treatment: Anticoagulation, with local thrombolysis in select patients

CYSTIC KIDNEY DISEASE
Renal — Medicine, Pediatrics

Autosomal Dominant PKD

General: AD genetic cystic kidney disease, commonly from PKD1 (chromosome 16) or PKD2 (chromosome 12) genes

Clinical: Hypertension, hematuria, renal insufficiency, or flank pain
- Extrarenal features include: Cerebral aneurysms, hepatic/pancreatic cysts, cardiac valvular disorders (ie MVP), and diverticulosis

Diagnosis: Ultrasound (multiple and bilateral renal cysts)

Management:
- No therapy has been shown to prevent disease progression
- BP Control (ACEi/ARB)
- ESRD: Renal replacement (dialysis/transplant)
- Consider screening for cerebral aneurysms

Autosomal Recessive PKD

General: Infantile inherited AR disorder characterized by cystic dilation of the renal collecting ducts

Clinical: (Patients can vary in severity and age of disease onset)
- Prenatal: Screening US shows enlarged kidneys
- Neonates: Renal dysfunction, +/- pulmonary hypoplasia (Potter syndrome)
- Infants/Children: Renal dysfunction, plus liver involvement (biliary dysgenesis, hepatic fibrosis, portal hypertension)

Diagnosis: Ultrasound (enlarged, echogenic kidneys) plus coexisting liver disease
- Genetic testing can confirm

Management: Supportive (no curative therapies)

Simple Renal Cyst

General: Typically benign renal cysts that can be bilateral and multiple. Rarely the cysts can rupture and bleed.

Diagnosis:

Features of Benign Cysts	Features of Malignant Cysts
- Thin walled, non-septated	- Thick walls, irregular, and multilocular
- Non-enhancing on CT/MRI	- Enhancing on CT/MRI
- Homogenous interior	- Heterogeneous interior

Management:
- Benign: No follow up required
- Suspicious: Requires further workup for malignancy

NEPHROLITHIASIS — Renal, Medicine, Surgery

Type	Radio	Shape	pH	Cause/Findings
Calcium oxalate (80%)	Dense	Envelope	< 5.5	- Hypercalciuria or hyperoxaluria (increased oxalate absorption in GI disorders [ie IBD, malabsorption], vitamin C abuse, and ethylene glycol)
Calcium phosphate (5%)	Dense		> 5.5	- Seen in hyperparathyroidism, proximal RTA, and thiazide use
Struvite (Ammonium magnesium phosphate) (10%)	Dense	Coffin lid	> 5.5	- UTI from urease producing organisms (*Proteus, Klebsiella, Serratia, Enterobacter*) - Most common composition for staghorn calculi
Uric Acid (10%)	Lucent	Diamond	< 5.5	- Hyperuricemia from gout or chemo - Risk factors also include low urine volume/acidic urine
Cystine (<1%)	Lucent	Hexagonal	< 5.5	- Cystinuria (see genetics)
Drug Stones				- Acyclovir, indinavir, sulfadiazine

Clinical: Flank pain (generally waxing/waning), gross or microscopic hematuria, nausea, urinary urgency

Diagnosis:
- Noncontrast CT
- Ultrasound (in those that you wish to limit radiation, ie pregnant/kids)

Management:

Scenario	Interventions
≤ 5 mm	- Pain Control: NSAIDs or opioids - Fluids - Antispasmodics: Tamsulosin or Nifedipine
5-10 mm	- Can initially monitor for spontaneous passage, but intervention generally required (see below)
> 10 mm	- Depending on size/location, one of the following is used: (1) Shock wave lithotripsy (2) Ureteroscopy w/ holmium laser lithotripsy
Staghorn	- Percutaneous nephrolithotomy
Septic Patients	- If obstructing stone if found, percutaneous drainage or ureteral stenting is required, plus antibiotics
Prevention	- Increase fluids (> 2L/day), low sodium diet, low protein diet, high citrate diet, normal calcium diet - Pharm: Thiazides, urine alkalinization, or Allopurinol (depending on stone etiology)

INCONTINENCE

Renal
Medicine, OB-GYN

Type	General	Clinical	Management
Urge	- Uninhibited and involuntary detrusor contraction - Causes: Idiopathic (elderly), dementia, CVA, DM, early MS, Parkinson's	- Characterized by sudden urge with loss of large volumes, nocturnal wetting - Dx: Clinical. Urodynamics can confirm (but typically not used).	- Lifestyle (Bladder training exercises, Kegel's) - Anticholinergics (Oxybutynin, Tolterodine, Solifenacin, TCA) - Neurostimulators (Sacral nerve modulation, posterior tibial nerve stim)
Stress	- Weakness of pelvic floor muscles, leads to proximal urethra below pelvic floor, transmitting intraabdominal pressure to bladder - Causes: Obesity, vaginal delivery (high parity), menopause	- Involuntary loss of urine with increase abdominal pressure (ie sneeze) - Lacks nocturnal urge/symptoms - Dx: Bladder stress test, Q-tip test	- Lifestyle (weight loss, caffeine limit, etc) - Kegels/Physical Therapy - Estrogen replacement (post menopause) - Pessary - Surgery (Midurethral sling: Tension free vaginal tape OR urethropexy) - ISD: Bulking agents injected at sphincter
Overflow	- Eventual overflow from urinary retention, from obstruction or lack of normal detrusor muscle contractility - Causes: Pelvic organ prolapse, mass, detrusor underactivity (idiopathic, neuropathy, MS)	- Persistent small volume leakage, with small volume voids - Dx: Elevated post-void residual volume	- Catheterization (for chronic retention) - Cholinergic (Bethanechol) - α-blockers (Doxazosin, Terazosin) - Surgery may be required for outlet obstruction
Irritative	- Inflammation, from bladder irritant (ie UTI, malignancy, stone)	- Presents similarly to urge	- Treat underlying
Functional	- Can't get to bathroom		- Bladder training
Fistula	- Fistula formation between vagina and urethra or bladder	- Persistent vaginal leakage of urine - Dx: Dye test, cystourethroscopy	- Surgical repair (must wait 3-6 months after the insulting surgery to correct)

URINARY TRACT INFECTIONS
Renal Medicine

Urinary Tract Infection

General: Infection of the lower genitourinary tract, synonymous with cystitis

Micro:
(1) *E. Coli* (most common)
(2) Enterobacteriaceae (*Proteus, Klebsiella*)
(3) *S. saprophyticus*
(4) *Pseudomonas* (if healthcare exposure)

Clinical: Dysuria, increased frequency/urgency, suprapubic pain

Diagnosis: Clinical (symptoms above) sufficient
- Urinalysis (+ nitrites, leuk esterase) can be supportive
- Culture generally not required, but used in those with persistent symptoms /high risk for drug resistant organism

Management	Criteria	Management
Simple Cystitis (uncomplicated)	- Infection confined to bladder in non-pregnant woman or man - Lacks systemic symptoms below	- First line: TMP-SMX, Nitrofurantoin, Fosfomycin
Complicated	(1) Systemic signs (ie Temp > 100°F) (2) Flank pain/CVA tenderness	See next page
Pregnancy	- [See: OB-GYN]	
Prophylaxis	- Recurrent UTI (≥ 2 infections in six months or ≥ 3 UTIs in one year) - Risks: Frequent sexual activity, spermicide use, post-menopause	- Behavioral modification (post-coital voiding, stop spermicide use) - Pharm: TMP-SMX or other drug can be used. Use can be daily ppx, post-coital ppx, or intermittent self treatment.

Interstitial Cystitis/Bladder Pain Syndrome

General: Chronic bladder pain and discomfort for > 6 weeks without clear underlying medical cause

Risk: More common in women, those with psychiatric history

Clinical: Dysuria, increased urinary frequency, dyspareunia, relief with voiding, pelvic pain (with palpation)

Diagnosis: Diagnosis of exclusion. Urinalysis (rule out UTI).

Management:
(1) Behavioral Modification (trigger avoidance)
(2) Pharm: Amitriptyline
(3) Analgesics (Phenazopyridine, Methenamine) for short term relief
(4) Surgical Interventions (bladder hydrodistention)

URINARY TRACT INFECTIONS
Renal Medicine

Complicated UTI/Pyelonephritis

General: Infection of the upper urinary tract (extending past the bladder), most commonly from ascending lower urinary tract infection

Micro: E. coli, enterobacteriaceae (*Proteus, Klebsiella*), other gram negative (*Pseudomonas*), Enterococcus, fungi (*Candida*)

Clinical:
- UTI symptoms, plus systemic signs (fever, chills, flank pain), CVA tenderness
- Urinalysis (pyuria/bacteriuria, WBC casts)
- Gram stain and culture often positive

Diagnosis:
- Clinical diagnosis (systemic symptoms plus pyuria and bacteriuria)
- Imaging (CT) reserved for cases when patient is not improving

Management:

	General	Empiric Management
Outpatient	- Young, otherwise healthy patients can receive ER care with close follow up	- IM Dose of Ceftriaxone plus TMP-SMX Amox-Clav, or 3rd gen PO cephalosporin - Fluoroquinolone (Ciprofloxacin) (especially in patients with risk for multi-drug resistant organism)
Inpatient	- Septic/critically ill patients - Urinary hardware/obstruction	- Ceftriaxone, fluoroquinolone, pip-tazo - Carbapenem (if risk factor for MDR organism)

Complications:

Renal/Perinephric Abscess
- Walled of cavity of necrosis. Can be
    (1) Renal or
    (2) Perinephric (perirenal fat to Gerota's fascia)
- Generally occurs as a complication of pyelo, but can be due to seeding
- Dx: CT or US
- Tx: Antibiotics +/- percutaneous drainage (> 5 cm renal and all perinephric)

Chronic Pyelonephritis
- Chronic interstitial disease due to recurrent/chronic infection
- Causes: Vesicoureteral reflux, chronic urinary obstruction (ie stone)

Xanthogranulomatous pyelonephritis
- Subtype of chronic pyelonephritis (generally from obstructive stone)
- Massive kidney damage from granulomatous inflammation and foamy macrophages

RENAL MALIGNANCY
Renal — Medicine, Surgery

Renal Cell Carcinoma

General: Most common cause of renal cancer (85%), usually composed of clear cell tumors of proximal tubule epithelium. Other subtypes include:
- Papillary tumors (proximal tubular cells)
- Oncocytomas (intercalated cell tumors, associated with tuberous sclerosis)

Risk:
- Cigarette smoking
- Polycystic kidney disease
- Occupational exposures
- Cytotoxic medications
- Genetic (including vHL)

Clinical: Variable presentation, including abdominal mass/pain, hematuria, systemic symptoms (fever, night sweats, weight loss), paraneoplastic syndromes, or symptoms from metastases
- Paraneoplastic syndromes include:
    - Hypercalcemia (PTHrP or lytic bone lesions)
    - Anemia OR Erythrocytosis (excess EPO production)

Diagnosis: Abdominal CT + Biopsy

Management:
- Localized: Radical or partial nephrectomy
- Advanced: Targeted immunotherapy +/- surgical nephrectomy/debulking
    - Immunotherapy includes checkpoint inhibitors (CTLA4 inhibitors, PD-1 inhibitors), anti-VEGF therapy

Von-Hippel Lindau

General: AD defect in vHL gene on chromosome 3, which codes for a tumor suppressor protein

Clinical:
- Hemangioblastomas (Retina, brain stem, cerebellum, spine)
- Renal cell carcinomas
- Pheochromocytoma
- Endolymphatic sac tumors of middle ear

Diagnosis: Suspected based on clinical features, but confirmed with genetic testing

Management:
- Screening (annual eye/retinal exam, abdominal MRI, urine metanephrines, brain/spinal MRI)

BLADDER MALIGNANCY
Renal
Medicine, Surgery

Subtype	Risk Factors
Transitional Cell	- Urothelial carcinogens (cigarette smoke, occupational chemical exposures, cyclophosphamide, phenacetin) - Jobs at risk for chemical exposure include painters, textiles, metal workers, rubber workers, leather workers, and electrical workers
Adenocarcinoma	- Urachal remnant - Non-urachal: *Schistosoma* infection, bladder exstrophy
Squamous Cell	- Chronic Inflammation (chronic/recurrent UTI, *Schistosoma* infection, radiation, bladder stone)

Clinical: Painless hematuria (generally age > 40)

Diagnosis: Cystoscopy + Biopsy

Management:
    - No muscle invasion: TURBT (transurethral resection of bladder tumor)
    - Muscle invasion: Radical cystectomy, plus neoadjuvant/adjuvant chemo
        - Intravesical BCG or Mitomycin

PROSTATE MALIGNANCY
Renal — Medicine, Surgery

Prostate Cancer

General: Adenocarcinoma of prostate. 2nd most common cancer in men.

Risk: ↑ Age, African-American, family history, genetics (ie BRCA, Lynch)

Clinical:
- Most often asymptomatic, picked up on routine screening
    - DRE showing nodularity, irregularity (is indication for biopsy)
    - PSA (no clear set criteria or threshold value, but major increases from prior PSA, PSA > 7, or ↑ PSA in conjunction with abnormal exam is indication for biopsy)
- Rarely, advanced disease can cause symptoms (hematuria, dysuria, or bone pain from metastasis)
    - Note: BPH can also cause hematuria/dysuria

Diagnosis: Transrectal biopsy (with aid of transrectal US)
- At least 12 samples, add together two worst to calculate Gleason score

Management:

Screening	- Controversial. Currently, advise discussion with patients over pros and cons of screening (ie small increased ability to diagnose cancer, balanced with risk of overdiagnosis and unnecessary invasive procedures) - In general, those between 50-70 with > 10 yr life expectancy should consider PSA screening. Other ages unlikely to get benefit, unless at especially high risk.
Initial Eval	- Local Staging (DRE + transrectal US +/- MRI) - Tech-99 Bone scan (if symptomatic or high risk for metastasis)
Initial Therapy (local dz)	- For very low and low risk (ie Gleason < 6) → Active surveillance (can consider radiation therapy or prostatectomy) - Intermediate risk (Gleason 7) → RT or prostatectomy - High/Very high risk (Gleason ≥ 8) → RT +/- brachytherapy or radical prostatectomy - Surveillance with PSA for all
Lymph Node Involvement/ Disseminated	- Androgen deprivation therapy: Medical (ie Leuprolide) or surgical orchiectomy - Possible chemotherapy

PEDIATRIC RENAL NEOPLASIA
Renal Pediatrics

Wilms Tumor

General: Most common childhood renal malignancy. Associated with WT1 mutation on chromosome 11.

Etiology: Can be idiopathic. 10% associated with congenital syndromes (below).

Clinical:
- Abdominal mass/swelling (usually smooth, rarely cross midline)
    - Often asymptomatic, discovered on routine health visit
- May be associated with abdominal pain, vomiting, hypertension
- Lung is most common metastatic site

Diagnosis:
- Imaging (Initially US, then CT/MRI to better characterize)
- Surgical excision/biopsy for definitive diagnosis

Management:
- Surgical resection
- Chemotherapy and/or radiation therapy (indications depend on stage)

Congenital Syndromes (associated with Wilms)

Beckwith-Wiedemann	- Wilms tumor - Macroglossia - Macrosomia, limb hemihypertrophy - Medial abdominal wall defects (omphalocele) - Hyperinsulinism (hypoglycemia) - Hepatoblastoma (monitor w/ abdominal US and AFP levels)
WAGR	- Wilms tumor - Aniridia - GU malformation - Retardation
Denys-Drash	- Wilms tumor - Progressive kidney failure - Male pseudohermaphroditism

CONGENITAL RENAL ABNORMALITIES

Renal Pediatric

Type	General	Clinical	Management
Potter	- Syndrome found in infants that suffer from severe oligohydramnios in utero	- Pulmonary hypoplasia - Limb deformities (club feet, hip dislocation) - Abnormal facies (flattened ears/nose, recessed chin, etc)	
Horseshoe Kidney	- Fusion of lower poles of the kidneys - Often found in pelvis with abnormal blood supply (trapped under IMA)	- Most often asymptomatic - Can result in hydronephrosis, recurrent infection, or stones	- Usually requires no intervention
Renal Agenesis	- Complete lack of kidney one or both kidneys - Ureteric bud fails to develop and induce differentiation of metanephric mesenchyme	- Bilateral renal agenesis is always fatal early in life - Unilateral renal agenesis is often asymptomatic	
Multicystic Dysplastic Kidney	- Congenital cystic renal dysplasia - Nonfunctional kidney consisting of cysts and connective tissue	- Picked up on prenatal ultrasound - Often asymptomatic if other kidney normal (which should hypertrophy in response to the abnormal kidney)	- Observation (abnormal kidney will naturally involute) - Monitor growth of other kidney
Ureteropelvic-junction Obstruction	- Blockage where ureter enters kidney, causing hydronephrosis - Caused by ureteral stenosis/compression	- Often picked up as hydronephrosis - Can present as abdominal mass, UTI, etc - Can also present after large volume intake (ie binge drinking) - Dx: US, followed by diuretic renography	- Symptomatic patients receive surgical correction - Can simply monitor if kidney function not severely affected
Ectopic Ureter	- Abnormal insertion of ureter into bladder (Note: Girls can also implant into vagina) - Often associated with duplex collecting system	- Associated with pediatric UTI, vesicoureteral reflux, and urinary incontinence - Dx: US (hydroureter/hydronephrosis)	- Surgical correction

Renal32

CHILDHOOD UROLOGIC ISSUES
Renal — Pediatrics, Surgery

Vesicoureteral Reflux

General: Retrograde passage of urine from bladder into upper urinary tract, most commonly due to inadequate closure of the ureterovesical junction. Leads to increased risk for recurrent upper urinary tract infections and possible CKD.

Etiology:
- Primary: Mechanical failure of the ureterovesical junction (most common)
- Secondary: Excess bladder pressure (from posterior urethral valve, bladder obstruction, etc)

Clinical:
- Can be picked up prenatally as hydronephrosis
- Diagnosed after febrile UTI in infants and young children

Grades

Grade 1	- Urine refluxes part way up ureter
Grade 2	- Urine refluxes all the way up ureter
Grade 3	- Grade 2, plus mild dilatation of ureter and blunting of calyces
Grade 4	- Severe dilatation or ureter/blunting of calyces
Grade 5	- Massive dilatation or ureter/blunting of calyces, plus loss of renal cortex

Diagnosis: Voiding cystourethrogram (VCUG)

Management:
- Grade 1/2: Watchful waiting. Antibiotic prophylaxis is an option.
  - 80% have spontaneous resolution
- Grade 3-5: Antibiotic prophylaxis. Surgery in grade 4-5 and refractory cases.

Complications:
- Recurrent pyelonephritis
- ESRD/renal scarring

Pediatric UTI

Clinical: Most commonly presents with fever
- Abdominal pain, dysuria, incontinence are all possible presentations

Diagnosis: Urinalysis/culture (must be clean sample, straight cath often necessary in neonates/infants)
- > 5-10 WBCs/HPF, + leuk esterase or nitrite indicative of UTI
- > 10,000 CFU on culture of straight cath (> 100,000 on clean catch)

Management:
- 1-2 weeks of antibiotics (3rd generation cephalosporins first line)
- Must workup for vesicoureteral reflux with:
  - Renal/bladder US
    - Indicated for any child < 2, recurrent UTI, or lack of symptom improvement
  - VCUG:
    - Used if positive US results, ≥ 2 y/o febrile UTIs

CHILDHOOD UROLOGIC ISSUES
Renal — Pediatrics, Surgery

Posterior Urethral Valves

General: Congenital posterior urethral obstruction due to membranous folds

Clinical:
- Most often identified prenatally on US (hydronephrosis, dilated bladder)
- Postnatally can present as UTI, poor urinary stream, abdominal distension
- ↑ Risk for CKD and bladder dysfunction

Diagnosis:
- VCUG (dilated posterior urethra with linear defect in the voiding phase)
- Confirm with cystoscopy

Management:
- Postnatal (initial): Urinary catheter for drainage. Correct fluids/lytes.
- After stabilized, surgical correction (cystoscopy + ablation)

Hypospadias/Epispadias

Hypospadias	- Congenital anomaly with abnormal ventral opening of male urethra - Often associated with abnormal foreskin/urethral meatus - Tx: Delay circumcision, with surgical closure weeks after birth
Epispadias	- Congenital opening of urethra on dorsal surface of penis - Associated with bladder exstrophy

CHILDHOOD UROLOGIC ISSUES
Renal — Pediatrics, Surgery

Cryptorchidism

General: Failure of descent of testicle by 4 months of age. If bilateral, must suspect endocrine or genetic disorder.

Risk: Prematurity/SGA/Low birth weight, genetic disorders, neural tube defects

Clinical:
- Empty, hypoplastic, poorly rugated scrotum
- Possible inguinal fullness (indicating testicle in inguinal canal)

Diagnosis: Clinical

Management:
- Orchiopexy (before year 1)
    - Indicated after 6 months, as unlikely to spontaneously descend after this point
    - Without intervention, high risk for testicular cancer, infertility, torsion, inguinal hernia

Phimosis/Paraphimosis

	Phimosis	Paraphimosis
Gen	- Tight foreskin that cannot be retracted to show glans - Normal (physiologic) in newborns, but should resolve by school age - Pathologic: Truly non-retractable foreskin due to distal scarring of prepuce (usually from trauma or inflammation)	- Retracted foreskin that cannot be returned to normal position - Usually occurs with forcible retraction of the foreskin
Clin	- Can be associated with irritation, dysuria, painful erections, recurrent infections	- Causes severe pain and swelling, focused on the glans
Tx	- Stretching exercises, topical corticosteroids - Circumcision (definitive)	- Pain control/manual reduction - Surgical correction for severe cases

PEDIATRIC FLUIDS/ELECTROLYTES

Renal Pediatrics

Pediatric Dehydration

Severity	Symptoms
Mild (3-5%)	- Sticky or slightly dry oral mucosa - Increased thirst - Normal vitals - Normal/slightly decreased urine output
Moderate (6-9%)	- Dry oral mucosa - Increased thirst, irritable - Sunken eyes/fontanelle, reduced skin turgor - Tachycardia, tachypnea, possible hypotension - Decreased urine output
Severe (>10%)	- Very dry oral mucosa - Lethargy, coma - Sunken eyes/fontanelle, reduced skin turgor - Cool skin, acrocyanosis - Tachycardia, tachypnea, hypotension - Anuria

Management:
- Emergent replacement (for moderate/severe dehydration)
    - 20 mL/kg bolus of isotonic saline
    - Repeat as necessary until replete
- Secondary fluid repletion (for mild/moderate dehydration, or after emergent replacement in severe cases)
    - Oral fluid replacement preferred

Proteinuria

General: Protein excretion > 100 mg/m^2 in children

Cause	Features
Transient Proteinuria	- Transient increases in urinary protein excretion - Induced by fever, strenuous exercise, seizures, hypovolemia - No intervention necessary
Orthostatic Proteinuria	- Benign increase in protein excretion when upright - Confirm with early morning urinalysis or P/Cr ratio - Requires no further workup or intervention once diagnosed
Persistent (Pathologic)	- Persistent on multiple occasions, concerning for glomerular or tubular pathology - Workup with 24 hour urine protein, US, and pediatric nephrology referral

PEDIATRIC FLUIDS/ELECTROLYTES

Renal Pediatrics

Pediatric Hypertension

Age	1-13 y/o	> 13 y/o
Normal	< 90th percentile	< 120/< 80 mmHg
Elevated	90th - 95th percentile	120-129/< 80 mmHg
Stage 1 HTN	> 95th percentile	130-139/80-89 mmHg
Stage 2 HTN	≥ 95th percentile + 12 mmHg	> 140/90 mmHg

Etiology:
- Primary: Idiopathic
    - More likely in overweight, family history, black/hispanic
- Secondary:
    - Renal (glomerulonephritis, CKD, polycystic kidney)
    - Endocrine (pheo/neuroblastoma, Cushing's, hyperthyroidism)
    - Cardiac (coarctation of the aorta)

Clinical: BP values found elevated on 3 consecutive visits
- Patients with secondary HTN often have other symptoms and findings associated with their underlying disorder

Workup:
- Electrolytes, renal function, lipid panel, urinalysis
- Renal US in younger children
- Consider ECHO to evaluate for LVH
- Consider 24 hour BP monitoring (many kids have white coat HTN)

Management:
- Primary: Lifestyle modification (weight loss, diet, exercise)
    - Pharm:
        - Indicated in Stage 2 HTN, symptomatic kids, or refractory Stage 1
            - ACEi/ARB, CCB, thiazide most common options
- Secondary: Evaluate and treat underlying disorder

TESTICULAR CANCER
Renal/Urology
Medicine, Surgery

Testicular Cancer

Subtype	Description/Features
Germ Cell (Seminomatous)	
Seminoma	- Most common subtype, with good prognosis - Highly sensitive to treatment (chemo/radiotherapy) - "Fried egg cell" histology (large cell, eccentric nucleolus, clear cytoplasm) - Serum biomarkers usually normal (but can have modest ↑)
Germ Cell (Non-seminomatous)	
Embryonal	- Malignant subtype with aggressive spread - Modest hCG production
Yolk sac	- Endodermal sinus tumor - Common child subtype, with characteristic AFP production
Choriocarcinoma	- Most malignant with rapid hematogenous spread - β-HCG production
Teratoma	- Can be benign (usually in kids) or malignant (usually in adults, associated with mixed-germ cell tumors) - Derived from multiple embryonic layers
Mixed germ cell	- Multiple types of germ cell tumor present
Sex-Cord Stromal	
Leydig	- Produce androgens or estrogen (precocious puberty, gynecomastia in kids, or ED/impotence/loss of libido in adults)
Sertoli	- Benign and usually clinically silent
Other	
Lymphoma	- Occurs in older males. Diffuse large B-cell

General: Generally seen in men between 15-35 y/o. Most commonly germ cell tumors.

Risk: Cryptorchidism, infertility, personal/family history of testicular cancer

Clinical: Most common clinical feature of testicular cancer is a painless testicular mass

Diagnosis:
- US (solid mass is highly concerning for cancer)
- Further evaluation with β-hCG, AFP, LDH, pelvic CT

Management:
- Radical inguinal orchiectomy (both diagnostic and therapeutic)
- Adjuvant chemotherapy or radiotherapy for higher risk local disease
- Chemotherapy (ie bleomycin, etoposide, cisplatin) for disseminated disease (ie lymph node or distant metastasis)

PROSTATE
Urology
Medicine, Surgery

Benign Prostatic Hyperplasia

General: Benign enlargement of the prostate from growth of the transitional zone (also known as periurethral zone)

Risk: > 50 y/o, black men

Clinical:
- Often asymptomatic (especially early on)
- Storage Symptoms (urgency, incontinence, ↑ frequency, nocturia)
- Voiding Symptoms (↓ urinary stream, hesitancy, straining to void, dribbling)
- Hematuria (both microscopic and gross) possible
- Diffusely enlarged, firm, nontender prostate on DRE

Diagnosis: Clinical (from history and physical). Check PSA.

Management:
- Behavioral Modification (avoid diuretics like caffeine/EtOH, avoid fluids at bedtime, etc)
- Pharm
    - Mild to moderate: α1 antagonists (ie Tamsulosin, Doxazosin)
    - Severe: α1 antagonists PLUS 5α Reductase Inhibitor (Finasteride)
- Surgery (Indicated if: Renal dysfunction, hydronephrosis, severe urinary retention, recurrent UTI)
    - Transurethral resection or ablation (TURP)

Bacterial Prostatitis

	Acute Bacterial Prostatitis	**Chronic Bacterial Prostatitis**
Gen	- Acute prostate infection, usually affecting younger men - E. Coli, Gonorrhea, Chlamydia	- Subtle, non-acute prostate infection seen in older men - More common than acute prostatitis - Gram negative rods (ie E. Coli) most common
Clin	- Fevers, chills, toxic appearing - UTI symptoms (dysuria, frequency) - Pelvic/perineal/low back pain - Exquisitely tender prostate on DRE - Cloudy urine/pyuria	- Recurrent UTI w/ same organism - Often chronically symptomatic, with mild lower UTI symptoms - Prostate may be tender on exam, but is often normal
Dx	- Clinical - Urine gram stain/culture	- Clinical (presumptive dx/treatment) - Urine gram stain/culture after prostatic massage
Tx	- TMP-SMX or fluoroquinolone	- Fluoroquinolone - If no improvement, suspect chronic prostatitis (ie chronic pelvic pain syndrome)

PROSTATE/PENIS
Urology
Medicine, Surgery

Chronic Prostatitis/Chronic Pelvic Pain Syndrome

General: Clinical noninfectious syndrome of urologic symptoms and pelvic pain, without clear pathophysiology or etiology

Clinical:
- Pain (in perineum/pelvis/genitalia)
- Voiding difficulty, dysuria
- Pain with ejaculation
- Minimal prostatic tenderness of DRE, sterile urine culture

Diagnosis: Clinical (diagnosis of exclusion)

Management:
- Initial: Tamsulosin + Fluoroquinolone
- Chronic: α blockers and 5α Reductase inhibitors

Penile Pathology

Disorder	Clinical Features
Balanitis/ Balanoposthitis	- Infection of head of penis and foreskin, respectively - Usually due to inadequate hygiene in uncircumcised men - Tx: Hygiene, saline irrigation, topical antifungals if severe
Priapism	- Persistent erection no associated with sexual stimulation (for at least 4 hours). - Risk for penile ischemia and permanent erectile dysfunction - Causes include ischemic (Low flow: PDE5 inhibitor use, sickle cell, Prazosin, Trazodone) or nonischemic (High-flow: Fistula between artery and corpus cavernosum, usually after trauma) - Dx: Clinical. Evaluate with US or cavernous aspiration/ABG. - Tx: Ischemic → Phenylephrine injection. Nonischemic → Observe, with arteriography/embolization if not improving.
Penile Fracture	- Occurs with erect penis during sex - Snapping sound, with rapid detumescence, and severe pain - Evaluate with US, followed by emergent surgical repair
Carcinoma of the Penis	- Most commonly SCC. Very rare in US/Europe. - Risk: Older men, third-world countries, phimosis, HPV infection - Presents as mass or ulceration, most commonly at glans, associated with local lymphadenopathy - Dx: Biopsy - Tx: Local excision, +/- lymph node dissection and chemotherapy
Erythroplasia of Queyrat	- Carcinoma in situ on glans, velvety red appearance
Bowen disease	- Carcinoma in situ, on penile shaft epithelium - Presents as single red plaque with crusting and oozing

TESTICULAR PAIN
Urology
Medicine, Surgery

Testicular Torsion

General: Inadequate fixation of the testes to the tunica vaginalis, allowing for twisting of testes around spermatic cord, with ischemia from vascular obstruction

Clinical:
- Acute severe testicular pain, can cause nausea, vomiting
- Profound swelling and diffuse tenderness
- Negative cremasteric reflex, "high-riding" testis oriented transversely
- Common scenarios include post trauma or physical activity, or waking up in the middle of night (in kids)
- Prehn's sign: Lifting of testes alleviates pain from epididymitis, not torsion

Diagnosis: Scrotal US

Management: Detorsion and fixation (of both testes)

Appendix Testis Torsion
- Most occurs in school age children
- Presents with gradual onset of pain. Cremasteric reflex is normal.
    - "Blue dot sign" (blue spot seen through scrotum in superior aspect of the testes)
- Dx: Scrotal US
- Tx: NSAIDs, ice, scrotal support

Epididymitis

General: Inflammation of the epididymis. Usually infectious, but can be autoimmune or traumatic.
- < 35: Gonorrhea/Chlamydia most common
- > 35: *E. Coli, Pseudomonas*, other gram negatives

Clinical:
- Localized testicular pain (tenderness/swelling over epididymis)
- Can spread to testis (orchitis), causing testicular pain
- Dysuria or other urinary symptoms are possible
- Fever/systemic symptoms rare, but possible

Diagnosis: Clinical. US to rule out torsion, and obtain urine culture/urinalysis.

Management:
< 35: Ceftriaxone/Doxycycline
> 35: Fluoroquinolone

TESTICULAR/SCROTAL PATHOLOGY
Urology — Medicine, Surgery

Disorder	General	Clinical	Management
Varicocele	- Dilation of venous pampiniform plexus - Usually left-sided (nutcracker effect on left renal vein, increases pressure) - Right-sided varicocele indicates possible venous thrombosis	- Soft, scrotal mass, "bag of worms" - Becomes less severe when lying down - Can cause aching pain, testicular atrophy, or infertility if severe - US can confirm dilated veins, retrograde flow	- Support/NSAIDs - Gonadal vein ligation or embolization (if severe)
Hydrocele	- Collection of fluid between parietal and visceral layers of tunica vaginalis (from lack of obliteration) - Can also be secondary to neoplasm or inflammation	- Presents as smooth, transilluminating mass - Generally nontender	- No intervention required, unless symptomatic (in which case the sac can be excised)
Spermatocele	- Cystic sac in the epididymis	- Soft, round mass in head of epididymis	- Usually require no treatment
Fournier's	- Necrotizing fasciitis of the scrotum and perineum - Mixed aerobic/anaerobic infection	- Causes sudden pain - Skin signs: Tense edema, blistering, crepitus - Possible odor, purulent discharge from tissue - Systemic signs (fever, weakness, shock, etc)	- IV Antibiotics PLUS surgical debridement

HEMATURIA

Renal/Urology Medicine, Surgery

General Hematuria

Definitions:
- Microscopic Hematuria: ≥ 3 RBC on microscopy
- Gross Hematuria: Grossly red urine
- Pseudohematuria: Red pigment in urine (from foods like beets, and drugs like rifampin)
- Other Pigments: Myoglobin, bilirubin (both can present with dark urine)

Hematuria Throughout	Terminal Hematuria	Initial Hematuria
- Glomerulonephritis - Pyelonephritis - Nephrolithiasis - Upper urinary cancers	- Cystitis - Bladder stones or cancer - BPH/prostate cancer	- Urethra injury (trauma, urethritis, etc)

Hematuria Workup

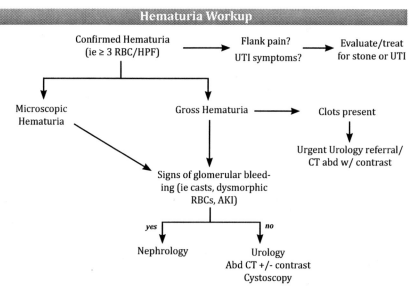

Imaging Options

Test	Indications
CT Urography (CT abdomen/pelvis with/without contrast)	- Unexplained hematuria
CT Abdomen (w/o contrast)	- Stones, masses
Ultrasound	- Stones, masses in someone with contraindication to radiation
Cystoscopy	- Evaluation of bladder (for mass, bleed, etc)

Renal43

RENAL PHARM

Renal Medicine

	Mechanism	Indication	Side Effects/Management
Acetazolamide	- Carbonic anhydrase inhibitor (HCO_3 diuresis)	- Glaucoma, Urinary alkalinization, Altitude sickness	- Sulfa drug - Proximal RTA
Loop Diuretics Furosemide Bumetanide Torsemide Ethacrynic acid	- Inhibit Na/K/2Cl transporter of thick ascending limb of the loop of Henle	- Edema - Hypercalcemia	- Sulfa drug (except ethacrynic acid) - Ototoxicity (high doses) - Hypokalemia, dehydration, alkalosis - Nephritis (interstitial) - Gout
Thiazides HCTZ Chlorthalidone Metolazone	- Inhibit NaCl cotransporter in distal convoluted tubule - Increases distal tubule Ca^{2+} resorption	- Hypertension - Hypercalciuria - Diabetes insipidus	- Sulfa drug - Hypokalemic metabolic alkalosis - Hyponatremia - Hyperglycemia - Hyperlipidemia - Hyperuricemia
K-Sparing Spironolactone Eplerenone Triamterene Amiloride	- Competitive aldosterone antagonists (spirono/eplerenone) - Na Channel blockers in collecting duct	- HF - Cirrhosis - Hyperaldosteronism	- Hyperkalemia - Anti-androgen (spirono): Gynecomastia
ACEi Captopril Enalapril Lisinopril	- Inhibits ACE (conversion of ANG to ANG-II) - Also inhibits breakdown of bradykinin	- HTN - CHF - Proteinuria	- Cough - Angioedema - Teratogen - ↑ Creatinine - Hyperkalemia
ARB Losartan Candesartan Valsartan	- Inhibits AR-1 (angiotensin receptor)	- HTN - CHF - Proteinuria	- Teratogen - ↑ Creatinine - Hyperkalemia
Aliskiren	- Direct renin inhibitor	- HTN	- Hyperkalemia, ↑ Creatinine

UROLOGY PHARM

Urology — Medicine, Surgery

	Mechanism	Indication	Side Effects/Management
Tamsulosin	- $\alpha1_A$ receptor antagonist	- BPH	- Hypotension (orthostasis, syncope)
Doxazosin Terazosin Doxazosin	- $\alpha1$ receptor antagonist	- Hypertension (second-line agent)	
Finasteride	- 5α-reductase inhibitor	- BPH - Prostate cancer - Male pattern baldness	- Sexual dysfunction
Flutamide	- Androgen receptor antagonist	- Prostate cancer	- Anti-androgen effects (gynecomastia, breast tenderness, sexual dysfunction)
Sildenafil Vardenafil Tadalafil	- Phosphodiesterase 5 inhibitor	- Erectile dysfunction	- Headache, flushing, nausea - Cyanopia (blue vision) - Hypotension (must avoid use with nitrates especially)
Alprostadil	- PGE1 agonist	- Erectile dysfunction (corporal injections or urethral suppositories)	

Renal46

HYPOTHALAMIC PITUITARY AXIS

Endocrine Medicine

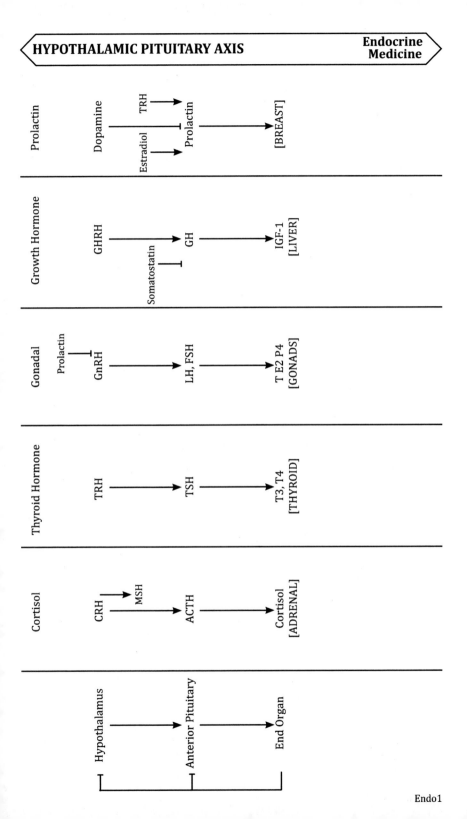

Endo1

THYROID OVERVIEW

Endocrine Medicine

Thyroid Hormone

Functions:
- Bone growth
- CNS maturation
- Increase metabolic rate (Na/K pumps)
- Increased β1 heart receptors (increased CO, contractility, HR, SV)

Regulatory:
- Wolff Chaikoff: Large iodine intake → Decrease T3/T4 level
- Jad Basedow: Excess T3/T4 production after iodine intake in someone with hyperthyroidism

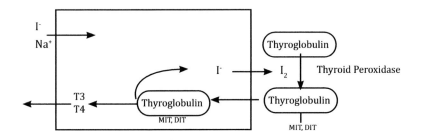

Clinical Features of Hypo/Hyperthyroidism

	Hypothyroid	**Hyperthyroid**
Sx	- Fatigue, weakness, lethargy - Cold intolerance - Slowed mentation, inability to concentrate - Weight gain - Constipation - Menorrhagia	- Anxiety, insomnia, irritability - Tremors, sweating, heat intolerance - Weight loss with normal appetite - Diarrhea - Palpitations
PE	- Dry skin - Hoarseness - Edema - ↓ DTR	- Goiter - Fine hair - Stare/lid lag - ↑ DTR
Lab	- Hyperlipidemia	- Hypercalcemia (↑ bone turnover) - Decreased lipid levels
Other	- Bradycardia - Hypertension	- Tachyarrhythmias (AF, sinus tachy) - CV (increased contractility, cardiac output, HR, and pulse pressure)

HYPOTHYROIDISM — Endocrine Medicine

Etiology	Clinical	Diagnostic Findings
Chronic Lymphocytic Thyroiditis (Hashimoto)	- Autoimmune lymphocytic thyroid invasion - Presents as gradual loss of thyroid function	- Elevated TPO auto-Ig, TG
Painless Thyroiditis	- Variant of Hashimoto - Transient hyper, then hypothyroid states - Generally resolves to euthyroid	- Low radioiodine uptake
Subacute Thyroiditis (de Quervain)	- Postviral inflammatory process - Generally initial hyperthyroid period, followed by hypothyroidism - Exam: Painful, tender thyroid	- Low radioiodine uptake - Elevated ESR/CRP
Fibrous Thyroiditis (Riedel's)	- Fibrous thyroid infiltration - Signs of extension (hoarseness, dyspnea, dysphagia) - Exam: Slowly growing, painless goiter	- Associated with IgG4 disorders
Subclinical	- High TSH with normal T3/T4 - Generally asymptomatic	
Euthyroid Sick	- Decreased T3/T4 in the setting of critical illness - TSH can be normal, increased, or decreased - Reverse T3 elevated - Intervention generally not indicated	
Other	- Postpartum thyroiditis - Iatrogenic (radioiodine therapy, thyroidectomy, drugs [lithium]) - Iodine deficiency - Infiltrative disease (sarcoid, hemochromatosis) - Secondary/tertiary hypothyroidism (anterior pituitary & hypothalamic disease)	

Diagnosis:
- Primary (Overt) Hypothyroidism: ↑ TSH, ↓ free T4
- TPO antibodies (don't have to check)

Management:
- Overt: Levothyroxine (check TSH in 6 weeks, titrate dose to TSH 0.5-5.0)
- Subclinical: TSH ≥ 10 or symptomatic receive levothyroxine

Myxedema Coma
- Rare, severe hypothyroidism leading to multiorgan dysfunction
- Clinical: Altered mentation, hypoventilation, hypothermia, hypotension, hyponatremia, bradycardia
- Tx: Levothyroxine/Liothyronine, mechanical ventilation, corticosteroids, fluids

HYPERTHYROIDISM — Endocrine Medicine

Etiology	Clinical Findings
Graves'	- Most common cause of hyperthyroidism - Due to production of TSH receptor Ig (specific finding) - Exam: Diffusely enlarged, symmetric nontender thyroid (+/- bruit) - Ophthalmopathy: Exophthalmos, periorbital edema, eye irritation, diplopia (due to orbital GAG buildup) - Pretibial Myxedema (due to dermal mucopolysaccharide buildup)
Multinodular Goiter	- Hyperfunctioning thyroid nodules, with atrophy of remaining thyroid
Thyroid Adenoma	- Rare - Single hyperfunctioning nodule
Thyroiditis	- All causes of thyroiditis can cause transient periods of hyperthyroidism
Other	- Iatrogenic (Levothyroxine), excess iodine, drugs

Diagnosis:
- TSH ↓ and T3/T4 ↑ in primary hyperthyroidism
- In general: Acute onset of hyperthyroidism with clinical features of Graves' is sufficient for diagnosis
- If unsure, TSH-R Ab, radioactive uptake, and thyroglobulin levels

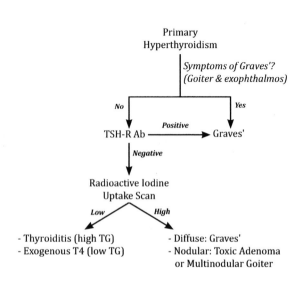

HYPERTHYROIDISM

Endocrine Medicine

Management: Graves'

Acute	Used for initial symptomatic control, prior to definitive therapy: - Beta-blocker (ie Atenolol, Metoprolol, Propranolol) - Thionamide (Methimazole)

Definitive	Indication	Drawbacks
Thionamide	- Mildly symptomatic - Older age (limited remaining life)	- Medication side effects (ie agranulocytosis)
Radioiodine Ablation	- Moderate or severely symptomatic hyperthyroidism	- Permanent hypothyroidism - Worsens orbitopathy
Surgery	- Moderate or severe orbitopathy - Large/obstructive goiter - Cancer	- Permanent hypothyroidism - Hypoparathyroidism - Recurrent laryngeal nerve damage

Note: Toxic adenoma/multinodular goiter follow the same above acute/chronic plan. Radioiodine ablation is typically utilized for definitive management.

Thyroid Storm

General: Acute, life-threatening complication of thyrotoxicosis, generally precipitated by stressor (sepsis, DKA, trauma, surgery, labor, acute iodine load [ie contrast])

Etiology: Occurs in those with chronic untreated hyperthyroidism, but generally triggered by one of the above stressors

Clinical:
- Hyperpyrexia (up to 106°F)
- Encephalopathy, psychosis, or coma
- CV: Tachycardia, hypertension, arrhythmia (ie AFib), HF
- GI: Diarrhea, nausea, vomiting, abdominal pain, jaundice

Diagnosis: Clinical features PLUS elevated T3/T4

Management:
- Beta-blocker (ie Propranolol)
- Corticosteroids (Hydrocortisone)
- Propylthiouracil
- Potassium Iodine
- Supportive ICU care

THYROID NODULE/MALIGNANCY
Endocrine — Medicine, Surgery

Thyroid Nodule

General: Cancer is found in ~5-10% of all investigated nodules. Malignancy is suggested by firm, fixed, irregular masses with associated lymphadenopathy. Nodules investigated with algorithm below.

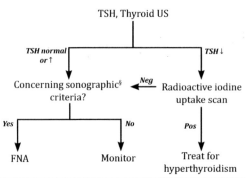

§Sonographic Criteria:
- Large nodules (≥ 2cm)
- Small nodules (≥ 1 cm) w/ irregular US features (ie micro calcifications, irregular margins, extrathyroidal invasion)
- Purely cystic lesions are almost always benign

FNA Result	Management
Benign	- Reassurance and periodic US monitoring
Indeterminate	- Repeat FNA - If still indeterminate, follow up with molecular testing or diagnostic surgery
Suspicious	- Surgery

Thyroid Malignancy

Subtype	Features	Management
Papillary	- Most common thyroid cancer - Risk: Radiation, family history	- Total thyroidectomy or lobectomy
Follicular	- Well-differentiated tumor of thyroid epithelium - Risk: Radiation, family history - Vascular spread	- Total thyroidectomy or lobectomy
Medullary	- Parafollicular cell tumor with characteristic calcitonin production - Risk: Sporadic, or MEN2 associated	- Total thyroidectomy with lymph node dissection
Anaplastic	- Poorly differentiated tumor found more commonly in elderly - Poor prognosis	- Chemoradiation + Surgery (for purely local disease)
Lymphoma	- Rare B-cell neoplasm associated with Hashimoto's - Presents as rapidly enlarging goiter with extra thyroid compression (dyspnea, dysphagia)	- Chemoradiation

Note: Choice of total vs lobectomy is based on size and lymph node involvement
Post-Surgery Management:
- Levothyroxine w/ TSH monitoring (want it suppressed)
- Radioiodine ablation (for those with regional extension/metastatic disease)

DIABETES INSIPIDUS

Endocrine Medicine

Nephrogenic and Central DI

General: Deficient secretion or response to ADH, resulting in polyuria and abnormal water balance

Etiology	Pathophysiology	Causes
Central	- Abnormal neurohypophyseal ADH secretion	- Idiopathic, trauma, surgery, ischemic lesions, infiltrative diseases
Nephrogenic	- Renal tubular ADH resistance	- Drugs (Lithium, Demeclocycline, Foscarnet, Amphotericin) - Hypercalcemia - Congenital (AQP-2 defects)

Clinical: Polyuria (> 3L/day), polydipsia, nocturia
- Note: Central DI can have impaired thirst mechanism, leading to higher Na^+

Diagnosis:
- High normal or elevated $[Na^+]$ is indicative of DI, but not always present
- Water restriction test (Patient water deprived, urine Osm measured)

	Water Deprivation Urine Osm (mOsm/kg)	+ Desmopressin Urine Osm (mOsm/kg)
Normal	> 800	No response
Central DI	< 300	> 300 mOsm/kg or > 50-100% increase in Uosm
Nephro DI	< 300	No or minimal response
Polydipsia	> 500	No response

Management:
- Nephrogenic DI: Sodium restriction, thiazide diuretics
- Central DI: Sodium restriction, thiazides, desmopressin

Polyuria DDx

Note: Polyuria is defined as > 3L of urine/day (different than urinary frequency seen with BPH, UTI, etc)

(1) Nephrogenic or Central DI
(2) Primary Polydipsia
(3) Solute Diuresis
- Glucose
- Sodium (ie after large volume expansion)
- Urea (azotemia)
(4) Diuretic Use
(5) Hypercalcemia

HYPERALDOSTERONISM

Endocrine Medicine

Primary Hyperaldosteronism

General: Elevated, unregulated, and inappropriate adrenal aldosterone production

Etiology:
- Adrenal hyperplasia (~66%)
- Adrenal adenoma (~33%) ("Conn's Syndrome")
- Adrenal carcinoma (~1%)

Clinical: Hypertension, hypokalemia, metabolic alkalosis, mild hypernatremia
- Euvolemic due to aldosterone escape

Diagnosis:
- Elevated aldosterone:renin ratio (> 20)
- If elevated, adrenal suppression test (see below)
    - Patient given sodium load via diet or saline infusion
    - Test is positive if urinary aldosterone is not suppressed after oral sodium load or saline infusion

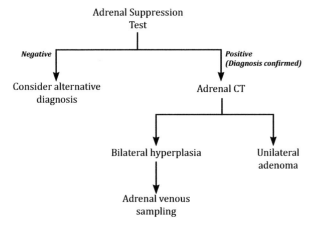

Note: Adrenal venous sampling can help to differentiate unilateral from bilateral disease, as the management differs as seen below

Management:
- Unilateral adenoma/hyperplasia: Adrenalectomy
- Bilateral hyperplasia: Medical therapy (Spironolactone or Eplerenone)

Secondary Hyperaldosteronism

General: Hyperreninemic hyperaldosteronism (ie elevated RAAS activity), typically due to limited renal perfusion

Etiology:
- Renal artery stenosis
- Edematous disorders (ie CHF, cirrhosis, nephrotic syndrome)
- Juxtaglomerular renin secreting tumor (very rare)

HYPERCORTISOLISM

Endocrine Medicine

Cushing's Disease and Syndrome

General: Hypercortisolism (Cushing's syndrome) results from elevated glucocorticoids

Etiology:
- Central pituitary tumor ACTH secretion ("Cushing Disease")
- Ectopic non-pituitary tumor ACTH production
- Iatrogenic (taking steroids)
- Adrenal production (adenoma or carcinoma)

Clinical:
- Changed appearance: Central obesity, hirsutism, moon facies, "buffalo hump," purple striae, acne, easy bruising
- Hypertension, hyperglycemia
- Menstrual irregularity or hypogonadism
- Proximal muscle weakness/wasting
- Depression, mania, or psychosis

Diagnosis:

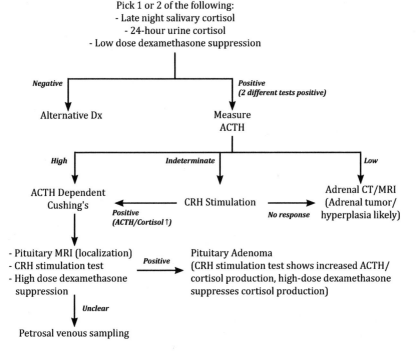

Management:
- Iatrogenic: Taper off steroids
- Pituitary adenoma: Transphenoidal resection
- Ectopic ACTH-secreting tumor: Surgical resection
- Medical therapy (if surgery fails or not an option) → Cabergoline
- Adrenal adenoma or hyperplasia: Unilateral or bilateral adrenalectomy
- Refractory disease (of any cause): Bilateral adrenalectomy

HYPOCORTISOLISM

Endocrine Medicine

Adrenal Insufficiency and Central Hypocortisolism

General: Hypocortisolism, plus hypoaldosteronism in primary disease

	Primary (adrenal)	Secondary/Tertiary (central)
Key Finding	Low cortisol + aldosterone	Low cortisol
ACTH	↑	↓
Na	Hyponatremia	Hyponatremia
K	Hyperkalemia	Normal
Other	- Hypotension - Hyperpigmentation	- Hypotension (less prominent)
Causes	- Autoimmune - TB - Metastatic disease - Hemorrhage or infarct	- Chronic steroids - Pituitary or hypothalamic disease

Clinical: Gradual onset of malaise, weakness, anorexia, orthostasis, GI symptoms
- Acute Adrenal Crisis
    - Seen in individual with subacute adrenal insufficiency, that undergoes stressor, triggering severe symptoms
    - Presents with shock, with nonspecific symptoms (nausea, vomit, abdominal pain, weakness)

Diagnosis:
(1) Basal (morning) Plasma ACTH/Cortisol
(2) 250 mcg ACTH (cosyntropin) Stimulation Test

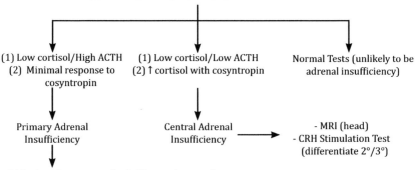

- 21-hydroxylase autoantibody (for autoimmune)
- CT Abdomen (look for hemorrhage/mets to adrenal)
- FNA (can establish infectious or malignancy diagnosis)

Management:
- Crisis: Fluids/ICU level support. Dexamethasone (not picked up on cortisol assay).
- Chronic:
    - Corticosteroids (Dexamethasone, Prednisone, or Hydrocortisone)
    - Fludrocortisone (in those with primary disease)
    - Increased steroids during minor illnesses or surgery

HYPOPITUITARISM

Endocrine Medicine

Hypopituitarism

General: Decreased secretion of pituitary hormones

Etiology:
- Masses (pituitary adenoma, craniopharyngioma, metastasis)
- Radiation, surgery, infiltrative diseases (ie sarcoid)
- Pituitary infarction (Sheehan) or hemorrhage

Clinical: Presents as a combination of each hormone deficiency
- Cortisol: Fatigue, anorexia, weight loss, etc
- Thyroid: All typical symptoms of hypothyroidism
- FSH/LH:
    - Premenopausal female: Amenorrhea, infertility, hot flashes
    - Postmenopausal female: Asymptomatic
    - Male: Decreased energy, libido, erectile dysfunction
- GH: ↓ lean mass, ↑ fat mass
- Prolactin: Asymptomatic, unless after birth (failure to lactate)

	Diagnosis	Management
ACTH	- Morning cortisol	- Glucocorticoids
TSH	- Free T4 levels (better than TSH, which can be variable)	- Levothyroxine
LH/FSH	- Male: Testosterone (↓), LH (↔) - Female: Estradiol (↓), FSH (↔)	- Testosterone (male) - Estrogen/progestin (female)
GH	- Serum IGF-1 - Hypoglycemia/arginine stim test	- GH not typically recommended

Specific Etiologies of Hypopituitarism

Sheehan Syndrome:
- Infarction of the pituitary after childbirth, due to severe postpartum hemorrhage
- Clinical presentation ranges from severe hypopituitarism, to subacute disease that presents as failure to lactate or failure for menses to return

Pituitary Apoplexy:
- Sudden hemorrhage into the pituitary, most often into an adenoma
- Presents as sudden onset headache, double vision, and hypopituitarism

PITUITARY ADENOMA/PROLACTINEMIA

Endocrine Medicine

Pituitary Adenoma

General: Benign tumor of the anterior pituitary
- Macroadenoma (> 10 mm) and microadenoma (< 10 mm)

Etiology: Generally idiopathic, but can be seen associated with MEN1. Subtypes below.

Lactotroph	- Usually cause hyperprolactinemia
Corticotroph	- Usually cause Cushing's
Somatotroph	- Usually cause acromegaly
Gonadotroph	- Generally non-functioning
Thyrotroph	- Generally non-functioning - Rarely produce TSH, leading to hyperthyroidism

Clinical:
- Mass Effect: Headache and Bitemporal Hemianopsia
- Effects from hormone production

Diagnosis: Pituitary MRI

Treatment: See each following section for specifics. Prolactinomas generally treated medically, while others treated surgically.

Prolactinemia

General: High prolactin levels

Etiology:
- Prolactinoma
- Drug (antipsychotics, SSRI)
- ↓ Dopamine inhibition (from mass effect or hypothalamic/stalk lesion)

Clinical:
- Male: Decreased energy, libido, erectile dysfunction, gynecomastia
- Premenopausal Female: Menstrual dysfunction, infertility, hot flashes
- Postmenopausal: Asymptomatic, unless tumor has compressive symptoms

Diagnosis:
- Serum prolactin level (5-20 is normal, > 200 is indicative of adenoma)
- MRI

Management:
- Asymptomatic Microprolactinoma: No treatment
- Symptomatic Microprolactinoma: Cabergoline
- Macroprolactinoma:
    - Cabergoline
    - Consider surgical resection if refractory/tumor growing

GROWTH HORMONE

Endocrine Medicine

Acromegaly

General: Clinical syndrome from excess growth hormone secretion

Etiology: GH secreting adenoma

Clinical: Insidious (ie > 10 year) onset of tissue overgrowth
- Macrognathia, coarse facies, spaced out teeth
- Thickened skin
- Visceral enlargement: LVH, OSA
- Increased colon cancer risk
- Adenoma compressive symptoms (headache, bitemporal hemianopsia)

Diagnosis:

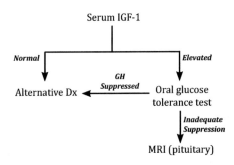

Management:
- Operable: Transsphenoidal resection
- Non-operable or refractory: Pharmacologic treatment
    - Octreotide (somatostatin analog) +/- Cabergoline
    - Pegvisomant (GH blocker) for refractory disease

Gigantism

General: GH excess that occurs during period of linear growth

Etiology: GH Adenoma (often associated with genetic syndromes like McCune-Albright or MEN-1)

Clinical:
- Rapid linear growth, +/- obesity
- Large hands/feet, coarse facies

Diagnosis: Serum IGF-1, with GH suppression test (oral glucose tolerance) for definitive diagnosis. Brain MRI to identify etiology.

Management:
- Transsphenoidal resection
- Radiation/Octreotide if refractory

CALCIUM HOMEOSTASIS

Endocrine Medicine

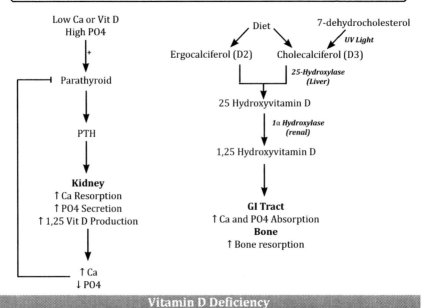

Vitamin D Deficiency

General: Vitamin D deficiency is generally asymptomatic, but can place patients at risk for falls, osteoporosis, and fractures

Etiology:
- Decreased intake or absorption (malabsorption, gastric bypass, dietary)
- Reduced sun exposure (winter time, certain areas of world)
- Defective hydroxylation (renal failure, cirrhosis, hypoparathyroidism)

Clinical: Generally asymptomatic, but can lead to osteomalacia (adults) or rickets (kids) if severe. Hypocalcemia and/or hypophosphatemia if moderate.

Osteomalacia	- Bone pain, muscle weakness, "waddling" gait, fractures - Classic radiology findings: Looser pseudofractures, fissures
Rickets	- Abnormal development of growth plates and bones - Presents with parietal and frontal bossing - Enlargement of the costochondral junction ("rachitic rosary") - Lateral bowing of the femur and tibia (bow legs)

Diagnosis: 25-hydroxyvitamin D level measurement (20 to 50 ng/mL normal)

Management:

Vitamin D	- Vitamin D3 (Cholecalciferol) is preferred - If mildly low (10-20 ng/mL): 600-800 IU/day - If very low (< 10 ng/nL): 50K IU weekly for 8 weeks, then 800 IU/day
Calcium	- 1000-1200 mg of calcium daily (between diet and any supplements)

HYPOPARATHYROIDISM

Endocrine Medicine

Hypoparathyroidism

General: Abnormal PTH secretion due to glandular destruction or abnormal PTH production

Etiology:
- Iatrogenic (surgical parathyroid removal)
- Autoimmune glandular destruction
- Infiltrative disease, radiation
- Genetic disorders

Clinical:
- Ranges from asymptomatic severely symptomatic from hypocalcemia

Diagnosis:
- Hypocalcemia PLUS Inappropriately Low/Normal PTH

Management:
Acute: Often post-thyroidectomy
- IV Calcium (when symptomatic or Ca < 7.5)
- Otherwise oral calcitriol/vitamin D sufficient

Chronic: Calcitriol and Vitamin D
- Recombinant PTH for those with refractory hypocalcemia

Pseudohypoparathyroidism (Type 1A)

General: AD genetic resistance to PTH due to inability to make cAMP when PTH binds its receptor (GNAS mutation). Defect inherited from mother.

Clinical:
- Hypocalcemia and hyperphosphatemia
- "Albright Hereditary Osteodystrophy": Round face, short stature, short fourth metacarpal, developmental delays, obesity

Pseudopseudohypoparathyroidism
- If abnormal GNAS is inherited from father, the child will have the physical abnormalities of Albright's above, but with normal calcium homeostasis.

HYPERPARATHYROIDISM

Endocrine
Medicine, Surgery

Etiology	Ca	PO4	PTH	Cause
Primary	↑	↓	↑	- Parathyroid adenoma (most common) - Parathyroid hyperplasia (~15%) - Parathyroid carcinoma (rare)
Secondary	↓	↑	↑	- CKD - Vitamin D deficiency - Calcium malabsorption or renal loss
Tertiary	↑	nl/↑	↑	- Dramatically ↑ PTH secretion, due to parathyroid dysregulation - Rare: Seen in patients with long-term CKD

Clinical:
- Asymptomatic hypercalcemia is most common
- If severe: "Stones, bones, groans, psych overtones" [See: Renal]

Diagnosis:
- Hypercalcemia with PTH inappropriately normal or elevated
- 24-Hour Urine Calcium
    - Differentiates 1° HPT from familial hypocalciuric hypercalcemia
    - Can predict potential renal damage from hypercalciuria
- Localization (only if surgery is to be performed)
    - Sestamibi scintigraphy (MIBI-SPECT), ultrasound, or CT

Management:

Primary	**Surgery:**
	- Indications: Age < 50, osteoporosis, CKD, very high calcium, or severely symptomatic
	
	- Procedure
	  - Adenoma: Resect single lesion
	  - Hyperplasia: Remove 3.5 glands, or all 4 and implant 0.5 of a gland in the arm
	
	Pharm: Bisphosphonates or cinacalcet
	  - Indicated if not a surgical candidate, but symptomatic or have side effect like osteoporosis
	  - Observe asymptomatic hypercalcemia in those that surgery is not indicated

Secondary	- Manage underlying renal disease - Correct vitamin D deficiency and hyperphosphatemia if present
Tertiary	- Cinacalcet - Surgery for refractory cases

MALE REPRODUCTIVE ENDOCRINE

Endocrine Medicine

Hypogonadism

General: Decreased sperm and testosterone production by the testes

	Findings	Etiology
Primary	↑ LH/FSH ↓↓ Testosterone/Sperm	- Radiation/Chemotherapy - Infection - Trauma - Varicocele - Klinefelter
Secondary	↓/↔ LH/FSH ↓ Testosterone/Sperm	- Pituitary (tumors, apoplexy, infiltrative disease, etc) - Hyperprolactinemia - Kallmann syndrome

Clinical:
- Decreased libido, energy, muscle mass, body hair
- Gynecomastia (usually seen in just primary)
- Infertility

Diagnosis:
- Morning (8-10am) serum total testosterone
    - Consider free testosterone levels if concern about SHBG
- If abnormal, obtain LH, FSH, semen analysis (if worried about fertility)
- Further workup to determine etiology (ie karyotype if primary, prolactin and brain MRI if secondary)

Management:
- Treat underlying condition
- Testosterone replacement
    - Transdermal gels/patch preferred method
    - Oral preparations associated with liver disease

Androgen Abuse

"Positive" Effects	Adverse Effects
- ↑ fat free mass/muscle strength	- ↓ Testicular function (atrophy) - Aggression/behavioral changes - Gynecomastia - Erythrocytosis (↑ HCT) - Hepatotoxicity (17α alk. androgens) - Virilization (women), acne, baldness - ↑ Clotting - ↓ HDL

Synthetic Androgens: Stanozolol, Nandrolone, Methandienone, Trenbolone, Boldenone

Androgen Precursors: Androstenedione, DHEA

Other performance enhancing drugs: GH, hCG (stimulates testes to produce T like LH), erythropoietin

MALE REPRODUCTIVE ENDOCRINE

Erectile Dysfunction

General: Inability to acquire or sustain a sufficiently rigid and durable erection for sexual intercourse

Risk: ↑ Age, obesity, smoking, comorbid/chronic medical problems. Also associated with atherosclerotic disease, previous pelvic disease/surgery, hypogonadism, drugs (antidepressants, beta blockers)

Etiology:
- Psychologic: Depression, stress. Note: If nighttime erections still occur, highly likely that ED is due to psychological factors.
- Medical ("Organic")
    - Endocrine: Hypogonadism
    - Neurologic: Perineal trauma, prostate surgery, etc
    - Cardiovascular: Atherosclerosis

Management:
- Identify/treat risk factors (ie testosterone for hypogonadism, lifestyle modifications for vascular disease, removal of possible drug causes)
- Pharm
    - PDE5 inhibitors (Sildenafil, Tadalafil, etc)
        - Contraindicated with nitrates
    - Second line: Alprostadil (intracavernosal), vacuum device
    - Penile implants if all else fails

ADRENAL NEOPLASIA

Endocrine Medicine

Adrenal Incidentaloma

General: Adrenal mass lesion > 1 cm found on CT or MRI imaging

Etiology: Benign adenoma (+/- functional hormone production), adrenal carcinoma, pheochromocytoma

Diagnosis:

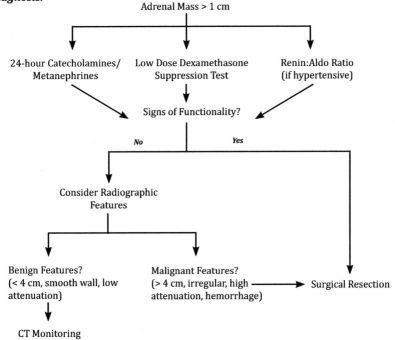

Management:
- Surgically Resect: Functional tumors, malignant appearing tumors, > 4 cm benign tumors (if the patient is a good surgical candidate)
- Serial CT/MRI monitoring for those with nonsurgical tumors
    - Consider surgery for those that grow by > 1 cm at follow-up

Adrenal Carcinoma

General: Rare, highly malignant neoplasm of the adrenal cortex. Poor prognosis.

Clinical: Generally found incidentally (see above)
- Associated with secretion of a variety of hormones, resulting in Cushing's, hyperaldosteronism, or androgen production (virilization)

Management: Surgical resection, followed by hormone therapy (Mitotane)

ADRENAL NEOPLASIA

Endocrine Medicine

Pheochromocytoma

General: Catecholamine-secreting tumors that arise from chromaffin cells of the adrenal medulla and the sympathetic ganglia. "Rule of 10's":
- ~10% are bilateral or malignant
- ~10% in children
- ~10% extra-adrenal

Etiology:
- Majority are sporadic
- Genetic conditions (MEN2, vHL, NF-1)

Clinical:
- Classic triad: Episodic headache, sweating, and tachycardia
- Most common: Sustained/paroxysmal hypertension
- Symptoms can be triggered by surgery (ie anesthesia) or some drugs

Diagnosis:
- 24-hour urinary fractionated catecholamines and metanephrines
  - Alternative: Use plasma fractionated metanephrines
- CT/MRI to localize the tumor

Management:
- Surgical Resection (laparoscopic adrenalectomy)
  - Preoperative: Alpha-blockade (Phenoxybenzamine) followed by beta-blockade (Propranolol)

PANCREATIC NEUROENDOCRINE TUMOR

Endocrine Medicine

Tumor	General/Clinical	Diagnosis	Management

Gastrinoma (Zollinger-Ellison)	- Excess gastrin secretion → Excess gastric acid secretion
	- Presents as chronic diarrhea, reflux, abdominal pain
	- Peptic ulcers (can be distal to duodenum, refractory to PPI therapy)
		- Suspect in: Multiple/refractory ulcers, enlarged gastric folds on endoscopy
		- Serum fasting gastrin level (off PPI)
		  > 1000 → Gastrinoma (diagnostic)
		  100-1000 → Elevated (but nonspecific)
		- Secretin Stimulation Test (secretin ↑↑ gastrin levels in gastrinoma cells)
		- Localization: CT, MRI
			- High Dose PPI
			- Resection

Insulinoma	- Islet-cell tumor that secretes insulin - Presents as fasting hypoglycemia, with neuroglycopenic/hypoglycemic symptoms	- High insulin during period of induced hypoglycemia (72 hour fast) - Localization: CT, MRI	- Surgical Resection - Diazoxide (↓ insulin secretion in those with refractory disease or not undergoing surgery)

Glucagonoma	- Secretes glucagon
	- Presents with GI symptoms (diarrhea, weight loss), glucose intolerance
	- Venous thrombosis, neuropsychiatric disturbance
	- Necrolytic Migratory Erythema: Erythematous plaques on face, perineum, extremities. Eventually develop central clearing/blistering, with surrounding scaling.
		- Elevated fasting plasma glucagon level (> 500 pg/mL)
		- Localization: CT, MRI
			- Pharm:
			  - Octreotide
			  - Insulin (if glucose ↑)
			  - Nutritional support
			- Surgical resection (if local), but most are metastatic (require chemoradiation)

PANCREATIC NEUROENDOCRINE TUMOR

Endocrine Medicine

	General/Clinical	Diagnosis	Management
VIPoma	- Neuroendocrine tumor secreting VIP - Presents as: Watery diarrhea (secretory, confirmed by low osmotic gap) - Hypochlorhydria (↓ gastric acid secretion) - Flushing, nausea/vomit, lethargy, weakness - Electrolyte abnormalities (hypokalemia, hypercalcemia, hyperglycemia)	- VIP > 75 pg/mL - Localization: CT, MRI	- Fluid replacement - Octreotide - Surgical resection
Somatostatinoma	- D-cell tumor secreting somatostatin - Presents as: Cholelithiasis (↓ CCK), glucose intolerance (↓ insulin), steatorrhea (↓ pancreatic enzymes)	- Somatostatin > 30 pg/mL - Localization: CT, MRI	- Surgical resection - Octreotide (for unresectable)

Multiple Endocrine Neoplasia

Patients with diagnosed MEN or with known family history should receive screening for malignancy as below.

MEN1 (AD MEN1 mutation)
- Screen using Ca, PTH, prolactin
- Imaging (controversial, but US, CT, MRI can be used)

MEN2a/2b (AD RET mutations)
- Screen for cancer using plasma metanephrines, serum calcium, calcitonin, thyroid US
- Note: 2b: Generally have associated gastrointestinal issues (chronic constipation/megacolon)

	MEN1	MEN2A	MEN2B
Pituitary (adenomas)	+		
Pancreatic (neuroendocrine tumor)	+		
Parathyroid (adenoma)	+	+	
Thyroid (medullary cancer)		+	+
Pheochromocytoma		+	+
Mucosal/Intestinal Neuroma			+
Marfanoid Habitus			+

HYPOGLYCEMIA

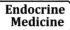
Endocrine Medicine

General: Abnormally low plasma glucose concentration, generally < 70 mg/dL OR based on Whipple's Triad (symptoms of hypoglycemia, low blood sugar, and resolution of symptoms with normalization of glucose)

Etiology:
- Vast majority of cases occur in diabetics using insulin or secretagogue
- Critical illness
- Hormone deficiency (hypocortisolism)
- Endogenous hyperinsulinemia (see differential table below)

Clinical:
- Neuroglycopenic symptoms: Cognitive impairment, psychomotor abnormalities, seizure, coma
- Autonomic symptoms: Tremor, palpitations, diaphoresis, increased anxiety

Diagnosis: Workup for a non-diabetic, healthy individual with hypoglycemia:
- Check glucose, insulin, C-peptide, proinsulin, and oral hypoglycemic agent screen. Must check during period of symptomatic hypoglycemia, either:
  - Spontaneous or
  - Induced (Short fast, mixed-meal, or 72-hour fast)

Etiology	Pathophys	Diagnostic Findings
Insulin	- Iatrogenic insulin therapy	↑ Insulin ↓ Proinsulin, C-pep
Insulin Secretagogue	- Sulfonylurea drugs, which stimulate endogenous insulin production	↑ Insulin, C-pep, proinsulin + secretagogue screen
Insulinoma	- Insulin producing malignancy	↑ Insulin, C-pep, proinsulin
Autoimmune Hypoglycemia	- Antibodies directed to endogenous insulin or to the insulin receptor	↑ Insulin, C-pep, proinsulin + Insulin Autoantibodies
NIPHS*	- Endogenous hyperinsulinemia due to islet hypertrophy and nesidioblastosis - Often postprandial (2-4 hours) - Similar pathophysiology also seen after gastric bypass surgery	↑ Insulin, C-pep, proinsulin
Non-islet Cell Tumor	- Increased insulin-like growth factor-2 (IGF-2) production	- C-pep, insulin, and proinsulin normal

* Noninsulinoma pancreatogenous hypoglycemia syndrome

DIABETES MELLITUS

Endocrine Medicine

Etiology and Clinical Features of Diabetes Mellitus

	Type 1	Type 2
Path	- Autoimmune B-cell destruction	- Insulin resistance
Inherit	- Multifactorial (increased risk, but still < 10% incidence in child of a type I diabetic)	- Multifactorial (2-3x increased risk if history in first degree relative)
Risk	- N/A	- Obesity, sedentary lifestyle, smoking, non-white
Insulin	- Low or absent	- Can be normal/elevated, especially early on - Eventual loss of insulin production
Onset	- Childhood (4-14 y/o)	- Generally adult
Clinical	- Polyuria, polydipsia, weight loss - Often presents in DKA	- Asymptomatic (picked up on screening) - Can develop polyuria/polydipsia

Diagnosis: One of the following sufficient:
- Fasting plasma glucose ≥ 126 mg/dL
- Plasma glucose ≥ 200 mg/dL, 2 hours post oral glucose tolerance test
- Symptoms of hyperglycemia with glucose ≥ 200 mg/dL
- Hemoglobin A1C ≥ 6.5% (typically used for Type II DM)

Other Causes of Diabetes

MODY (Mature onset diabetes of the young)
- Non-insulin dependent diabetes from AD mutation in one of the following:
  - Glucokinase (increased glucose required for insulin secretion)
  - Hepatic nuclear factor 1-alpha (low insulin secretion)
  - Presents in 20's

Destruction of Pancreatic Tissue
- Chronic pancreatitis
- Cystic fibrosis
- Hemochromatosis

Endocrinopathies
- Cushing's syndrome or exogenous glucocorticoids

DIABETES MELLITUS

Endocrine Medicine

Glycemic Control in Diabetes Mellitus Type I

Glucose Control (Goal A1C < 7):

Multiple Daily Injection	- Once/twice injected long acting insulin plus pre-meal short acting bolus - Multiple different combinations available, but common one is evening long acting Detemir/Glargine, with premeal Lispro/Aspart/Glulisine
Insulin Pump	- Continuous infusion of short-acting insulin, with pre-meal bolus

*Multiple daily glucose checks (either multiple sticks, or continuous monitoring)

Glycemic Control in Diabetes Mellitus Type II

Glycemic Control
- Goal A1C < 7 in average adult
- Goal A1C < 8 in higher risk adults (older, high risk for hypoglycemia)

Initial Therapy	- Aggressive lifestyle modifications - Metformin (started concurrently in most) - If severe hyperglycemia (ie A1C > 9.5%), consider starting insulin
Failure of One Agent	- Add additional oral agent (any can be chosen from any class, weighing pros and cons; glitazone, sulfonylurea, GLP-1, DPP-4, SGLT-2)

Failure of Two Agent	- Add additional oral agent OR
	- Consider starting insulin
	  - Start with basal insulin (ie Glargine/Detemir/Degludec)
	  - Add premeal rapid acting if fails on basal alone

- Bariatric surgery in BMI ≥ 40 or BMI 35 to 39.9 when hyperglycemia is inadequately controlled with therapy

Inpatient Management of Blood Sugar

Goal: Preprandial blood sugars < 140, with all glucose checks ideally < 180

Therapy:
- If on home oral meds, can continue if patient is overall well (eating, no contraindications to home med, not critically ill)
- All others → Insulin
  - Basal insulin (Detemir or Glargine) PLUS
  - Prandial insulin (rapid acting Lispro/Aspart/Glulisine with meals)
  - Correctional insulin (based on a graded scale)

DIABETES MELLITUS

Endocrine Medicine

Complication	Clinical	Management	Screening
Macrovascular			
Accelerated Atherosclerosis	- CAD (MCC death) - PAD - CVA	- ASA/Statin	- Initial lipid screen at time of diagnosis
Microvascular			
Nephropathy	- Efferent arterial glycosylation leads to glomerular hyperfiltration, with eventual GBM and mesangial disease, resulting in albuminuria - Long-term damage can lead to glomerulosclerosis and nephrotic syndrome	- ACE/ARB - BP control < 130/80	- Annual urine albumin:Cr

Peripheral Neuropathy	- Peripheral symmetric distal "stocking-glove" sensory neuropathy
	  - Large Fiber: Proprioception/pressure
	  - Small Fiber: Pain, paresthesia
	- CN III Palsy (eye pain, diplopia, ptosis)
		- If painful: Amitriptyline, Venlafaxine, Duloxetine, or Pregabalin	- Annual physical exam, sensory testing

Autonomic Neuropathy	- GU: Neurogenic bladder, erectile dysfunction - GI: Gastroparesis - CV: Postural hypotension, tachycardia, silent ischemia	- Bladder: Urination schedule, or intermittent catheterization - ED: PDE-5 inhibitor - Gastroparesis: If severe, give Metochlopromide or Erythromycin	
Retinopathy	- Generally nonproliferative, but can progress to proliferative - Hemorrhages, exudates, microaneurysms, venous dilatation	- Photocoagulation for proliferative disease	- Annual slit-lamp exam
Foot	- Wounds (lack of sensation predisposes to injury)	- Frequent self-foot checks	- Annual podiatric check
Infection	- ↑ infection risk/wound healing		

Endo26

DIABETES MELLITUS

Endocrine Medicine

Diabetic Ketoacidosis/Hyperosmolar Hyperglycemic State

General: Diabetic states in which insulin deficiency leads to severe hyperglycemia, ketogenesis, and electrolyte/fluid abnormalities. Both states are generally triggered by a precipitating factor (ie infection) and/or inadequate insulin therapy. HHS and DKA are on a spectrum.

Criteria	DKA	HHS
Glucose	> 250 mg/dL	> 600 mg/dL, and often > 1000
pH	< 7.30, and near 7.0 if severe	> 7.30
HCO3	< 18 mEq/L	> 18 mEq/L
Ketones	Present in urine and serum	Negative or mild
AG	> 10-12	Normal
Serum Osm	Variable	> 320 mOsm/kg
Pathophys	- More common type I DM - Insulin deficiency and glucagon excess, leading to hyperglycemia, and production of ketoacids	- More common type II DM - Insulin deficiency and glucagon excess, leading to hyperglycemia, osmotic diuresis, and extreme hyperosmolarity - Insulin present in sufficient amounts to prevent ketone production
Clinical	- Rapid onset of polyuria/polydipsia, abdominal pain, nausea/vomiting - Kussmaul respiration - "Fruity" breath (acetone)	- Gradual onset of polyuria/polydipsia and weight loss - Neurologic symptoms (lethargy, mental obtundation, coma) as state progresses (usually Osm > 320)

Management:

Fluids	- Normal Saline @~1 L/hr initially, transition to ½ NS once volume status improves - Add 5% glucose once glucose < 200-250
Insulin	- Initial: IV Insulin (bolus plus continuous drip) - Once glucose < 200 mg/dL, can switch to SQ insulin or lower dose drip
Potassium	- Give IV KCl if ≤ 5.3 mEq/L (and hold insulin if K < 3.3) (Most patients have severe K depletion from renal loss, but current dehydration/insulin deficiency/acidosis has K shifted extracellularly)
Other lytes	- Monitor and replace Mg, Ca - Replace PO4 if < 1 mg/dL or signs of cardiac dysfunction
HCO_3	- Generally not given, unless pH < 6.9
Monitoring	- Monitor q2-4 hour chemistries, β-hydroxybutyrate until stable

Crisis Resolved When:
- DKA: Gap closes, β-hydroxybutyrate normalizes, patient can eat
- HHS: Osm drops < 315, mentation normalizes

PEDIATRIC THYROID DISEASE

Endocrine Pediatrics

Congenital Neck Mass DDx

Thyroglossal Duct Cyst	- Cystic expansion of remnant of thyroglossal duct tract - Anterior midline neck mass that moves with swallowing or protrusion of the tongue. Often asymptomatic. - Can become tender if infected/inflamed - Dx: US or CT - Tx: Antibiotics (if infected), followed by surgical excision
Branchial Cleft Cyst	- Failure of obliteration of one of the branchial clefts in embryonic development (most commonly 2nd) - Presents as lateral neck mass, usually anterior to the sternocleidomastoid muscle, no movement with swallowing - Dx: US or CT - Tx: Can treated conservatively or surgically excise

Congenital Hypothyroidism

Etiology:
- Thyroid dysgenesis (most common)
- Defective thyroid hormone synthesis, transport, or ↓ TSH-R sensitivity
- Maternal iodine deficiency or excess iodine exposure

Clinical:
- Usually asymptomatic at birth (maternal T4 crosses over)
- If not picked up with neonatal screens, over the first few months of life:
    - Lethargy, hypotonia
    - Hypothermia, jaundice
    - Poor feeding, constipation
    - Puffy/coarse facies, macroglossia
    - Umbilical hernia, large fontanelles
    - Risk for mental retardation, severe bone/growth delay

Diagnosis: TSH/T4

Management: Levothyroxine (10 mcg/kg then titrate)

Neonatal Thyrotoxicosis

General: Transplacental passage of TSH-R IgG (from maternal Graves disease), causing excessive release of T4 in the neonate

Clinical:
- Low birth weight, preterm birth, microcephaly
- Warm moist skin, tachycardia
- Poor feeding, irritability, failure to thrive

Diagnosis: ↑ TSH-R IgG in mother

Management:
- Resolves months after birth
- Methimazole, beta-blocker (ie Propranolol)

PEDIATRIC REPRODUCTIVE ENDOCRINE

Endocrine Pediatrics

Precocious Puberty

General: Onset of puberty at age > 2 SD lower than normal onset (Boys ≤ 9, Girls ≤ 8)

Subtype	Definition	Examples
Central	- Early maturation of the hypothalamic-pituitary-gonadal axis	- Idiopathic (constitutional, 90% of cases in girls, ~60% of cases in boys) - CNS lesions (hamartomas, tumors, etc)
Peripheral	- Sex hormone secretion/exposure (GnRH independent)	- Ovarian cysts/tumors - Leydig tumor - β-HCG secreting mass - Exogenous sex steroids - Congenital adrenal hyperplasia - Adrenal tumor - McCune Albright
Benign Variants	- Premature isolated thelarche, pubarche, adrenarche - Note: These are isolated findings and do not require intervention	

Clinical:
- Signs of estrogen excess: Breast development and possibly vaginal bleeding
- Signs of androgen excess: Pubic and/or axillary hair, enlarged clitoris, acne

Diagnosis:
- Basal LH (most important, see algorithm below), FSH, E2/T
- Bone Age
    - Within normal limits in benign variants
    - Advanced with central and peripheral etiologies
- Workup (once precocious puberty diagnosed)
    - Pelvic or testicular US
    - Head MRI (especially in boys)

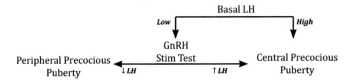

Management:
- Central: GnRH agonists (ie Leuprolide)
- Peripheral: Remove underlying cause
    - Surgically excise tumors
    - Remove exogenous sex steroids
    - CAH: Treat with glucocorticoids

Endo29

PEDIATRIC REPRODUCTIVE ENDOCRINE

Endocrine Pediatrics

Delayed Puberty

General: Puberty delayed past normal range (Boys: No testicular enlargement by age 14. Girls: Absence of breast development by age 12)

Etiology:

Primary Hypogonadism	- Lack of gonadal sex hormone production (LH/FSH ↑, T/E2 ↓) - Causes include Turner's, Klinefelter's, Gonadal injury
Secondary Hypogonadism	- Due to failure of GnRH release (causes seen below) - LH/FSH ↓, T/E2 ↓
Constitutional Delay of Puberty	- Most common cause of delayed puberty - Transient, idiopathic delay in GnRH release
GnRH Deficiency	- Occurs with Kallmann syndrome
Others	- Excess exercise or poor nutrition - Chronic illnesses (ie IBD, hypothyroidism, etc)

Diagnosis:
- LH, FSH, E2, T levels (help to determine primary vs secondary hypogonad)
- Workup for underlying cause (ie TSH, prolactin, imaging)

Management:
- Treat underlying cause if present
- Constitutional Delay
    - Observation
    - Can consider short term hormonal (E2 or T) therapy

PEDIATRIC ADRENAL DISEASE

Endocrine Pediatrics

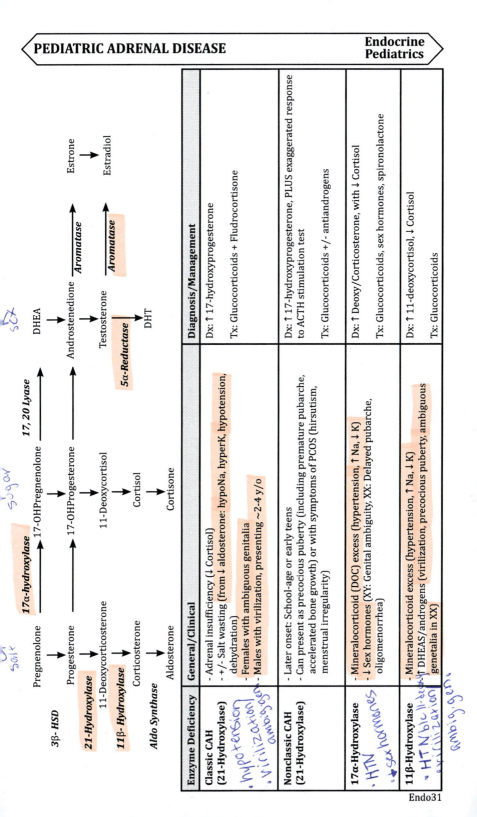

Enzyme Deficiency	General/Clinical	Diagnosis/Management
Classic CAH (21-Hydroxylase)	- Adrenal insufficiency (↓ Cortisol) - +/- Salt wasting (from ↓ aldosterone: hypoNa, hyperK, hypotension, dehydration) - Females with ambiguous genitalia - Males with virilization, presenting ~2-4 y/o	Dx: ↑ 17-hydroxyprogesterone Tx: Glucocorticoids + Fludrocortisone
Nonclassic CAH (21-Hydroxylase)	- Later onset: School-age or early teens - Can present as precocious puberty (including premature pubarche, accelerated bone growth) or with symptoms of PCOS (hirsutism, menstrual irregularity)	Dx: ↑ 17-hydroxyprogesterone, PLUS exaggerated response to ACTH stimulation test Tx: Glucocorticoids +/- antiandrogens
17α-Hydroxylase	- Mineralocorticoid (DOC) excess (hypertension, ↑ Na, ↓ K) - ↓ Sex hormones (XY: Genital ambiguity, XX: Delayed pubarche, oligomenorrhea)	Dx: ↑ Deoxy/Corticosterone, with ↓ Cortisol Tx: Glucocorticoids, sex hormones, spironolactone
11β-Hydroxylase	- Mineralocorticoid excess (hypertension, ↑ Na, ↓ K) - ↑ DHEAS/androgens (virilization, precocious puberty, ambiguous genitalia in XX)	Dx: ↑ 11-deoxycortisol, ↓ Cortisol Tx: Glucocorticoids

| MISC ENDOCRINE | Endocrine Pediatrics |

Neuroblastoma

General: Tumor that arises from primitive sympathetic ganglion cells, most commonly adrenal or paravertebral. Most common neoplasm in infants; more than half of patients present before age 2.

Clinical:
- Often asymptomatic
- Abdominal mass +/- pain, constipation
- Bone pain, periorbital ecchymosis ("raccoon eyes")
- Horner's syndrome, back pain
- Paraneoplastic syndromes
    - Opsoclonus-Myoclonus: Rapid, dancing eye movements, rhythmic jerking (myoclonus) involving limbs or trunk, and/or ataxia

Diagnosis:
- Imaging (ie US) to confirm mass
- Urine/serum catecholamines (↑ VMA/HVA)
- Biopsy (small basophilic cells in rosettes)

Management:
- Surgical resection
- +/- Chemoradiation, immunotherapy, others (depending on how high-risk)
- Prognosis: Highly varied, depends on histology, genetic factors (ie NMyc)

Adrenoleukodystrophy

General: Peroxisome disorder resulting in long chain fatty acid accumulation in the body (XR-ABCD1 gene)

Clinical:
- Neurologic deficits: Intellectual disability/behavioral abnormalities, followed by development of quadriplegia, blindness, and other CNS defects
- Sexual dysfunction
- Adrenal insufficiency

Diagnosis:
- Elevated VLCFA levels
- Brain MRI (showing areas of demyelination)
- Genetic analysis

Management:
- HCT
- Glucocorticoid replacement

GROWTH/SHORT-STATURE

Endocrine Pediatrics

Definitions of Short Stature

General: Short stature is anyone < 2 SD below the mean height (< 3rd percentile)
- Normal Variant: < 2 SD, but normal linear growth curve
- Pathologic: < 2 SD, growing with abnormal growth velocity (ie < 2 inch/yr)

Mid-Parental Height
- Can be used to help reassure those with normal variant short stature
- Child should fall +/- 4 inches of the following calculations
- Female MPH= 0.5 x [(Father's Height - 5 inch) + Mother's Height]
- Male MPH= 0.5 x [(Mother's Height + 5 inch) + Father's Height]

Differential of Short Stature

Type	Findings
Normal Variant (see definition above)	
Familial (Genetic)	- Normal bone age/onset of puberty
Constitutional	- Delayed bone age/onset of puberty
Pathologic (see definition above)	
Proportionate	- Normal upper to lower body segment ratio DDx: - Endocrine (hypothyroidism, GH deficiency, Cushing's) - Genetic (Turner's, Prader-Willi, etc) - Systemic (ie malnutrition, glucocorticoids, severe cardiac/pulmonary/renal disease, etc)
Disproportionate	- Abnormal upper to lower body segment ratio - DDx includes Rickets, skeletal dysplasia (ie osteogenesis imperfecta, achondroplasia, SHOX mutations)

Common Causes of Dwarfism

Achondroplasia	- Sporadic AD mutation in FGFR3 (Failure of longitudinal bone growth/endochondral ossification) - Clinical: Short limbs relative to body, trident hands, large head with frontal bossing, rhizomelia, genu varum - Cervical spinal compression serious potential complication - Mental function, life span, fertility not affected
Laron Dwarfism	- Defective GH receptor (decreased linear growth, increased GH, decreased IGF-1) - Clinical: Short height, small head, characteristic facies with saddle nose and prominent forehead, delayed skeletal maturation, small genitalia - Increased insulin sensitivity (resistant to diabetes and cancer) - Tx: IGF-1

ENDOCRINE PHARM

Endocrine Medicine

		Mechanism	Indication	Side Effects/Management
Insulin	*Rapid Insulin* Lispro Aspart Glulisine	- 1 hour peak action	- Diabetes Mellitus	- Hypoglycemia - Injection site reactions (immediate or long term lipodystrophy) - Weight gain
	Short Insulin Regular	- 2-4 hour peak		
	Int. Insulin NPH	- 8 hour peak		
	Long Insulin Degludec Detemir Glargine	- 24 hour activity		
Oral Hypoglycemic Agents				
	Biguanides Metformin	- ↓ gluconeogenesis - ↑ glycolysis - ↓ peripheral glucose uptake	- Diabetes Mellitus (first line agent)	- GI Disturbances (diarrhea, nausea, vomiting) - Lactic acidosis (contraindicated in CKD) - Modest weight loss
	Sulfonylurea Glimepiride Glyburide Glipizide	- Stimulates insulin release from pancreatic β-cells	- Diabetes Mellitus	- Hypoglycemia - Weight gain - Old agents (ie chlorpropamide): SIADH
	Thiazolidinedione Pioglitazone Rosiglitazone	- Activator of PPAR (↓ insulin resistance)	- Diabetes Mellitus	- Edema (especially in HF) - Hepatotoxicity - Weight gain - Possible ↑ bladder cancer risk

ENDOCRINE PHARM

Endocrine Medicine

	Mechanism	Indication	Side Effects/Management
Oral Hypoglycemic Agents			
GLP-1 Agonists Dulaglutide Exenatide Liraglutide	- Agonists of the GLP-1 receptor (stimulate insulin release, ↓ glucagon release)	- Diabetes Mellitus	- GI upset - Injection site reactions - Weight loss
DPP-4 Inhibitor Linagliptin Saxagliptin Sitagliptin	- Inhibits DPP-4 enzyme that deactivates GLP-1	- Diabetes Mellitus	- Nasopharyngitis - Weight neutral
SGLT-2 Inhibitor Canagliflozin Empagliflozin	- Inhibit SGLT-2 channel in proximal tubule responsible for glucose resorption	- Diabetes Mellitus (possible benefit in patients with CV disease)	- Glycosuria, dehydration from osmotic diuresis - UTIs/Vaginal yeast infections
Meglitinide Nateglinide Repaglinide	- Stimulates insulin release from pancreatic β-cells (similar mechanism to sulfonylurea)	- Diabetes Mellitus	- Hypoglycemia - Weight gain
α-glucosidase inh. Acarbose Miglitol	- Inhibits intestinal brush border glucosidases, decreasing glucose uptake	- Diabetes Mellitus	- GI upset (flatulence and diarrhea)
Glucocorticoids			
Beclomethasone Dexamethasone Hydrocortisone Methylprednisolone Prednisone	- Inhibit production of cytokines associated with inflammation (via NF-KB)	- Adrenal insufficiency - Immunosuppression - Autoimmune conditions - Asthma/COPD	- Cushing-type symptoms (with long term use) - Adrenocortical atrophy - Peptic ulcers - Glucose intolerance - Steroid psychosis - Cataracts - Myopathy

ENDOCRINE PHARM

Endocrine Medicine

	Mechanism	Indication	Side Effects/Management
Fludrocortisone	- Aldosterone analog (without glucocorticoid effect)	- Mineralocorticoid replacement	- Sodium/water retention, edema, hypertension
Conivaptan Tolvaptan	- ADH V2 receptor antagonist	- SIADH	- Thirst, dry mouth - Hypotension
Demeclocycline	- ADH antagonist (TCA structure)		
Desmopressin	- ADH agonist	- Diabetes insipidus - Clotting disorders - Bed wetting	- Hyponatremia - Headache, facial flushing
Octreotide	- Somatostatin analog	- Carcinoid syndrome - Pancreatic neuroendocrine tumor - Cirrhosis (variceal bleeds, hepatorenal syndrome)	- Hypothyroidism (suppresses TSH) - Cholelithiasis - Increased insulin resistance
Cinacalcet	- CaSR receptor potentiator	- Hyperparathyroidism	- Hypocalcemia

Thionamides
Propylthiouracil
Methimazole
	- Inhibits thyroperoxidase
	- PTU also blocks 5-deiodinase
		- Hyperthyroidism
		- Pregnancy (PTU used in 1st trimester, methimazole in 2nd/3rd)
			- Rash, itching, hives
			- Aplastic anemia
			- Hepatotoxicity
			- ANCA+ Vasculitis
			Agranulocytosis
			- If fever + sore throat (within 90 days of starting):
			  - Stop drug immediately
			  - Check WBC (< 1 → Confirmed agranulocytosis)

Levothyroxine	Thyroid hormone replacement	- Hypothyroidism	- Hyperthyroid symptoms if dose too high

ESOPHAGEAL DISEASE
Gastrointestinal Medicine, Surgery

Gastroesophageal Reflux Disease (GERD)

General: Retrograde flow of gastric contents from decreased lower esophageal tone or anatomic disruption of GE junction

Risk:
- Smoking, obesity
- Dietary: Certain food (chocolate, peppermint, fat), coffee/caffeine, alcohol
- Structural abnormalities (hiatal hernia)

Clinical:
- Classic symptoms are heartburn, regurgitation, dyspepsia
- Others: Chest pain, dysphagia, pulmonary symptoms (wheeze/cough)

Diagnosis:
- Initial diagnosis is purely clinical in those with classic symptoms
- If alarm symptoms, disease > 5 years, cancer risk factors: Should receive endoscopy (helps to rule out malignancy, Barrett's, erosive esophagitis)

Management:

Severity	Definition	Intervention
Mild	- < 2 episodes/week - Mild symptoms	- Lifestyle (weight loss, smoking cessation, raise head of bed) - Avoid dietary triggers (if correlation) - Low dose H2R Antagonist - Step up therapy if refractory
Severe	- Esophagitis on endoscopy OR > 2 episodes per week - Severe symptoms	- Daily PPI therapy - For refractory, see algorithm below

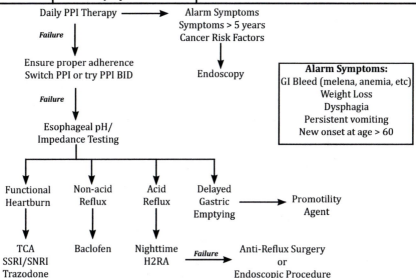

GI1

ESOPHAGEAL DISEASE
Gastrointestinal Medicine, Surgery

Complications of GERD

Erosive Esophagitis: Erosions and ulcerations of the esophageal mucosa

Barrett's: Metaplastic transformation of esophageal epithelium to columnar
- Predisposes patient to esophageal adenocarcinoma
- Screening guidelines are controversial
    - In general, those at high risk for Barrett's/cancer should be screened with endoscopy
    - Risk factors include age > 50, long-term GERD, smoking, obesity

Strictures: Fibrous narrowing of the esophageal lumen, often causing dysphagia

Extraesophageal Manifestations:
- Asthma
- Laryngitis
- Dental disease
- Pneumonia

Hiatal Hernia

General: Herniation of GI elements through the diaphragmatic esophageal hiatus. Generally a congenital abnormality, but can develop post-surgery or trauma.

Subtype	Definition	Appearance
Sliding	- GE Junction displaced above the diaphragm	
Paraesophageal	- Upward displacement of gastric fundus through defect in phrenoesophageal membrane	

Clinical:
- Often asymptomatic
- High association with GERD. Can also cause nonspecific abdominal pain.

Diagnosis:
- Generally discovered incidentally with barium swallow, endoscopy, or some other imaging

Management:
- Sliding Hiatal Hernia: Manage GERD
- Paraesophageal: Surgery in those with gastric complication from the hernia

ESOPHAGEAL DISEASE

Gastrointestinal Medicine, Surgery

Esophageal Cancer

	Squamous Cell	Adenocarcinoma
Risk	- Smoking/EtOH Use - Achalasia, strictures - Dietary factors (N-nitroso)	- Barrett's/GERD
Location	- Mid-esophagus	- Distal Esophagus (GE Junction)
Metastasis	- Cervical or mediastinal nodes	- Celiac/gastric nodes

Clinical:
- Progressive dysphagia (initially solids, then liquids)
- Systemic symptoms (weight loss, anorexia)

Diagnosis:
- Endoscopic biopsy
- Metastasis workup (endoscopic US, and CT/PET)

Management:

	Definition	Treatment
Superficial	- Limited to mucosa/submucosa	- Esophagectomy or - Endoscopic resection
Localized	- Local invasion/node spread	- Surgical resection - Chemoradiation
Advanced	- Distant mets - Local invasion of trachea, aorta, or other vital structures	- Palliative chemoradiation

ESOPHAGEAL DISEASE

Gastrointestinal Medicine, Surgery

Disorder	General	Clinical	Diagnosis	Management
Achalasia	- Degeneration of myenteric ganglion cells → Failure of LES relaxation and lower esophagus peristalsis - Can be idiopathic, or associated with autoimmune, malignancy, or infiltrative disease	- Dysphagia for solids and liquids - Regurgitation or heartburn	- Endoscopy (can't pass scope past LES) - Manometry (confirms) - Barium esophagram (if other tests equivocal)	- Pneumatic dilation or surgical myotomy - Nonsurgical candidates: Botulinum toxin, nitrates, Ca-channel blockers
Hypertensive Peristalsis (Nutcracker Esophagus)	- Overactive excitatory innervation, resulting in normal timing of peristalsis, but excess amplitude of contractions	- Dysphagia for solids and liquids - Chest pain - Heartburn, regurgitation	- Endoscopy (to rule out structural pathology) - Manometry	- Treat GERD (PPI) - Diltiazem (preferred first line agent) Alternative options: - Botulinum toxin - Isosorbide dinitrate - Sildenafil
Diffuse-Esophageal Spasm	- Impaired inhibitory esophageal innervation, causing increased simultaneous contractions of the esophagus			
Zenker's Diverticulum	- Herniation at Killian's triangle, (area of muscular weakness between cricopharyngeus and lower inferior constrictor muscles) - Thought to be due to abnormal esophageal motility	- Dysphagia - Aspiration/regurgitation - Foul breath, gurgling, neck mass	- Barium esophagram - Endoscopy	- Surgical or endoscopic resection
Esophageal Rings and Webs	- Thin membrane/tissue esophageal obstruction, often from chronic inflammation - Plummer-Vinson: Iron deficiency anemia, web, dysphagia, glossitis	- Often asymptomatic - Can cause dysphagia, or food impaction	- Barium esophagram - Endoscopy	- Endoscopic rupture or dilatation

GI4

ESOPHAGEAL DISEASE

Gastrointestinal Medicine, Surgery

Disorder	General	Clinical	Diagnosis	Management
Mallory-Weiss Tear *"mucosa"*	- Longitudinal mucosal laceration due to ↑ abdominal pressure - Most commonly due to vomiting, strain, cough, or iatrogenic (NG/scope)	- GI Bleed +/- abdominal pain	- Clinical symptoms - Endoscopy (to rule out other causes of upper GI bleed)	- PPI - Endoscopic intervention for active bleeds (coag, clip, ligate, epinephrine)
Esophageal Perforation *"blown all the way through"*	- Boerhaave syndrome → Effort based esophageal rupture - Can result in mediastinal contamination with gastric contents - Note: Traumatic rupture discussed in surg/trauma	- High-grade chest pain - Hoarseness, dysphagia - Subcutaneous emphysema	- Contrast esophagram	- Medical: NPO, antibiotics, PPI, parental nutrition - Surgical Repair (if septic, highly symptomatic)
Eosinophilic Esophagitis	- Immune-mediated esophageal disease with eosinophilic infiltrate and inflammation	- Dysphagia - Chronic GERD → PPI, then oral fluticasone - Food impaction	- Endoscopy with biopsy	- Dietary modification - Fluticasone (swallowed) *PPI if not already on*
Medication Esophagitis	- Tetracycline, KCl, NSAIDs, iron, bisphosphonate	- Odynophagia, dysphagia - Chest pain — *no bleeding — no abd pain*	- Clinical - Endoscopy if uncertain	- Discontinue medication
Infectious Esophagitis	- Often occurs in immunosuppressed patients Etiology: - Candida *→ fluconazole* - HSV (round ulcers) *→ val-/acyclovir* - CMV (linear ulceration) *→ ganciclovir*	- Odynophagia - Dysphagia - Oral thrush (Candida) - Oral ulcers (HSV)	- Upper endoscopy w/ biopsy (if viral) - KOH prep for suspected Candida	- Candida → Fluconazole - HSV → Val-/acyclovir - CMV → Ganciclovir

ESOPHAGEAL DISEASE
Gastrointestinal Medicine, Surgery

Dysphagia Workup

General: Subjective sense of difficulty or abnormal swallowing

Class	Clinical Features	Etiologies
Oropharyngeal	- Difficulty initiating a swallow - Associated with choking, coughing, aspiration and globus sensation	- Variety of neurologic, structural, infectious, and iatrogenic etiologies

Esophageal	- Difficulty swallowing seconds after initial swallow
	- Sensation of food in esophagus
	  - Solids/liquids → Motility
	  - Solids alone → Structural
		- Motility disorders
		- Structural lesions
		- Esophagitis

Acute-Onset	- Sudden onset inability to swallow food/liquids	- Food impaction

Diagnosis:
    Esophageal Dysphagia
        - Upper Endoscopy (generally first test, to rule out structural lesions)
        - Barium swallow
    Oropharyngeal
        - Modified barium swallow (investigates oral, pharyngeal, and esophageal phases)

Globus Sensation

General: Sensation of lump or food bolus in oropharynx, that is not due to any clear underlying pathology

Risk: Higher occurrence in those with psychiatric disease

Diagnosis: Barium swallow (rule out other disorders)

Management: Reassurance

GASTRIC DISEASE

Gastrointestinal Medicine, Surgery

Gastritis/Gastropathy

General: Gastritis and gastropathy refer to states of gastric damage from mucosal barrier dysfunction or mucosal inflammation

	Gastropathy	Gastritis
Pathophys	- Mucosal barrier breakdown, leading to mucosal damage	- Mucosal inflammation from an autoimmune or infectious etiology - Inflammation can be either acute or chronic
Histologic Findings	- Foveolar hyperplasia, edema - Lack of inflammatory cells	- Acute: Mucosal damage, hemorrhage, and neutrophilic infiltrate - Chronic: Lymphocytic infiltration, with atrophy and metaplasia
Etiology	- Chemicals (EtOH, bile, NSAIDs) - Hypoperfusion (sepsis, burns, hypovolemia, trauma) - Chemotherapy - Portal hypertension	- *H. Pylori* infection - Autoimmune (autoantibody against parietal cells, resulting in gastritis and pernicious anemia)
Other Findings		- Can lead to atrophy/metaplasia, increased cancer risk - Hypochlorhydria, leading to elevated gastrin secretion

Clinical: Can present as epigastric pain, nausea, vomiting, anorexia, weight loss

Diagnosis: Endoscopy with mucosal biopsy
- Macroscopic features (erythema, mucosal erosions, lack of rugal folds) suggestive, but not diagnostic. Biopsy is diagnostic.

Management: Treat underlying etiology

GASTRIC DISEASE
Gastrointestinal Medicine, Surgery

Peptic Ulcer Disease

General: Defect in the gastric or duodenal mucosa that extends through the muscularis mucosa

	Gastric	Duodenal
Etiology	- H. pylori - NSAID	- H. pylori - NSAID - Zollinger Ellison
Cancer	- Increased risk	- Generally benign
Location	- Type I: Lesser curvature (most common) - Type II: Gastric and duodenal - Type III: Prepyloric - Type IV: Near EG junction	- Posterior duodenum (generally 1-2 cm distal to pylorus)

Clinical:
- Epigastric pain
- Nausea, early satiety, feeling of fullness

Curling - burn victims
Cushing - steroids + brain trauma
Gastrinoma - diarrhea

Diagnosis:
- Endoscopy (with biopsy of ulcer margin)
- Barium esophagram (suggestive, but not confirmatory like endoscopy)
- Etiology: Assess NSAID history, work up for H. pylori (see next section)

Management:
- Treat underlying cause (avoid NSAIDs, treat H. pylori)
- PPI (regardless of etiology)
- Endoscopic surveillance of gastric ulcers

↳ *Triple tx: clarithromycin, amox (or metronidazole), PPI*
x EtOH
x smoking

Complications:

	Clinical	Management
Perforation	- Acute onset, severe abdominal pain with signs of peritonitis	- Surgical repair
Bleed	- Either acute or subacute upper GI bleed	- Endoscopic intervention
Outlet Obstruction	- Epigastric fullness, early satiety, weight loss, nausea, vomit	- Surgical

GASTRIC DISEASE — Gastrointestinal Medicine, Surgery

Helicobacter pylori

General: Gram negative gastric bacteria that is associated with gastritis and PUD

Diagnosis:
- If upper endoscopy is indicated: biopsy with urease testing + culture
- Noninvasive Testing:
    - Stool antigen assay
    - Urea breath test
    - Serology is avoided (low spec/sens, does not differentiate active from previous infection)

Management:
- Triple Therapy (First Line): Amoxicillin, Clarithromycin, PPI
- Quad Therapy: Metronidazole, Tetracycline, PPI, Bismuth
    - Used if local macrolide resistance
- After treatment, test for eradication (same tests as diagnosis)

Gastric Outlet Obstruction

General: Mechanical obstruction of the gastric outlet

Etiology:
- Peptic ulcer disease (causes scar formation)
- Caustic ingestion (stricture)
- Malignancy
- Gastric bezoar (accumulation of ingestion material, like hair)

Clinical: Nausea/vomiting, epigastric pain, early satiety, abdominal distension
- Succussion splash: Hear gastric contents splash > 3 hours after eating

Diagnosis: CT or Endoscopy

Management:
- NPO, NG tube decompression, PPI
- Treat underlying (surgically remove masses, dilate strictures, etc)

Misc. Gastric Pathology

Dieulafoy's Lesion: Dilated submucosal blood vessel that, in the absence of ulceration, invades through the gastric mucosa. Rare cause of upper GI bleed.

Menetrier Disease: Rare acquired stomach disease in which gastric hyperplasia results in rugal hypertrophy. Can cause chronic epigastric pain, weight loss, nausea, vomiting. May have increased cancer risk.

GASTRIC DISEASE
Gastrointestinal Medicine, Surgery

Gastric Cancer

	Clinical Features	Risk Factors
"Intestinal" Adenocarcinoma	- Well-differentiated, glandular proliferation	- *H. pylori* - Chronic gastritis - Diet (N-nitroso) - Obesity, smoking, EtOH - Family history - Genetic syndrome (ie BRCA, HNPCC, etc)
"Diffuse" Adenocarcinoma	- Poorly-differentiated proliferation of tumor cells, due to loss of cadherin intercellular adhesions - Signet ring cells - Rapidly progressive/bad prognosis	
GIST	- Tumor from interstitial cells of Cajal	- Usually sporadic - Familial syndromes
Lymphoma	- Marginal or diffuse large B-cell lymphoma of the MALT tissue	- *H. pylori* - Autoimmune gastritis - IBD/Celiac

Clinical: Abdominal pain, weight loss, nausea, early satiety
- Signature metastatic findings:
  - Krukenberg tumor: Metastasis to the ovary
  - Sister-Mary-Joseph node: Subcutaneous periumbilical lesion
  - Virchow node: Metastasis to supraclavicular node

Diagnosis:
- Endoscopy with biopsy
  - Intestinal masses can look like polypoid mass or ulcer
  - Diffuse may appear diffusely thick/rigid ("linitis plastica")
- Staging: CT, PET, Endoscopic US

Management:

Adenocarcinoma	- Partial or total gastrectomy with neoadjuvant/adjuvant chemotherapy - If metastatic: Palliative chemoradiation
GIST	- Local resection +/- Imatinib
Lymphoma	- Radiation therapy, Rituximab, treat underlying *H. pylori*

GASTRIC DISEASE — Gastrointestinal Surgery

Bariatric Surgery

Procedure Type	Features
Roux-en-Y Gastric Bypass	- Stomach is divided into a small upper pouch, and the small bowel is divided 40 cm below the gastric outlet. The small stomach pouch is than connected with the distal small bowel. - Weight loss through smaller gastric pouch and diversion of nutrients around a long stretch of small bowel - Can be complicated by gastric remnant distention/rupture, stomal stenosis, marginal ulcers, dumping syndrome
Sleeve Gastrectomy	- Removal of 80% of the stomach, leaving a sleeve like pouch - Decreases total amount of food able to eat, and alters gut hormones (responsible for hunger, satiety, etc) - Can be complicated by GI bleeding, gastric leaks, and stenosis of the gastric outlet
Gastric Band	- Inflatable band placed around upper stomach, creating a small upper pouch of the stomach that holds less food - Allows less food to be consumed and seems to decrease hunger - Can be complicated by band erosion, slippage, and port infection/ malfunctioning
Biliopancreatic Diversion with Duodenal Switch	- Gastrectomy, plus division of the duodenum at the gastric outlet, reconnection of the stomach to distal small bowel, reanastomosis of the bypassed small bowel to the distal small bowel (to deliver bile, pancreatic enzymes, etc) - Weight loss through smaller stomach, diversion of nutrients, and malabsorption due to less time of food being contacted by digestive pancreatic enzymes - Can cause serious protein-calorie malnutrition, and high risk for fat soluble vitamin deficiency

Indications:
    (1) BMI ≥ 40 kg/m² without comorbidity
    (2) BMI ≥ 35 kg/m² with at least one comorbidity
        - Includes Type II DM, OSA, HTN, HLD, NAFLD/NASH, others

Complications:
    - Nutrition:
        - Must supplement and monitor the following: Thiamine, folate, B12, iron, vitamin A/D/E/K, copper, zinc
    - Anastomotic leak or obstruction (usually < 30 days postoperative)
    - Marginal or gastrojejunal ulcers
    - Dumping syndrome
        - Severe diarrhea, nausea, vomiting and abdominal pain after eating from rapid gastric emptying of certain foods (usually high sugar)

SMALL BOWEL DISEASE

Gastrointestinal Medicine, Surgery

Malabsorption

General: Impaired nutrient absorption, due to acquired or congenital defects in the absorptive epithelium of the small intestine, or improper digestion of nutrients

Etiology: See following pages

Clinical: Diarrhea with fatty, large-volume, foul-smelling stools and weight loss
- Vitamin and mineral deficiencies if severe

Diagnosis:
- Fecal fat malabsorption (Sudan III stain)
- Carbohydrate absorption tests (D-xylose → Absorbed normally in chronic pancreatitis)
- Variety of tests for specific etiologies (fecal elastase, hydrogen breath test, etc, explained on next pages)

Celiac Disease

General: Hypersensitivity to gluten, a protein found in wheat, resulting in small bowel mucosal inflammation

Risk: Family history, HLA-DQ2/DQ8

Clinical: Malabsorption (diarrhea, weight loss, vitamin/mineral deficiency)
Associated with:
- Dermatitis Herpetiformis
- Autoimmune disorders (Type I DM, Hashimoto Thyroiditis)

Diagnosis:
- tTG-IgA levels (Alternative test: Deamidated gliadin peptide [DPG] IgG or anti-endomysial IgA)
  - Note: ↑ risk of IgA deficiency, so if IgA is low, check tTG or DPG IgG
  - Check HLA-DQ2/DQ8 (high NPV)
- Endoscopy with duodenal biopsy
  - Villous atrophy, crypt hyperplasia, intraepithelial lymphocytosis

Management: Gluten free diet
- Ensure proper vitamin and mineral levels (ie Fe)

Pancreatic Insufficiency

General: Loss of exocrine pancreas function

Etiology: Chronic pancreatitis, cystic fibrosis, duct obstruction, small bowel resection (↓ secretin/CCK production), advanced hemochromatosis

Clinical: Steatorrhea, malabsorption

Diagnosis: ↑ Fecal fat, elevated fecal elastase, decreased duodenal pH
- Plus features of underlying etiology

Management: Pancreatic enzyme replacement
- Supplementation of fat soluble vitamins

SMALL BOWEL DISEASE
Gastrointestinal Medicine, Surgery

	General	Clinical	Diagnosis	Treatment
Lactose Intolerance	- Lactase deficiency, resulting in lactose transit to colon, with production of hydrogen gas and fatty acids - Primary: Congenital or acquired non-persistence of enzyme - Secondary: GI disease (ie after infectious gastroenteritis)	- Abdominal pain, bloating, flatulence	- Hydrogen breath test (diagnostic) Other signs: - Stool: Osm gap > 125 - pH < 6	- Dietary lactose restriction - Lactase enzyme supplements
Whipple Disease	- Rare, SI overgrowth of *T. whipplei*, resulting in buildup of macrophages with PAS+ intracellular material	- Chronic diarrhea - Progressive onset of arthralgia, weight loss - Other: Cardiac (myocarditis), neurologic dysfunction	- Endoscopy with biopsy (classic macrophages, or use molecular test like PCR)	- Antibiotics (Penicillin or Ceftriaxone, followed by 1 year of TMP-SMX)
Tropical Sprue	- Chronic diarrheal disease with unclear etiology - Occurs in those that have spent ≥ 1 month in endemic area (band of countries ~30° latitude, including India, Haiti, DR, PR, cuba)	- Chronic diarrhea and malabsorption, in someone with consistent travel history	- Endoscopy with biopsy	- Tetracycline and folate
SIBO (Small Intestinal Bacterial Overgrowth)	- Overgrowth of colonic bacteria in the SI, resulting in enterocyte damage and malabsorption - Risks: Pancreatic insufficiency, anatomic abnormalities (ie post surgery), small-intestinal motility disorders	- Watery diarrhea, bloating, flatulence, abdominal pain	- Carbohydrate breath test - Jejunal culture (>10^3 CFU) Note: Low levels of many vitamins possible, but elevated folate/vitamin K	- Antibiotics (Rifaximin)

SMALL BOWEL DISEASE
Gastrointestinal Medicine, Surgery

Acute Mesenteric Ischemia

General: Sudden onset intestinal hypoperfusion, in the superior mesenteric artery

Etiology:
- Arterial Embolization (AFib, valvular disease, etc)
- Arterial Thrombosis (over an atherosclerotic plaque)
- Venous Thrombosis (rare)

Clinical:
- Classic presentation is acute severe abdominal pain disproportionate to physical findings
- Peritonitis, sepsis, and shock if severe ischemia/perforation

Diagnosis:
- CT Angiography (if hemodynamically stable)
- Laparotomy for those hemodynamically unstable

Management:

Type	Indication	Intervention
Surgical	- Peritonitis, sepsis, pneumatosis intestinalis	- Mesenteric embolectomy or bypass - Bowel resection for necrotic bowel
Endovascular	- Stable - No advanced intestinal ischemia	- Pharm thrombectomy - Balloon angioplasty/stent
Medical	- All patients	- NPO, fluids - Antibiotics, PPI - Heparin

Chronic Mesenteric Ischemia

General: Atherosclerotic disease of mesenteric vessels (celiac artery, superior and inferior mesenteric arteries), resulting in hypoperfusion

Clinical: Postprandial dull pain. Weight loss or nutritional deficiency.

Diagnosis: CT Angiography

Management: Endovascular revascularization (for those with severe symptoms)

SMALL BOWEL DISEASE
Gastrointestinal Medicine, Surgery

Appendicitis

General: Inflammation of the appendix, a common cause of acute abdomen. Secondary to obstruction (fecalith, lymph node hyperplasia, tumors, etc), leading to distension, vascular compromise, and eventual bacterial invasion.

Risk: Age (most common in 2nd/3rd generations of life)

Clinical:
- Abdominal pain: Periumbilical (visceral), followed by RLQ (peritoneal) at McBurney's point
- Nausea, vomiting, anorexia
- Variety of signs:
    - Rovsing: RLQ pain with LLQ palpation
    - Iliopsoas: RLQ pain with active right hip flexion
    - Obturator: RLQ pain with internal rotation of the hip

	Diagnosis	Management
Child	- Purely clinical (if classic), can go straight to surgery - US preferred imaging test	- Laparoscopic appendectomy - Antibiotics (ie Cefoxitin, Ceftriaxone/Metronidazole)
Adult	- CT with contrast preferred	- Laparoscopic appendectomy - Antibiotics (ie Cefoxitin, Ceftriaxone/Metronidazole)
Pregnant	- US	- Laparoscopic appendectomy - Antibiotics

Note: Some evidence points towards purely antibiotic management of appendicitis, but this is not widely accepted in the US at this time, as many of these patients require surgery within a few years.

Complications:

Perforation:
- Perforation of the appendix, generally contained in a phlegmon or abscess
Tx:
- Unstable (peritoneal signs, septic, etc): Emergent appendectomy
- Stable: IV antibiotics, percutaneous drainage of any abscess
- Some perform appendectomy in 6-8 weeks

SMALL BOWEL DISEASE
Gastrointestinal Medicine, Surgery

Small Bowel Obstruction

General: Obstruction of normal flow in the small bowel. Subtypes:
    Complete: No passage of stool or gas (but can be residual post-obstruction)
        - Compromised blood supply can result in ischemia or necrosis
    Partial: Some gas still passes, much lower risk for strangulation

Etiology:
- Adhesions (prior GI surgery or inflammation)
- Hernias
- Malignancy
- IBD (strictures)
- Intussusception, volvulus, gallstone ileus
- SMA syndrome (intermittent obstruction of the 3rd portion of the duodenum between the SMA/aorta)

Clinical:
- Abdominal pain, bilious emesis, nausea/vomiting
    - Borborygmi (high tympanic bowel sounds) initially as peristalsis increased in attempt to bypass obstruction
    - Followed by decreased bowel sounds as distension increases and peristalsis declines

Diagnosis:
- Abdominal XR (dilated loops, air-fluid levels)
- CT with oral + IV contrast

Management:
- Stable patients should undergo trial of nonoperative management, which includes NPO, NG tube decompression, IVF, and PO water-soluble contrast
- Surgery indicated for any with peritoneal signs, hemodynamic instability, or evidence of bowel ischemia/necrosis on imaging

Paralytic Ileus

General: Decreased or absent peristalsis, resulting in obstipation and intolerance of oral intake

Etiology: Commonly occurs post-operatively (2-3 days is normal). Other causes include narcotics, electrolyte abnormalities.

Clinical: Abdominal pain/distension, nausea/vomiting, failure to pass flatus, inability to tolerate oral diet

Diagnosis: Clinical. Plain abdominal XR show dilated bowel loops.

Management: Supportive care (IVF, pain control without narcotics, dietary restriction)

SMALL BOWEL DISEASE

Gastrointestinal Medicine, Surgery

Hernias

General: Protrusion of bowel through a weak spot in the abdominal fascia. Can be reducible (able to be pushed back inside the abdominal wall) and irreducible.

Subtype	Definition	Risk
Indirect Inguinal	- Protrusion of hernia sac through internal inguinal ring, lateral to the inferior epigastric artery	- Congenital defect (patent processus vaginalis)
Direct Inguinal	- Protrusion of hernia sac through Hesselbach's triangle, medial to the inferior epigastric artery	- Acquired abdominal wall defect (ie chronic straining)
Femoral	- Peritoneal hernia sac passing through the femoral canal	- More common in women
Ventral	- Anterior abdominal wall hernia - Includes incisional, umbilical, epigastric, and Spigelian hernias	- Prior surgery for incisional - Obesity or ascites for umbilical

Clinical: Physical bulge in abdominal wall, with varying degrees of pain and discomfort

Diagnosis: Generally a clinical diagnosis. US/CT can be used in uncertain situations.

Management:

	Definition	Management
Strangulated	- Necrotic tissue from ischemia	- Emergency surgery
Incarcerated	- Compromised blood supply, without necrotic bowel - Richter's hernia is special subtype with incarceration of only part of the bowel wall	- Urgent surgery (especially if SBO or not reducible) - Can attempt to reduce (but surgery is generally preferred)
Minimal Symptoms	- No evidence of incarceration or strangulation	- Elective surgery OR - Watchful monitoring

SMALL BOWEL DISEASE — Gastrointestinal Medicine, Surgery

Subtypes of Small Intestinal Cancer

Neuroendocrine (Carcinoid)	- Secrete serotonin and other bioactive products
Adenocarcinoma	- Rare. Generally seen in someone with chronic inflammation (ie Crohn's).
Lymphoma	- Primary GI lymphoma most often associated with autoimmune conditions and immunosuppressed
GIST	- Malignant mesenchymal tumors (sarcomas)

Carcinoid Tumor

General: Well-differentiated neuroendocrine tumors arising from enterochromaffin cells. Most commonly found in small bowel, but can be found in the lungs and stomach.

Clinical: Vague symptoms, generally relating to the impacted organ

Diagnosis: Often discovered incidentally (ie imaging like CT). Confirmed with biopsy.

Management: Surgical resection

Carcinoid Syndrome

General: Carcinoid tumor that metastasizes to liver, allowing for systemic serotonin release (normally degraded by MAO in liver)

Clinical:
- GI: Diarrhea, abdominal pain
- Pulmonary: Bronchospasm/wheeze
- Skin: Flushing, telangiectasias
- CV: Right-sided valvular lesions (fibrosis, collagen deposition)

Diagnosis:
- Elevated urinary 5-HIAA
- CT/MRI to localize

Management:
- Octreotide
- Hepatic resection (of metastasis)

FUNCTIONAL BOWEL DISORDERS
Gastrointestinal Medicine, Surgery

Overview of Functional GI Disorders

General: Disorders of the GI tract producing symptoms (ie pain, nausea, etc) without any clear anatomical or biochemical basis

Disorders include functional abdominal pain (commonly in children), heartburn, dyspepsia, diarrhea, etc.

Irritable Bowel Syndrome (IBS)

General: Functional GI disorder characterized by chronic abdominal pain and altered bowel habits. Unclear pathophysiology, but theories include gut visceral hypersensitivity, motility disorder, abnormal immune system functioning, and altered microbiome.

Risk: Associated with psychiatric disorders

Clinical: Periodic cramping pain, constipation, and/or diarrhea
- Patients can have predominantly diarrhea, constipation, or mixed features

Diagnosis: ROME IV Criteria
- Recurrent abdominal pain (≥ 1 day/week), for the last three months PLUS two of the following:
    (1) Related to defecation
    (2) Change in stool frequency
    (3) Change in stool appearance

Management:
- Initial: Dietary and lifestyle modification
    - Exclude gas-producing foods, lactose, gluten, etc
    - Psyllium if constipation predominant
- Refractory Constipation
    - Polyethylene Glycol, Lubiprostone, Linaclotide
- Refractory Diarrhea
    - Loperamide
- Refractory Abdominal Pain
    - Dicylcomine/Hyoscyamine or TCA

Cyclic Vomiting Syndrome

General: Recurrent episodes of vomiting with intervening periods of normal health. High association with migraine headaches.

Clinical:
- Up to a week long episode of daily morning vomiting
- Intermittent (months long) periods of normal health

Management:
- Abortive: Anti-migraine (ie Sumatriptan) plus antiemetic (Ondansetron)
- Prophylactic: Anti-migraine prophylaxis (Amitriptyline, Propranolol)

INFLAMMATORY BOWEL DISEASE

Gastrointestinal Medicine, Surgery

	Crohn's Disease	Ulcerative Colitis
Gen	- Areas of transmural inflammation found throughout the GI tract - Terminal ileum involvement is classic, but can involve anywhere from mouth to anus, with "skip lesions"	- Recurring episodes of mucosal inflammation in the colon (spares rest of GI tract)
Path	- Microscopy: Transmural inflammation, noncaseating granulomas - Cobblestoned mucosa, creeping fat, bowel wall thickening ("string sign"), linear ulcers and fissures	- Microscopy: Inflammation, crypt abscess, architectural distortion - Friable mucosal pseudopolyps, loss of haustra ("lead pipe")
Risk	- Peak age is bimodal (15-40, 50-80) - More common in Caucasians - Family history - Smoking (↑ Crohn's risk, ↓ UC risk [quitting smoking ↑ risk for UC flare])	
Clin	- Diarrhea (usually nonbloody) - Abdominal pain (often RLQ) - Malabsorption, weight loss - Complications include abscess, fistula, strictures	- Hematochezia or bloody diarrhea - Abdominal pain - Tenesmus - Greatly increased colon cancer risk - Associated with primary sclerosing cholangitis
	Extraintestinal Manifestations: - Skin: Rash (pyoderma gangrenosum, erythema nodosum) - Eye: Uveitis, episcleritis - Joints: Arthritis	
Dx	- Colonoscopy (for colon/ileum) - Capsule or CT/MR enterography (for SI)	- Colonoscopy
Tx	Initial Induction of Remission: - Steroids (Budesonide or Prednisone) +/- early initiation of anti-TNF Maintenance of Remission: - Low Risk: May require no medication or only monotherapy - High Risk: Dual pharm therapy with anti-TNF and thiopurine	Initial Induction of Remission: - Oral/Topical 5-ASA - Steroid course if severe Maintenance of Remission: - Oral/Topical 5-ASA - Thiopurine or anti-TNF used for moderate-severe disease Surgical (Colectomy): - Severe, debilitating, refractory disease, increased colon cancer risk, or severe complication (megacolon, hemorrhage)
	Drug Options: - 5-ASA: Sulfasalazine or Mesalamine - Thiopurines: 6-Mercaptopurine, Azathioprine - Anti-TNF: Adalimumab, Infliximab - Others: Ustekinumab, Natalizumab	

COLORECTAL DISEASE
Gastrointestinal Medicine, Surgery

Colon Cancer

General: Majority of tumors are endoluminal adenocarcinoma, typically arising from adenomatous polyps. The typical molecular pathway involves the loss of APC, KRAS, and p53. *FAP*

Risk: Age > 50, prior history of colon cancer, adenomatous polyps, IBD, family history, genetic conditions

Clinical: Often asymptomatic (picked up on normal screen), but can present as abdominal pain, hematochezia (more common right-sided), partial bowel obstruction (more common left-sided), iron deficiency anemia, thin stools

Diagnosis: Colonoscopy (with biopsy)

Management:
- Localized Disease: Colonic resection (partial colectomy)
    - Adjuvant chemotherapy for node-positive disease
- Metastatic Disease: Palliative chemotherapy
    - Some patients with limited mets can have aggressive surgery with chemotherapy (attempt at cure)
- Follow patients in remission with annual CT, colonoscopy, and CEA level

Colon Cancer Screening/Polyps

	Features	Malignancy Potential
Hyperplastic	- Simple glandular hyperplasia - ~ 90% of polyps found	- None
Hamartoma	- Normal colonic mucosa cells, with distorted architecture - Most common juvenile polyp - Associated with Peutz-Jeghers	- Sporadic hamartomas are rarely malignant - If associated with genetic syndrome, ↑ malignancy risk
Adenoma	- Tubular (most common) - Tubulovillous - Villous: Greatest risk of malignancy	Increasing risk with: - Villous - Increasing size - Sessile polyp - Cellular atypia

Screening Methodology

Colonoscopy	- q10 years
Flex Sigmoidoscopy	- q5 years or q10yr + annual FIT
CT Colonography	- q5 years
FIT (fecal immunochemical test)-DNA	- q1 year
FOBT	- q1 year

GI21

COLORECTAL DISEASE
Gastrointestinal Medicine, Surgery

Colorectal Cancer Screening

Population	Timing of Onset	Freq	Notes
General	- 50-75 y/o > 75 depends on preference	10 yr	- Frequency can be increased to 3-5 years if the patient is found to have adenomas (exact timing depends on type and quantity of adenomas)
Family Hx	- 40 y/o, or 10 years prior to cancer diagnosis	5 yr	- 1° relative < 60 y/o OR - Two 1° relatives with colon cancer at any age
IBD	- 8 years post diagnosis	1-2 yr	
FAP	- 10-12 years old	1 yr	
HNPCC	- 20-25, or prior to first family colon cancer diagnosis	1-2 yr	

Hereditary Conditions

Syndrome	Characteristics
FAP (Familial Adenomatous Polyposis)	- AD defect in the APC gene → KRAS → P53 - > 100 pancolonic adenomatous polyps arise starting around puberty, in addition to upper GI (duodenal) cancer - Management: Colectomy (once polyps are found), with upper endoscopy monitoring for duodenal adenomas [prophylactic] Subtypes (FAP + the following): - Gardner: Osteoma [jaw], dental issues, desmoid tumor, hypertrophy of retinal pigment epithelium, cutaneous lesions (cysts, fibromas) - Turcot: Brain tumors [brain] (medulloblastoma or glioma)
Peutz-Jeghers	- AD defect in STK11 gene - Mucocutaneous macules (lips, hands feet), gastrointestinal hamartomatous polyps (which can bleed, obstruct, become malignant) - Increased risk of cancer (colon, pancreatic, breast) - Management: Early onset screening for cancer (colonoscopy, mammography, and pancreatic MRI)
Juvenile Polyposis	- Genetic syndrome of childhood onset of gastrointestinal polyposis (hamartomas), with increased CRC risk - Early onset colonoscopy screening is indicated
HNPCC (Lynch or Hereditary Nonpolyposis Colon Ca)	- AD DNA mismatch repair gene defect (MSH/MLH), causing microsatellite instability - Greatly increased colon and endometrial cancer risk - Also at risk for ovarian, stomach, small bowel and other cancers - Amsterdam Criteria: Suspect in those with 3 relatives, 2 generations, and 1 diagnosed < 50 and 1 first degree relative - Colon screening (see above), endometrial/upper GI screening [Colorectal, Endometrial, Ovarian]

COLORECTAL DISEASE — Gastrointestinal Medicine, Surgery

Diverticulosis

General: False outpouching of the colonic mucosal layers, commonly occuring where the vasa recta penetrate the colonic muscularis. Most commonly found in the sigmoid colon. Increased intraluminal pressure (ie constipation) predisposes this condition.

Risk: Diet (low fiber, high fat/meat), obesity

Clinical: Asymptomatic, but very common cause of GI bleed (painless hematochezia)

Diagnosis: Often picked up incidentally on colonoscopy, CT, or barium enema study

Management:
- Asymptomatic: Monitor
- Bleeds: Resuscitation, colonoscopy (with intervention on active bleeders)

Diverticulitis

General: Inflammation and/or infection of a colonic diverticulum

Risk: Diverticular disease risk listed above. Note: Nuts/seeds not associated.

Clinical: LLQ abdominal pain, diarrhea/constipation, fever

Diagnosis: CT (with oral/IV contrast): Look for bowel wall thickening, inflamed pericolic fat, phlegmons/abscesses. Note: Colonoscopy/enema are contraindicated during active inflammation.

Management:

Type	Indication	Therapy
Outpatient Medical	- Uncomplicated disease (ie no complications seen below)	Antibiotics: - Cipro/Metronidazole - TMP-SMX/Metronidazole - Amox-Clavulanate
Inpatient Medical	- Uncomplicated disease, but high risk due to comorbidities (ie old age) or sepsis	- IV Pain control, fluids, NPO - IV Antibiotics (many regimens, just ensure anaerobes covered)
Complications		
Frank Perforation	- Microperforations medically treated, but large perforations need surgical correction	- Emergent surgery
Fistula		- Surgery
Obstruction		
Abscess	> 3 cm	- Percutaneous drainage - Surgery if refractory
	< 3 cm	- IV antibiotics

Follow-up: Colonoscopy ~ 6 weeks after episode resolves
- Those with complicated disease, > 2 episodes or smoldering symptoms should receive an elective colectomy

COLORECTAL DISEASE
Gastrointestinal Medicine, Surgery

	General	Clinical	Diagnosis	Treatment
Ischemic Colitis	- Malperfusion of large bowel, resulting in colonic ischemia - Can be transient to full-blown necrosis - Impacts "watershed" areas - Risks: Aortic instrumentation, CP bypass, any cause of hypotension	- Mild to severe abdominal pain - Hematochezia	- Clinical - Colonoscopy can confirm	- Medical: Antibiotics, NPO, NG tube - If evidence of necrosis: Surgical exploration/resection
Sigmoid Volvulus	- Sigmoid colon twisting about its mesentery, causing obstruction - Risk: Long sigmoid, narrow mesentery	- Progressive abdominal pain, nausea, bloating, and constipation	- Abd XR: Coffee bean sign - CT (preferred confirmatory test)	- Sigmoidoscopic detorsion + rectal tube placement - Surgery if signs of necrosis or endoscopy fails - Elective sigmoid resection (high risk for recurrence)
Angio-dysplasia	- Sporadic, aberrant blood vessels that have a tendency to bleed - Risk: Old age, CKD	- Generally asymptomatic, unless they bleed	- Colonoscopy	- GI Bleed: Endoscopic intervention (ie cautery) - Incidentally found: Do nothing
Large Bowel Obstruction	- Causes: Cancer, volvulus, inflammation (ie IBD, diverticulitis), stricture (prior surgical anastomosis)	- Acute or subacute presentation of pain, bloating, obstipation	- Abdominal XR or CT	- Supportive: IVF, NPO, gastric decompression - Surgical intervention often required
Ogilvie's Syndrome	- Acute nonstructural obstruction of colonic flow - Occurs in acutely ill and hospitalized patients	- Abdominal distension - Pain, nausea, vomit, constipation	- Abdominal CT (rule out mechanical obstruction)	- Initially conservative/supportive measures (IVF, stop offending medications) - Neostigmine - Colonoscopic decompression

APPROACH TO GI BLEEDS
Gastrointestinal Medicine, Surgery

Location	Clinical	Etiology
Upper (Proximal to Ligament of Treitz)	- Hematemesis - Melena - Brisk upper GI bleed can present with hematochezia	- PUD - Mucosal tears - Esophagitis/Gastritis - Esophageal varices
Lower GI (Distal to Ligament of Treitz)	- Hematochezia	- Diverticulosis - Neoplasm - Colitis (infectious, ischemic, IBD, radiation) - Angiodysplasia - Anal (hemorrhoid, fissure)

Initial Workup:
- CBC, type and screen, coags, and platelets
- Nasogastric lavage (can rule in or out upper GI bleed)

Initial Management:
- Two 16 gauge IVs with IVF (crystalloid)
- NPO
- Transfuse
    - Blood (if Hgb < 7, or Hgb < 9 in certain high risk patients)
    - Platelets (if count is < 50k)
    - FFP or prothrombin complex for coagulopathy
- Pharm Therapy
    - IV high dose PPI
    - Octreotide/IV antibiotics if likely variceal bleed

Localization of Bleed:
- Endoscopy (either upper or lower, based on clinical suspicion)
    - Alternative: Arteriography with IR embolization (used in rapid bleeds when acute intervention required)

- If cause of bleeding not identified:
    - Capsule enterography (examines small bowel)
    - Tagged RBC scan (for slow, occult bleeding)
    - CT angiography (can pick up faster, active bleeding)
    - Push enteroscopy (for cases of small bowel bleeding)

ANAL/RECTAL DISEASE
Gastrointestinal Medicine, Surgery

Hemorrhoids

General: Dilated submucosal veins in the anal mucosa

	Internal	External
Gen	- Dilated submucosal vein of superior rectal plexus - Above dentate line	- Dilated vein arising from inferior to the hemorrhoidal plexus - Distal to dentate line
Clin	- Painless bleeding with bowel movement - Irritation, pruritus	- Painless bleeding/irritation - Severe pain if thrombosed
Dx	- Rectal exam, anoscopy	
Tx	- All: Dietary modification, high fiber diet - Supportive: Topical analgesics, topical steroids, sitz bath - Refractory: Rubber band ligation or sclerotherapy	- All: Dietary modification, high fiber diet - Supportive: Topical analgesics, topical steroids, sitz bath - Refractory or Thrombosed: Surgical hemorrhoidectomy

Anal Fissure

General: Tear in the lining of the anal canal distal to the dentate line. Most commonly in the posterior midline, possibly with associated skin tag.

Etiology:
- Primary (local trauma, straining)
- Secondary (IBD, infection)

Clinical: Anal pain, worse after defecation. Bloody stools.

Diagnosis: Rectal exam (visualize, or reproduce pain)

Management:
- Supportive: High fiber diet, stool softener, sitz, topical analgesic
- Nifedipine or Nitroglycerine (relaxes anal sphincter)
- Refractory: Botulinum toxin injection or lateral internal sphincterotomy

ANAL/RECTAL DISEASE
Gastrointestinal Medicine, Surgery

Perianal Abscess

General: Infected anal crypt gland, likely due to obstruction
- Perianal: Simple abscess of the superficial anus
- Perirectal: Deep abscess (ie ischiorectal, supraelevator, intersphincteric)

Clinical: Severe pain in anal or rectal area, +/- fever

Diagnosis: Clinical exam (perianal erythema, fluctuant mass)
- Deeper abscesses may require imaging (ie CT/MRI)

Management: I&D, plus antibiotics (Amox-Clav or Ciprofloxacin)

Complications: Anal fistula (requires fistulotomy)

Pilonidal Cyst

General: Soft tissue disorder of the upper gluteal cleft, in which debris plugs hair follicles, resulting in possible infection

Risk: Obesity, trauma, prolonged sitting

Clinical: Can be asymptomatic, but acute flares present as tender mass with possible pus or bleeding

Diagnosis: Clinical exam

Management:
- Asymptomatic: Supportive, encourage perianal hygiene
- Acute Infection: I&D, plus antibiotics
- Chronic: Excision of sinus tracts and skin pores

Anal Cancer

General: Cancer of the anal mucosa, most commonly SCC

Risk: Men who have sex with men, HPV (16, 18), HIV

Clinical: Rectal bleed, +/- palpable mass

Diagnosis: Biopsy. CT/MRI for staging.

Management: Chemoradiotherapy (ie 5-Fluorouracil/Mitomycin + Radiation therapy)

BILIARY DISEASE
Gastrointestinal Medicine, Surgery

Cholelithiasis

Type	Risk Factors
Cholesterol	- Obesity, female, fertile (pregnancy, OCP), Native Americans, Crohn's, rapid weight loss
Bilirubin ("black pigment")	- Hemolysis
Mixed ("brown pigment")	- Biliary stasis and infection - β-glucuronidase increased amount of unconjugated bilirubin in the bile

Clinical: Can cause biliary colic (colicky RUQ pain that generally occurs after meals)
- Many cases asymptomatic and can be detected on routine imaging workups

Diagnosis: RUQ US

Management:
- Asymptomatic: Reassurance, monitor
- Biliary colic: Elective cholecystectomy

Cholecystitis

General: Stones obstructing the biliary duct, resulting in gallbladder distension, with eventual ischemia, bacterial invasion, and necrosis. Organisms are typical enteric:
- *E. Coli, Bacteroides, Enterobacter, Enterococcus, Klebsiella*

Clinical: Constant RUQ pain, with fever and leukocytosis. + Murphy's sign.

Diagnosis:
- RUQ US (thickened wall, pericholecystic fluid, sonographic murphy, stones)
- HIDA scan (second line, if RUQ US is not diagnostic)

Management:
- Initial: Fluids, pain control
- Antibiotics (Ceftriaxone-Metronidazole, or Amp-Sulbactam or Pip-Tazo)
- Surgical
    - Emergent cholecystectomy (can be delayed if patient stable with supportive measures), percutaneous cholecystostomy

Complications:
- Gallbladder gangrene, perforation, abscess
- Emphysematous cholecystitis (Air in gallbladder wall from gas producing bacterial organism. Worse prognosis, need for emergent surgery higher)

Surgical Complications:
- Postcholecystectomy Syndrome: RUQ pain or dyspepsia that continues after surgery. Typically due to residual stone, biliary dysfunction, or other GI pathology.
- CBD Injury: Blood/bile leakage into the peritoneal space. Dx with US or CT. Presents as fever, pain, bilious ascites. Requires T-Tube repair or Roux-en-Y hepaticojejunostomy.

BILIARY DISEASE
Gastrointestinal Medicine, Surgery

Handwritten note: 2) ampicillin, gentamicin, + metronidazole etc

	General	Clinical	Diagnosis	Treatment
Acalculous Cholecystitis	- Biliary stasis, resulting in ischemia, infection, and necrosis - Risk: Critically ill, hospitalized	- Sepsis - Jaundice - RUQ pain	- US (CT is alternative)	- Antibiotics - Percutaneous cholecystostomy
Choledocholithiasis	- Stone in the common bile duct - Presents as obstructive jaundice (↑ bilirubin, LFTs, alk phos, etc)	- RUQ pain - Nausea, vomiting	- US - Labs (LFTs, bili, etc)	- ERCP - Followed by cholecystectomy
Cholangitis	- Stone in CBD, with ascending infection - Can also be caused by strictures, parasitic infections, and biliary instrumentation	- Charcot: RUQ pain, fever, jaundice + Hypotension and altered mentation (Reynaud's pentad)	- US (bile duct dilatation) - MRCP/ERCP is alternative for negative US with high suspicion	- Antibiotics, IVF, supportive care - ERCP (emergent) - Followed by cholecystectomy
Biliary Dyskinesia	- Sphincter of Oddi spasm/dysfunction - Dilated biliary system without evidence of stones	- RUQ pain (mimics cholecystitis)	- HIDA scan - Sphincter manometry	- Endoscopic sphincterotomy
Gallstone Ileus	- Stone passes through enteric fistula, lodges in ileum	- Intermittent obstructive symptoms (ie nausea/vomit), with eventual small-bowel obstruction	- CT (pneumobilia, obstructing stone)	- Enterolithotomy - Cholecystectomy (and fistula repair)
Chronic Cholecystitis	- Fibrosis, inflammation of gallbladder from chronic cholelithiasis/cystitis - Can lead to calcified "Porcelain" gallbladder	- Can have symptoms of gallbladder disease (ie RUQ pain)	- CT	- Cholecystectomy (possible ↑ gallbladder cancer risk)

GI29

BILIARY DISEASE
Gastrointestinal Medicine, Surgery

Biliary Cysts

General: Cystic dilatation of the biliary tree. Associated with cholangiocarcinoma, as well as rupture, stricture, cholangitis, and stone formation. Variety of subtypes, but type I cysts (most common) are single, extrahepatic dilations of the bile duct.

Clinical: Abdominal pain, jaundice, nausea, vomiting, pruritus. Palpable mass.

Diagnosis: US, CT, ERCP/MRCP can all pick up cysts

Management: Surgical excision (reduces malignancy risk) +/- Roux-en-Y hepaticojejunostomy

Cholangiocarcinoma

General: Adenocarcinoma arising from anywhere within the biliary tree (outside of the gallbladder or ampulla)

Risk: Majority occur without underlying risk factor, but risk includes primary sclerosing cholangitis, cystic liver/biliary disease, parasite infection, chronic liver disease (intrahepatic cholangiocarcinoma)

Clinical: Jaundice (+ pruritus/dark urine), RUQ pain, systemic signs (weight loss, fever)

Diagnosis: MRI/MRCP preferred for intrahepatic lesions, while ERCP/endoscopic US are preferred for extrahepatic

Management: Chemotherapy, radiotherapy, with surgery for purely local disease. Prognosis is generally poor.

Gallbladder Cancer

General: Adenocarcinoma of the gallbladder

Risk: Chronic gallbladder inflammation (ie gallstones, chronic infection, biliary cysts)

Clinical: Nonspecific and vague presenting symptoms. May present as biliary obstruction (jaundice, biliary colic, weight loss, RUQ mass).

Diagnosis: Often picked up on histology of removed gallbladders. If looking for cancer, first line imaging includes US, MRI/MRCP.

Management: Cholecystectomy, adjuvant chemotherapy/chemoradiation. Poor prognosis.

BILIARY DISEASE

Gastrointestinal Medicine, Surgery

Bilirubin Metabolism (Overview)

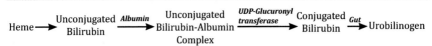

Jaundice occurs when total bilirubin is > 2 mg/dL

	Unconjugated Hyperbilirubinemia	Conjugated Hyperbilirubinemia
Features	- Water insoluble, neurotoxic - Elevated urobilinogen excretion	- Water soluble, nontoxic - Excreted in urine (dark urine)
Etiology	- Hemolysis - Decreased conjugation (Gilbert's, Crigler-Najjar, neonatal jaundice) - Cirrhosis - Impaired hepatic bilirubin uptake	- Extrahepatic biliary obstruction (stones, malignancy, stricture, etc) - Decreased intrahepatic secretion (cirrhosis, PBC/PSC, Dubin-Johnson/Rotor)
Clinical	- Elevated risk of pigmented stones	- Dark urine with pale stools - Pruritus (elevated serum bile salt) - Steatorrhea: Impaired fat digestion

Genetic Causes of Hyperbilirubinemia

Gilbert	- Inherited disorder of bilirubin glucuronidation (UDP-glucuronyltransferase) - Mild unconjugated hyperbilirubinemia/jaundice, exacerbated by periods of stress (ie illness, surgery)

Crigler-Najjar	- Type 1: Complete absence of UDP glucuronyltransferase in hepatic tissue
	    - High risk of kernicterus. Requires phototherapy daily.
	- Type 2: Reduced UDP glucuronosyltransferase activity. Not as severe as Type 1.
	    - Managed with daily phenobarbital

Dubin-Johnson	- Defective excretion of conjugated bilirubin from hepatocytes into bile - Mild icterus, conjugated hyperbilirubinemia. Liver is grossly black.
Rotor	- Defect in hepatic conjugated bilirubin storage, which leaks into the plasma - Mild icterus, conjugated hyperbilirubinemia

BILIARY DISEASE
Gastrointestinal Medicine, Surgery

	General	Clinical	Diagnosis	Treatment
Primary Sclerosing Cholangitis	- Chronic, progressive fibrosis, and stricturing of intra/extrahepatic bile ducts - Strong association with ulcerative colitis, P-ANCA, and human leukocyte antigen DRw52a	- Pruritus, jaundice, dark urine, light stool - Hepatosplenomegaly - Cholestatic LFT pattern (increased bili/AlkPhos) <u>Complications:</u> - Cholangiocarcinoma (PSC) - Cirrhosis/HCC - Malabsorption - Osteoporosis	- MRCP/ERCP (usually diagnostic) - Liver biopsy (if imaging not definitive)	- Strictures: Endoscopic stent and dilatation - Liver transplant (for cirrhosis) - Screen for cholangiocarcinoma
Primary Biliary Cirrhosis	- Progressive, autoimmune intrahepatic bile duct destruction - Autoimmune condition, commonly seen in middle age women (with other autoimmune disease)		- US (to rule out extra hepatic obstruction) - AMA antibodies - Liver biopsy (definitive)	- Ursodeoxycholic acid - Obeticholic acid/fibrates - Liver Transplant (last line)
Secondary Biliary Cirrhosis	- Extrahepatic biliary obstruction, causing bile stasis - Caused by cancer, strictures, or gallstones		- US, CT, MRI, MRCP, ERCP depending on etiology	- Treat underlying

PANCREATIC DISEASE
Gastrointestinal
Medicine, Surgery

Acute Pancreatitis

General: Inflammation of the pancreas from inappropriately activated pancreatic digestive enzymes, resulting in autodigestion. Subtypes:
- Interstitial Edematous (~85%): Enlarged pancreas w/ inflammatory edema
- Necrotizing (~15%): More severe, areas of pancreatic necrosis

Etiology:
- Gallstones   HART
- Ethanol   ↓
- Hypertriglyceridemia
- Tumors (obstructing outflow)
- Hypercalcemia
- Post-instrumentation (ie ERCP)
- Trauma
- Infections (Mumps, *Mycoplasma*, Coxsackie, HIV, others)
- Toxins (brown recluse, certain scorpions)
- Drugs
- Hereditary (SPINK mutations)

Clinical:
- Severe epigastric pain, may radiate to back
- Nausea, vomiting
- Fever, tachypnea, tachycardia
- Associated (rare) clinical signs — you "turn-her" on her flank"
    - Grey Turner (flank hemorrhage)
    - Cullens (blue discoloration at umbilicus)
    "umbill-Cullens"

Diagnosis: (2/3 of the following)
(1) Epigastric pain
(2) Elevation of amylase/lipase ≥ 3x the upper limit of normal
(3) Characteristic imaging findings
    - CT/MRI can reveal edema and areas of necrosis

* Multiple criteria (Ranson's, APACHE) can be used to prognosticate

Management:
- IVF, pain control (Morphine/Fentanyl), electrolyte correction, NPO
- Nutritional support (if NPO > 7 days, provide NJ tube)
- Provide ICU level care for those with severe disease

- Use CT to look for complication if septic, severe pancreatitis, or deterioration after > 72 hours

GI33

PANCREATIC DISEASE
Gastrointestinal Medicine, Surgery

Complications of Acute Pancreatitis

Necrosis	- Necrotic pancreatic tissue with high risk for infection	- Can diagnose infection with CT or CT guided FNA - Treat with broad spectrum antibiotics +/- necrosectomy (debridement of pancreatic necrosis, reserved for severe cases)
Pancreatic Pseudocyst	- Encapsulated collection of fluid with a well-defined wall - Usually occurs > 3-4 weeks after acute episode	- Asymptomatic: Monitor - Symptomatic or Enlarging: Endoscopic or surgical drainage
Abdominal Compartment Syndrome	- Intra-abdominal pressure > 20 mmHg, causing organ failure - Screen in ICU using bladder pressure	- Surgical decompression

Chronic Pancreatitis

General: Progressive and chronic disease of fibrosis and inflammation of the pancreas, resulting in structural damage, and impaired exocrine and endocrine function

Risk: Chronic alcoholism, cystic fibrosis, malignancy, stones/obstructions

Clinical: Chronic, recurrent bouts of epigastric pain, nausea, vomiting
- Weight loss, malabsorption

Diagnosis:
- Imaging (CT, plain films showing pancreatic calcifications)
    - MRCP or ERCP if unclear
- Secretin stimulation test
- Fecal elastase

Management:
- Small volume meals, quit alcohol/tobacco use
- Pain control, PPI
- Pancreatic enzyme supplementation (Lipase)
- Surgery (if all else refractory)
    - Pancreaticojejunostomy and/or pancreatic resection

Complications:
- Pseudocyst, duct stricture
- Diabetes mellitus (usually late in disease course)
- Malabsorption, steatorrhea
- Pancreatic adenocarcinoma
- Splenic vein thrombosis
- Pleural effusion or ascites

PANCREATIC DISEASE
Gastrointestinal Medicine, Surgery

Pancreatic Adenocarcinoma

General: Adenocarcinoma of the pancreatic exocrine ducts

Risk: Male smokers, chronic pancreatitis, high-fat diet, Jewish, Black

Clinical: Pain, jaundice, and weight loss
- Migratory thrombophlebitis (Trousseau syndrome)
- Palpable gallbladder (Courvoisier sign)

Diagnosis:
- If jaundiced: Perform US. MRCP/CT are 2nd line if US not diagnostic.
- Biopsy for definitive diagnosis
- CT for staging/disease extent (FNA or during surgery)

Management:
- Surgery (only if no mets or local vascular invasion)
    - Head Tumor: Pancreaticoduodenectomy (Whipple)
    - Tail Tumor: Distal pancreatectomy + splenectomy
- Chemotherapy
- Monitor CEA for prognosis/recurrence
- Palliative care for complications:
    - Abdominal pain
    - Biliary obstruction
    - Gastric outlet obstruction

Other Pancreatic Masses

<u>Benign Masses</u>
- Serous or Mucinous Cystadenomas
- Treatment: Resection

<u>Intraductal Papillary Mucinous Neoplasm</u>
- Produce mucin that obstructs ducts, causing recurrent pancreatitis
- Diagnosis with CT
- Treatment: Resection

<u>Periampullary Cancers</u>
- Cancer that obstructs the ampulla of vater, which can arise from the ampulla itself, pancreas, or duodenum
- Clinical: Obstructive jaundice, possible GI bleed
- Diagnosis: CT, with ERCP/biopsy for definitive diagnosis
- Treatment: Pancreaticoduodenectomy

< **CIRRHOSIS** | **Gastrointestinal Medicine** >

Cirrhosis Overview

General: Chronic liver disease characterized by hepatic fibrosis, distortion of architecture, and formation of regenerative nodules

Etiology: Most common in the US include alcohol abuse, hepatitis C, and non-alcoholic fatty liver disease, but many other causes (hemochromatosis, autoimmune hepatitis, others covered on the following pages)

Clinical:
- Nonspecific: Anorexia, weight loss, fatigue
- Portal HTN: Ascites, HSM, variceal bleeding
- Neurologic: Hepatic encephalopathy, asterixis
- Skin: Jaundice, palmar erythema, spider angiomas, terry nails
- Heme: Thrombocytopenia, anemia, coagulopathy
- Reproductive: Testicular atrophy, gynecomastia

- Poor synthetic function: ↓ albumin, ↑ INR, ↑ bilirubin

Diagnosis: Combination of clinical presentation and below diagnostic testing
- RUQ US is typically used to evaluate liver/extrahepatic manifestations
- Evaluation of Hepatic Fibrosis:
    - Hepascore (serologic scoring system of fibrosis)
    - Elastography (US that measures "stiffness" of liver)
- Biopsy (definitive diagnosis, but not always necessary)

Management:
- Slow progression of disease by treating underlying cause (ie alcohol abstinence, treat hepatitis, adjust drug doses, etc)
- Protect the liver: Vaccines, avoid hepatotoxic drugs
- Manage the complications seen on the following pages
- Monitor for HCC (AFP + US q6 months)
- Consider liver transplantation

Classifications:
- Scoring systems to monitor severity of disease

Child Pugh	1	2	3
Ascites	Absent	Mild	Moderate
Bilirubin	< 2	2-3	> 4
Albumin	> 3.5	2.8-3.5	< 2.8
PT (INR)	< 1.7	1.7-2.3	> 2.3
Encephalopathy	None	Grade 1 or 2	Grade 3 or 4

Class A (5-6 points), Class B (7-9 points), Class C (10-15 points)

- MELD score is alternative scoring system

CIRRHOSIS
Gastrointestinal Medicine

Ascites (from Portal Hypertension)

General: Accumulation of fluid in the peritoneal cavity due to portal hypertension (increased hydrostatic pressure) and hypoalbuminemia (reduced oncotic pressure)

Clinical: Abdominal distension, fluid wave, shifting dullness

Diagnosis: RUQ US, with paracentesis showing SAAG > 1.1

Management:
- Salt restriction (< 2000 mg)
- Combination Furosemide-Spironolactone therapy
- For tense ascites: Large volume paracentesis (+/- supplemental albumin)
- Refractory: TIPS procedure or transplant

Spontaneous Bacterial Peritonitis

General: Ascitic fluid infection without an evident intra-abdominal surgical source. Thought to be due to bowel translocation. Organisms include *E. Coli, Klebsiella, Strep, Staph*.

Clinical: Abdominal pain, fever (> 100°F), altered mental status

Diagnosis: Paracentesis
- PMN > 250 /mm^3
- SAAG > 1.1
- Positive ascites culture/gram stain

Management:
- 3rd Generation Cephalosporin or Fluoroquinolone
- Albumin
- Watch for and manage renal failure (common complication)
- Prophylaxis: Ciprofloxacin or TMP-SMX
    - Indicated if high-risk (history of SBP, current GI bleed)

Hepatic Encephalopathy

General: Reversible neuropsychiatric abnormalities from toxic effect of ammonia and other substances on CNS function

Risk: Precipitated by alkalosis, hypokalemia, drugs, GI bleed, infection, hypovolemia, medication non-adherence

Clinical:
- Decreased mental function (may be subtle or overt, depending on severity)
- Neuromuscular abnormalities: Hyperreflexia, rigidity, bradykinesia, myoclonus, and asterixis

Diagnosis: Clinical diagnosis of exclusion
- Ammonia levels frequently elevated but not helpful/diagnostic

Management:
- Acute: Supportive care, treat underlying cause, give Lactulose +/- Rifaximin
- Prophylaxis: Lactulose and or Rifaximin therapy for recurrent episodes

CIRRHOSIS

Gastrointestinal Medicine

Variceal Bleeding

General: Portal hypertension results in venous variceal formation in the following areas (between portal and systemic venous systems)

Esophagus	High risk for bleeding	Left Gastric ↔ Azygous
Rectum	Anorectal varices	Superior ↔ Inferior Rectal
Umbilicus	Caput Medusae	Paraumbilical ↔ Epigastric

Esophageal Variceal Bleeds

Clinical: Upper GI bleed (hematemesis, melena)

Diagnosis: Urgent endoscopy

Management:
    Acute:
    - Initial resuscitation with IV access, IVF, antibiotics, and Octreotide
    - Balloon tamponade can be used in patients with severe bleeding
    - Urgent upper endoscopy (with variceal ligation or sclerotherapy)
    - Severe Rebleeding: Endoscopy preferred, but TIPS or surgery if refractory

    Chronic Prophylaxis
    - Most cirrhotics should undergo screening for varices (upper endoscopy)
    - Smaller, lower risk varices receive beta-blocker (ie Nadolol) for prophylaxis
    - Larger, higher risk varices receive endoscopic variceal ligation

Hepatorenal Syndrome

General: Progressive renal failure in advanced liver disease, secondary to renal hypoperfusion (decreased vasodilatory molecules, with subsequent RAAS activation, and worsening renal perfusion)

Risk: Advanced cirrhosis. Often precipitated by GI bleed, vomiting, overdiuresis.

Clinical: Azotemia, oliguria, hyponatremia, hypotension

Diagnosis: Elevated BUN/Cr, with FeNa < 1 % and absence of other cause
    - No response to fluids (differentiates from prerenal)

Management:
    - Midodrine, Octreotide, Albumin
        - Norepinephrine used if in ICU. Terlipressin in Europe.
    - Transplant is only definitive therapy

ACUTE LIVER FAILURE
Gastrointestinal Medicine

Acute Liver Failure

General: Defined as severe acute liver injury with encephalopathy and impaired synthetic function in someone without prior liver disease

Etiology:
- Viral (Hepatitis A, B, D, E, CMV, HSV)
- Drug/Toxin (most commonly Acetaminophen)
- Ischemia (shock liver)
- Vascular (Budd-Chiari)
- Autoimmune hepatitis

Clinical:
- Fatigue, weakness, lethargy, confusion
- Jaundice, hepatomegaly, RUQ pain, and thrombocytopenia

Diagnosis:
- Clinical diagnosis with the combination of:
    - Encephalopathy
    - INR ≥ 1.5
    - Elevated AST/ALT (often marked elevation > 1,000)
- Other Findings: Elevated bilirubin, thrombocytopenia

Management:
- ICU level supportive care, treat underlying cause
- IV N-acetylcysteine
- Monitor for cerebral edema (complication of hepatic encephalopathy)
- Liver transplant in those unlikely to recover

Interpretation of LFTs

AST/ALT	< 500	> 1,000	> 10,000
Etiology	- Chronic Viral Hepatitis - EtOH - NAFL/NASH	- Acute Viral Hepatitis - Autoimmune Hepatitis - DILI (drug induced liver injury) - Ischemia	- Severe Shock Liver - Severe Viral Hepatitis - Severe Acetaminophen Toxicity

Note: ALT/AST elevations are a sign of hepatocellular injury

Alkaline Phosphatase:
- Can come from other parts of body (ie bone, intestines, etc)
    - Can differentiate with GGT
- True hepatic elevation indicates cholestasis. Differential includes:
    - Biliary epithelial damage (cirrhosis, hepatitis)
    - Intrahepatic cholestasis
    - Biliary obstruction

ETIOLOGIES OF LIVER DISEASE — Gastrointestinal Medicine

	General	Clinical	Diagnosis	Treatment
Non-Alcoholic Fatty Liver	- Hepatic Steatosis without history of alcohol abuse - NAFL: Steatosis - NASH: Steatosis + inflammation	- Asymptomatic or mild RUQ discomfort - Associated with obesity, HTN, insulin resistance, dyslipidemia	- Steatosis (on US/CT imaging or biopsy) - History (absence of EtOH use, but features of metabolic syndrome)	- Lifestyle modification (ie weight loss, control of comorbidities)
Alcoholic Hepatitis	- Hepatic steatosis and inflammation from EtOH abuse	- RUQ tenderness - Anorexia, jaundice	- Hx of EtOH abuse, with other causes of hepatitis ruled out - AST:ALT > 2, ↑ GGT	- Supportive care - Prednisolone (if discriminant function > 32) - Alcohol abstinence
Autoimmune Hepatitis	- Chronic autoimmune hepatitis	- Variable, ranging from asymptomatic to acute liver failure	- + ANA/Anti-SM Ab - Hypergammaglobulin - Liver biopsy	- Prednisone - Azathioprine or 6-MP for severe or refractory cases
Wilson's Disease	- Impaired copper excretion into bile (AR mutation in ATP7B gene)	- Acute or chronic hepatitis - Yellow corneal rings (Kayser-Fleischer) - Renal damage - CNS (psychiatric changes, Parkinsonian features, chorea, dysarthria)	- ↓ Serum ceruloplasmin - ↑ Urinary copper - Slit lamp exam - Biopsy/genetics if above are equivocal	- D-penicillamine or Trientine
Congestive Hepatopathy	- Any cause of right heart failure, resulting in elevated central venous pressure and thus hepatic venous pressure	- Evidence of LFT elevation and right heart failure - Generally asymptomatic	- RUQ US with doppler	- Treat CHF

GI40

ETIOLOGIES OF LIVER DISEASE — Gastrointestinal Medicine

Hereditary Hemochromatosis

General: AR disorder of iron absorption (HFE gene on chromosome 6), which causes increased iron absorption, with buildup of storage in tissues
- Note: Secondary hemochromatosis can occur from iron overload due to chronic blood transfusions

Clinical: Asymptomatic until ~age 40 (women delayed due to menses)
- GI: Transaminitis, progressively worsen to cirrhosis. ↑ HCC risk.
- Skin: Hyperpigmentation
- MSK: Arthralgias, chondrocalcinosis
- Endocrine: Diabetes mellitus, hypogonadism, hypothyroidism
- CV: Cardiomyopathy, conduction issues
- Infection Risk (*Vibrio vulnificus, Yersinia enterocolitica, Listeria*)

Diagnosis:
- Elevated ferritin/transferrin saturation
- Genetic testing (used for definitive diagnosis), liver biopsy (alternative)

Management:
- Asymptomatic patients with ferritin < 500 ng/mL are typically monitored
- Scheduled phlebotomy (generally weekly or biweekly)
    - Initiated if symptomatic, or labs progressively worsening
- Avoid EtOH, Fe, vitamin C, and uncooked seafood
- Screen for HCC
- Iron chelation (only required if contraindication to phlebotomy)

Budd-Chiari

General: Hepatic venous outflow obstruction, either due to clot (primary) or infiltrative lesion (secondary)

Etiology:
- Primary: Hypercoagulable state, OCP use, myeloproliferative disorder (ie polycythemia vera)
- Secondary: Malignancy, benign liver lesions, or structural abnormality

Clinical:
- Presentation ranges from acute liver failure to chronic liver disease
- Symptoms include abdominal pain, ascites, jaundice, edema, GI bleed, or hepatic encephalopathy

Diagnosis: US (with doppler). CT/MRI are used as alternatives.

Management:
- Correct underlying disorder
- Anticoagulation (LMWH, Warfarin)
- Thrombolytic therapy or angioplasty with stenting
- TIPS, shunting, or transplant for those that do not improve

VIRAL HEPATITIS

Gastrointestinal Medicine

	General	Clinical	Diagnosis	Treatment
Hepatitis A	- Picornavirus (ss-RNA) - Fecal-oral spread - Risk: Travel to endemic areas, MSM, drug use	Acute Hepatitis - Initial signs of RUQ pain, fever, anorexia, nausea - Hepatosplenomegaly, jaundice (~1 month, self-limiting) - Never chronic, fulminant disease is rare	- LFT elevation (can be > 1000) - Bilirubin elevation - Confirmed via serology (Hep A IgM)	- Supportive Care - PPX: Hep A Vax (use prior to travel, high risk individuals, post-exposure)
Hepatitis B	- Hepadnavirus (ds-DNA) - Sexual spread, blood, body fluids	See next page		
Hepatitis C	- Flavivirus ssRNA - Transmitted by blood (IVDU, transfusions prior to 1992) - Rarely sexual transmission	Acute - Either asymptomatic or symptoms of acute hepatitis Chronic (> 50% develop) - Generally asymptomatic or vague findings	- HCV RNA - Anti-HCV Ab (ELISA)	- Antivirals (see next page) ↳ ribavirin + INF-2α
Hepatitis D	- Incomplete ssRNA - Requires hepatitis B infection - Often spread with Hep B (ie via sex/blood)	- Acute hepatitis (more likely to be severe/result in liver failure compared to hep B alone)	- Serum HDAg and/or HDV RNA	- Peg-interferon
Hepatitis E	- Calicivirus (ss-RNA) - Enteric transmission	- Acute Hepatitis [See: Hep A] - Acute liver failure more likely in pregnant woman	- HEV IgM/ HEV RNA	- Supportive - Ribavirin if prolonged/chronic

VIRAL HEPATITIS

Gastrointestinal Medicine

Hepatitis B

	HBsAg	HBeAg	Anti-HBc IgM	Anti-HBc IgG	Anti-HBs	Anti-HBe	HBV DNA
Acute Early HBV	↑	↑	↑				↑↑
Acute Window			↑				↑
Acute Recovery				↑	↑	↑	
Chronic	↑			↑			
Acute on Chronic	↑	↑	↑	↑			↑
Vaccine					↑		
Cleared Infection				↑	↑		

Clinical:
- Acute Infection
  - Many are asymptomatic or anicteric, but ~30% get symptoms
  - Symptomatic patients suffer from prodrome of arthralgia, rash
  - Followed by acute hepatitis (RUQ pain, jaundice, etc)
  - Fulminant disease is rare
- Chronic Infection (~5% adults, but 50% of young kids, and 90% of neonates)

Diagnosis: See hepatitis serology/DNA chart above

Management:
- Acute: Supportive, monitor serology to evaluation for clearance
- Chronic
  - Antivirals (Tenofovir or Entecavir) first line

Hepatitis C (Management)

Check the HCV genotype (which directs therapy)
- Genotype 1 (most common): Glecaprevir-Pibrentasvir, Ledipasvir-Sofosbuvir, or Sofosbuvir-Velpatasvir
- Genotype 2-3: Glecaprevir-Pibrentasvir effective

*In General: Regimens are a combination of a NS3/4A protease inhibitor with NS5A inhibitor (both proteins are required for RNA replication)
- Antivirals now standard of care (interferon/ribavirin almost entirely out)

Class	Drug Options
Protease (NS3/4A) Inh.	- Boceprevir, Glecaprevir, Paritaprevir, Simeprevir, Telaprevir
NS5A Inhibitors	- Daclatasvir, Ledipasvir, Pibrentasvir, Velpatasvir
NS5B Inhibitors	- Dasabuvir, Sofosbuvir

LIVER MALIGNANCY — Gastrointestinal Medicine

Hepatocellular Carcinoma

Risk: Cirrhosis (of any cause)
- Increased risk with chronic hepatitis B/C, hereditary hemochromatosis
- Toxins (aflatoxin, alcohol, smoking)

Clinical: Generally asymptomatic, but have signs of chronic liver disease
- Can present as decompensated cirrhosis
- Other symptoms possible (weight loss, abdominal pain, palpable mass)
- Paraneoplastic:
    - Hypoglycemia (high metabolic demand, IGF-II secretion)
    - Erythrocytosis (EPO secretion)
    - Watery diarrhea

Diagnosis:
- Often picked up on US (screening, or incidental)
- CT/MRI can better characterize the type of lesion
- AFP
- Biopsy if diagnosis uncertain

Management:
- Surgery (resection)
    - Often not possible due to underlying cirrhosis/invasion of tumor
- Ablation, TACE (transarterial chemoembolization), radiotherapy
    - Used for local unresectable disease
- Extrahepatic metastasis
    - Systemic therapy (Sorafenib)

Other Liver Masses

Hepatic Adenoma	- Benign epithelial liver tumors tumors found in young woman - Associated with OCP, anabolics, pregnancy - Generally asymptomatic, but can present with RUQ fullness - Dx: US/CT/MRI - Tx: Surgically resect if > 5 cm or symptomatic tumors. Others can be monitored. Risk for rupture/hemorrhage.
Cavernous Hemangioma	- Common, congenital vascular tumor - Generally asymptomatic, but can cause RUQ pain/mass - Dx: US/CT/MRI - Tx: Large (> 5 cm) or symptomatic are resected. Others observed.
Focal Nodular Hyperplasia	- Benign liver mass without malignant potential - Occurs in reproductive age women (no OCP correlation) - US/CT/MRI (central scar, hyperattenuation on arterial phase CT) - Management: Reassurance
Angiosarcoma	- High-grade malignant vascular neoplasm - Associated with vinyl chloride, arsenic, thorium, anabolic steroids

LIVER MASSES

Gastrointestinal Medicine

Liver Cysts

Etiology	Characteristics
Simple Cyst	- Simple, uniform, clear fluid containing cystic lesions - Generally asymptomatic, but can cause RUQ fullness if large - US and CT (w/ contrast) can help characterize - Tx: Conservative monitoring if asymptomatic. Larger cysts can receive needle drainage with injection of sclerosing agent (ie EtOH).
Polycystic Liver	- Multiple liver cysts seen in patients with ADPKD
Hydatid Liver Cyst	- Acquired from *Echinococcus granulosus*, a dog tapeworm - Humans ingest eggs ⟶ Hatch and migrate to liver - Generally asymptomatic, but as cyst grows can cause mild RUQ pain, nausea, hepatomegaly - Dx: US/CT/MRI (see cyst with internal septa and calcifications). Serologic (ELISA) testing also used. - Tx: Albendazole, plus percutaneous or surgical drainage of lesions > 5 cm

Liver Abscess

Etiology	Characteristics

Pyogenic	- Bacterial liver abscess, seen in patients with spread from bacterial peritonitis or systemic infection
	- Clinically presents as abdominal pain, fever, and other nonspecific findings (nausea. vomit, etc)
	- Diagnosis: US/CT, followed by aspiration gram stain/culture
	- Management:
	   Antibiotics: Ceftriaxone plus Metronidazole or beta-lactam/inhibitor
	   Drainage: Percutaneous needle, catheter, or surgical drainage

Amebic	- Caused by intestinal amebiasis (*Entamoeba histolytica*), which invades the portal vein - Presents as weeks of RUQ pain, fever, nausea, vomiting - Possible concurrent or prior history of dysentery - Dx: US/CT/MRI. Plus serology (ELISA IgG). - Tx: Metronidazole + Paromomycin (for intraluminal cysts) *Surgical aspiration dangerous due to rupture risk

DIARRHEA — Gastrointestinal Medicine

Acute Diarrhea

General: Most cases of acute diarrhea are infectious/viral, but bacterial causes can result in more severe presentations requiring hospitalization
- "Dysentery" is diarrhea plus visible blood and mucous

Clinical: > 3 loose, watery bowel movements per day for < 14 days

Diagnosis: Clinical diagnosis
- Further workup (ie stool cultures) if:
  - Severe illness (hospitalized for any reason, hypovolemic, etc)
  - Blood, mucous, or fevers > 100.4°F present
  - High risk (age > 70, immunocompromised, etc)
- Consider *C. diff*, Ova/Parasite testing if indicated by clinical scenario

Management:
- Supportive (fluids, Ondansetron, Loperamide, etc) for most
- Antibiotics (Azithromycin or fluoroquinolone) if sick, including:
  - Severe disease, bloody or mucoid stool, immunocompromised, or age > 70

DDx of Infectious Diarrhea

Bug	Source	Clinical Clues
Watery Diarrhea		
Norovirus	- Fecal-oral (food or water)	- Outbreaks in health care, restaurants, schools, military
Rotavirus	- Fecal-oral (food or water)	- Daycare, young children
ETEC	- Fecal-oral (food or water)	- Travel to endemic areas (usually resource-limited areas)
Clostridium perfringens	- Infected meats and poultry	
Staph aureus	- Spoiled mayo, dairy	
Bacillus cereus	- Reheated rice	
Listeria	- Processed meats, cheeses	- Immunocompromised, pregnancy
Giardia	- Fecally contaminated water	- Travel, hiking, camping, pools
Cryptosporidium	- Infected fruit/vegetables	- Immunocompromised
Inflammatory Diarrhea		
Salmonella	- Meats, eggs, fish, produce	- Animal contact (especially petting zoos, reptiles)
Shigella	- Raw vegetables	- Daycare, resource-limited settings
Campylobacter	- Meats, unpasteurized milk	- Animal contact (puppies/kittens) - Resource-limited settings
EHEC	- Meats, unpasteurized milk	- Daycare, Nursing homes
Yersinia	- Pork	
Vibrio	- Raw shellfish	- Cirrhosis
Entamoeba	- Fecally contaminated food or water	- Resource-limited settings

DIARRHEA
Gastrointestinal Medicine

Clostridioides difficile Infection

General: Nosocomial infection from overgrowth of *C. difficile*, most commonly after alteration of normal gut flora. Produce toxins (A/B) which mucosal inflammation and injury. NAP1/BI/027 hypervirulent strain gaining increased recognition for outbreaks.

Risk: Recent antibiotic therapy, increased age, chronic PPI
- Commonly implicated: Fluoroquinolone, Penicillin, and Clindamycin

Clinical:
- CDAD (*C. diff* associated diarrhea): Diarrhea (> 3 watery stools a day), LLQ abdominal cramping/pain, fever, leukocytosis
- Fulminant Colitis: Above, plus severe pain, distension, hypovolemia

Diagnosis: (Controversial and varies between institution)
- ELISA for GDH, Toxin A/B
- PCR can be used for equivocal toxin results
- Endoscopy generally not required (but can find classic pseudomembranes)

Management:

Class	Criteria (no consensus)	Treatment
Nonsevere	- Otherwise healthy patients	- Oral Vancomycin (alternative agent Fidaxomicin) - For recurrent disease, can taper prolonged oral vancomycin course
Severe	- WBC > 15 K - Albumin < 3 - Cr ≥ 1.5x baseline	- Oral Vancomycin For Refractory/Recurrent: - Fidaxomicin - Vancomycin (PO) + Metronidazole - Fecal transplant
Fulminant	- Peritoneal signs, signs of megacolon, etc - WBC > 15 K and ↑↑ Lactate	- Vancomycin (PO) + Metronidazole - Colectomy

Toxic Megacolon

General: Nonobstructive colonic dilatation and systemic toxicity

Etiology: Complication of IBD or infectious colitis

Clinical: Severe, bloody diarrhea and systemic toxicity (see criteria below)

Diagnosis: Typically diagnosed with the following:
- Radiographic colonic distension (plain XR) PLUS (3 of the following)
    - HR > 120, Temp > 38°C, Anemia, Neutrophils > 10.5K
- Dehydration/altered mentation/hypotension also common

Management:
- Supportive (fluids, NPO, antibiotics, NG decompression)
- If supportive care fails → Subtotal colectomy

DIARRHEA — Gastrointestinal Medicine

Chronic Diarrhea

Clinical: ≥ 3 loose or watery stools daily lasting ≥ 4 weeks

Etiology	Clinical	Workup
Secretory (stool osmotic gap < 50 mOsm/kg)		
Microscopic Colitis	- Chronic inflammatory disease of colon resulting in chronic, watery secretory diarrhea - Confirmed via biopsy	- Exclude infection (stool culture, O/P) - Exclude structural causes (CT, colonoscopy) - Cholestyramine trial (to rule out bile acid malabsorption) - Plasma peptides (gastrin, VIP) - Urine 5-HIAA
Neuroendocrine Tumor	- Includes VIPoma and gastrinoma	
Bile Acid Malabsorption	- Associated with diseases of the terminal ileum (ie Crohn's) or surgical removal of the ileum	
Postsurgical (post-cholecystectomy)	- Excess bile acids entering GI tract, irritating colon, resulting in secretory diarrhea - Improves with bile acid resins	
Non-osmotic Laxatives	- Senna, docusate	
Osmotic (stool osmotic gap > 125 mOsm/kg)		
Lactose Intolerance	- Carbohydrate malabsorption leading to osmotic diarrhea	- Stool osmotic gap - Fasting (should correct issue if truly osmotic)
Osmotic Laxatives	- PEG	
Inflammatory		
IBD	- See IBD section - Fecal calprotectin can suggest diagnosis, confirm with colonoscopy with biopsy	- Stool culture, O/P - Fecal WBCs - Fecal calprotectin
Chronic Infection	- *C. difficile, Campylobacter, Giardia, Cryptosporidium*, etc	
Malabsorption		
Chronic Pancreatitis	- All present with greasy, floating stools	- Quantitative stool fat - Fecal elastase
SIBO		
Celiac Sprue		
Functional		
IBS	- Chronic crampy abdominal pain and diarrhea	- Diagnosis of exclusion
Medications		
Drug Side Effects	- Antibiotics, SSRIs, PPIs	

CONSTIPATION
Gastrointestinal Medicine

Constipation

Etiology:
- Primary (functional): From slow transit, dyssynergic defecation, or IBS
- Secondary:
    - Mechanical (mass, cancer, stricture, etc)
    - Drugs (opiates, antihypertensives)
    - Lifestyle (low fiber, dehydration)
    - Neurologic (spinal cord injury, MS, parkinsonism, others)

Clinical: Defined by ≥ 2 of the following
- Hard lumpy stools
- Sensation of incomplete evacuation
- Need to use digital maneuvers
- Straining with bowel movements
- Decrease in stool frequency

Management:
- Lifestyle Modification (all): Defecate when motility the highest (after meals, mornings), increase dietary fiber
- Laxatives (see below)

Class	Examples
Bulk Forming	- Psyllium - Methylcellulose
Osmotic	- Polyethylene glycol - Lactulose - Magnesium-based
Stimulant	- Bisacodyl - Senna - Docusate (poor efficacy)
Severe Constipation	
Suppositories	- Bisacodyl
Enema	- Warm water - Mineral oil
Manual Disimpaction	

NEONATAL/CONGENITAL GI

Gastrointestinal
Pediatrics, Surgery

Meconium

General: Meconium is normally passed within 24 hours after birth. If passed in the uterus, risk for fetal meconium aspiration. If passed > 24 hours, concerning for one of the following conditions:

	Meconium Ileus	**Hirschsprung's**
Gen	- Obstruction from inspissated meconium in the ileum - Highly associated with CF	- Megacolon due to lack of ganglion cells in distal segment of colon (failed neural crest migration) - Associated with trisomy 21, but most often an isolated finding
Clin	- Delayed meconium, feeding intolerance, biliary vomiting	- Delayed meconium (> 48 hours), signs of complete bowel obstruction (abdominal distension, vomiting) (+) Squirt sign: Rectal exam relieves obstruction with rapid emptying - Associated with GU/CV anomalies, hearing/visual defects
Dx	- XR (to rule out dangerous pathology), followed by contrast enema (generally shows microcolon throughout colon)	- Contrast enema (Transition zone: Aganglionic area thin, dilated area proximally, generally in rectosigmoid) - Rectal suction biopsy (full thickness): Confirmatory
Tx	- Gastrografin enema (diagnostic/therapeutic)	- Colonic resection with anastomosis

Necrotizing Enterocolitis

General: Ischemic necrosis of GI mucosa, with transmural inflammation, infection with gas producing organisms, and dissection of gas

Risk: Preterm, low birth weight, antibiotics, early exposure to non-human milk. If term, associated with congenital heart disease, sepsis, hypotension.

Clinical:
- Feeding intolerance, abdominal distension, hematochezia
- Lethargy, respiratory failure, other hemodynamic changes all possible
- XR: Pneumatosis intestinalis

Diagnosis: Clinical (based on findings above)

Management:
- Supportive: NPO, GI decompression, parenteral nutrition, fluid/electrolytes
- Broad spectrum IV antibiotics (ie Amp + Gentamicin + Metronidazole)
- Surgery (bowel resection): Indicated if perforation or deteriorating

NEONATAL/CONGENITAL GI
Gastrointestinal Pediatrics, Surgery

Bilious Emesis DDx/Workup

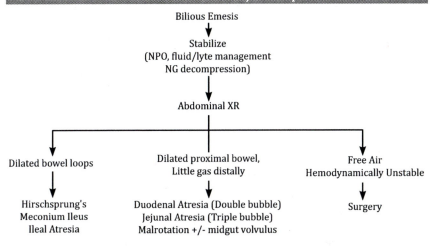

Intestinal Atresia

General: Congenital obstruction of the normally hollow GI tract. Can occur anywhere, but most frequently occurs at level of duodenum.

	Duodenal	Jejunal/Ileal
Gen	- Failure of duodenum to recannulate during embryogenesis	- Vascular disruption, leading to ischemic necrosis, with "apple peel" appearance
Risk	- Down's, other chromosomal abnormalities	- Cystic fibrosis, malrotation
Clin	- Emesis (+/- bilious), abdominal distension	- Bilious emesis, distension
Dx	- XR: Double-bubble (dilated stomach/proximal duodenum) - Upper GI series (rule out annular pancreas, malrotation, other similarly presenting pathologies)	- XR: Multiple dilated bowel loops, air-fluid levels - "Triple bubble" sign in jejunal atresia - Upper GI series/contrast enema
Tx	- Surgery within few days of birth (Duodenoduodenostomy)	- Surgery (resection/anastomosis)

GI51

NEONATAL/CONGENITAL GI
Gastrointestinal — Pediatrics, Surgery

Malrotation/Midgut Volvulus

General: Failure of the embryonic gut to complete normal rotation, with resulting improper positioning of bowel, and formation of fibrous adhesions ("Ladd's bands"). Often insidious until development of volvulus.

Risk: Often idiopathic, but can be associated with abdominal wall defects, intestinal atresia, diaphragmatic hernia, and other congenital GI malformations

Clinical:
- Highly variable and can present during infancy or early childhood
- Mild, nonspecific symptoms include vomiting, abd pain, failure to thrive

- Midgut Volvulus (bowel twists along SMA, causing ischemia/necrosis)
    - Presents with vomiting, severe abdominal pain, distension
    - Complicated by hematemesis/hematochezia, peritonitis, shock
    - Urgent surgery indicated if above complications present
- Duodenal obstruction also possible (from Ladd band adhesions)

Diagnosis:
- XR (initial, to rule out perforation)
- Upper GI series w/ contrast: Misplaced/corkscrew/obstructed duodenum

Management:

Malrotation	- Elective surgical correction (controversial, some recommend supportive care/observation)
Volvulus	- NG Decompression, broad spectrum antibiotics - Emergent surgery (Ladd's procedure: Remove adhesions, appendix, put small bowel on right and colon on left)

Biliary Atresia

General: Idiopathic, progressive, fibro-obliterative degeneration of the extrahepatic biliary system

Clinical:
- Initially normal, but development of conjugated hyperbilirubinemia at 1-8 weeks after birth
- Jaundice, acholic stools/dark urine, hepatomegaly

Diagnosis:
- Abdominal US (gallbladder often abnormally shaped)
- Hepatobiliary scintigraphy (tracer excretion rules out biliary atresia)
- Liver biopsy (expanded portal tracts with bile duct proliferation)
- Intraoperative cholangiogram (definitive diagnosis)

Management: Hepatoportoenterostomy (Kasai procedure)
- Postoperative ursodeoxycholic acid

NEONATAL/CONGENITAL GI
Gastrointestinal — Pediatrics, Surgery

Esophageal Atresia/Tracheoesophageal Fistula

General: Esophageal narrowing, which most often occurs with fistula formation between esophagus/trachea. Often occurs as part of VACTERL series of abnormalities.

Subtypes:
- A: Pure esophageal atresia
- B: Esophageal atresia with proximal TEF (rare)
- C: Esophageal atresia with distal TEF (most common)
- E: Pure TEF ("H-type")

Clinical:
- Polyhydramnios (if any degree of esophageal atresia)
- Excess secretions, drooling, choking, respiratory distress
- Air in stomach with TEF
- Cyanosis from laryngospasm

Diagnosis:
- Place NG tube ⟶ CXR
    - EA: Tube curled in chest
    - TEF: Air in stomach
- Contrast esophagram if unsure
- Screen for other VACTERL abnormalities

Management: Surgical (TEF ligation, with esophageal anastomosis)

Anorectal Malformations

General: Heterogenous group of disorders, ranging from stenosis of the anus, to completely imperforate anus with blind rectal pouch. Associated with VACTERL malformations.

Clinical:
- Failure to pass meconium
- Usually obvious on first physical examination

Diagnosis: Clinical, but pelvic XR can be used as an aid in uncertain cases

Management: Surgery (perineal anoplasty or colostomy)

NEONATAL/CONGENITAL GI
Gastrointestinal — Pediatrics, Surgery

Congenital Diaphragmatic Hernia

General: Congenital diaphragm defect in which abdominal contents herniate into the chest, compressing lung tissue, resulting in varying degrees of pulmonary hypoplasia. Defects most commonly left sided and posterior.

Clinical:
- Respiratory distress soon after birth
- Decreased left sided breath sounds, barrel-shaped chest

Diagnosis:
- In utero: US
- After birth: CXR (with abdominal contents in chest)

Management:
- Initial supportive care/stabilization
    - Intubation, NG decompression, fluid/electrolyte management
- Surgery: Surgical reduction + primary or patch repair
    - Delayed until medically stabilized (hope for some lung maturity)

Hypertrophic Pyloric Stenosis

General: Hypertrophy of the pylorus, resulting in stenosis of the gastric outlet

Risk: Family history, erythromycin use during pregnancy

Clinical:
- Projectile, nonbilious vomiting in healthy 4–8 week-old male
- "Olive shaped" mass RUQ
    - Possible retrograde peristaltic stomach waves
- Hypochloremic, hypokalemic metabolic alkalosis, dehydration

Diagnosis: Abdominal US
- Long, thick pylorus. Causes "doughnut sign."

Management:
- Volume resuscitation/electrolyte replacement
    - Medical stabilization vital before surgery
- Surgery: Pyloromyotomy (Ramstedt)
    - Mild vomiting/regurgitation common after surgery, but patients should start feeds

NEONATAL/CONGENITAL GI

Gastrointestinal — Pediatrics, Surgery

	General	Clinical	Management
Omphalocele	- Midline abdominal wall defect - Associated with trisomy 13/18/21, Turner's, and other chromosomal abnormalities	- Membranous herniation sac containing abdominal contents, most commonly at the site of cord insertion (cord inserts into membrane) - Easily diagnosed on prenatal US - Liver herniation/damage biggest concern	- Prenatal: Careful observation, C-section, with careful dressing at birth Surgical Closure - Small (2-3 cm) can be reduced and closed soon after birth - Larger (> 5 cm) should be placed in silo, allowed to naturally reduced, then surgically closed
Gastroschisis	- Full-thickness abdominal wall defect - ↑ risk for inflammation, bowel wall thickening, NEC	- Evisceration of bowel contents - Located periumbilically, usually on right, with normal cord insertion - ↑ Maternal AFP during pregnancy, picked up on fetal US	- Careful fetal monitoring during pregnancy. Deliver if signs of bowel ischemia/necrosis. - At birth: Sterile dressing, antibiotics, gastric decompression - Primary surgical closure (use silo if too large to reduce initially)
Bladder Exstrophy	- Embryological defect in abdominal wall development, resulting in outside exposure of bladder	- Exposure of bladder and urethra on the surface of the lower abdomen - Diagnosis made on prenatal US (or apparent at birth on PE)	- Properly dress opening at birth - Surgical repair weeks after birth
Umbilical Hernia	- Herniation through fascial opening that allows passage of umbilical vessels - Associated with hypothyroidism, prematurity, Beckwith-Wiedemann, Ehlers-Danlos	- Reducible paraumbilical sac - Usually asymptomatic - Very rarely rupture/strangulate	- Monitor (most spontaneously close) - Consider closing if > 5 years old or symptomatic - Surgical reduction if incarcerated or strangulated

NEONATAL/CONGENITAL GI
Gastrointestinal — Pediatrics, Surgery

Meckel's Diverticulum

General: True diverticulum (all bowel wall layers) of the small intestine, due to failure of obliteration of Vitelline duct
- Can contain heterotopic gastric tissue (most common) or pancreatic. HCl secretion can result in substantial amounts of bleeding.
- Rule of 2's
    - 2% prevalence, 2:1 boy:girls
    - 2 feet from ileocecal valve
    - 2 inches long
    - 2% get complications, usually before 2 y/o

Clinical:
- Most often asymptomatic
- Painless hematochezia is most common presentation
- Intussusception, volvulus, obstruction all possible

Diagnosis: Technetium-99 Scan ("Meckel's Scan")
- Other: Mesenteric arteriography (used especially during acute GI bleeds)

Management:
- Symptomatic: Surgery (diverticulectomy or small bowel resection)
- Asymptomatic (incidentally found): Controversial. Can either monitor or remove electively.

Intussusception

General: Telescoping of a part of the intestine into itself. Common pediatric issue (ie < 2 y/o), with decreased frequency at older ages.

Risk: Usually idiopathic, but can be associated with certain lead points, including mesenteric lymphadenopathy (postviral or rotavirus vax), Meckel's diverticulum, or tumor/mass

Clinical:
- Waxing/waning, cramping, severe abdominal pain
- 15 minute painful episodes, followed by asymptomatic periods
- Palpable mass, "currant jelly" stools (uncommon but pathognomonic)

Diagnosis: Abdominal US ("Bull's Eye" or "Target sign")

Management:
- Reduction with air enema (alt: water soluble contrast enema)
- Surgery: If evidence of perforation or refractory to multiple attempts at non-operative reduction

NEONATAL/CONGENITAL GI

Gastrointestinal
Pediatrics, Surgery

Pancreatic Malformations

Annular Pancreas	- Ring of pancreatic tissue surrounding the descending duodenum - Caused by failure of the ventral bud to rotate with the duodenum - Risk for pancreatic duct obstruction (pancreatitis) and duodenal obstruction - Dx: GI series or abdominal CT - Tx: Duodenoduodenostomy (ie bypass the annulus, do NOT resect)
Pancreatic Divisum	- Failure of fusion of the ventral and dorsal ducts - Usually asymptomatic. Possible ↑ risk for pancreatitis. - Picked up with abdominal imaging (ie CT or MRCP) - If severely symptomatic, can consider endoscopic sphincterotomy

Short Bowel Syndrome

General: Shortened small intestine, resulting in malabsorption/malnutrition and abnormal bowel function

Etiology: Any congenital lesion that requires small bowel resection (ie gastroschisis, volvulus, or intestinal atresia)

Clinical: Diarrhea, malabsorption, failure to thrive

Management: Long term TPN

Food Protein-Induced Enterocolitis Syndrome (FPIES)

General: Infantile food hypersensitivity, most commonly induced by protein in milk or soy (but rarely solid food)

Clinical: Often starts weeks after birth, either acutely with repetitive vomiting, diarrhea, dehydration, or more insidiously with weight loss/failure to thrive

Diagnosis: Clinical, plus confirmed improvement after withdrawal of suspected trigger

Management: Dietary elimination of triggering substance, generally resolves by 3 y/o

Gastroesophageal Reflux

General: Normal spit-up caused by short esophagus, immature gastroesophageal sphincter. Note: Not called "disease" because no pathologic consequences, such as weight loss, esophagitis, etc.

Clinical: Frequent regurgitation events after feeding
- No warning signs, such as failure to thrive, GI bleeding, forceful vomiting

Management: Education/reassurance
- Frequent small volume feeds, upright position for 20-30 min after
- Thickening formula/breast milk if symptoms bothersome
- Should resolve spontaneously by 1 y/o
- PPIs only indicated if some degree of esophagitis

GI PHARM

Gastrointestinal Medicine

	Mechanism	Indication	Side Effects/Management
Anti-ulcer			

PPIs
Omeprazole
Lansoprazole
Esomeprazole
Pantoprazole
Dexlansoprazole
	- Irreversible inhibition of the H+/K+ ATPase	- GERD
		- Gastritis/PUD
		- Esophagitis
		- *H. pylori* eradication
			- Short Term: Generally well tolerated, can cause diarrhea
			- Long Term:
			  - Hypomagnesemia, other nutrient malabsorption
			  - Increased risk of *C. Difficile* infection, pneumonia
			  - ↓ Calcium absorption, ↑ fracture risk

H₂ Antagonist Cimetidine Ranitidine Famotidine	- Competitive antagonist of the H₂ receptor, resulting in decreased stomach acid	- GERD - Gastritis/PUD - Esophagitis	- Cimetidine (CYP450 inhibitor, anti-androgen, headache, mental status changes) - Others are well tolerated
Bismuth	- Binds to ulcers, may suppress *H. pylori* growth	- Quadruple therapy (*H. Pylori*)	- Blackens stool
Sucralfate	- Binds to areas of mucosal damage and promotes healing	- GERD, PUD (second line agent)	- Can bind other drugs
Al hydroxide Ca carbonate Mg hydroxide	- Neutralize gastric acid and reduce acid delivery to the duodenum	- GERD (used for short-term symptomatic management of mild disease)	- Hypophosphatemia - Hypercalcemia, Milk-alkali syndrome - Diarrhea
Antiemetics			
Ondansetron	- 5-HT3 antagonist	- Antiemetic	- Headache - QT Prolonging
Metoclopramide Prochlorperazine Droperidol	- D2 antagonist	- Antiemetic - Gastroparesis (metoclopramide)	- QT prolonging - Dystonia, parkinsonism
Aprepitant Fosaprepitant	- NK1 antagonists	- Antiemetic	- CYP inhibitor

GI58

GI PHARM — Gastrointestinal Medicine

	Mechanism	Indication	Side Effects/Management
Anti-constipation (see laxatives in constipation section)			
Lubiprostone	- Chloride channel activator that increases intestinal fluid secretion	- Constipation predominant IBS	
Linaclotide	- Guanylate cyclase agonists that stimulates intestinal fluid secretion	- Constipation predominant IBS	
Methylnaltrexone	- Mu receptor antagonist, limited blood brain barrier penetrance	- Constipation associated with opiate use	
Anti-diarrheal			
Loperamide Diphenoxylate	- Mu-receptor opiate agonists	- Diarrhea	- QT prolonging
Others			
Ursodiol	- Non-toxic bile acid (increases bile secretion)	- Primary biliary cirrhosis - Gallstone prevention	

GI59

ANEMIA

Hematology/Oncology Medicine

Anemia Overview

Definition: Hgb < 12 g/dL in women, < 13.5 g/dL in men

Clinical: Varies from asymptomatic to vague symptoms (weakness, fatigue, dyspnea)
- Skin or conjunctival pallor

Diagnostic Tests:
- MCV (average volume of RBC, see below)
- MCH (mean corpuscular hemoglobin)
- MCHC (mean corpuscular hemoglobin concentration)
- Reticulocyte Count
  - Correction= Retic % x (Pts Hematocrit/Normal Hematocrit)
- Blood smear (look for morphologic abnormalities)
  - Hypochromia: Iron deficiency
  - Spherocytes: Spherocytosis, autoimmune hemolytic anemia
  - Targets: Thalassemia
  - Dacrocytes (tear-drop): Marrow fibrosis
  - Acanthocytes: Liver disease
  - Schistocytes: Hemolysis

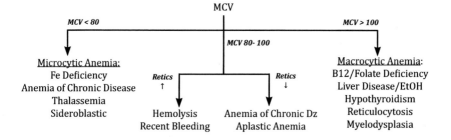

Evaluation of Iron Studies

	Serum Fe	Ferritin	TIBC	Smear
Fe Deficiency	↓	↓	↑	Hypochromic Cells
Chronic Disease	↓	↑	↓	
Thalassemia	↔/↑	↔/↑	↔	Target Cells
Sideroblastic	↑	↑	↔	Ringed Sideroblasts

Heme1

MICROCYTIC ANEMIA

Hematology/Oncology Medicine

	General/Etiology	Clinical	Diagnosis	Treatment
Fe Deficiency	- Bleeding - ↓ Fe Absorption (ie Celiac's, bariatric surgery, gastritis) - Redistribution (post EPO) - Poor diet (mostly kids) - ↑ utilization (pregnancy)	- Pica, ice-craving - Associated with restless leg	- See Fe studies chart - ↑ RDW, ↓ MCH/MCHC	- PO iron supplements (watch for GI side effects) - IV iron (now utilized with increased frequency)
Sideroblastic	Acquired: - EtOH, Isoniazid, lead - Myelodysplastic syndromes Genetic: - Most commonly XL-SA from mutation in ALA-Synthase (part of heme synthesis)	- Nonspecific	- Bone marrow biopsy (ringed sideroblasts) - Genetic tests if suspect genetic basis	- Acquired: Correct underlying etiology - Genetic: Vitamin B6, manage anemia/iron overload
Anemia of Chronic Inflammation	- Chronic anemia from increased hepcidin (acute phase reactant) Seen in those with: - Malignancy - Infection - Chronic inflammation	- Generally mild and asymptomatic	- Normocytic or slight microcytic anemia - Low reticulocyte count - Nl/↑ ferritin, ↓ serum Fe	- Treat underlying condition - EPO can be attempted in those with low Hgb (< 10) and no malignancy

MICROCYTIC ANEMIA
Hematology/Oncology Medicine

Alpha-Thalassemia

General: Abnormality in the alpha globin gene on chromosome 16

Gene	Name	Clinical
aa/a-	Trait or Minima	- Silent carrier, normal H/H
aa/-- or a-/a-	Minor	- Minor, asymptomatic anemia
a-/--	HbH (β4 tetramers form, causing hemolysis)	- Hemolytic anemia, with ineffective RBC production - Jaundice, splenomegaly - Skeletal abnormalities
--/--	Barts (γ4 tetramers)	- Fetal hydrops/incompatible with life

Diagnosis:
- Suspected with hypochromic, microcytic anemia, with abnormal smears
    - Target cells, poikilocytosis, on smear
- Confirmed with hemoglobin analysis and/or genetic testing

Management:
- Folate supplementation
- HbH disease can have moderate to severe anemia that requires transfusions

Beta-Thalassemia

General: Abnormality in the beta-globin gene on chromosome 11

Gene	Name	Clinical
β / β°	Minor	- Mild microcytic anemia
β+/β+	Intermedia	- Moderate microcytic anemia
β°/β° β°/β+	Major	- Severe anemia, transfusion dependent - Skeletal deformities (bossing, premature fusion, osteopenia, marrow expansion) - Hepatosplenomegaly - Growth abnormalities

*Presentation delayed until ~6 months due to fetal hemoglobin (vs alpha thal)

Diagnosis:
- Suspected with hypochromic, microcytic anemia, with abnormal smears
- Confirmed with hemoglobin analysis and/or genetic testing
    - $HgA_2 > 4\%$

Management:
- Folate supplementation
- For Major: Chronic transfusions (watch for secondary iron overload)
    - Splenectomy and stem cell transplant can be considered

Heme3

MACROCYTIC ANEMIA
Hematology/Oncology Medicine

B12/Folate Deficiency

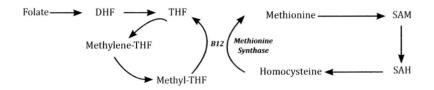

	Folate	B12
Source	- Many meat and vegetables - Fortified in food (first world)	- Meat products (meat, eggs, dairy)
Absorp	- Jejunum	- Haptocorrin in saliva binds B12 - Acid knocks off haptocorrin in stomach - Intrinsic factor binds in duodenum - B12-IF absorbed in ileum
Etio	- Malnutrition (EtOH, elderly) - Increased use (pregnancy, hemolysis) - Malabsorption (celiac, bypass) - Meds (MTX, TMP, etc)	- Pernicious anemia - Poor diet (year long stores, but can develop in alcoholism or serious vegans) - Bariatric surgery - Fish tapeworm

Clin	- Megaloblastic anemia	- Megaloblastic anemia
		- CNS (subacute combined degeneration)
		  - Neuropathy
		  - Neuropsychiatric changes

Dx	- Measure B12/folate levels - If equivocal, use MMA/homocysteine (Both ↑ in B12 deficiency, just homocysteine in folate deficiency)	
Tx	- Oral folate	- Oral B12 - IV/IM B12 for severe disease

Other Causes of Macrocytosis

- Hypothyroidism
- EtOH
- Liver disease
- Reticulocytosis
- Drug-induced (Dapsone, Methotrexate, Phenytoin)
- Myelodysplasia
    - Note: Isolated macrocytosis without anemia is often a sign of MDS

NORMOCYTIC ANEMIA
Hematology/Oncology Medicine

Aplastic Anemia

General: Pancytopenia secondary to bone marrow hypoplasia

Etiology:
- Cytotoxic drugs/radiation
- Drugs (Carbamazepine, Methimazole)
- Virus (EBV, HIV, parvo [RBC only], hepatitis A-E)
- Autoimmune disease (ie SLE)

Clinical: Symptoms from pancytopenia
- Bleeding/bruising
- Infection
- Anemia (normocytic)

Diagnosis: Confirmation with bone marrow biopsy (hypocellular BM)
- If likely reversible cause is present, can correct and monitor prior to biopsy

Management:
- Stop offending agent
- Transfuse as necessary
- Bone marrow stimulation
- If severe:
    - HCT (if < 50 y/o and otherwise healthy)
    - Immunosuppression (if not qualified for HCT)

Anemia as a Complication of CKD

General: Normocytic anemia from the lack of EPO production from the peritubular capillaries

Management:
- EPO: Generally given to CKD patients with Hgb < 10
    - Hgb goal is 10-11.5 g/dL

NORMOCYTIC ANEMIA

Hematology/Oncology Medicine

Hemolysis (Overview)

General: Premature destruction of RBCs, resulting in normocytic anemia with elevated reticulocyte count

Etiology:

Extrinsic	Intrinsic
- Autoimmune hemolytic anemia - Microangiopathic HA - Mechanical (mechanical valve, AS)	- Sickle Cell - Spherocytosis - PNH - G6PD Deficiency

Clinical:

	Intravascular	Extravascular
Pathophys	- Vascular RBC destruction	- Splenic destruction of RBC
LDH	↑	↑
Haptoglobin	↓↓	↓/↔
Indirect Bili	↑	↑
Urine	Hemoglobinuria ↑ Urobilinogen	↑ Urobilinogen

Note: Features often overlap as these disorders have components of both intravascular and extravascular hemolysis

Autoimmune Hemolytic Anemia

	IgG ("warm")	IgM ("cold")
Etio	- SLE - CLL, lymphoma - Drug (Penicillins, Methyldopa)	- Infection (Mycoplasma, EBV) - Lymphoproliferative disorders
Clin	- Various degrees of anemia - Spherocytes on smear	- Various degrees of anemia - Livedo reticularis - Acral cyanosis
Dx	- Direct Coombs (positive for IgG +/- C3)	- Direct Coombs (positive for C3 or IgM)
Tx	- Corticosteroids (first-line) - Rituximab, cytotoxic immunosuppression (next line) - Splenectomy if refractory	- Avoidance of cold (mild disease) - Rituximab

NORMOCYTIC ANEMIA

Hematology/Oncology
Medicine, Pediatrics

	General	Clinical	Diagnosis	Treatment
Hereditary Spherocytosis	- AD defects in RBC structural proteins (ie ankyrin, spectrin, band-3) - Causes spherocytosis and chronic extravascular hemolysis	- Hemolytic anemia - Jaundice - Splenomegaly - ↑ MCHC, reticulocytes, RDW, spherocytes on smear	- Eosin-5-maleimide binding test (confirmatory) - Osmotic fragility no longer used	- Folate - Transfusions as necessary - Splenectomy
G6PD Deficiency	- XR disorder in the glucose-6 phosphate dehydrogenase enzyme - Hemolysis precipitated by oxidant stress (Infection, drugs [sulfonamides, primaquine], fava beans)	- Episodic hemolytic anemia - Blood smear with "bite cells" and Heinz bodies	- G6PD enzyme assay (fluorescent spot test screen, followed by quantitative NADPH calculation) (Note: Can be negative during acute episode)	- Avoidance of triggers - Supportive care (ie transfuse as necessary) during episodes
Paroxysmal Nocturnal Hemoglobinuria	- Acquired defect in the GPI molecule (a phospholipid anchor for surface proteins) - Results in lack of CD55 (blocks splenic extravascular hemolysis) and CD59 (blocks complement) on RBCs	- Chronic hemolysis with normocytic anemia - Pancytopenia - Thrombosis - Smooth muscle dystonia (abdominal pain, erectile dysfunction, pulm HTN) - Renal insufficiency	- Flow cytometry (for CD55/59)	- Eculizumab (complement inhibitor) - HCT

Heme7

NORMOCYTIC ANEMIA
Hematology/Oncology — Medicine, Pediatrics

Sickle Cell Anemia

General: AR condition in Hgb beta chain, which results in HbS replacing HbA. Point mutation (Glutamic acid → Valine) which promotes Hgb polymerization, especially under conditions of stress (ie acidemia, hypoxia, dehydration, infection).

Clinical: Chronic hemolytic anemia
- Variety of complications (see next page)

Diagnosis:
- Hgb Analysis (via HPLC, gel electrophoresis, or isoelectric focusing)
    - Provides information about Hgb distribution (see chart below)
- Prenatal diagnosis made by genetic testing

Management:
- Avoid crisis precipitators (ie stay hydrated, avoid high altitudes, etc)
- Vaccinations (including pneumococcal, flu, HIB, meningococcal)
- Folate supplementation
- Antibiotic PPX (until at least age 5): Penicillin (alt: Erythromycin)
- Hydroxyurea (↑ HgbF) is recommended in most children and adults that suffer from recurrent occlusive crises
- Selective use of RBC transfusion
- Severe, refractory disease: Consider HCT

Sickle Cell Trait

General: Carrier of one mutated Hgb beta gene. Patients have significant amounts of both HgbA and HgbS.

Clinical: Generally asymptomatic, but the following complications can occur:
- Hematuria (due to renal papillary infarcts)
- Hyposthenuria (abnormal urinary concentration, leading to polyuria)
- Renal medullary carcinoma
- Splenic infarct (esp at high altitude)

Hemoglobin Distribution (> 5 y/o)

Disorder	Hgb	HgbA	HgbA2	HgbF	HgbS	HgbC
Normal	AA	95%	3%	< 2%	-	-
Sickle Cell Disease	SS	0	3%	5-15%	> 85%	-
Sickle Trait	AS	> 50%	3%	< 2%	30-40%	
HgbSC Disease	SC	0%	3%	< 5%	45%	45%
β-Thalassemia Minor	Aβ	90%	> 3.5%	< 2%	-	-
β-Thalassemia Major	ββ	0%	> 3.5%	> 90%	-	-
Sickle-Beta Thal	Sβ	0%	> 3.5%	10-15%	> 80%	-

NORMOCYTIC ANEMIA
Hematology/Oncology
Medicine, Pediatrics

Complications of Sickle Cell

	Clinical	Management
Pain Crisis	- Acute episode of severe pain due to vaso-occlusion - Can occur anywhere in body, but dactylitis is common (especially in kids) - Often preceded by trigger - Purely clinical diagnosis	- Hydration (oral or IV) - Opioid pain medication
Splenic Sequestration Crisis	- Occlusion in the spleens of kids that have not undergone complete fibrosis - Traps large volumes of blood in the spleen - Presents as LUQ pain, splenomegaly, worsening anemia, hypovolemic shock	- Transfusion - Elective splenectomy after episode has resolved
Aplastic Crisis	- Acute drop in reticulocyte %, leading to worsening anemia - Most commonly due to parvo B19, but other etiologies possible	- Supportive transfusions
Acute Chest Syndrome	- New pulmonary infiltrate, along with fever/respiratory symptoms - Multifactorial etiology, but likely due to some combination of ischemia, infarction, atelectasis, and infection	- Fluids, pain control - Broad spectrum antibiotics (to cover for pneumonia, which often can't be ruled out) - Bronchodilator treatments - Transfusion

Other Complications:

GI	- Bilirubin gallstones
ID	- ↑ infection risk (due to hyposplenism, progressive splenic autoinfarction)
MSK	- Avascular necrosis (chronic, progressive pain compared to acute pain episodes) - Osteomyelitis (*Salmonella*) - Chronic leg ulcers
Renal	- Renal insufficiency, hematuria
GU	- Priapism
CNS	- Stroke (cerebral thrombosis) - Can screen with transcranial doppler

DISORDERS OF HEME SYNTHESIS

Hematology/Oncology
Medicine, Pediatrics

Lead Poisoning

General: Exposure to lead, leading to systemic toxicity, including abnormal heme synthesis (via inhibition of ferrochelatase and ALA-dehydratase)

	Children	Adults
Etio	- GI Exposure (paint, food/water, breast milk if mom has ↑ lead)	- Pulmonary Exposure (gas, paint, gun powder, moonshine, etc)
Clin	- Neurologic/behavioral changes - Encephalopathy/hearing loss at extremely high levels - Abdominal pain, renal insufficiency	- Abdominal pain - Neurologic (poor concentration, memory problems) - Anemia (+/- basophilic stippling) - Nephropathy
Dx	- Measure blood lead level (> 5mcg/dL abnormal)	
Tx	< 45 mcg/dL: Confirm level, removal from exposure, family education 45-70 mcg/dL: Above, plus chelation with succimer > 70 mcg/dL: Succimer + EDTA	< 40 mcg/dL: Remove exposure 40-80 mcg/dL: Remove exposure, consider chelation > 80 mcg/dL: Chelation

Chelation agents: DMSA (Succimer) generally preferred. CaNa2EDTA/Penicillamine are alternative agents. EDTA and Dimercaprol used if child has encephalopathy.

Porphyria

	Acute Intermittent Porphyria	Porphyria Cutanea Tarda
Gen	↓ porphobilinogen deaminase activity - Episodes triggered by stress, fasts, EtOH, smoking, estrogen, certain drugs	↓ uroporphyrinogen decarboxylase activity - Associated with HIV, Hep C, smoking, EtOH, estrogen use
Clin	- Neurologic dysfunction (peripheral neuropathy, autonomic dysfunction [tachycardia, tremors, sweating]) - Abdominal pain - Dark urine	- Blisters, bullae to photoexposed skin - Scarring, with pigmentation changes - Transaminitis
Dx	- Urinary porphobilinogen	- Increased plasma/urine porphyrin
Tx	- Supportive care during episodes - Hemin administration - Avoid triggers	- Phlebotomy plus low dose hydroxychloroquine

THROMBOCYTOPENIA — Hematology/Oncology Medicine

Overview of Thrombocytopenia

General: Platelet count < 150K/mm^3. Generally asymptomatic, but severe (< 50K) have elevated risk for bleeding. Can be due to increased destruction, decreased production, or sequestration.

Etiology:

Autoimmune	- ITP - SLE, RA
Consumption	- HUS/TTP, DIC, HIT
Production	- Bone marrow failure (presents as pancytopenia) - Myelodysplasia - B12/Folate deficiency
Drug Induced	- NSAIDs - Sulfa drugs - IIb/IIIa inhibitors - Heparin - Quinine - EtOH
Infection	- HIV, Hep C, EBV
Genetic	- Bernard Soulier (AR Defect in GPIb-IX) - Glanzmann Thrombasthenia (AR Defect in GPIIb-IIIa)
Sequestration	- Seen with hypersplenism, portal hypertension
Pseudo	- Pseudothrombocytopenia (platelet clumping, resulting in abnormal test)

Special Scenarios:
- Malignancy (bone marrow invasion or DIC)
- Pregnancy (gestational thrombocytopenia, preeclampsia, HELLP)
- Liver failure (↓ TPO, splenic sequestration)

Clinical:
- Superficial bleeding (petechiae, purpura, mucosal bleeding)
- Epistaxis, menorrhagia

Management:
- Avoidance of aspirin/NSAIDs
- Generally want platelets > 50K prior to procedure
- Platelet transfusion
  - Active bleeding with count < 50K OR any person < 10K

THROMBOCYTOPENIA
Hematology/Oncology
Medicine, Pediatrics

Immune Thrombocytopenic Purpura

General: Auto-antibody formation against host platelet glycoproteins, resulting in removal of platelets by splenic macrophages. The disorder tends to be acute and self-limited in children, but chronic and relapsing in adults.

Etiology:
- Primary: Idiopathic, generally occurs after viral infection
- Secondary: HIV, HCV, SLE, CLL

Clinical: Generally asymptomatic, but can develop bleeding (purpura, petechiae, and mucosal bleeding like epistaxis)

Diagnosis: Isolated thrombocytopenia with normal smear (+ for megakaryocytes)
- Primary ITP: Diagnosis of exclusion
- Secondary ITP: Thrombocytopenia in someone with associated condition

Management:

Adult	
Acute	
Platelets > 30K	- Observe
Platelets < 30K or Severe Bleeding	- Glucocorticoids (alt: IVIG) - Severe bleeds should receive combo of steroids, IVIG, platelet transfusion
Chronic	
Refractory to initial therapy	- Rituximab - Romiplostim or Eltrombopag - Splenectomy
Children	
Life-threatening/severe-bleeding OR Desire for rapid rise in platelets	- Steroids, IVIG +/- platelet transfusion
Asymptomatic or minimal symptoms	- Monitor

THROMBOCYTOPENIA
Hematology/Oncology Medicine

Thrombotic Microangiopathy

	Thrombotic Thrombocytopenic Purpura	Hemolytic Uremic Syndrome
Gen	- Deficiency or autoantibody to ADAMS T13, which normally cleaves VWF multimers	- Released toxin promotes thrombogenesis over the endothelium
Etio	- Often idiopathic, can be related to SLE, HIV, drugs, and pregnancy - Rarely hereditary	- Shiga-toxin *E. Coli* (90%) - Acquired complement deficiency, pneumococcus rarer causes
Clin	- Microangiopathic HA - Thrombocytopenia - Neurologic dysfunction (HA, confusion, focal deficits) - AKI less common	- Microangiopathic HA - Thrombocytopenia - AKI - STEC: Prodrome of bloody diarrhea and abdominal pain
Dx	- Clinical diagnosis (hemolysis, thrombocytopenia, etc) - ADAMS T13 activity assay	- Clinical diagnosis (classic prodrome followed by above triad)
Tx	- Urgent plasma exchange w/ FFP - Glucocorticoids - Variety of immunosuppressants used for refractory disease	- Supportive care (fluids, electrolyte management) - Transfusions (RBC, platelets if severe bleeding) - Dialysis for severe renal failure

Heparin Induced Thrombocytopenia

General: Immune-mediated complication of Heparin, due to autoantibodies against platelet factor-4 (in type 2)
- Type 1: Transient drop in platelet count, self-limited (can continue Heparin)
- Type 2: More severe form, with the clinical manifestations seen below

Clinical: "4 T's"
- Timing: > 5 days from exposure (can be sooner with previous heparin use)
- Thrombocytopenia: Platelet reduction > 50% from baseline
- Thrombosis: Arterial or venous thrombosis
- Other causes not apparent
- Necrotic skin lesions at injection sites

Diagnosis:
- Clinical diagnosis (stop Heparin if suspicion)
- ELISA immunoassay (alt: Serotonin release assay)

Management:
- Stop Heparin products
- Start direct thrombin inhibitor (ie Argatroban)

| COAGULOPATHY | Hematology/Oncology Medicine, Pediatrics |

von Willebrand Disease

General: AD disorder characterized by deficiency or defect of vWF. Most common inherited coagulopathy. Subtypes:
- Type 1 (most common): Decreased levels of vWF
- Type 2 (less common): Qualitative abnormalities of vWF
- Type 3 (least common): Absent vWF (most severe form)

Clinical:
- Superficial bleeding (mucosal/cutaneous bleeds, epistaxis, easy bruising)
- Menorrhagia
- Bleeding time prolonged, normal or mildly increased PTT

Diagnosis:
- Screen with: vWF:Ag assay, vWF activity assay (ie ristocetin cofactor), or factor VIII activity assay

Management:
- Therapy only indicated when patients develop bleeding/hemostatic stress
- Mild bleed, minor surgery: Desmopressin
- Major bleed, big surgery: vWF replacement therapy
- Other options: Antifibrinolytics, topical agents

Hemophilia A/B

General: Inherited XR disorder in factor VIII (A) or factor IX (B). Female carriers generally asymptomatic, but can have mild symptoms.

Clinical:
- Prolonged bleeding (after trauma or surgery)
- Hemarthrosis, leading to chronic arthropathy
- Mucosal bleeding (ie GI bleeds), intracranial bleeds
- Hematoma formation (intramuscular, retroperitoneal)
- Prolonged PTT (normal platelets, bleeding time, PT)

Diagnosis: Factor VIII or IX activity assay (< 40% of expected)

Management:

	Indication	Intervention
Acute	- Bleeding - Surgical procedure	- Desmopressin (mild disease) - Factor replacement
Chronic PPX	- High risk (< 1% factor activity) - Recurrent bleeding	
Hemarthrosis		- Analgesia, immobilization, ice - Arthrocentesis

| COAGULOPATHY | Hematology/Oncology Medicine |

Disseminated Intravascular Coagulation

General: Abnormal activation of the coagulation pathway, leading to microthrombi throughout the vasculature, with consumption of platelets, coagulation factors, and fibrin

Etiology:
- Sepsis
- Malignancy
- Trauma
- OB Complications (amniotic fluid embolism)

Clinical:
- Bleeding/oozing from catheter sites
- Thrombocytopenia, prolonged PT/PTT, prolonged bleeding time
- Low fibrinogen, elevated D-Dimer
- Schistocytes on peripheral smear

Diagnosis: Clinical PLUS Laboratory diagnosis (no single definitive test)

Management:
- Supportive care (fluids, hemodynamic support)
- Treat/manage underlying cause
- Manage active bleeding with transfusions (FFP, platelets, RBC)

Warfarin Toxicity/Vitamin K Deficiency

General: Vitamin K is required for the γ-carboxylation of clotting factors II, VII, IX, X, C, and S

Etiology:
- Warfarin/liver failure (not true deficiency, rather lack of factor synthesis)
- Malabsorption (CF, pancreatic insufficiency), malnutrition, antibiotic use

Clinical: Elevated risk for severe hemorrhage
- PT/INR prolonged (more sens/spec), PTT prolonged

Diagnosis: Clinical features plus PT/PTT

Management:

Indication	Intervention
Active Bleeding (w/ INR > 2) or Surgery (emergent reversal)	- Prothrombin complex or FFP
INR > 10	- Hold Warfarin, give vitamin K
INR > 4.5	- Hold Warfarin, consider vitamin K

THROMBOPHILIA
Hematology/Oncology
Medicine, Pediatrics

Differential Diagnosis of Hypercoagulability

General: Risk for thrombus formation is increased in those with features of Virchow's Triad: (1) Endothelial Injury (2) Hypercoagulability (3) Stasis

Etiology	Findings
Acquired	
- Stasis (immobilization, surgery) - Malignancy - Hormonal (OCPs, pregnancy, tamoxifen) - Other Syndromes: Antiphospholipid syndrome, PNH, myeloproliferative neoplasms	
Genetic	
Factor V Leiden	- Most common inherited coagulopathy among Caucasians - Mutated factor V that is resistant to cleavage by protein C
Antithrombin Deficiency	- Can be inherited or acquired (from cirrhosis, nephrotic, DIC) - Lack of antithrombin results in unregulated thrombin activity
Protein C/S Deficiency	- Unregulated protein V/VIII activity - Associated with warfarin skin necrosis (protein C deficiency)
Prothrombin Mutation	- G20210A mutation, resulting in ↑ prothrombin production

Diagnosis: Protein activity assay (C/S, antithrombin deficiency) or genetic testing

Management: If recurrent thrombotic episodes, patients generally require chronic anticoagulation (warfarin/LMWH/DOAC)

Antiphospholipid Syndrome

General: Prothrombotic state induced by the presence of an antiphospholipid antibody

Risk: Occurs in those with autoimmune predisposition, especially SLE

Clinical:
- Thrombosis (venous/CVA), pulmonary emboli
- Pregnancy complications (recurrent abortions)
- Thrombocytopenia and prolonged PPT
- Derm: Livedo reticularis, superficial venous thrombosis, skin ulcers

Diagnosis: *(At least 1 of clinical and lab criteria below)*

Clinical	Laboratory

(1) Vascular Thrombosis (arterial/ venous)
(2) Pregnancy Morbidity
   - ≥ 3 straight abortions prior to week 10
   - Premature birth (< 34 weeks) with pre-eclampsia
- Unexplained fetal demise > 10 weeks
	(1) Lupus Anticoagulant (dilute russell venom viper test, mixing study)
	(2) Anti-cardiolipin (ELISA IgM/IgG)
	(3) Anti-β-2 glycoprotein (ELISA IgM/IgG)

Management:
- Acute Thromboembolism: Anticoagulation
- Chronic PPX: Warfarin +/- Aspirin (indicated if history of arterial thrombus)

ONCOLOGY BASICS

Hematology/Oncology Medicine

Cancer Definitions

Neoplastic Progression

Dysplasia	- Abnormal growth of cells with abnormal shape/orientation
Carcinoma in situ	- Neoplastic cells, but contained within basement membrane
Carcinoma	- Neoplastic cells invade basement membrane of normal tissue
Metastasis	- Spread to distant organ

Nomenclature

Carcinoma	- Malignancy of epithelial cell origin Adenocarcinoma: Glandular epithelium Angiocarcinoma: Endothelial cells
Sarcoma	- Malignancy of connective tissue origin Liposarcoma: Adipose Chondrosarcoma: Cartilage Osteosarcoma: Bone Myosarcoma: Muscle
Leukemia	- Leukocyte malignancy found in blood and bone marrow
Lymphoma	- Leukocyte malignancy found in lymphoid tissue

Grade/Stage

Grade	- Pathologic description of differentiation
Stage	- Classifying cancer based on extent of invasion/spread

Cancer Therapy

Surgery	- Often part of treatment for non-hematologic malignancies
Radiation	- Ionizing radiation to disrupt DNA and result in death of cells
Chemotherapy	- Cytotoxic drugs which inhibits growth of all rapidly dividing cells
Targeted Therapy	- Drugs that target deregulated proteins specific to cancer cells
Immunotherapy	- Using own immune system's cells, cytokines, etc to target cancer

Heme17

ONCOLOGIC EMERGENCIES — Hematology/Oncology Medicine

	General	Clinical	Management

Tumor Lysis Syndrome	- Massive tumor cell lysis, with release of intracellular contents
	- Can occur with the initiation of cytotoxic chemo (especially with aggressive leukemia/lymphoma), but can also occur spontaneously with certain high risk malignancies
		- Electrolyte abnormalities (↑ PO4, uric acid, K⁺; but ↓ Ca)
		- AKI (deposition of uric acid or CaPhos crystals)
		- Arrhythmias
			- Acute Episode: Supportive care (aggressive fluids/lytes repletion, telemetry), Rasburicase
			- PPX:
			  IV fluid hydration
			  Hypouricemic drug (Rasburicase/ Allopurinol)

Febrile Neutropenia	- Patients undergoing cytotoxic chemo therapy can develop translocation of GI flora across the compromised GI mucosa, potentially resulting in severe infection - Fever may be only sign due to blunted neutrophil response	- Fever (temp > 100.4°F) - Neutropenia (ANC < 1500, but especially at risk if ANC < 500)	- Infectious workup (cultures, etc) - Empiric Abx: Gram-negative coverage (ie Cefepime) +/- gram-positive coverage
Hypercalcemia	- Either from osteolytic mets, PTHrP production, or vitamin D production	- Bones, stones, groans, psychiatric overtones	- Acute: Normal hypercalcemia management - PPX: Bisphosphonates
Hyperviscosity	- Most commonly occurs with high protein disorders (Waldenström's macroglobulinemia, multiple myeloma) or acute leukemia	- Visual blurring, headache - Vertigo, nystagmus, diplopia - Ataxia - Can measure serum viscosity to confirm dx	- Plasmapheresis
SVC Syndrome	- Obstruction of SVC, resulting in facial/ UE edema	- Edema - Severe manifestations include CNS edema and laryngeal edema	- Endovenous stenting or radiation therapy (for emergencies) - Chronic: Treat underlying malignancy
Spinal Cord Compression	- Tumor compressing the dural sac	- Back pain, focal neurologic deficits (weakness, incontinence, sensory loss) - Dx: MRI	- Corticosteroids
Other Complications			
Cachexia	- Multifactorial weight loss from muscle catabolism, systemic inflammation, and poor caloric intake		- Tx: Progesterone or corticosteroids (increase appetite)

Heme18

OVERVIEW OF LIQUID ONCOLOGY

Hematology/Oncology Medicine

Hematopoiesis

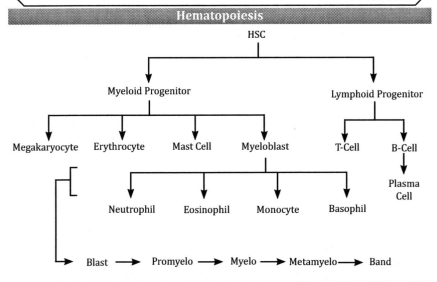

Origin of Liquid Malignancies

Subtype	Cell of Origin
Myeloid Neoplasms	
AML	Myeloid progenitor
CML	Hematopoietic stem cell or myeloid progenitor
Myelodysplasia	Myeloid progenitor
Lymphoid Neoplasms	
ALL	B or T-Cell progenitor
CLL	Post-germinal center B-cell
Mantle Cell Lymphoma	Naive B-cell
Follicular Lymphoma	Germinal center B-cell
Burkitt Lymphoma	Germinal center B-cell
DLBCL	Germinal center or post-germinal center B-cell
Hodgkin Lymphoma	Germinal center or post-germinal center B-cell
Multiple Myeloma	Post-germinal center B-cell

Heme19

PLASMA CELL DYSCRASIAS
Hematology/Oncology Medicine

Monoclonal Gammopathy of Uncertain Significance (MGUS)

General: Asymptomatic, premalignant clonal plasma cell proliferative disorder. Risk to progress to:
- Multiple myeloma (if IgA/IgG producing)
- Waldenström macroglobulinemia (if IgM producing)

Clinical: Asymptomatic, no end-organ damage like that seen with myeloma

Diagnosis:
- Serum/Urine protein electrophoresis (monoclonal Ig at < 3 g/dL)
- Serum FLC (free light chain) and Immunoglobulin

Note: Patients must have no clinical symptoms consistent with MM or WM, and < 10% clonal plasma cells on bone marrow biopsy (if performed)

Management: Monitor patients (progress to malignancy at ~1% per year)
- Annual serum and urine M-protein, CBC, calcium, etc

Multiple Myeloma and Waldenstrom Macroglobulinemia

	Multiple Myeloma	Waldenström Macroglobulinemia
Gen	- Plasma cell neoplasm with monoclonal Ig production	- Clonal lymphoplasmacytic proliferation with IgM production
Clin	"CRAB" Features - Hypercalcemia - Renal Failure (bence jones protein) - Anemia (BM infiltrate/renal failure) - Bone (osteolytic lesions with increased fracture risk) - Increased infection risk (due to monoclonal Ig production)	- Hyperviscosity (CNS symptoms: blurred vision, HA, stroke, etc) - Neuropathy (paresthesia, weakness) - Organomegaly (LA, HSM) - Anemia - Bleeding
Dx	- SPEP: Non-IgM serum monoclonal protein ≥ 3 g/dL - ≥ 10% clonal plasma cells in bone marrow aspirate	- SPEP: IgM serum monoclonal protein ≥ 3 g/dL - ≥ 10% clonal lymphoplasmacytic cells in bone marrow aspirate
Tx	- Chemotherapy (first line) - Bortezomib, Lenalidomide, low-dose Dexamethasone (first line) - HCT - Bisphosphonates for bone lesions	- Asymptomatic: Monitor - Symptomatic: Chemotherapy (Rituximab, Dexamethasone, others) - Acute Hyperviscosity: Plasmapheresis

MYELOPROLIFERATIVE DISEASE — Hematology/Oncology Medicine

Myelodysplasia

General: Malignant hematopoietic stem cell disorder characterized by dysplasia and ineffective red and white blood cell production

Risk: Old age, prior chemotherapy/radiation exposure

Clinical:
- Pancytopenia (can present as anemia, thrombocytopenia, leukopenia, or combination of each)
- Increased infection risk
- Blood smear shows dysplasia in RBC/WBC lineages
- Risk to progress to AML

Diagnosis: Bone marrow aspirate
- Significant dysplasia (> 10%)
- Blasts < 20% (> 20% would be leukemia)

Management:
- Symptomatic cytopenias treated with blood product transfer
- Depending on risk, these patients can be simply monitored, or started on chemotherapy or undergo HCT if higher risk

Myeloproliferative Neoplasms

General: Group of myeloid neoplasms that have terminal myeloid cell expansion in the peripheral blood (see next page for classic MPNs). Often associated with JAK-2 gene mutations.

Clinical: Depending on the disorder, various degrees of erythrocytosis, leukocytosis, thrombocytosis, bone marrow hypercellularity/fibrosis, and splenomegaly

Differential of Polycythemia

	Etiology	RBC Mass	EPO	Other Findings
Primary	- Polycythemia Vera	↑	↓	- Hypervolemia
Appropriate Absolute	- Lung disease - Cyanotic heart defects - High altitude	↑	↑	- Hypoxemia
Inappropriate Absolute	- Ectopic EPO production (ie malignancy)	↑	↑	
Relative	- Volume loss	↔	↔	- Hypovolemia

MYELOPROLIFERATIVE DISEASE
Hematology/Oncology Medicine

	General	Clinical	Management
Essential Thrombocytosis	- Excessive clonal platelet production, often due to JAK2 mutation	- Unexplained, persistent thrombocytosis - Vasomotor symptoms (syncope, headache, dizziness, erythromelalgia) - Thrombosis/hemorrhage risk	Diagnosis: - Thrombocytosis > 450k/mm3 - Bone marrow biopsy (proliferation of enlarged, mature megakaryocytes) - Classic mutation or clear clonal marker Treatment: - Aspirin or anticoagulation - Cytoreduction (Hydroxyurea or Anagrelide)

Polycythemia Vera	- Acquired disorder characterized by primary polycythemia, most commonly associated with JAK2 V617F mutation in myeloid progenitor	- Elevated hemoglobin
		- Thrombocytosis, leukocytosis possible
		- Hyperviscosity
		  - Erythromelalgia (burning cyanosis in hands/feet)
		  - Blurry vision
		- Aquagenic pruritus
		- Thrombosis (Budd-Chiari, portal/splenic thrombosis)
		- Can progress to AML or myelofibrosis
			Diagnosis:
			- ↑ Hgb, ↓ EPO level (should be suppressed)
			- JAK2 or other classic mutation
			Treatment:
			- Phlebotomy (goal Hct < 45%)
			- Aspirin
			- If refractory: Cytoreductive therapy (ie Hydroxyurea or others)

Myelofibrosis	- Clonal myeloid proliferation, resulting in fibroblast hyperactivity and fibrosis of the bone marrow - Can be primary or secondary (due to "burnout" of myeloproliferative disorder like PV or essential thrombocytosis)	- Systemic symptoms (fatigue, fever, weight loss) - Splenomegaly (key finding in disease), hepatomegaly - Extramedullary hematopoiesis - Anemia (teardrop RBCs on smear) - WBC/platelet counts are variable	Diagnosis: - Bone marrow biopsy (fibrotic marrow) Treatment: - Hydroxyurea for mild disease - Ruxolitinib (JAK 2 inhibitor) - HCT for severe disease

LEUKEMIA
Hematology/Oncology — Medicine, Pediatrics

Acute Lymphoblastic Leukemia

General: Neoplasm of early lymphocytic precursors. Subtypes:

B-Cell ALL	- Markers: CD10+, 19+, 22+, TdT+ - t(12;21) common mutation, favorable prognosis - t(9;22) BCR-ABL also possible (can use TK inhibitors)
T-Cell ALL	- CD 2-8 +

Risk: Most common malignancy in kids (usually 2-5 y/o), increased risk in Down's
- Second peak in those ~60 y/o

Clinical:
- Systemic symptoms (fevers, chills, fatigue, lymphadenopathy, bone pain)
- Cytopenias (bleeding, recurrent infections)
- T-Cell can present with mediastinal mass in teenager, with possible dysphagia, stridor, SVC syndrome

Diagnosis:
- Bone marrow biopsy
  - > 25% lymphoblasts diagnostic
- Specialized immunophenotype and cytogenetic testing (supportive)

Management:
- Induction Chemotherapy: Cytotoxic regimens
  - Commonly 1st Line: Vincristine, corticosteroids, Asparaginase
  - Localized chemotherapy for CNS/Testes ("sanctuary sites")
- HCT for high risk patients

LEUKEMIA

Hematology/Oncology Medicine

Hairy Cell Leukemia

General: Clonal B-cell neoplasm, almost universally from BRAF (serine/threonine kinase) mutation

Clinical:
- Cytopenias (anemia, thrombocytopenia, neutropenia)
    - Risk for infection, bleeding
- Significant splenomegaly, often causing abdominal pain
- Circulating mononuclear cells with hairy appearance

Diagnosis:
- Bone marrow biopsy: Hypercellularity with hairy cell infiltrate
    - + TRAP stain (historically)
    - "Dry-Tap" from bone marrow fibrosis
- Flow cytometry: Mature B cell markers

Management:
- Asymptomatic: Monitor
- Symptomatic: Cladribine (or Pentostatin), possibly followed by Rituximab

Chronic Lymphocytic Leukemia

General: Chronic lymphoproliferative disorder with production of mature malfunctioning lymphocytes. Same disorder as small lymphocytic lymphoma.

Risk: Generally idiopathic, occuring in elderly (ie age > 70)

Clinical:
- Generally asymptomatic, and found on routine labs
- Painless, waxing/waning cervical lymphadenopathy or hepatosplenomegaly
- Bloodwork shows lymphocytosis, with possible cytopenias
    - Smear reveals mature lymphocytes with possible "smudge cells"

Diagnosis:
- Flow cytometry: Clonal population of CD19, CD20, CD23, or CD5 + cells
- Bone marrow biopsy: Not required for diagnosis, but shows > 30% lymphocytes

Management:
- Asymptomatic: Monitor
- Symptomatic, Advanced Stage: Localized radiation, systemic chemo (variety of regimens, but Fludarabine/Rituximab commonly used)

Complications:
- Infection (patients can have hyper or hypogammaglobulinemia, but the Ig produced not useful for fighting infection)
- Autoimmune hemolytic anemia
- Progression to diffuse large B-cell lymphoma (Richter transformation)

LEUKEMIA
Hematology/Oncology Medicine

Acute Myeloid Leukemia

General: Clonal expansion of malignant hematopoietic precursor cells of myeloid lineage. Median age 65 (can occur earlier).

Risk: Associated with prior chemo/radiation, myelodysplasia, Down's

Clinical:
- Weakness, fatigue, other nonspecific symptoms
- Anemia, thrombocytopenia, neutropenia (dyspnea, bleeds, infections)
- High risk for DIC

Diagnosis:
- > 20% blasts in peripheral blood and/or bone marrow biopsy
- Flow cytometry: Confirms myeloid lineage
    - Other signs: Auer rods, + myeloperoxidase

Management: (for AML other than promyelocytic)
- Intensive induction chemotherapy: Daunorubicin plus Cytarabine
    - Followed by consolidation, maintenance chemotherapy
- Allogeneic HCT for high risk patients

Acute Promyelocytic Leukemia	- PML-RARA translocation t(15;17) - Highly associated with DIC - Responds to ATRA, arsenic +/- anthracycline-based chemo

Chronic Myeloid Leukemia

General: Myeloproliferative neoplasm of maturing granulocytes (ie neutrophils) with fairly normal differentiation. Most commonly due to fusion of BCR (on chromosome 22) and ABL1 (on chromosome 9).

Clinical: Multiple phases.
- Chronic
    - Asymptomatic or nonspecific symptoms (fatigue, night sweats)
    - Hepatosplenomegaly
    - Leukocytosis (> 100k), thrombocytosis, anemia all possible
- Accelerated: Increasing leukocytosis, often difficult to control
- Blast crisis: Phase of blast and promyelocyte production (AML, rarely ALL)

Diagnosis:
- Peripheral smear: Myelocyte lineage proliferation
    - Increased amounts of immature cells ("myelocyte bulge")
    - Low leukocyte alkaline phosphatase activity
    - Eosinophilia/basophilia possible
- Bone marrow biopsy (similar to smear above: granulocyte hyperplasia)
- Confirmation of t(9;22) via cytogenetics

Management:
- Chronic: Imatinib (or alternative tyrosine kinase inhibitor like Nilotinib)
- Accelerating/Blast: TKI plus HCT
- HCT for treatment resistant disease

LYMPHOMA

Hematology/Oncology
Medicine, Pediatrics

Hodgkin Lymphoma

General: B-cell lymphoma. Subtypes below:

Subtype	Pathologic Findings
Nodular Sclerosing	- Nodular growth pattern, with fibrous bands
Mixed Cellularity	- Reed-Sternberg cells, pleomorphic background, eosinophilia
Lymphocyte Rich	- Few Reed-Sternberg cells and many B cells
Lymphocyte Deplete	- Paucity of inflammatory cells, poor prognosis

Risk: Bimodal age distribution (15-30 y/o, then > 65), EBV, Immunosuppression

Clinical:
- Painless lymphadenopathy (often cervical)
- B-symptoms sometimes present (fever, night sweats, weight loss)
- Possible mediastinal mass on X-ray or CT imaging

Diagnosis: Lymph Node Biopsy (Reed-Sternberg cells)
- Large cell with two or more nuclei ("owl's eyes"), CD 15, 30+
- Inflammatory infiltrate around RS cells (plasma cells, eosinophils, fibroblasts, and lymphocytes)

Management: Chemotherapy + Radiation Therapy
- ABVD Regimen (Doxorubicin, Bleomycin, Vinblastine, Dacarbazine)

Non-Hodgkin Lymphoma

General: Heterogeneous group of lymphoid malignancies from B or T cell lineages

Risk: Radiation, chemo, immunosuppression, viruses (HIV, HTLV-1, EBV)

Clinical:
- Indolent (Follicular, CLL/SLL, marginal zone)
  - Present as slow growing lymphadenopathy, hepatosplenomegaly, cytopenias
- Aggressive (DLBCL, Burkitt's, T-cell)
  - Certain subtypes present rapidly systemic B symptoms (fever, night sweats, weight loss), mass/lymphadenopathy, ↑ LDH

Diagnosis: Excisional biopsy (with histology, immunologic/molecular assessment)

Management:
- Dependent on underlying subtype, but the majority are treated with combined systemic, cytotoxic chemotherapy
- Rituximab (anti-CD-20 monoclonal antibody) is added to many regimens for B-cell lymphomas

LYMPHOMA

Hematology/Oncology
Medicine, Pediatrics

Subtype	Clinical Features and Management
B-Cell Non-Hodgkin Lymphomas	
Burkitt	- Highly aggressive B cell neoplasm, commonly in adolescents, either endemic (typically seen in Africa, associated with EBV), sporadic, or immunodeficiency associated - Endemic: Presents as rapidly enlarging facial or bone lesions - Sporadic: Presents as abdominal mass, often with tumor lysis - Dx: Biopsy ("starry sky" pattern, t(8,14) C-myc/heavy chain Ig)
Diffuse Large B-Cell	- Most common NHL subtype - Presents as rapidly enlarging mass in neck/abdomen, +/- B symptoms - Dx: Excisional Biopsy (diffuse proliferation of mature B-cells)
Follicular	- Germinal-center B-cell proliferation - Presents as indolent, waxing/waning painless peripheral lymphadenopathy - Can progress to DLBCL - Dx: Lymph node biopsy (nodular growth pattern, often expressing BCL2, t(14;18))
Mantle Cell	- Aggressive, mature B-cell lymphoma - Presents as lymphadenopathy, often with extranodal disease at the time of presentation, with possible B-symptoms - Dx: Biopsy (often has t(11;14), overexpression of cyclin D1)
Marginal Zone	- Can be nodal or extranodal (MALToma, associated with chronic inflammation, as seen with autoimmune disease or *H. pylori* infection) - Presents with nonspecific/variable symptoms, typically based on the organ that is affected - Dx: Biopsy of affected site or lymph node
T-Cell Lymphoma	
Peripheral T-Cell	- Variety of different T-Cell based lymphomas - Dx: Lymph node biopsy (w/ CD2-8 + cells)
Adult T-Cell Leukemia-Lymphoma	- Associated with HTLV-1 - Presents with lymphadenopathy, hepatosplenomegaly, lytic bone lesions, and skin lesions
Mycosis Fungoides	- Extranodal nHL of T-cell origin - Presents as skin plaques and lesions - Dx: Skin biopsy (CD4 cells with cerebriform nuclei)

OTHER HEMATOLOGIC MALIGNANCIES
Hematology/Oncology, Medicine, Pediatrics

Langerhans Cell Histiocytosis

General: Rare disease of histiocytic infiltration of tissues, most commonly bone. Occurs commonly in age 1-3.

Clinical:
- Lytic bone lesions ("Eosinophilic Granuloma")
    - Can present as pathologic fracture
- Skin lesions: Can present as rash or ulcerative lesions
- Lung cysts/nodules (can lead to spontaneous pneumothorax)
- CNS: Diabetes insipidus

Diagnosis: Biopsy of lesion (CD1a+, or Birbeck granules on EM)

Management: Chemotherapy

Mastocytosis

General: Rare, excessive mast cell proliferation and accumulation in dermal tissue (cutaneous) or extradermal tissue (systemic). Generally due to activating mutation in KIT gene.

Clinical:
- Dermal: Flushing, pruritus, urticaria pigmentosa (tan macules)
    - Can be episodic, mimicking anaphylaxis
- Systemic
    - GI: Steatorrhea, malabsorption, hepatosplenomegaly
    - Skeletal lesions (lytic or sclerotic)
    - Heme: BM invasion (mild anemia, other cytopenias)

Diagnosis:
- Tryptase level (elevated if systemic)
- Biopsy (bone marrow if systemic, skin if cutaneous)

Management:
- Epinephrine pens (many experience anaphylaxis)
- Antihistamines and other therapy for allergic mediators
- For advanced disease: HCT or Midostaurin (kinase inhibitor)

AMYLOIDOSIS

Hematology/Oncology Medicine

Primary and Secondary Amyloidosis

General: Extracellular tissue deposition of conformationally abnormal protein fibrils, most commonly in beta-pleated sheets

Etiology	Clinical Features
Primary AL	
Ig Light Chain	- Generally derived from plasma cell dyscrasias
Secondary AL	
AA	- Secondary to chronic inflammation (RA, IBD, vasculitis, chronic infection, lymphoma) Familial Mediterranean Fever - Chronic hereditary serosal inflammation - Recurrent attacks of fever and serosal inflammation - Increased risk for AA amyloid - Tx: Colchicine
Dialysis	- $\beta 2$ microglobulin from ESRD patients - Tx: Change renal replacement methodology
Heritable	- Variety of different inherited mutated proteins Examples: - Mutated transthyretin (causing cardiomyopathy)
Senile	- Transthyretin (wild-type) deposition most commonly in heart
Organ-Specific	Examples: - Alzheimer's (Beta-amyloid)

Clinical: Variable multisystem infiltration
- Derm: Waxy skin, easy bruising, nodules
- MSK: Enlarged tongue, muscles, arthropathy
- GI: Hepatomegaly, splenomegaly
- CV: Cardiomyopathy
- CNS: Neuropathy, dementia
- Renal: Insufficiency, proteinuria, nephrotic syndrome
- Heme: Increased hemorrhage risk

Diagnosis: Tissue Biopsy (either fat pad or of specific organ)
- Hyaline material, stains with Congo red, apple green birefringence under polarized light

Management: Treat underlying condition (ie plasma cell dyscrasia or inflammation)

BLOOD PRODUCT TRANSFUSIONS

Hematology/Oncology Medicine

Blood Product Transfusion

Product	Indication
Packed RBCs	- Transfuse to maintain hemoglobin at > 7 g/dL - Transfuse when Hgb < 8 g/dL in acute coronary syndrome - Transfuse when Hgb < 10 g/dL in symptomatic anemia
Platelets	- Bleeding with a platelet count < 50,000 - Any patient < 10,000 (Exceptions: Platelet consuming disorder)
FFP	- Elevated INR (> 2) with major bleeding or preparation for surgery
Prothrombin Complex Concentrate	- Recombinant 4 factor concentrate (factors II, VII, IX, and X) - Similar indications to FFP, and becoming preferred
Cryoprecipitate	- Contains fibrinogen, factor VIII, XIII, and VWF - Now used less commonly, but can be used in disorders of fibrinogen or with DIC

Specialty RBC Treatments

Irradiated	- Radiation to disrupt donor T lymphocytes (prevents graft-versus host disease) - Indications: Bone marrow transplant/immunosuppressed
Leukoreduced	- Eliminates leukocyte debris and cytokines, prevent CMV transmission - Most hospitals leukoreduce all blood - Indications: Prevent CMV in immunosuppressed, chronically transfused, transplant recipients
Washed	- Removes any residual plasma/plasma proteins from RBC - Indications: IgA deficiency, recurrent allergic reaction to transfusion

Bone Marrow Stimulating Agents

Neutrophils	- Filgrastim
Platelets	- Romiplostim - Eltrombopag
Red Blood Cells	- Erythropoietin - Epoetin alfa

BLOOD PRODUCT TRANSFUSIONS
Hematology/Oncology Medicine

	Mechanism	Clinical	Treatment
Acute Hemolytic	- ABO incompatibility - Immediate onset	- Fever, flank pain, renal failure - DIC - Positive direct Coombs test - ↑ plasma hemoglobin/hemoglobinuria	- Stop transfusion - IV Fluids - Supportive
Delayed Hemolytic	- Revival of Ig against minor RBC Ag that was at low levels (thus missed on screen) - 3-10 day onset	- Low-grade hemolysis/mild fever - Positive direct Coombs	- Generally self-limited
Febrile Nonhemolytic	- Cytokine accumulation in stored blood - Risk reduced with leukoreduction - Hours after transfusion	- Fevers, chills, headache, flushing	- Stop transfusion - Antipyretics
Anaphylactic	- Associated with IgA deficiency - Immediate onset	- Acute onset shock, urticaria, edema, and respiratory distress	- Stop transfusion - Epinephrine
Allergic (urticarial)	- IgE/Mast cell activation - Hours after transfusion	- Urticarial rash, pruritus, flushing - Angioedema	- Diphenhydramine - *Can administer remainder of blood product*
TRALI (Transfusion-related acute lung injury)	- Antibodies to human leukocyte antigens, which results in inflammatory activation and pulmonary capillary leakage - Hours after transfusion	- Acute hypoxemic respiratory failure - Noncardiogenic pulmonary edema	- Stop transfusion - O_2/ventilatory support
TACO (Transfusion-associated circulatory overload)	- Volume overload from infusion	- Acute dyspnea and signs of volume overload, pulmonary edema	- Supplemental O_2 - Fluid diuresis

TRANSPLANT
Hematology/Oncology Medicine

General Principles

General: Organs that can be transplanted include heart, kidney, liver, lungs
- Bone marrow transplants are a special type of transplant, in which the transplanted cells are used for their anti-host effect in an attempt to cure certain types of leukemia or lymphoma

Subtypes:
- Autograft: Transplant of graft from same person
- Allograft: Transplant of an organ or tissue between two humans
- Xenograft: Transplant of organ or tissue between two different species

Management:
- Require chronic immunosuppression to prevent graft rejection
    - Options include steroids, Tacrolimus, Mycophenolate, others
- Infection Prophylaxis
    - PCP (TMP-SMX, Atovaquone, others)
    - HSV (Acyclovir)
    - CMV (High risk: Valganciclovir)
    - Fungal (required for some)

Transplant Rejection

Type	Clinical Findings	Management
Hyperacute (within hours)	- ABO/ lymphocytotoxic mismatch (rarely seen clinically) - Results in immediate vascular thrombosis	- Explant tissue
Acute (weeks to months)	- CD8 cells activated against donor MHC - Graft vasculitis and lymphocytic infiltration	- Corticosteroids - Should not occur if proper immunosuppression is initiated
Chronic (years)	- CD4 cells respond to recipient APCs presenting donor peptides - Results in proliferation of vascular smooth muscle, atrophy, interstitial fibrosis	- Poor prognosis - Re-transplant

Graft vs Host	- Immune cells from donor recognize the recipient as foreign, initiating an immune reaction
	- Utilized for its anti-leukemia/ lymphoma effect, but too much can result in the systemic issues below:
	  - Skin: Maculopapular rash
	  - Liver: ↑ bilirubin, hepatomegaly
	  - GI: Diarrhea
	  - Lung: Bronchiolitis obliterans
		- Corticosteroids

IMMUNOLOGIC REACTIONS — Hematology/Oncology Medicine

Hypersensitivity Reactions

	Clinical Features	Examples
Type I	- Anaphylaxis/atopy - IgE response to antigen (ie food, sting, drug) - Rare IgE independent causes	- Atopic dermatitis - Asthma - Urticaria - Anaphylaxis
Type II	- Cytotoxic reaction of IgM or IgG against antigen	- Myasthenia gravis - Graves - Many others
Type III	- Immune complex formation - Serum sickness (fever, skin rash, and arthralgias weeks after exposure to Ag) - Arthus reaction (local inflammatory reaction to injected antigen)	- SLE - Post-Strep GN - Acute Hepatitis B
Type IV	- Delayed T-Cell mediated reaction to antigen	- Contact dermatitis - Multiple sclerosis - Transplant rejection

Complement Disorders

Disorder	Clinical Features
Hereditary Angioedema	- Deficiency of C1 esterase inhibitor, resulting in elevated bradykinin levels - Presents as recurrent episodes of angioedema (without pruritus or urticaria) - No response to steroids or antihistamines - Dx: Low C4 levels and C1INH - Tx: Replace serum C1INH, Icatibant (bradykinin inhibitor) for acute episodes
C1 Deficiency	- C1q, C1r, C1s deficiency most common complement deficiency - Associated with increased SLE risk, recurrent infections
C3 Deficiency	- Severe/recurrent infections with encapsulated bacteria - Presents very early in life
C5-C9 Deficiency	- Increased risk of meningococcal infection

IMMUNODEFICIENCIES

Hematology/Oncology
Medicine, Pediatrics

B-Cell Disorders

	Mechanism	Clinical	Diagnosis/Treatment
Bruton's Agammaglobulinemia	- X-Linked disorder in BTK, which prevents B-cell maturation	- Recurrent bacterial and enteroviral infections after age ~6 months (not before then because maternal IgG) - Scanty lymph nodes and tonsils	Dx: ↓ Ig/B-Cells with molecular defect in BTK Tx: IVIG
Selective IgA Deficiency	- Selective deficiency of serum IgA	- Generally asymptomatic - Complications can include increased risk for AI disease, atopic reaction, anaphylaxis to blood products	Dx: ↓ IgA, Normal IgM/IgG Tx: Education/monitoring
Common Variable Immunodeficiency	- Impaired B-cell differentiation, defective production of Ig - Can present in ages 20-40 - Increased risk for autoimmune disease	- Bacterial sinopulmonary infection - Pulm: Bronchiectasis - GI: Chronic diarrhea - ↑ risk for non-Hodgkin lymphoma	Dx: ↓ IgA, IgM, IgG Tx: IVIG

T-Cell Disorders

	Mechanism	Clinical	Diagnosis/Treatment
DiGeorge	- Deletion of 22q11, resulting in thymic and parathyroid abnormalities	- Conotruncal cardiac anomalies - Hypoplastic thymus/parathyroid (↓Ca) - Recurrent viral/fungal infections - Facial abnormalities (ie cleft palate)	Dx: ↓ CD3+ T-cells, confirmed 22q11 mutation Tx: Surgical correction of structural abnormalities, HCT for severe immunodeficiency
Job Syndrome	- AD STAT3 mutation, causing impaired neutrophils chemotaxis	- Recurrent skin and pulmonary infections - Eczematous dermatitis	Dx: ↑ IgE, eosinophilia Tx: PPX antibiotics
Chronic Mucocutaneous Candidiasis	- Heterogeneous group of genetic defects (including AIRE) resulting in chronic *Candida*	- Chronic skin/mucosal candidiasis - Endocrine disorders: Hypoparathyroidism, adrenal insufficiency, etc	Dx: Clinical Tx: Antifungals

IMMUNODEFICIENCIES

Hematology/Oncology — Medicine, Pediatrics

	Mechanism	Clinical	Diagnosis/Treatment
Combined T and B-Cell Disorders			
Severe Combined Immunodeficiency	Several Causes: - Defective IL-2R gamma chain (XR) - ADA deficiency (AR)	- Recurrent severe infections, diarrhea, and failure to thrive in infants - Often leads to early death	Dx: ↓ T-cells, genetic defect Tx: IVIG, infection prophylaxis, HCT or ADA enzyme replacement
Ataxia-Telangiectasia	- AR defect in DNA double strand break repair (ATM gene)	- Progressive cerebellar ataxia/atrophy - Immunodeficiency - Telangiectasia	Dx: ↓ IgA, IgM, IgG. ↑ AFP. Tx: Poor prognosis. Support with IVIG and treatment of infections.
Wiskott-Aldrich	- X Linked disorder of WASP, responsible for actin cytoskeleton rearrangement	- Recurrent bacterial, viral and fungal infections - Thrombocytopenia - Eczema - ↑ Risk for autoimmune disease, malignancy	Dx: Genetic analysis, ↓/↔ IgG and IgM. ↑ IgA and IgE. Tx: IVIG/antibiotics, platelet transfusions for active bleeds, HCT only definitive therapy
Hyper IgM Syndrome	- Defective class-switch recombination, most often from CD40 ligand deficiency	- Recurrent sinopulmonary and GI infections	Dx: ↑ IgM, ↓ IgA, IgG, IgE. Flow cytometry for CD40L, genetic testing confirms. Tx: IVIG/prophylactic antibiotics

Heme35

IMMUNODEFICIENCIES

Hematology/Oncology
Medicine, Pediatrics

Phagocyte Disorders

	Mechanism	Clinical	Diagnosis/Treatment
Chronic Granulomatous Disease	- X-linked defect in phagocyte NADPH oxidase	- Recurrent bacterial and fungal infections (ie PNA, soft tissue, adinitis, osteomyelitis) - Common organisms: *Staphylococcus aureus, Pseudomonas, Burkholderia, Serratia, Nocardia, Aspergillus*	Dx: Dihydrorhodamine 123 test Tx: Chronic PPX with TMP-SMX, Itraconazole - IFN-g injections if severe - HCT for definitive cure
Chediak-Higashi	- AR defect in vesicle trafficking proteins, resulting abnormal neutrophil digestion and neurologic dysfunction	- Recurrent pyogenic infections - Hypopigmentation - Neurologic deficits (neuropathy, ataxia) - Accelerated phase: Lymphohistiocytic infiltration of all organ systems (fatal)	Dx: Smear (characteristic granules in leuks/platelets) Tx: HCT
Leukocyte Adhesion Deficiency (Type I)	- Defect in beta-2 integrin (CD18), impairs chemotaxis/migration	- Recurrent bacterial infections - Absent pus - Impaired wound healing - Omphalitis is classic presentation	Dx: Absent CD18 on flow cytometry Tx: HCT if severe
Leukocyte Adhesion Deficiency (Type II)	- Defect in fucosylation of macromolecules on leukocytes, preventing binding to selectin molecules (impaired chemotaxis)	- Less severe and fewer infections than those with LAD Type I	Dx: Flow cytometry (absent CD15 [ie Sialyl-Lewis X]) Tx: Prophylactic antibiotics, fucose supplementation

Heme36

CRYOGLOBULINEMIA

Hematology/Oncology Medicine

Cryoglobulinemia

General: Proteins that precipitate from serum and plasma when cooled

	Type 1	**Type II/III**
Path	- Monoclonal Ig	- Mixed monoclonal Ig or polyclonal Ig
Risk	- Lymphoproliferative disease (ie multiple myeloma)	- HCV - SLE and other connective tissue disease - Other infections (ie HBV, HIV)
Clin	- **Hyperviscosity** (blurry vision, HA or focal neuro deficits) - Thrombosis - Reynaud - Livedo reticularis or purpura	- **Immune-complex vasculitis** - Palpable purpura - Arthralgias - LA and HSM - Renal disease (glomerulonephritis, usually years later)
Dx	- Normal complement - Test for cryoglobulins	- ↓ C4 Levels, CH50 - Test for cryoglobulins - Biopsy (can confirm vasculitis)
Tx	- Treat underlying malignancy - Manage hyperviscosity	- Glucocorticoids PLUS - Cyclophosphamide or Rituximab - Plasma exchange (if severe)

HEMATOLOGY PHARM — Hematology/Oncology Medicine

	Mechanism	Indication	Side Effects/Management
Antiplatelet			
Aspirin	- Irreversible inhibition of COX - ↓ prostaglandin and TXA$_2$ synthesis	- Analgesia, antipyretic - Anti-inflammatory (high doses) - Primary/secondary MI/Stroke PPX	- Bleeding - Gastritis, GI bleeds - Reye's Syndrome (Kids)
Clopidogrel Prasugrel Ticagrelor	- ADP receptor (P2Y$_{12}$) inhibitor (↓ GPIIb/IIIa activation)	- Acute coronary syndrome - Vascular stenting	- Bleeding
Cilostazol Dipyridamole	- Phosphodiesterase inhibitor (↓ platelet aggregation)	- Claudication (Cilostazol) - Coronary vasodilation (Dipyridamole)	- Headache, flushing, heat intolerance, palpitations
Abciximab Eptifibatide Tirofiban	- Direct GPIIb/IIIa inhibitor	- Acute coronary syndrome - Vascular stenting	- Bleeding - Thrombocytopenia
Anticoagulants			
Heparin Enoxaparin Fondaparinux	- ↓ activity of thrombin and factor Xa	- DVT/PE treatment and prophylaxis - AF - ACS	- Bleeding - HIT
Apixaban Rivaroxaban	- Factor Xa inhibitor	- DVT/PE - Atrial fibrillation (non-valvular)	- Bleeding - Contraindicated in CKD
Bivalirudin Dabigatran	- Direct thrombin inhibitor	- DVT/PE - Atrial fibrillation	- Bleeding
Warfarin	- Inhibits γ-carboxylation of vitamin K dependent clotting factors (II/VII/IX/X C, S)		- Bleeding - Teratogenic - Skin/tissue necrosis (seen with protein C deficiency)
Fibrinolytics			
Alteplase Reteplase	- Tissue plasminogen activator (tPA), catalyzes conversion of plasminogen to plasmin	- Ischemic stroke - PE - STEMI	- Extremely high risk for bleeding - Long list of contraindications [See: Neuro]

TRANSPLANT PHARM — Hematology/Oncology Medicine

	Mechanism	Indication	Side Effects/Management
Cyclosporine	- Calcineurin inhibitor (↓ IL-2 production, prevent T-cell activation)	- Transplant rejection prophylaxis	<table><tr><th>Side Effect</th><th>Cyclosporine</th><th>Tacrolimus</th></tr><tr><td>Nephrotoxicity</td><td>++</td><td>+</td></tr><tr><td>Hypertension</td><td>++</td><td>+</td></tr><tr><td>NODAT (new onset diabetes)</td><td>+</td><td>+</td></tr><tr><td>Thrombotic Microangiopathy</td><td>+</td><td>+</td></tr><tr><td>Neurotoxicity</td><td>-</td><td>+</td></tr><tr><td>GI Side Effects</td><td>-</td><td>+</td></tr><tr><td>Alopecia</td><td>-</td><td>+</td></tr><tr><td>Gingival Hyperplasia</td><td>+</td><td>-</td></tr><tr><td>Hirsutism</td><td>+</td><td>-</td></tr><tr><td>Hyperlipidemia</td><td>+</td><td>-</td></tr></table>
Tacrolimus			
Sirolimus	- mTOR inhibitor	- Transplant rejection prophylaxis	- Pancytopenia - NODAT (New-onset diabetes) - Hyperlipidemia
Mycophenolate Mofetil (MMF)	- Inosine monophosphate dehydrogenase inhibitor, blocking purine synthesis, preventing proliferation of B/T cells	- Transplant rejection prophylaxis	- Pancytopenia (especially anemia and leukopenia) - GI side effects (nausea, vomiting, diarrhea, gastritis, GI bleed, GI ulcerations)
Azathioprine	- Inhibitor of purine synthesis, preventing proliferation of B/T cells	- Transplant rejection prophylaxis	- Pancytopenia

CYTOTOXIC CHEMOTHERAPY — Hematology/Oncology Medicine

	Mechanism	Side Effects (Selected)
Nucleotide analogs		
Azacitidine	- Purine or pyrimidine analogs that inhibit DNA synthesis	- Myelosuppression - Hepatotoxicity
Azathioprine		
Cladribine		
Cytarabine		
Gemcitabine		
Mercaptopurine		
5-Fluorouracil	- Inhibition of thymidylate synthase, ↓ DNA production	- Myelosuppression
Methotrexate	- Folic acid analog, inhibiting dihydrofolate reductase, ↓ DNA production	- Myelosuppression (reversible with use of Leucovorin) - Hepatotoxicity - Stomatitis - Pneumonitis/fibrosis
Alkylating Agents		***Myelosuppression (all)**
Busulfan	- Cross link DNA (triggers cellular apoptosis)	- Pulmonary fibrosis - Hyperpigmentation
Cyclophosphamide		- Hemorrhagic cystitis (reversed with Mesna), bladder cancer
Dacarbazine		- Severe nausea
Nitrosoureas		- Neurotoxicity
Anthracyclines		
Daunorubicin Doxorubicin	- Intercalates DNA, preventing DNA replication	- Myelosuppression - Cardiotoxicity (dilated CM)
Taxanes		
Paclitaxel Docetaxel	- Microtubule inhibitor (hyperstabilize mitotic spindles)	- Myelosuppression - Neuropathy
Topoisomerase Inhibitors		
Topotecan	- Topoisomerase I inhibitor	- Myelosuppression, severe GI side effects
Etoposide	- Topoisomerase II inhibitor	
Peptide Antibiotics		
Actinomycin	- Inhibits RNA transcription	- Myelosuppression, alopecia
Bleomycin	- Induces DNA strand breaks	- Pulmonary fibrosis
Platinum Agents		
Carboplatin Cisplatin	- DNA cross linker, inhibiting replication	- Myelosuppression - Nephrotoxicity - Neuropathy/ototoxicity
Vinca Alkaloids		
Vincristine Vinblastine	- Inhibit microtubule proliferation	- Peripheral neuropathy

TARGETED THERAPEUTICS — Hematology/Oncology Medicine

	Mechanism	Side Effects (Major, if important)
Alemtuzumab	- Antibody against CD-52	- Precipitates autoimmune disease
Bevacizumab	- Antibody against VEGF	- ↑ risk of bleeding
Bortezomib	- Inhibitor of proteasome	
Cetuximab	- Antibody against EGFR	
Eculizumab	- Antibody against C5	- Infection (meningococcus)
Imatinib	- Inhibitor of BCR-ABL	- Hepatotoxicity
Nivolumab	- Antibody against PD-1	
Pembrolizumab	- Inhibitor of PD-1	- Pneumonitis, endocrine issues
Rituximab	- Antibody against CD-20	- Opportunistic infections - Progressive multifocal leukoencephalopathy
Trastuzumab	- Antibody against HER-2 tyrosine kinase receptor	- Cardiotoxicity
Ustekinumab	- Antibody against IL-12, 23	
Vemurafenib	- Inhibitor of BRAF oncogene	

Heme42

ARTHRITIS

Rheumatology/MSK Medicine

Differential Diagnosis for Joint Pain

	Monoarticular	Polyarticular
Non-inflammatory	- Osteoarthritis - Trauma - Malignancy - Avascular necrosis - Charcot joint - Internal derangement	- Osteoarthritis
Inflammatory	- Gout/pseudogout - Septic arthritis	- Infection (viral, Lyme) - Rheumatoid arthritis - Spondyloarthropathy - SLE

Arthrocentesis

Indications:
- Signs of joint inflammation (septic arthritis or gouty arthritis)
- Relief of moderate or large sized effusion

Interpretation:

	Color	WBC	PMN	Other Findings
Normal	Clear	< 200	< 25%	
Non-inflam	Clear/yellow	< 2,000	< 25%	
Inflammatory	Cloudy/yellow	> 2,000	> 50%	- Crystals seen with gout
Septic	Turbid purulent	> 20,000	> 75%	- Culture often positive
Hemorrhagic	Bloody	Variable	50-75%	

Charcot Joint

General: Progressive degeneration of a bony joint due to repetitive trauma in the setting of loss of sensation from neuropathy

Etiology: Diabetic neuropathy, vitamin B12 deficiency, tertiary syphilis, any cause of peripheral neuropathy or spinal cord injury with sensory deficit

Clinical:
- Insidious onset of erythema and swelling of joint (most often foot/ankle)
- Lack of sensation in same extremity
- Deformity of joint
- Degenerative joint disease or fractures on x-ray

Management:
- Manage underlying condition
- Acute inflammation: Casting (off-loading) and immobilization
- Chronic: Mechanical devices (ie braces) to protect and support from further damage

ARTHRITIS

Rheumatology/MSK Medicine

	Osteoarthritis	Rheumatoid Arthritis
Gen	- Degeneration of cartilage, hypertrophy of bone at articular margins - Most commonly affects weight bearing joints (hips, knees, lumbar spine)	- Chronic inflammatory autoimmune arthritis involving the synovium
Risk	- Age - Obesity - Excessive joint loading - Trauma (major injuries or micro-trauma over time)	- Family history/genetics (HLA-DR4) - Smoking - Females
Clin	- Insidious onset of joint pain - Morning stiffness < 30 min - Limited ROM - Joint crepitus - Bouchard/Heberden nodes (PIP/DIP) - XR (joint space narrowing, osteophytes, subchondral cysts) - Can support, but not diagnostic	- Insidious joint pain, stiffness, and swelling - Morning stiffness > 1 hour, improving with activity - Typically symmetric joint involvement - MCP, PIP joints in hands, wrists common early in disease (spares DIP) - Ulnar deviation, swan neck deformities - Cervical instability (C1/C2): Spine subluxation, spinal cord compression Extra-articular Manifestations: - Skin: Rheumatoid nodules - Ocular: Scleritis - Pulm: ILD - Heme: Anemia of chronic inflammation Felty's: Splenomegaly, neutropenia, RA
Dx	- Clinical diagnosis	Clinical criteria: > 3 joint involvement, > 6 weeks + RF or anti-citrullinated peptide Ab ↑ ESR/CRP
Tx	Nonpharmacologic - Weight loss - PT (strengthening exercises) - Canes/crutches, braces Pharmacologic - Topical NSAID, Capsaicin - Oral NSAIDs, Acetaminophen Injections - Steroids: Every 3-4 months, but effect is short term - Hyaluronic acid: Does not have great evidence yet Surgery - Total joint replacement	Initial Treatment: - Initiate DMARD (see options below) - Bridge with NSAIDs or steroids Flares: - Steroids Refractory Cases: - Add additional DMARD agents, or consider adding biologic DMARD Options: - Methotrexate (first line) - Alternatives: Leflunomide, Hydroxychloroquine, Sulfasalazine Biologics: TNF-α inhibitors, others

ARTHRITIS
Rheumatology/MSK
Medicine, Pediatrics

Juvenile Idiopathic Arthritis (JIA)

General: Child-onset inflammatory arthritis (JIA is a heterogeneous entity that likely includes multiple distinct disorders)
* Previously called Still's disease or juvenile rheumatoid arthritis

Subtype	Clinical Findings
Oligoarticular	- Symmetric arthritis for > 6 weeks - Arthritis with < 4 joints involved
Polyarticular	- Symmetric arthritis for > 6 weeks - Arthritis with ≥ 5 joints involved
Systemic	- Arthritis (as above) - Daily high spiking fever (so-called "quotidian fever" pattern) - Rash (salmon pink, macular rash)

Diagnosis: Purely clinical diagnosis of exclusion
- The following labs can be associated (but not specific)
    - Elevated ESR/CRP
    - Elevated ferritin
    - Hypergammaglobulinemia
    - Thrombocytosis, leukocytosis, anemia

Management:
- NSAIDs
- Glucocorticoids (intraarticular or oral)
- Biologics (anti Il-1 agents, anti Il-6, anti-TNFα)

Adult-Onset Still's Disease

General: Inflammatory polyarthritis that presents similarly to systemic JIA but occurs in adults

Clinical:
- Polyarthritis
- Daily high spiking fever
- Salmon pink macular rash
- Other nonspecific findings: LA, splenomegaly, leukocytosis, etc

Diagnosis: Diagnosis of exclusion
- Ferritin often extremely elevated
- ANA/RF generally not positive

Management:
- NSAIDs
- Corticosteroids
- Methotrexate, or other DMARD or biologic agent

CRYSTAL ARTHROPATHY
Rheumatology/MSK Medicine

Gout

General: Inflammatory monoarticular arthritis caused by the crystallization of monosodium urate in joints

Etiology/Risk:

Decreased Uric Acid Excretion	- > 90% of those with gout - Can be associated with renal disease, diuretic/NSAID use, EtOH use (uses same excretion site in kidney as urate)
Increased Uric Acid Production	- Chemotherapy - Hematologic malignancy - Chronic hemolysis
Genetic Enzyme Defects	- Lesch-Nyhan (HGPRT deficiency) - PRPP Synthetase overactivity (ie Von Gierke)

Clinical:
- Asymptomatic hyperuricemia (typically years before first episode)
- Acute Flare: Acute, painful monoarthropathy with edema and erythema
    - Podagra (1st MTP) is classic
- Intercritical Periods (asymptomatic time between gout flares)
    - > 50% have recurrence in a year, < 10% never have flare again
- Tophaceous gout: Chronic pain in joint
    - From packed uric acid crystals causing joint inflammation
    - Can visualize tophi (nodules of uric acid collection)

Diagnosis:
- Arthrocentesis (during acute flare)
    - Needle-shaped, negatively birefringent urate crystals
      (Yellow → Parallel, Blue → Perpendicular)
- Imaging can reveal articular destruction in advanced, chronic disease

Management:

Acute	- Oral glucocorticoids - NSAIDs (Naproxen/Indomethacin) - Colchicine (both NSAID and Colchicine contraindicated with CKD) - Intra-articular steroid injection (if only 1 or 2 joints affected)
Chronic	Urate lowering medication (indicated for recurrent gout flares) - Allopurinol (alt: Probenecid or Febuxostat) - Uric acid goal is < 6 mg/dL - Colchicine used concurrently for first few months to prevent flares
Lifestyle	- Weight loss - Reduce dietary animal/seafood protein consumption - Reduce EtOH intake

CRYSTAL ARTHROPATHY/REYNAUD
Rheumatology/MSK Medicine

Pseudogout

General: Calcium pyrophosphate crystal deposition, causing inflammatory arthritis

Risk:
- Majority idiopathic
- Hyperparathyroidism
- Hemochromatosis
- Joint trauma/osteoarthritis

Clinical:
- Often asymptomatic up until flare
- Acute flare: Acute/subacute arthritis of single extremity joint
    - Large joints (ie knees) most commonly affected
- Can result in polyarticular inflammatory arthritis (looks like RA)

Diagnosis:
- Weakly positively birefringent rod-shaped and rhomboidal crystals
    - Inflammatory synovial fluid findings
- Joint XR: Chondrocalcinosis (cartilage calcification)

Management: Managed similar to gout (steroids/NSAID/Colchicine or intra-articular steroid injection)

Reynaud's

General: Abnormal vascular reactivity in distal extremities, characterized by exaggerated vasoconstriction in response to cold temperatures or stress

Clinical: Classic attack includes acute onset coldness in the distal extremity, followed by pallor ("white attack"), ischemia/cyanosis ("blue attack"), and eventual reperfusion (back to pink/red)

	Primary	Secondary
Etio	- Idiopathic	- Connective tissue disease (SLE, RA, scleroderma) - Drugs (amphetamines, others) - Cryoglobulinemia, cold agglutinin disease - Trauma (ie use of vibrating tools)
Clin	- Minimal systemic symptoms - No tissue injury - ESR/CRP, ANA and other tests typically normal	- Symptoms of underlying autoimmune disease - Distal extremity ulcerations and tissue damage + Nailfold capillary microscopy
Tx	- Avoid triggers - Ca-Channel Blockers	- Treat underlying condition - Ca-Channel Blockers (alt: Sildenafil) - Aspirin (for ulcerations)

CONNECTIVE TISSUE DISEASE — Rheumatology/MSK Medicine

Systemic Lupus Erythematosus

General: Autoimmune disorder characterized by auto-antibody formation against intracellular proteins/material (ie DNA), which results in immune complex formation and subsequent multiorgan inflammatory damage

Risk: Middle aged women. Black, Hispanic women at increased risk.

Clinical:
- Constitutional symptoms (fatigue, fever, and weight loss)
- Dermatologic/mucous membrane
    - Malar* "butterfly" rash (erythematous rash over cheeks/nose)
    - Discoid* lesions (erythematous raised patches with scaling)
    - Photosensitivity, oral or nasopharyngeal ulcers*, alopecia*
- Polyarthritis*
- Serositis* (pleuritis, pericarditis)
- Vascular disease (vasculitis, Raynaud's, VTE)
- Renal* (glomerulonephritis, proteinuria)
- Hematologic (hemolytic anemia*, leukopenia*, thrombocytopenia*)
- Immunologic dysfunction (impaired immune response, ↑ infection risk)
- Neuropsychiatric* dysfunction
- Ophthalmologic (scleritis)
- Cardiovascular (Libman-Sacks endocarditis: Thrombi on both sides of valve)

Diagnosis:
- ANA* (initial screening test of choice)
- Anti-dsDNA*, Anti-Smith*, Antiphospholipid*
- Positive Direct Coombs*
- Low Complement* (Low C3, C4, or CH50)

SLICC Diagnostic Criteria: ≥ 4/17 of the above (starred) features, with at least one clinical and one lab feature

Management:
- Lifestyle Management: Sun protection, proper immunizations, pregnancy and contraception counseling

Severity	Definition	Intervention
Mild	- Skin, joint, and mucosal involvement	- Hydroxychloroquine +/- course of NSAIDs/low dose steroids
Moderate	- Significant symptoms, but no evidence of organ failure	- Hydroxychloroquine + short course of Prednisone
Severe	- Severe/life threatening organ involvement	- High dose IV Methylprednisolone - Immunosuppression (ie Azathioprine, Mycophenolate, Cyclophosphamide, or Rituximab)

CONNECTIVE TISSUE DISEASE — Rheumatology/MSK Medicine

Systemic Sclerosis (Scleroderma)

General: Autoimmune condition characterized by immune activation, vascular damage, and systemic tissue fibrosis (collagen deposition)

	Limited	Diffuse

Clin	- Cutaneous fibrosis, most commonly of distal extremities
	  - Morphea: Fibrotic plaques
	  - Linear fibrotic bands
	  - Sclerodactyly
	Other Findings:
	- Raynaud's
	- Telangiectasias
	
	- Some have CREST syndrome (Calcinosis of fingers, Raynaud, Esophageal dysmotility, Sclerodactyly, and Telangiectasia)
		- Cutaneous fibrosis more widespread (versus limited), Raynaud's, telangiectasias
		
		Organ Involvement
		- GI: Esophageal dysmotility, reflux, dysphagia, dyspepsia
		- Pulm: Interstitial fibrosis and pulmonary hypertension
		- CV: Myocardial fibrosis, pericarditis
		- Renal: HTN, scleroderma renal crisis (MAHA, oliguria, thrombocytopenia)

Dx	Clinical features plus auto-antibodies: - ANA (positive in most) - Anti-topoisomerase I (anti scl-70, most commonly diffuse) - Anti-centromere antibodies (most commonly limited)	
Tx	- No effective cure, manage problems of each individual organ system - Immunosuppression (Methotrexate, Mycophenolate, Cyclophosphamide, etc) used for severe skin disease or multi-organ involvement	

Skin	- Topical/intralesional steroids, or other topical agents
Raynaud's	- Ca-Channel Blockers
Arthritis	- NSAIDs
Renal	- ACEi
GI	- PPI
Pulm	- Immunosuppression for fibrosis, vasodilators for PAH

CONNECTIVE TISSUE DISEASE
Rheumatology/MSK Medicine

Sjogren Syndrome

General: Autoimmune lymphocytic infiltration and destruction of lacrimal and salivary glands. Can be primary or secondary to other AI disease (ie SLE, RA).

Clinical:
- Dry eyes (keratoconjunctivitis sicca): Burning/red eyes, blurred vision
    - Can be confirmed objectively via Schirmer test
- Dry mouth (xerostomia): Tooth decay, parotid enlargement
- Extraglandular manifestations:
    - Reynaud
    - Arthritis
    - Vasculitis, interstitial lung disease, interstitial nephritis

Diagnosis:
- Autoantibody: Ro/La (SS-A/B) positive
    - Can cross placenta, causing neonatal heart block
- ANA and RF often also positive
- Lip biopsy is highly specific (lymphocytic glandular infiltrate)

Management:

Mouth	- Behavioral modification (good oral hygiene, regular oral hydration) - Artificial saliva or pilocarpine can be used if necessary
Eyes	- Artificial tears
Systemic	- DMARDs (ie Hydroxychloroquine, Methotrexate), steroids, or other systemic agents

Mixed Connective Tissue Disease

General: Overlap syndrome of SLE, systemic sclerosis, and polymyositis

Clinical:
- Raynaud's
- Myositis, sclerodactyly
- Polyarthritis
- Pulmonary hypertension (major cause of death) and interstitial fibrosis
- GI dysmotility
- Lack of renal, CNS disease

Diagnosis: Positive anti-U1 ribonucleoprotein (RNP) antibodies is characteristic

Management: Glucocorticoids

SERONEG SPONDYLOARTHROPATHY

Rheumatology/MSK, Medicine, Pediatrics

	General/Clinical (*All associated with HLA B27)	Diagnosis	Management
Psoriatic Arthritis	- Inflammatory polyarthritis seen in up to 30% of people with psoriasis - Asymmetric and polyarticular arthritis, generally years after skin findings - Characteristic finger edema, "sausage digits" (dactylitis) - Onycholysis (separation of nail) and nail pitting	- Clinical diagnosis (no specific laboratory tests) - XR (joints show erosive changes and new bone formation, which is defining)	- Mild arthritis (without evidence of joint damage) → NSAIDs - Refractory arthritis, or evidence of joint damage → DMARD (Methotrexate, Leflunomide, etc) - Biologics often required (ie TNF-α inhibitors) to control severe disease

Ankylosing Spondylitis	- Inflammatory arthritis of the spine, typically presenting in young adult males
	- Bilateral sacroiliitis
	- Spinal involvement (loss of lordosis, restricted chest mobility)
	- Peripheral arthritis, dactylitis, enthesitis
	- Extra-articular: Uveitis, IBD, psoriasis, aortitis/aortic root disease
		- Clinical diagnosis
		- Lumbar imaging (XR/MRI)
		  - Erosions, ankylosis, or sclerosis
		  - "Bamboo spine"
		- No labs specific (ESR/CRP generally elevated)
			- NSAIDs, plus regular exercise/PT
			- If not effective: Biologic agents used (ie TNF-α inhibitors)
			*DMARDS not effective

Reactive Arthritis	- Inflammatory arthritis associated with recent extra-articular infection Presents weeks after infection with: - Asymmetric arthritis, enthesitis, dactylitis - Eye: Conjunctivitis or uveitis - Oral ulcers - Keratoderma blennorrhagica (scaly foot rash) - Circinate balanitis (ulcerative genital lesions)	- Clinical diagnosis - Associated with recent GI/GU infection with the following: *Salmonella, Shigella, Campylobacter, Chlamydia, Yersinia*	- NSAIDs - Refractory: Intra-articular/oral steroids
IBD Associated Arthritis	- Peripheral arthritis, spondylitis, or sacroiliitis associated with IBD (UC/Crohn's)	- Clinical diagnosis	- Treat IBD appropriately (usually helps arthritis) - NSAIDs

SARCOIDOSIS

Rheumatology/MSK Medicine

Sarcoidosis

General: Chronic granulomatous inflammation characterized by the presence of noncaseating granulomas in multiple different organ systems

Risk: Most commonly affects young adult, black females

Clinical:

Pulm	- Most common clinical manifestation (> 90%) - Cough, dyspnea, chest pain - Bilateral hilar LA and interstitial infiltrates (restrictive lung disease)
Derm	- Papules, nodules, plaques, and atrophic or ulcerative lesions
MSK	- Acute and/or chronic polyarthritis
Ophtho	- Anterior or posterior uveitis
CNS	- Central DI, cranial mononeuropathy, other focal defects
CV	- Restrive or dilated cardiomyopathy, pericarditis, conduction disease
Misc Findings	- Peripheral lymphadenopathy, splenomegaly - Elevated serum ACE levels - Hypervitaminosis D (↑ 1α hydroxylase activity) → Hypercalcemia - ↑ CD4/CD8 ratio in bronchoalveolar lavage
Lofgren Syndrome	- Hilar LA, fever, polyarthritis, and erythema nodosum

Diagnosis:
- Imaging
    - CXR: Bilateral hilar adenopathy (+/- pulmonary infiltrate)
    - Chest CT: Provides higher resolution
- Biopsy of lesion (noncaseating granulomas)
    - Use most accessible (cutaneous lesions, superficial lymph node)
    - If not available, use lung lesion (via bronchoscopy/endobronchial biopsy)
- Diagnosis is confirmed when imaging and biopsy is consistent with sarcoid, and other possible diagnoses are ruled out

Management:
- Pulmonary disease
    - Asymptomatic: Observe/monitor. Often spontaneous remission.
    - Symptomatic: Glucocorticoids
- Derm: Topical/intralesional/systemic corticosteroids
- Arthropathy: NSAIDs, corticosteroids

MYOPATHY
Rheumatology/MSK Medicine

Myopathy Differential Diagnosis

	Clinical	Abnormal Labs
Inflammatory Myopathy (DM/PM)	- Proximal muscle weakness	↑ ESR/CRP, ↑ CK
Inclusion Body Myositis	- Muscle weakness and atrophy without pain	Normal ESR, ↔/↑ CK
Glucocorticoid Induced	- Proximal muscle weakness without pain or tenderness	
Statin Induced	- Muscle pain/tenderness	↑ CK
Hypothyroidism	- Proximal muscle pain, tenderness, and weakness	↑ CK, ↑ TSH
Myasthenia Gravis	- Progressive weakness with activity	Anti-BM antibodies
Polymyalgia Rheumatica	- Proximal muscle pain and stiffness, without weakness	↑ ESR/CRP

Others:
- Muscular dystrophy (including adult onset types like limb-girdle)
- Myotonic dystrophy
- Inherited metabolic myopathy
- Infiltrative disorders (amyloid, sarcoid, trichinellosis)

Inclusion Body Myositis

General: Rare sporadic adult-onset disorder of muscle weakness

Clinical:
- Insidious onset (years long) of muscle weakness
    - More often distal (compared to PM/DM)
- Muscle atrophy
- Dysphagia, facial muscle involvement possible
- Normal or modest CK elevations

Diagnosis: Clinical features above PLUS
- Muscle biopsy (shows CD8 infiltration as in polymyositis, but with inclusions on electron microscopy)

Management:
- Nonpharmacologic: Physical, speech, occupational therapy
- Poor response to any pharmacologic agents

MYOPATHY
Rheumatology/MSK Medicine

Polymyositis/Dermatomyositis

	Polymyositis	Dermatomyositis
Gen	- Immune-mediated myocyte injury - Endomysial CD8 T cells (surround and invade myofiber fascicles)	- Immune-mediated myocyte injury - Unclear pathophysiology, but CD4+ T cells are visualized perifascicularly and perivascularly *Associated with occult malignancy (including lung, breast, ovary, GI, kidney, lungs)
Clin	- Subacute onset of proximal, symmetric muscle weakness - Neck flexors, deltoids, hips commonly affected - Dysphagia/aspiration (upper esophageal muscle weakness) - Muscle atrophy in advanced disease Extramuscular: - Interstitial lung disease - Myocarditis	- Muscle weakness (similar to polymyositis) Skin Findings: - Gottron papules (papular, erythematous scaly lesions over the knuckles) - Heliotrope rash (periorbital rash) - Photodistributed erythema ("shawl sign") Extramuscular: - Interstitial lung disease - Myocarditis

Dx	- ↑ CK, LDH, Aldolase, AST/ALT
	
	- Autoantibodies:
	  - Anti Jo-1 (anti t-RNA synthetase)
	  - Anti-SRP
	  - Anti Mi-2
	- Electromyography (often abnormal but not specific)
	- Muscle biopsy
	
	* Diagnosis can be made with classic muscle weakness, elevated muscle enzymes, and classic rash (for PM). Biopsy and myography may be required in those with partial features.	

Tx	- Glucocorticoids (for acute episode) PLUS DMARD for chronic management - Additional DMARDs or Rituximab used for refractory disease	

MYOPATHY
Rheumatology/MSK Medicine

Polymyalgia Rheumatica

General: Common inflammatory rheumatologic condition of unclear etiology

Risk: Almost exclusively in those > 50 y/o, associated with temporal arteritis, HLA-DR4

Clinical:
- Symmetrical pain and morning stiffness in the shoulders, hip, neck, torso
- Decreased range of motion on exam, but no weakness
- Constitutional symptoms may be present (fever, weight loss)
- ESR/CRP elevated

Diagnosis: Clinical diagnosis (suspected in someone with > 2 weeks of pain/morning stiffness, elevated ESR/CRP, and response to glucocorticoids)

Management:
- Glucocorticoids (start at initial episode, then slowly taper as long as patient remains asymptomatic)
    - Disease is self-limited. Steroids can often be stopped in 1-2 years.

Fibromyalgia

General: Chronic pain caused by CNS/PNS hyperirritability

Risk: Most common in middle aged women

Clinical:
- Chronic, diffuse musculoskeletal pain (for > 3 months)
    - Exam demonstrates tenderness in specific anatomic locations
- Fatigue, abnormal sleep patterns
- Cognitive and psychiatric disturbances
- Headache
- Paresthesias

Diagnosis:
- Clinical diagnosis of exclusion
- Labs (ESR, CRP, CBC, TSH, etc) all normal
- Current guidelines focus on symptoms (widespread pain index and symptom severity scale) for diagnosis rather than tender point count

Management:
- Nonpharm: Patient education, regular exercise
- Pharm (if nonpharm does not sufficiently relieve symptoms)
    - TCA (Amitriptyline)
    - SNRI (Milnacipran/Duloxetine), Pregabalin
- Severe, refractory cases: Combine drugs, try CBT (with biofeedback training)

VASCULITIS — Rheumatology/MSK Medicine

Large Vessel Vasculitis

	General/Clinical	Diagnosis	Management
Giant Cell "Temporal" Arteritis	- Chronic inflammatory response of large and medium vessels - Classically temporal arterial involvement, but can also involve carotid and aorta - Seen almost exclusively in > 50 y/o Clinical: - Constitutional symptoms (fever, malaise, etc) - Severe HA - Visual impairment (25-50%) (Optic neuritis, amaurosis fugax, anterior ischemic optic neuropathy, can lead to blindness) - Jaw pain with chewing (intermittent claudication of jaw/tongue) - Tenderness over temples, possible nodules - Arm claudication with possible bruits, decreased pulses	- ESR/CRP ↑↑↑ - Temporal artery biopsy gold standard (for confirmation) *High association with PMR, aortic aneurysm/dissection	Acute: - High dose prednisone early (40-60 oral, unless visual symptoms → 1000mg IV methylpred) - Do not wait for lab/biopsy results to initiate treatment Chronic: - Taper steroids - ESR to monitor effectiveness of therapy - Ultimately is self-limited and rarely refractory, but can use MTX or Tocilizumab (Il-6 inhibitor) for recurrent disease
Takayasu	- Granulomatous vasculitis of aortic arch and major branches, potentially leading to stenosis - Risk: Young adult (20-40 y/o), Asian, women Clinical: - Constitutional (fever, weight loss) - Arterial-occlusive disease in UE (claudication) - Pain, bruits over involved vessels - Absent pulses in carotid, radial, ulnar - MI/stroke - Aortic aneurysms, regurgitation	- MRA (or CTA) - ESR/CRP often elevated	- Corticosteroids - Other immunosuppressives (ie MTX, Azathioprine, Mycophenolate, Tocilizumab) in refractory cases - Severe stenosis may require angioplasty/stenting

Rheum14

VASCULITIS
Rheumatology/MSK — Medicine, Pediatrics

Medium Vessel Vasculitis

	General/Clinical	Diagnosis	Management
Polyarteritis Nodosa	- Medium vessel vasculitis of adults - Risk: Often idiopathic, but increased risk with Hepatitis B/C, hairy cell leukemia Clinical: - Constitutional: Fever, fatigue, weight loss - Derm: Livedo reticularis, tender nodules, purpura - GI: Abdominal pain (mesenteric artery involvement) - Renal: Insufficiency, HTN (renal artery stenosis) - CNS: Mononeuritis multiplex	- Biopsy (inflammation of fibrinoid necrosis of medium vessels) - Mesenteric angiography (see multiple aneurysms and irregular constrictions)	- Glucocorticoids +/- Cyclophosphamide (if severe)
Kawasaki's	- Seen in 1-5 years old, especially Asians Clinical Criteria: - Fever (> 5 days) - Bilateral nonexudative conjunctivitis - Erythema of the lips/tongue/oral mucosa - Rash (polymorphous) - Extremity edema, erythema - Cervical lymphadenopathy Others: Leukocytosis, thrombocytosis, ↑ESR	- Clinical diagnosis (fever > 5 days, plus 4 more of the clinical signs, plus no other possible underlying etiology) * Risk for coronary artery aneurysms (can thrombose/rupture)	- IVIG plus Aspirin - ECHO (at time of diagnosis, and at weeks ~2 and 6, to rule out coronary involvement)
Buerger's Disease (Thromboangiitis obliterans)	- Small and medium vessel vasculitis that occurs in middle aged male smokers - Inflammatory thrombotic vessel occlusions - Clinical: Superficial thrombophlebitis, migratory phlebitis, ischemic ulceration	- Clinical diagnosis (age < 45, hx of tobacco use, extremity ischemia - Angiography used to image vessels	- Smoking cessation - Iloprost, Ca-Channel Blockers, and pneumatic compression (improve pain)

VASCULITIS

Rheumatology/MSK
Medicine, Pediatrics

Small Vessel Vasculitis

	General/Clinical	Diagnosis	Management
Granulomatosis w/ Polyangiitis [GPA] (Wegener's)	- Small vessel necrotizing vasculitis with granulomatous inflammation - Risk: Older, white men Clinical: - Constitutional: Fever, anorexia, and weight loss - Upper Resp: Sinusitis, otitis, discharge, ulcers - Lower Resp: Nodules, infiltrates, hemoptysis - Renal: Pauci-immune rapidly progressive GN - Derm: Ulcers, purpura - Eye: Conjunctivitis, scleritis, uveitis	- c-ANCA/PR3-ANCA (but other is possible) - Biopsy (for definitive diagnosis)	- Glucocorticoids PLUS Cyclophosphamide, Rituximab, or Methotrexate - Plasma Exchange (in severe renal or pulmonary disease)
Microscopic Polyangiitis	- Vasculitis without granuloma formation - Clinical: Very similar to GPA, but with decreased likelihood for upper respiratory disease	- p-ANCA/MPO-ANCA (but other is possible) - Biopsy (for definitive diagnosis)	
Eosinophilic Granulomatosis w/ Polyangiitis [EGPA] (Churg Strauss)	- Vasculitis with allergic features Clinical: - Chronic rhinosinusitis - Asthma (pulmonary infiltrates/fibrosis) - Peripheral neuropathy (mononeuritis multiplex) - Skin (palpable purpura, nodules) - Cardiac, renal disease	- ANCA positive (~50%) - Peripheral eosinophilia - CT chest (pulm infiltrates, ground glass, nodules) - Biopsy (generally lung or skin) for definitive diagnosis	- Glucocorticoids +/- other immunosuppression (Cyclophosphamide, Azathioprine)
Henoch-Schonlein Purpura	- IgA vasculitis, most common childhood vasculitis Clinical: (Often occurs within days of viral URI) - Skin: Palpable purpura - Arthralgias - Abdominal pain - Renal (hematuria, IgA nephropathy)	- Clinical - Biopsy (would be definitive, but often not required)	- Supportive care (fluids, NSAIDs for pain control, rest, etc) as disease generally self-limited - Corticosteroids if severe

Rheum16

VASCULITIS — Rheumatology/MSK Medicine

Behcet's disease

General: Syndrome of recurrent ulcers due to systemic vasculitis of all sized vessels

Risk: Young adults of Middle-Eastern (ie Turkish) and Eastern Asian descent

Clinical:
- Recurrent aphthous ulcers
- Urogenital ulcers
- Derm: Acne-like eruptions, pustules, erythema nodosum, pseudofolliculitis
    - Pathergy (erythematous papular response to local skin injury)
- Eye: Uveitis
- Vascular disease and thrombosis

Diagnosis: Clinical diagnosis (recurrent ulcers, plus some of the other above features and positive pathergy test)

Management:
- Topical steroids for ulcers
- Colchicine for chronic prevention of ulcers
- System immunosuppression for organ system involvement

Hypersensitivity Vasculitis

General: Also known as cutaneous leukocytoclastic vasculitis or cutaneous small vessel vasculitis, hypersensitivity vasculitis is a small vessel vasculitis that characteristically results in purpura

Risk: Idiopathic often, but can be caused by drugs, infection, or autoimmune disease

Clinical:
- Non-blanching, palpable purpura
    - Rash can cause pain or pruritus
- Postinflammatory hyperpigmentation (after lesions resolve)
- Systemic symptoms (fever, myalgias, arthralgias)
- *No organ system involvement (ie glomerulonephritis, etc)

Management:
- Treat underlying (remove drug, treat infection if present)
- Generally self-limited (just manage symptoms like pain/itching)
- Glucocorticoids if severe

< BONES >					< Rheumatology/MSK Medicine >

Osteoporosis

General: Disorder of low bone mass, abnormal bone structure, and fragility, resulting in decreased bone strength and increased fracture risk. Can be:
- Primary: Idiopathic or age-related
- Secondary:
    - Drugs (Glucocorticoids, Heparin, Cyclosporine, Phenytoin)
    - Endocrine (Cushing, hyperthyroidism, hyperparathyroidism, hypogonadism)
    - Nutritional (Vit D/Ca deficiency, malabsorption, other GI)

Risk:
- Modifiable: Smoking, EtOH, sedentary, low dietary Ca
- Non-modifiable: ↑ Age, low weight, post menopause, white or Asian

Clinical:
- Asymptomatic until fracture occurs
- All clinical manifestations (pain, deformity, loss of height, disability) associated with fracture
    - Vertebral Fx (most common, often asymptomatic, can lose height)
    - Hip and distal radius (Colles) Fx also common

Diagnosis: History of fragility fracture OR DEXA Scan

Normal	T Score between -1 and 1
Osteopenia	T score between -1 and -2.5
Osteoporosis	T score between < -2.5
Severe Osteoporosis	T score < -3.5 OR < -2.5 plus fragility fracture

Management:
- Lifestyle (exercise, smoking cessation, prevent falls, ↓ EtOH)
- Vitamin D (800 IU/day) and Calcium (1200 mg/day if diet not enough)

Pharmacologic
- Indicated if: Osteoporosis (DEXA < -2.5) OR Osteopenia plus high risk (↑ FRAX score)
- Agents:
    - Bisphosphonate (Alendronate, Risedronate)
    - Second line: Denosumab or Teriparatide

Screening: DEXA scan screening q3-5 years
- All women > 65, women < 65 with risk factors
- Only men with clinical manifestations of osteoporosis or risk factors

BONES — Rheumatology/MSK Medicine

	General/Clinical	Diagnosis	Management
Osteomalacia	- Defective mineralization of osteoid - Most commonly caused by vitamin D deficiency Ricket's (kids) - Bow legs, bead-like costochondral junctions, Craniotabes (soft skull), frontal bossing Osteomalacia (adults) - Bone pain, muscle weakness, cramps, difficulty walking	↓ Ca, PO4, 25-Vit D ↑ PTH, Alk Phos XR: Thin cortex, decreased density, pseudofractures	- Vitamin D if deficient (50k IU for 6-8 weeks, followed by standard 800 mg supplement)
Osteopetrosis	- Increased bone density from failure of proper osteoclastic bone resorption - AR (defect in carbonic anhydrase) is severe childhood form, while AD disease affects adults - Cranial nerve impingement from skull sclerosis	- XR: Sclerotic bone, or "bone within bone" appearance	- Bone marrow transplant (if genetically based)
Paget's (Osteitis Deformans)	- Disorder of excessive bone remodelling, from osteoclastic dysfunction Clinical - Most often asymptomatic - Bone pain and deformities - Skull (HA, hearing loss) & Spinal (radiculopathy) - Increased risk for bone tumors (osteosarcoma)	↑ Alk Phos. Normal Ca/PO4. ↑ Urine hydroxyproline, PINP - XR: Osteolytic and/or sclerotic lesions - Bone Scintigraphy: Assess extent of disease	- Bisphosphonates
Osteonecrosis (Avascular Necrosis)	- Death of bone marrow due to disruption of vasculature - Most commonly hip (medial circumflex femoral artery) - Risk: Trauma, corticosteroids, sickle cell, SLE, Legg-Calve-Perthes, SCFE - Presents as joint pain	- XR: Density changes, sclerosis, cysts, "crescent sign" (subchondral collapse) - MRI (provides much higher sensitivity)	- Try to spare joint for as long as possible (bisphosphonates or joint sparing procedures) - Joint replacement if severe

BONE AND JOINT INFECTIONS
Rheumatology/MSK
Medicine, Pediatrics

Septic Arthritis

General: Bacterial infection of a joint, most commonly due to:
- Hematogenous spread
- Contiguous spread from another locus of infection (osteomyelitis)
- Direct inoculation (trauma, surgery, bites)

Organisms include *Staphylococcus aureus* and *Streptococci*, and gram negatives (if immunocompromised). In prosthetic joints, organisms include *Staph aureus* and gram negatives (< 3 months post surgery), *Staph epidermidis* and *Enterococcus* (3-12 months post surgery), *Staph aureus* and beta-hemolytic *Streptococci* (> 12 months post surgery).

Risk: Pre-existing arthritis (especially RA, but also OA, gout, and diabetic arthropathy), immunocompromised, IV drug use

Clinical:
- Monoarticular, severely painful arthritis. Erythema, edema, swelling of joint.
- Constitutional (fever, chills, malaise)

Diagnosis:
- Arthrocentesis (definitive)
    - Gram stain, culture, cell counts
    - Septic fluid counts (> 20K WBC, > 75% neutrophils)
- Imaging (can rule in/out bone infection, help examine tough-to-tap joints)

Management:
Antibiotic Therapy (based on initial gram stain). Generally ~4 weeks required.
- Gram stain (+) bacteria: Vancomycin
- Gram stain (-) bacteria: 3rd Gen Cephalosporin (or Cefepime if concern for *Pseudomonas*)
- Gram stain not revealing: Vancomycin
    - Vanc + Ceftriaxone if immunocompromised
- Adjust to culture results

Drainage (needle, arthroscopic, or open), indicated:
- If abscess, refractory to initial treatment, or high risk joint (ie prosthesis)

Gonococcal Arthritis

General: Arthritis secondary to disseminated gonococcal infection

Clinical:
- Purulent monoarthritis or migratory, asymmetric polyarthritis
- Tenosynovitis
- Skin lesions (erythematous papules/pustules)

Diagnosis:
- Arthrocentesis (with gram stain/fluid analysis, NAAT)
- GU gonorrhea NAAT

Management:
- Ceftriaxone + Azithromycin/Doxycycline

BONE AND JOINT INFECTIONS
Rheumatology/MSK — Medicine, Pediatrics

Transient Synovitis

General: Self-limited inflammatory joint pain, most commonly after viral URI infection. Common cause of hip pain in children.

Clinical:
- Joint pain
- Systemic symptoms (low grade fever, malaise, etc)

Diagnosis:
- Clinical diagnosis (must rule out septic arthritis, but can simply follow clinically if T < 101.4°F, WBC < 12K, ESR < 20)

Management: NSAIDs

Osteomyelitis

General: Bacterial infection of bone, most commonly due to:
- Hematogenous spread (most commonly one organism)
    - Most common cause of osteomyelitis in children
- Contiguous spread from another locus of infection (ie soft tissue infection)
- Direct inoculation (trauma, like open fractures)

Micro: Most commonly *Staphylococcus aureus, Streptococcus*, gram negatives
- Puncture wound: *Staph, Pseudomonas*
- Prosthetic joint: Coagulase-negative *Staphylococci*
- Diabetic foot ulcer: Polymicrobial organisms
- IV drug abuse/Immunocompromise: Fungal species, *Pseudomonas*
- Sickle cell disease: *Salmonella*

Risk: IV drug use, open fractures, diabetes mellitus (ie ulcers), bacteremia

Clinical:
- Gradual onset of local pain with possible erythema, swelling at site
- Constitutional symptoms (fever, malaise) may be present. ESR ↑.
- Can become chronic with waxing/waning pain +/- draining sinus tract

Diagnosis:
- Imaging
    - XR: Periosteal thickening or elevation
    - MRI: Most sensitive
    - If hardware present: PET scan or triple phase bone scan
- Bone biopsy is definitive (may not need if + blood cx and image findings)

Management:
- Empiric Antibiotics (Vancomycin and Ceftriaxone)
    - Tailor to specific organism/sensitivities once available
- Surgical debridement often required (depending on response to antibiotics)

BONE AND SOFT TISSUE MALIGNANCY
Rheumatology/MSK Medicine, Pediatrics

	General/Clinical	Diagnosis/Management
Osteochondroma	- Benign bony exostosis with cartilaginous cap, seen in children and young adults - Most common at end of long bone (ie femur) - Presents as painless mass (but can rarely cause pain, deformity)	XR Tx: Observation. Resect if remains symptomatic. *Small chance of progression to osteochondrosarcoma
Giant Cell Tumor	- Benign, locally aggressive bone tumor most commonly seen in young adults - Presents as a lytic lesion in the epiphysis of long bones (most commonly distal femur) - Clinically presents as pain, swelling, decreased ROM of joint, pathologic fracture	XR: Soap bubble appearance (eccentric, locally aggressive lesions), CT/MRI used for better definition Biopsy: Multinucleated giant cells Tx: Surgery
Osteoid Osteoma	- Benign bone-forming tumor; seen most commonly in teens, with characteristic prostaglandin-producing central nidus - Presents as progressive night time pain, most commonly in long bone (femur) or spine	XR (or CT/MRI if required): Well-defined round lesion Tx: NSAIDs for pain. Surgical resection if symptomatic.
Osteosarcoma	- Malignant, primary tumor of bone, with bimodal onset of presentation (10-20 y/o, and > 65) - Associated with hereditary retinoblastoma, Li-Fraumeni syndrome, Paget's, other bone lesions - Presents with local bone pain with onset over months	XR (sunburst, Codman triangle [elevated periosteum]) Biopsy (for definitive diagnosis) Tx: Chemotherapy and surgical resection
Ewing Sarcoma	- Malignant, anaplastic small cell tumor, found in long bones - Seen most commonly in boys < 15 y/o - Presents with subacute presentation of localized pain and swelling	XR (moth eaten appearance, onion skin periosteal reaction) CT/MRI for better definition. Biopsy for definitive diagnosis. Tx: Chemoradiation (neoadjuvant) + Surgery

MUSCULOSKELETAL: BACK
Rheumatology/MSK, Medicine, Surgery

Overview of Low Back Pain

General: 85% of back pain cases are due to idiopathic, nonspecific, presumably musculoskeletal pain that is self-limited in nature
- Acute (< 4 weeks)
- Subacute (4-12 weeks)
- Chronic (> 12 weeks)

Etiology:
- Mechanical
    - Strain, spondylosis, osteoarthritis, spondylolisthesis, disc herniation, spinal stenosis, compression fx, kyphosis/scoliosis
- Nonmechanical
    - Neoplasia, infection (osteomyelitis, epidural abscess), rheumatic disease (ie ankylosing spondylitis, psoriatic spondylitis, etc)
- Visceral
    - Kidney pain (PKD), AAA, pancreatitis, PID

Diagnosis:
- Imaging not generally indicated within 4 weeks
    - Exceptions: Image patients with severe neurologic deficits, cancer hx, constitutional symptoms, osteoporosis, IV drug use
- After 4-6 weeks of conservative therapy, consider further workup
    - Plain XR (if nonspecific)
    - CT/MRI (if concerned about radiculopathy or spinal stenosis)
    - ESR/CRP (if concerned about cancer)

Management:

Acute	- Moderate activity levels - Trial of heat, massage, acupuncture, or spinal manipulation (if desired) - NSAIDs/Acetaminophen - Adjuncts (for refractory cases): Muscle relaxants, short opioid course
Subacute	- Similar to acute - Consider physical therapy and/or exercise therapy at this time
Chronic	- Treat underlying disease (ie surgery if necessary, etc) - Intermittent NSAID/Acetaminophen use (can consider adding muscle relaxant, Tramadol, or Duloxetine in severe cases) - Exercise/physical therapy

Lumbosacral Radiculopathy

General: Herniations usually occur posterolaterally, affecting nerve root below level of disc herniation

L3-L4	- Weakness of knee extension, weak patellar reflexes
L4-L5	- Weak dorsiflexion, difficulty heel walking, lateral leg/dorsal foot sensory loss
L5-S1	- Weakness of plantarflexion, difficulty toe walking, decreased Achilles reflex

MUSCULOSKELETAL: BACK — Rheumatology/MSK Medicine, Surgery

	General/Clinical	Diagnosis/Management
Lumbar Strain	- Common cause of acute low back pain. Due to stretching injury to muscles/tendons/ligaments. - Presents as paraspinal muscle tenderness, spasms	Dx: Clinical Tx: Conservative (see prior page). Self-limited.
Disc Herniation	- "Slipped disc." Protrusion of inner nucleus pulposus through outer fibrous ring - Herniation often caused by trauma - Presents as acute lumbosacral radiculopathy (including sciatica), +/- back pain. Exacerbated by ↑ pressure/valsalva.	Dx: Clinical. Imaging indicated if severe neurologic deficit or signs of infection or malignancy. Tx: Conservative (see prior page). Surgery if refractory (only required in ~ 10% of cases).
Spinal Stenosis	- Narrowing of spinal canal from degenerative spinal disease - Causes: Osteophytes (OA), ligamentum flavum hypertrophy, disc bulging, or spondylolisthesis - Presents with pain, neurogenic claudication (numbness/paresthesias in legs) - Worse with walking, relieved with sitting/leaning forward (+ leg raise test in ~ 10%)	Dx: MRI confirms diagnosis Tx: Conservative (if not severe/not progressive). Consider surgical therapy if conservative therapy fails.
Spondylolisthesis	- Anterior or posterior translation of vertebral body compared to adjacent vertebral body - Causes spinal stenosis (and its associated symptoms)	Dx: MRI Tx: Conservative initially. Surgical fusion if fails.
Compression Fractures	- Most commonly seen with osteoporosis, but also chronic steroid use, infection, spinal metastasis, Paget disease - Presents as acute back pain, often post minor trauma in person with osteoporosis or risk factors - Severe pain with palpation of site - Note: Can be chronic, which do not present with pain, but rather progressive kyphosis/loss of stature	Dx: XR Tx: Conservative (pain control, activity modification, etc). If pain extremely severe, or neurologic symptoms, consider surgery (kyphoplasty or vertebroplasty).

MUSCULOSKELETAL: BACK — Rheumatology/MSK Medicine, Surgery

Epidural Abscess

General: Abscess formation in the epidural space, from bacterial hematogenous spread, direct extension, or iatrogenic inoculation. *Staph aureus* responsible for most cases.

Risk: IV drug use, spinal procedures

Clinical:
- Classic triad: Fever, back pain, neurologic findings
    - Motor/sensory deficits, bowel/bladder dysfunction
- ↑ ESR

Diagnosis:
- Spinal MRI (with contrast)
- Blood culture or aspiration (for organism identification)

Management:
- Broad antibiotics (Vancomycin + 3rd/4th generation cephalosporin)
- Urgent surgical decompression/drainage (in most cases)

Vertebral Osteomyelitis/Discitis

General: Infection of vertebrae or disc, from hematogenous spread, direct extension, or iatrogenic inoculation. *Staph aureus* most commonly responsible.

Clinical:
- Back pain, tenderness upon palpation of spine
- Fever, ↑ ESR/CRP

Diagnosis:
- MRI (confirms diagnosis)
- Tissue biopsy/culture (Note: If blood culture positive, likely unnecessary)

Management:
- Antibiotics (Vancomycin + 3rd/4th generation cephalosporin)
- Surgery not usually necessary (unless complication, like abscess)

MUSCULOSKELETAL: BACK
Rheumatology/MSK Medicine, Surgery

Spinal Cord Compression

General: External compression of the spinal cord from vertebrae/abscess/neoplasm

Risk:
- Direct spinal cord injury (trauma)
- Infection (abscess)
- Malignancy

Clinical:
- Progressive, lower back pain
- Pain worse lying down
- Neurologic deficits
  - Lower extremity weakness, ↓ DTR, decreased rectal tone
  - Long term: Eventual (+) Babinski, increased DTR

Diagnosis: MRI

Management:
- IV glucocorticoids for acute cases
- Consider neurosurgical intervention

Cauda Equina/Conus Medullaris Syndrome

	Cauda Equina Syndrome	**Conus Medullaris Syndrome**
Gen	- Compression of one of the many cauda equina nerve roots	- Compression of the tapered, lower end of the spinal cord (conus)
Risk	- Herniated disc, spondylosis, spinal trauma, infection (abscess)	
Clin	- Gradual low back pain with bilateral lower extremity radiation (radicular pain)	- Acute, severe back pain (radicular pain less common)
	- Sensory loss ("saddle" distribution)	- Sensory loss (perianal)
	- Asymmetric weakness (ie of plantar flexion, or higher up depending on lesion)	- Symmetric motor weakness (mild/less marked compared to cauda equina)
	- Hyporeflexia - Erectile dysfunction rare - Possible bladder/bowel dysfunction (late in disease)	- Hyperreflexia - Erectile dysfunction common - Possible bowel/bladder dysfunction (early in disease)
Dx	- Emergent MRI	
Tx	- Urgent surgical decompression	

MUSCULOSKELETAL: BACK	Rheumatology/MSK Medicine, Surgery

Cervical Back Pain

Etiology	Features
Nonspecific Pain (ie cervical sprain)	- Most common cause of acute neck pain - Nonspecific paraspinal muscle tenderness - Treated similarly to general low back pain
Osteoarthritis (spondylosis)	- Common cause of chronic neck pain - Can result in myelopathy/radiculopathy
Cervical Radiculopathy	- Compression of spinal nerve leads to arm pain, numbness, weakness. Usually with unilateral neck pain. - Dx: MRI - Tx: Conservative initially (NSAIDs, PT, etc). Surgery if refractory.
Cervical Myelopathy	- Cervical spinal cord compression, most commonly from stenosis - Presents with gait disturbance, loss of motor function, and possible bowel/bladder findings - Dx: MRI - Tx: Surgical

Atlanto-axial Instability

General: Excessive laxity of the posterior cervical ligament, allowing for increased susceptibility to movement at the C1-C2 junction, with potential spinal cord injury

Risk:
- Genetic predisposition (Down's Syndrome, Osteogenesis imperfecta)
- Rheumatoid Arthritis

Clinical:
- Presents as acute spinal cord injury (neck pain, loss of motor function, loss of bowel/bladder function)

Diagnosis: Plain cervical XR

Management: Surgical correction

MUSCULOSKELETAL: UPPER EXT.
Rheumatology/MSK Medicine, Surgery

Shoulder

	General	Clinical	Management
Rotator Cuff Impingement	- Compression of rotator cuff tendons/subacromial bursa between head of humerus and acromion, causing pain	- Shoulder pain with overhead activity, localized to lateral deltoid - Exam: Tenderness over rotator cuff muscles, with pain upon abduction/external rotation	Dx: Clinical. Ultrasound can support. Tx: - Rest, Ice, NSAIDs, PT - Referral to orthopedics for failed conservative therapy for greater than 3 months for impingement/6 months for tendinopathy
Rotator Cuff Tendinopathy	- Inflammation of rotator cuff tendons - Can be caused by chronic shoulder impingement or repetitive overhead activity in sport or work	Special Tests for Impingement: - Neer's: Passive flexion of straight, internally rotated arm - Hawkin's: 90° Shoulder/elbow flexion → Quick internal rotation	
Rotator Cuff Tear	- Risk: Acute traumatic injury or chronic degeneration with eventual rupture	- Shoulder pain, weakness, especially with over head activity - Exam: Extreme weakness with external rotation - Positive empty can test (supraspinatus)	Dx: US or MRI Tx: Surgery for acute tears, conservative treatment for chronic (ie PT/steroid injections)
Adhesive Capsulitis	- "Frozen Shoulder" (chronic inflammation and fibrosis of joint capsule) - Risk: Either idiopathic or associated with prior shoulder injury	- Painful, stiff shoulder joint - Extreme limitation of active/passive ROM	Dx: Clinical Tx: Mobility exercises. Steroid injection/physical therapy if not improving.
Labral Tear	- SLAP tear most common (injury to superi- or portion of glenoid labrum) - Risk: Labor or athletics involving high intensity overhead activity	- Anterior shoulder pain, "clicking" in shoulder, decline in shoulder strength - Can occur with acute traumatic event - Positive O'Brien's active compression test, crank test, anterior glide test	Dx: MRI or MR arthroscopy Tx: Conservative preferred, but surgery in some athletes

Rheum28

MUSCULOSKELETAL: UPPER EXT.
Rheumatology/MSK Medicine, Surgery

Shoulder

	General	Clinical	Management
Ant. Shoulder Dislocation	- Most common type of dislocation - Occurs with traumatic blow to abducted/externally rotated arm	- Extreme pain/discomfort, with refusal of any movement - Shoulder abducted/externally rotated - Grossly abnormal appearance of shoulder - Often complicated by fractures or axillary nerve damage	Dx: Clinical, confirmed with XR Tx: Manual reduction, followed by shoulder immobilization
Post. Shoulder Dislocation	- Occurs with severe blow to anterior shoulder or extreme muscle contractions (classically seizure or lightening strike)	- Extreme pain/discomfort - Shoulder adducted/internally rotated - Prominent posterior shoulder (grossly) - Often associated with fractures, labrum/rotator cuff injuries	Dx: Clinical, with XR confirmation ("light bulb sign") Tx: Manual reduction
AC Joint Sprain	- Caused by trauma to adducted shoulder (ie direct blow/fall)	- Tenderness over the AC joint - Positive crossover test (pain with cross-body arm adduction)	Dx: XR (shows widened AC joint, possible ant/post shift of clavicle) Tx: Minor → Rest/Ice/Compression, Severe → Surgical
Biceps Tendinopathy	- Repetitive stress to the proximal long head of biceps, resulting in tendon injury/inflammation - Associated with other mechanical shoulder issues (ie impingement)	- Anterior shoulder pain, worse with pulling/lifting activities	Dx: Clinical Tx: Analgesia (NSAIDs, local steroid injections), physical therapy
Biceps Tendon Rupture	- Most commonly anterior biceps tendon rupture - Occurs with clear traumatic event/associated "pop"	- Acute, severe, anterior shoulder pain, edema, and ecchymosis - Gross deformity of biceps	Dx: US (alt. MRI) Tx: Conservative in some, surgical repair in athletes/workers that require strength

MUSCULOSKELETAL: UPPER EXT.
Rheumatology/MSK Medicine, Surgery

Elbow

	General	Clinical	Management
Medial Epicondylitis	- "Golfer's Elbow" - Risk: Repetitive, forceful flexion movements of elbow	- Localized pain of medial elbow and proximal wrist flexor muscles - Pain with passive wrist extension (with elbow extended)	Dx: Clinical Tx: Counter force bracing, NSAIDs, PT, activity modification
Lateral Epicondylitis	- "Tennis Elbow" - Risk: Repetitive, forceful extension movements of elbow	- Localized pain of lateral elbow and proximal wrist extensor muscles - Pain with passive wrist flexion (with elbow extended)	
Radial Head Subluxation	- "Nursemaid's Elbow" (occurs in kids) - Axial traction on forearm with arm extension, resulting in a torn or displaced annular ligament of the radiohumeral joint	- Arm held in extension and pronation - Should have no signs of fracture, such as focal bone tenderness/deformity/swelling (if they do, XR to rule out fracture)	Dx: Clinical Tx: Manual reduction (hyperpronation of arm)
Ulnar Collateral Ligament Injury	- Occurs in long term, competitive baseball players (can occur with acute injury or accumulated chronic trauma)	- Medial elbow tenderness, worse with the motion of throwing	Dx: MRI Tx: Tommy John surgery (UCL tendon repair)
Olecranon Bursitis	- Inflammation of bursa posterior to ulna - Becomes inflamed from trauma, chronic injury/overuse, or arthritis	- Swollen, tender, inflamed areas on the back of the elbow	Dx: Clinical Tx: NSAIDs, joint protection, fluid aspiration (Note: Fluid has high chance of recurring)

MUSCULOSKELETAL: UPPER EXT.

Rheumatology/MSK, Medicine, Surgery

	General	Clinical	Management
Hand (Nerve Issues)			
Carpal Tunnel Syndrome	- Increased pressure in the carpal tunnel, causing abnormal functioning of the median nerve - Risk: Obesity, diabetes, pregnancy, RA, connective tissue disease, chronic/repetitive movements of the wrist	- Painful paresthesias in median nerve distribution (first 3.5 digits) - Symptoms often occur at night - Provoked by movements of the wrist - Severe, chronic disease can lead to weakness or atrophy of thenar eminence - Exam: Phalen and Tinel signs, or manual carpal compression (reproduces symptoms)	Dx: Clinical - Nerve conduction studies and electromyography can support Tx: - Mild-Moderate → Splinting, glucocorticoid injections - Severe → Surgical (cut the transverse carpal ligament)
Ulnar Neuropathy	- Compression can occur either at the elbow or the wrist (Guyon's canal)	- Paresthesias/pain in ulnar nerve distribution (4th/5th digits) - Symptoms worse with elbow flexion or compression of the wrist - Chronic disease can cause weakness/atrophy	Dx: Clinical, with confirmation by nerve conduction studies Tx: Conservative (splinting, activity modification). Surgery (for severe or refractory cases).
Hand			
Felon	- Infection of the pulp of the finger tip	- Painful, red, swollen distal phalanx	- Surgical drainage
Paronychia	- Infection of the nail fold	- Painful, red, swollen nail fold	- Oral antibiotics, warm soaks
Gamekeeper Thumb	- Also known as Skier's Thumb - Ulnar collateral ligament injury, from forced hyperextension/abduction of the MCP joint	- Pain/swelling on ulnar side of MCP joint at base of thumb - Laxity of MCP joint - XR to rule out associated fractures	- Splinting, ice, rest (assuming no bony injury, in which case ortho referral)

MUSCULOSKELETAL: UPPER EXT.

Rheumatology/MSK Medicine, Surgery

Hand

	General	Clinical	Management
Jersey Finger	- Injury to flexor digitorum profundus tendon at insertion in phalanx - Due to hyperextension of DIP joint	- Pain and swelling at DIP joint - Inability to flex DIP	- Surgical correction
Mallet Finger	- Injury to extensor tendon at insertion into DIP	- Pain and swelling at dorsal surface of DIP - Inability to extend DIP joint	- Splinting, consider surgical intervention
Trigger Finger	- Flexor tendon catching in stenotic A1 pulley over the MCP joint	- Painless catching of the finger during flexion/extension of the finger	- Activity modification/splinting - Glucocorticoid injection (if refractory)
De Quervain Tenosynovitis	- Thickening of abductor pollicis longus and extensor pollicis brevis tendons at the styloid of the radius - Risk: Repetitive movements (ie mother carrying baby)	- Radial sided wrist pain, worse with movement - Medial wrist edema/tenderness over the radial styloid (worse with stretching of the thumb, called Finkelstein test)	Dx: Clinical Tx: Splinting, NSAIDs, Steroid injection if severe/persistent.
Dupuytren's Contracture	- Benign fibrous proliferative growth of palmar fascia - Risk: EtOH, northern Europeans, older age, men	- Stiff nodule over the palmar aspect of the hand, +/- tenderness - Decreased ROM of the fingers	Dx: Clinical Tx: Conservative (hand padding, intralesional steroids). Surgery if severe/persistent.

Rheum32

MUSCULOSKELETAL: LOWER EXT.

Rheumatology/MSK Medicine, Surgery

	General	Clinical	Management
Hip			
Trochanteric Bursitis	- Now called greater trochanteric pain syndrome	- Lateral hip pain with tenderness upon palpation	Dx: Clinical Tx: NSAIDs. Self-limited.
Osteoarthritis	- Degenerative hip disease	- Groin pain, worse with activity, improves with rest - Limited ROM, with pain elicited by movement (especially internal rotation)	Dx: Clinical. XR (not always needed, shows degenerative changes) Tx: [See: OA] NSAIDs, steroid injections, surgical hip replacement
Knee			
IT-Band Syndrome	- Overuse injury of lateral knee - Seen with athletes, runners, cyclists	- Pain over lateral femoral epicondyle where IT band inserts - Insidious onset, occurring only during activity, becoming more persistent	Dx: Clinical Tx: NSAIDs, rest, ice, PT
Pes Anserine Bursitis	- Pain at site of insertion of conjoined tendon (sartorius, gracilis, semitendinosus), associated with obesity/OA	- Tenderness over upper/medial tibia	Dx: Clinical. XR (to look for OA) Tx: PT, analgesia, weight loss
Prepatellar Bursitis	- Inflamed patellar bursa - Risk: Trauma, infection, or arthritis	- Focal swelling, erythema, and tenderness anterior to the patella/patella tendon	Dx: Aspiration (r/o infection) Tx: NSAIDs, activity modification, and bracing
Patellofemoral Pain	- Common cause of knee pain, especially in young adults	- Pain located behind patella, worse with weight bearing - (+) Patellofemoral compression test	Dx: Clinical Tx: Physical therapy (strength training for quads/hip muscles)
Baker Cyst	- Fluid buildup in semimembranosus/gastroc bursa - Risk: Knee trauma, arthritis	- Bulge behind knee, that may cause posterior knee pain/stiffness - Can dissect into calf (presents like DVT) - Rupture: Calf pain, warmth, erythema	Dx: Clinical (US if unsure) Tx: Treat underlying knee disease, steroid injection

MUSCULOSKELETAL: LOWER EXT.
Rheumatology/MSK Medicine, Surgery

Knee (Ligament injuries)

	General	Clinical	Management
ACL Tear	- Non-contact injury, commonly with change of direction, with planting of leg and accidental lateral bending (valgus stress) on the knee - "Unhappy Triad": ACL/MCL/Medial meniscus injuries	- "Pop" in knee, instability, and pain - Effusion/swelling quickly after injury - Lachman test (30° of flexion) has highest sens/spec. Anterior drawer classically used.	Dx: MRI Tx: - Can treat conservatively (but ↑ risk of OA, ligamentous injury) - Surgery (for athletes, or multi-ligament tears)
PCL Tear	- Posterior force directed at flexed knee, seen with MVC or sports (but rare)	- Can present with pain, swelling, instability (highly variable, because often have multiple other associated injuries) - Posterior drawer test (+)	Dx: MRI Tx: RICE, physical therapy/rehab
Meniscus Tear	- Can occur from acute, twisting trauma to the knee, or due to chronic degenerative process in older individuals	- Pain along the medial or lateral aspect of the knee, worse with twisting movements - Popping/catching or instability (knee "giving out") - McMurray's test (+)	Dx: MRI Tx: Can be treated conservatively or surgically corrected (if bad symptoms or athlete)
MCL Injury	- Injured by valgus stress to knee - Ranges from minor injury (grade I) to complete tear (grade III)	- Tenderness over MCL, pain, instability - Increased joint space opening upon valgus stress test	Dx: MRI Tx: RICE, physical therapy/rehab
LCL Injury	- Rare, often occur with other knee injuries - Due to blow to the medial part of knee	- Tenderness over LCL, pain, instability - Increased joint space opening upon varus stress test	Dx: MRI Tx: RICE, physical therapy/rehab

MUSCULOSKELETAL: LOWER EXT.   —   Rheumatology/MSK Medicine, Surgery

	General	Clinical	Management
Shin/Ankle			
Medial Tibial Stress Syndrome	- "Shin Splints" - Risk: Excessive physical activity (running)	- Pain along the inside edge of the tibia (diffuse, vs point tenderness of stress fracture) - Worse with activity	Dx: Clinical Tx: Activity reduction/modification, ice
Ankle Sprain	- Most commonly injury to ATFL, from inversion injury (medial sided deltoid ligaments rarely damaged) - Classifications: Grade 1: Partial ATFL rupture Grade 2: Complete ATFL/partial CFL Grade 3: Complete rupture of both	- Swelling, ecchymosis, tenderness over lateral ankle - History of traumatic mechanism consistent with strain	Dx: Clinical. XR requirement determined by Ottawa ankle rules (focal bony tenderness over distal 6 cm of either malleolus or unable to weight bear) Tx: RICE, physical therapy
Achilles Tendinopathy/ Rupture	- Tendinopathy is from chronic overuse - Rupture occurs acutely, with explosive movement	- Pain or stiffness in area 2-5 cm superior to the calcaneus - Worse with activity, improves with rest - Rupture: Acute pain, swelling, and complete loss of plantar flexion	Dx: Clinical Tx: Physical therapy, stretching for tendinopathy. Surgery for ruptures.
Foot			
Plantar Fasciitis	- Pain caused by the plantar fascia, possibly due to the development of bone spurs - Risk: Obesity, excessive standing, flat feet	- Pain in heel, worse with walking - Point tenderness over the heel on exam	Dx: Clinical Tx: Activity modification, shoe inserts, stretching, short course of NSAIDs
Morton Neuroma	- Benign interdigital growth from chronic nerve entrapment	- Numbness/burning pain between 3rd/4th distal metatarsal - Clicking sensation when palpating this space	Dx: US Tx: Orthotics or other pressure unloading devices

MUSCULOSKELETAL: NEUROVASCULAR
Rheumatology/MSK Medicine, Surgery

Brachial Plexus Lesions

Roots	Clinical Manifestation
Upper Trunk (C5-C6) Erb Palsy	- Often occurs during infant delivery (lateral traction on neck) or due to trauma in adults - Presents as adduction/internal rotation of the arm (supra/infraspinatus, deltoid weakness), flexion/supination of arm (biceps weakness) - Tx: PT/observation for recovery, with surgery if no improvement
Lower Trunk (C8-T1) Klumpke Palsy	- Risk: Traumatic birth, trying to catch something while falling - Paralysis of intrinsic hand muscles, resulting in claw like grasp, +/- Horner syndrome
Entire Plexus (C5-T1)	- Complete arm paralysis

Thoracic Outlet Syndrome

General: Collection of syndromes from neurovascular compression in thoracic outlet (area between first rib/behind clavicle). Can have different presentations depending on nerve, arterial, or venous involvement.

Risk: Rib/muscle abnormalities (trauma, congenital, repetitive movements)

Clinical:
- Neuro: UE pain, weakness, paresthesias. Muscle atrophy (if chronic).
- Arterial: Presents with thromboembolism to extremity (pain, pallor, cool)
- Venous: UE venous thrombosis, swelling, cyanosis

Diagnosis: CT/MRI, US, or electrodiagnostic testing (depending on subtype)

Management:
- Nerve: Conservative (PT). If refractory → Thoracic decompression.
- Arterial: Embolectomy, thoracic decompression, anticoagulation
- Venous: Thrombolysis, thoracic decompression, anticoagulation

MUSCULOSKELETAL: NEUROVASCULAR
Rheumatology/MSK Medicine, Surgery

Specific Nerve Lesions

Nerve	Clinical Manifestation
Upper Extremity	
Axillary	- Sensory loss over lateral shoulder - Risk: Shoulder trauma (dislocation, humeral head fracture)
Radial	- Wrist drop, weakness of wrist/finger extensors, sensory loss over back of hand - Risk: Compression of nerve in spinal groove ("Saturday night palsy"), or injury with midshaft humeral fracture
Long Thoracic	- Winged Scapula (ask to press arms against wall) - Risk: Trauma, or iatrogenic (breast surgery)
Lower Extremity	
Lateral Femoral Cutaneous	- Meralgia paresthetica (paresthesias/pain radiating down lateral thigh) - Risk: Compression (under inguinal ligament)
Superior Gluteal	- Trendelenburg gait (Pelvis tilts on downward on the side contralateral to the lesion) - Risk: Iatrogenic (surgery or injection in upper medial gluteus)
Common Peroneal	- Foot drop, steppage gait, sensory loss over dorsum of foot/lateral shin - Risk: Compression at point nerve wraps around fibula (at knee), most commonly from prolonged immobilization/pressure or casting
Posterior Tibial	- Tarsal tunnel syndrome (compression of nerve at ankle as it passes under tarsal ligament). Presents as paresthesias/sensory loss over the plantar surface of foot/toes. - Risk: Trauma (fracture/dislocation), arthritis

RHEUM PHARM — Rheumatology/MSK Medicine

	Mechanism	Indication	Side Effects/Management
Anti-inflammatory			
Acetaminophen	- COX inhibitor of CNS (mostly inactivated peripherally)	- Analgesia - Antipyretic	- Hepatotoxic (at high doses)
NSAID Ibuprofen Naproxen Indomethacin Ketorolac Diclofenac Meloxicam	- Reversibly inhibit COX1/COX2	- Analgesia - Antipyretic - Anti-inflammatory	- Gastritis/PUD (resulting in GI bleeds) - Renal: Interstitial nephritis, ischemia, prerenal AKI (vasoconstriction of afferent arteriole) - Increased risk of cardiovascular events
Celecoxib	- Reversibly inhibits COX2, spares COX1 (platelet effects)	- Analgesia, anti-inflammatory	- Increased risk of cardiovascular events
Colchicine	- Inhibit microtubule polymerization (↓ neutrophil chemotaxis and degranulation)	- Anti-inflammatory (gout, familial mediterranean fever)	- GI Disturbances (diarrhea, nausea, vomiting) - Agranulocytosis
Hypouricemic			
Allopurinol	- Inhibits xanthine oxidase	- Gout - Tumor lysis syndrome	- Hypersensitivity reactions (SJS/TEN) - Myelosuppression, hepatitis
Febuxostat	- Inhibits xanthine oxidase		- Increased death/MI (compared to allopurinol)
Probenecid	- Inhibits tubular resorption of uric acid in PCT		- Inhibition of renal tubular anion channels (reduces excretion of many drugs) - Uric acid nephrolithiasis
Pegloticase Rasburicase	- Recombinant uricase that catalyzes uric acid to water soluble product	- Tumor lysis syndrome	- Methemoglobinemia (if G6PDH deficiency)

Rheum38

RHEUM PHARM — Rheumatology/MSK Medicine

	Mechanism	Indication	Side Effects/Management
Bones			
Bisphosphonate Alendronate Ibandronate Risedronate Zoledronate (IV)	- Pyrophosphate analog that inhibits osteoclastic activity, induce apoptosis	- Osteoporosis - Hypercalcemia - Paget's of bone - Metastatic bone disease	- Esophagitis (drink with water, stay upright 30 min, empty stomach) - Jaw osteonecrosis (in those with high doses, most commonly cancer patients) - ↑ risk for atypical femur fractures - Bone/joint pain
Teriparatide	- Recombinant PTH analog given subcutaneously daily	- Osteoporosis	- Transient hypercalcemia
Calcitonin	- Antagonizes parathyroid hormone effects (inhibits osteoclastic bone resorption) - Administered intranasally	- Hypercalcemia - Osteoporosis (second line agent)	- Hypocalcemia - Rhinitis
Denosumab	- RANK-L antagonist	- Hypercalcemia (of malignancy) - Osteoporosis - Prevention of skeletal events from bone metastasis or multiple myeloma	- ↑ Infection risk - Jaw osteonecrosis - ↑ risk for atypical femur fractures - Bone/joint pain

RHEUM PHARM — Rheumatology/MSK Medicine

	Mechanism	Indication	Side Effects/Management
DMARD (Disease-Modifying Anti-Rheumatic Drugs)			
Methotrexate	- Folic acid analog, inhibiting dihydrofolate reductase, ↓ DNA production	- Rheumatoid arthritis - Other autoimmune conditions	- Myelosuppression (reversible with use of leucovorin) - Hepatotoxicity - Stomatitis - Pneumonitis/fibrosis
Leflunomide	- Inhibits pyrimidine synthesis		- Hepatotoxicity - Teratogen
Hydroxychloroquine	- Immunosuppression via impaired neutrophil chemotaxis and complement activity		- Retinal toxicity
Sulfasalazine	- Unclear MOA, but known immunosuppressive effects		- Hypersensitivity (sulfa drug) - Megaloblastic anemia/↓ folate absorption - Hemolytic anemia (G6PDH deficiency)
Biologic Anti-Rheumatic Agents			
Adalimumab Certolizumab Etanercept Infliximab	- TNF inhibitors	- Rheumatoid arthritis - Severe psoriasis - IBD	- Opportunistic infections (including reactivation of TB, fungal infections)
Anakinra	- IL-1 receptor antagonist	- Rheumatoid arthritis	- ↑ infection risk - Neutropenia
Tocilizumab	- IL-6 receptor antagonist	- RA/juvenile idiopathic arthritis - Temporal arteritis	- ↑ infection risk (including increased URIs)
Abatacept	- T-cell costimulation modulator	- Rheumatoid arthritis	- ↑ infection risk

DERMATOLOGY BASICS — Dermatology Medicine

Physical Exam

Morphology	Features	Examples
Macule	- Flat lesion < 1 cm in diameter	- Freckle
Patch	- Flat lesion > 1 cm in diameter	- Cafe-au-lait spot
Papule	- Elevated lesion < 1 cm in diameter	- Acne
Plaque	- Elevated lesion > 1 cm in diameter	- Psoriasis
Vesicle	- Fluid containing lesion < 1 cm	- Chickenpox
Bullae	- Fluid containing lesion > 1 cm	- Bullous pemphigoid
Nodule	- Solid, round, raised dermal lesion	- Erythema nodosum
Pustule	- Vesicle containing purulent fluid	- Folliculitis
Wheal	- Transient, edematous papule or plaque	- Urticaria
Petechiae	- Flat, non-blanching red spot < 3 mm	- Thrombocytopenia
Purpura	- Flat, non-blanching red spot 3-10 mm	- Thrombocytopenia
Ecchymosis	- Flat, non-blanching red spot > 10 mm	- Bruise
Scale	- Flaking off of skin	- Eczema
Crust	- Dry exudate	- Impetigo
Hyperkeratosis	- Increased thickness of stratum corneum	- Callus
Parakeratosis	- Hyperkeratosis + retained nuclei in corneum	- Psoriasis
Acanthosis	- Epidermal hyperplasia	- Acanthosis nigricans
Acantholysis	- Loss of adhesion of epithelial cells	- Pemphigus vulgaris

Topical Steroid Ladder

Group	Class	Drugs
Mild	Class 6 & 7	- Hydrocortisone acetate 1% (OTC)
Intermediate	Class 4 & 5	- Triamcinolone acetonide 0.1%
Potent	Class 2 & 3	- Betamethasone dipropionate 0.05%
Super Potent	Class 1	- Clobetasol propionate 0.05%

General Rules:
- Steroids prescribed for 14 day course BID

HYPERPIGMENTATION

Dermatology, Medicine, Pediatrics

Hyperpigmented Lesions

	Clinical Presentation	Diagnosis/Management
Freckle (Ephelides)	- Hyperpigmented macule from ↑ melanosome production - Seen in fair-skinned children	- Benign - Often fade with time
Lentigo	- Hyperpigmented macule from ↑ melanocytes - Can be simple (idiopathic, seen in kids) or solar ("liver spots," associated with sun exposure)	- Benign
Cafe-au-lait Spot	- Hyperpigmented macule from ↑ melanogenesis - Congenital or acquired at young age - Associated with McCune-Albright, NF1	- Benign
Melasma	- Acquired hyperpigmentation of sun exposed skin of face - Associated with pregnancy	- Sunscreen - Hydroquinone/steroid cream

Derm2

HYPOPIGMENTATION

Dermatology, Medicine, Pediatrics

	Clinical Presentation	Diagnosis/Management
Hypopigmented Lesions		
Albinism	- Group of AR inherited disorders of abnormal melanin biosynthesis - Presents with lack of skin, hair, and eye pigmentation - Abnormal vision	- Skin sun protection - Eye care
Vitiligo	- Acquired disorder of hypopigmentation from loss of melanocytes - Asymptomatic depigmented patches throughout the body - Associated with AI hypothyroidism, IBD, alopecia, psoriasis	- UVB light, plus topical or systemic steroids
Tinea Versicolor	- Common fungal skin infection seen in young adults (*Malassezia*) - Often seen with hot/humid climates - Well demarcated hyper or hypopigmented lesions of trunk and extremities	Dx: KOH prep of skin scraping (hyphae and yeast balls) Tx: Topical azoles, selenium sulfide, or zinc pyrithione * Lesions take months to resolve
Idiopathic Guttate Hypomelanosis	- Common acquired hypopigmentation disorder of older adults - Presents with diffuse small, round white macules - Asymptomatic other than cosmetic change	- Benign condition, but generally progressive - No clear treatment
Post-Inflammatory Hypopigmentation	- Acquired loss of skin pigmentation, occurring after the resolution of an inflammatory skin condition OR laser/cryo procedure	- Self-limited (resolves over time)

BENIGN/MISC DISEASE
Dermatology — Medicine, Pediatrics

		Clinical Presentation	Diagnosis/Management
Pityriasis	Pityriasis rosea	- Exanthematous skin condition believed due to HSV-7 - Presents with herald patch (single, large oval shaped pink lesion), followed in days by smaller lesions on the trunk and proximal extremities ("Christmas tree" pattern) - Itching commonly present	- Self-limited (resolves in 6-8 weeks) - Topical steroids for itching
	Pityriasis alba	- Dermatitis (often post inflammatory) with decreased melanocyte activity - Presents with asymptomatic, fine scaled patches of hypopigmentation on the trunk, face, and proximal extremities	- Self-limited - Topical steroids
Dry Skin/Scaling Disorders	Xerosis (Dry skin)	- Common condition of dry skin, seen in winter months (with cold and low humidity) - Presents with scaling rash, pruritus, and fissures	- Topical emollients
	Ichthyosis	- Chronic inherited skin disorder (most commonly of filaggrin gene). Large spectrum of severity depending on gene mutation identified. - Presents as rough, scaly dry skin	- Topical emollients *If severe: keratolytics (coal tar, salicylic acid) or topical retinoids

Derm4

BENIGN/MISC DISEASE — Dermatology Medicine

	Clinical Presentation	Diagnosis/Management
Cysts		
Epidermoid Cyst ("Sebaceous Cyst")	- Benign keratin producing squamous epithelium nodule - Dome shaped freely mobile nodule, with central punctum - Can produce cheesy white discharge - Can become irritated and infected	- Often resolves spontaneously. Can be excised (cosmetic) or I&D if infected.
Pilar Cyst	- Arise from hair follicle - Firm subcutaneous nodules on the scalp	- Excision if bothersome
Nodules		
Dermatofibroma	- Idiopathic, benign nodule from fibroblast proliferation - Firm, hyperpigmented nodule, +/- central buttonhole	- No treatment indicated
Erythema Nodosum	- Delayed-type hypersensitivity resulting in panniculitis (inflammation of all dermal layers) - Associated with sarcoid, IBD, TB, strep, Behcet's, coccidiomycosis - Painful, erythematous, tender nodules on the legs	- Self-limited (resolves over weeks)
Acrochordon (Skin Tag)	- Benign outgrowth of normal skin - Presents as nodule on stalk	- Excision if bothersome

BENIGN/MISC DISEASE — Dermatology Medicine

Common Skin Lesions

	Clinical Presentation	Diagnosis/Management
Seborrheic Keratosis	- Common benign epidermal lesion caused proliferation of immature keratinocyte - Round, hyperpigmented, warty lesions with stuck-on appearance (can be pink or brown) - Generally asymptomatic, but can get irritated, itch, or bleed - Leser-Trelat Sign: Appearance of multiple SK's associated with underlying malignancy	- No treatment required - Cryo or excision if cosmetic concern
Actinic Keratosis	- Proliferation of atypical epidermal keratinocytes, see with excessive sun exposure - Premalignant (SCC) - Scaly, erythematous papules in area of chronic sun exposure	- Surgical excision or cryotherapy - Topical 5-FU for multiple lesions
Acanthosis Nigricans	- Epidermal hyperplasia causing symmetric, velvety hyperpigmented thickening of skin - Associated with insulin resistance (ie DM, Cushings) and occult malignancy	- Workup and treat underlying cause
Lipoma	- Benign proliferation of mature adipocytes (most common benign soft-tissue neoplasms) - Presents with mobile subcutaneous nodule	- Treatment not required - Can excise if bothersome

INFLAMMATORY DISEASE
Dermatology Medicine

Acne Vulgaris

General: Acne is a common inflammatory disorder of the pilosebaceous unit. Pathogenesis involves follicular hyperkeratinization (obstructs sebaceous follicles), increased sebum production, *Propionibacterium acnes* proliferating in follicle, and inflammation within follicle.

Risk: Young adults, hyperandrogenism

Clinical: Most common on face, neck, chest, back
- Open comedones (blackheads)
- Closed comedones (whiteheads)
- Inflammatory papules, pustules, or nodules

Diagnosis: Clinical. Work up for hyperandrogenism if clinical signs.

Management:

Subtype	Description	Intervention
Comedonal	- Closed or open comedones	- Topical retinoids - Benzoyl peroxide - Salicylic or azelaic acid
Inflammatory	- Inflamed, red papules/pustules	- Topical antibiotics, topical retinoid, and benzoyl peroxide - Oral antibiotics if severe
Nodular	- Large, cystic appearing nodules	- Same as inflammatory - Refractory: Oral Isotretinoin

Rosacea

General: Chronic condition with unknown pathophysiology that classically causes facial redness in middle aged individuals

Clinical:
- Erythematous skin over the cheeks with flushing, telangiectasias
- Phymatous changes (thick skin, rhinophyma, bulbous appearance of nose)
- Papules, pustules
- Burning, stinging sensations, edema, and dryness
- Ocular involvement (in about half of patients)
    - Conjunctival injection, lid telangiectasias, scleritis

Diagnosis: Clinical

Management:
- Behavioral modification (avoid triggers like EtOH, use gentle cleansers, sun protection)
- Facial erythema: Topical Brimonidine or laser therapy
- Papules/pustules: Topical antibiotics (Metronidazole) or PO Tetracycline if severe

INFLAMMATORY DISEASE

Dermatology, Medicine, Pediatrics

	Clinical Presentation	Diagnosis/Management
Seborrheic Dermatitis	- Chronic, relapsing dermatitis - Associated with *Malassezia* Clinical - Mild: Scaly, flaky scalp rash (dandruff) - Severe: Yellowish, oily, thick flakes at hairline, near ears and skin folds - "Cradle Cap" in infants	- Mild: Ketoconazole (or zinc pyrithione/selenium sulfide) shampoo - Severe: Ketoconazole shampoo + topical high potency corticosteroid - Infants: Emollients
Allergic Dermatitis (Eczema)	- Common childhood pruritic inflammatory skin disease - Risk: Personal/family history of atopy, low humidity - Clinical: Presents as pruritic, scaly dry erythematous rash - Extensor surface at young age, flexor surfaces when older - Lichenified plaques at older ages	- Topical corticosteroids and emollients. Topical calcineurin inhibitor if severe. - Complications: Superimposed cellulitis, eczema herpeticum (vesicular eruption over eczema, requiring Acyclovir)
Allergic Contact Dermatitis	- Type IV hypersensitivity reaction against allergen (poison ivy, oak, iodine, rubber, nickel, other metal) - Acute: Erythematous papules and vesicles with oozing - Severe pruritus - Chronic: Skin thickening, excoriations	- Identify/avoid allergen - Topical corticosteroids - Oral corticosteroids if > 20% of body surface OR need rapid improvement
Irritant Contact Dermatitis	- Local inflammatory skin response to chemical or physical agent - Agents include detergents, acids, alkalis, metal, wood - Skin erythema, edema, vesicle formation, most commonly on hands	- Topical corticosteroid, emollient; avoid irritant exposure

Derm8

| INFLAMMATORY DISEASE | Dermatology Medicine |

Psoriasis

General: Chronic inflammatory skin disease causing plaques, from epidermal hyperproliferation and immune dysregulation

Clinical:
- Well-demarcated, erythematous plaques with silver scale
    - Auspitz sign: Pinpoint bleeding after removing scale
- Most common on extensor surface of knee/elbow, scalp, gluteal cleft
- Certain subtypes can result in pustules, nail involvement, or "reverse" psoriasis (involvement of intertriginous areas rather than extensors)

Diagnosis: Clinical. Biopsy (if uncertain) reveals epidermal hyperplasia, parakeratosis, and neutrophils in the stratum corneum.

Management:

Mild-Moderate	- Topical steroids, emollients - Alternative: Topical vitamin D, topical retinoids, tar
Moderate-Severe	- UV light therapy PLUS topical therapy (as above) - Systemic therapy (for refractory cases) - Agents used include Methotrexate, Cyclosporine, biologics

Lichen Planus

General: Chronic inflammatory disorder with mucocutaneous involvement. Associated with Hepatitis C infection, certain meds (beta-blocker, thiazides, Hydroxychloroquine).

Clinical:
- Cutaneous lesions: Pruritic, polygonal, purple, papules/plaques
    - White, lace-like pattern (Wickham's striae)
    - Often cause pruritus
- Can also involve scalp (alopecia), oral mucosa (ulcers or Wickham's striae), or genitals

Management: High potency topical steroids. Systemic steroids or phototherapy if widespread.

INFLAMMATORY DISEASE — Dermatology Medicine

Drug Eruptions

General: Adverse reactions to drugs can cause a diverse set of dermatologic eruptions, which are covered here or throughout this chapter. The differential includes:
- Drug-Induced Exanthems
- Erythema Multiforme or SJS/TEN
- Erythroderma
- Urticaria/angioedema/anaphylaxis
- Cutaneous small vessel vasculitis/serum sickness
- DRESS
- Photosensitivity

Condition	Clinical Features	Management
Drug-Induced Exanthem	- Also called morbilliform or maculopapular drug eruption - Most common adverse drug reaction - Presents within 3-14 days of med use with diffuse maculopapular rash, predominantly on trunk/proximal extremities	- Withdraw offending drug - Antihistamines and topical corticosteroids for symptoms
Serum Sickness	- Immune complex formation from exposure to, and antibody formation against, nonhuman protein (type III hypersensitivity) - Common causes include monoclonal/chimeric antibodies (ie Rituximab, anti-thymocyte globulin) - Serum sickness "like" reactions seen with a variety of drugs (Penicillins, TMP-SMX, Cefaclor, others) - Presents with fever, rash, and polyarthritis within 1-2 weeks of drug exposure	- Withdraw offending agent - Supportive care - Systemic steroids if severe
DRESS (Drug Reaction with Eosinophilia and Systemic Symptoms)	- T-Cell mediated hypersensitivity to certain drugs (most commonly sulfa, antiepileptics, and Allopurinol) Presents with: (2-6 weeks after med) - Constitutional: Fever/malaise/LA - Skin: Morbilliform skin eruption - Heme: Eosinophilia, atypical lymphocytosis - Lung: Pneumonitis - Renal: Interstitial nephritis - Liver: Drug-induced liver injury	- Withdraw offending drug - Topical steroids (for skin) - Systemic steroids (for lung/kidney involvement)

INFLAMMATORY DISEASE — Dermatology Medicine

Erythema Multiforme

General: Immune-mediated disorder (type IV hypersensitivity) against an infectious or drug antigen that causes cutaneous/mucosal lesions

Etiology:
- HSV (most common cause)
- Other infections: *Mycoplasma*, HIV, VZV, EBV
- Drugs: NSAIDs, sulfa drugs, antiepileptics, antibiotics

Clinical:
- Cutaneous: Erythematous papules, vesicles, target lesions
    - Target lesions have dusky center, red inflammatory zone, surrounding ring of edema, and an erythematous halo
- Generally starts on extremities with centripetal spread
- Mucosal lesions common

Diagnosis: Clinical. Biopsy if unsure.

Management:
- Self-limited (resolves in ~ 2 weeks)
- Supportive care (topical corticosteroids, antihistamines, etc)
- Withdraw offending agent (if known)

Stevens-Johnson Syndrome/Toxic Epidermal Necrolysis

General: Mucocutaneous reaction with extensive necrosis and epidermal sloughing
- SJS: < 10% of body surface involved
- SJS/TEN Overlap: 10-30% of body surface involved
- TEN: > 30% of body surface involved

Etiology:
- Drugs (Allopurinol, sulfa drugs, NSAIDs, Sulfasalazine, anticonvulsants)
- *Mycoplasma* infection
- Idiopathic (in many cases)
* Risk is increased in those with malignancy or HIV

Clinical: Generally within 1 month of exposure to above
- Influenza-like prodrome (high fever, myalgias, malaise)
- Cutaneous lesions: Erythematous macules and vesicles
    - Very painful skin to touch
- Skin sloughing (within days of onset)
- Mucosal erosions
- Ocular: Conjunctivitis, bullae, corneal ulceration, uveitis all possible
- Urogenital ulcers

Diagnosis: Clinical. Biopsy (can help to rule out other disorders if unclear diagnosis).

Management:
- Withdraw offending agent (once identified)
- Supportive care (wound care, fluids, treat pain, infection prevention)
- Adjunctive corticosteroids or cyclosporine

INFLAMMATORY DISEASE — Dermatology Medicine

Allergic Skin Reactions

Condition	Clinical Features	Management
Urticaria	- Edematous, fleeting wheals that cause intense pruritus or stinging Caused by: - IgE response to antigen (latex, food, insect bite, drugs, etc) - Direct mast cell activation (IV contrast, certain drugs like narcotics) - Certain viral or bacterial infections	- Antihistamines - Oral glucocorticoids if severe
Angioedema	- Edematous swelling of lips, tongue, throat, larynx, etc - Can also affect GI tract (nausea, vomit, abdominal pain) - Life threatening if airway compromised Subtypes: - Mast-Cell Mediated (allergic reaction) - Bradykinin Mediated (ACEi)	- Protect airway - Antihistamines (mild cases) - Glucocorticoids - Epinephrine (severe) - If Bradykinin mediated: C1 inhibitor concentrate OR FFP

Erythroderma (Exfoliative Dermatitis)

General: Diffuse erythema and scaling of ≥ 90% of body surface area, caused by a variety of underlying conditions (Note: Erythroderma is not a diagnosis, but rather a manifestation of an underlying condition)

Etiology:
- Exacerbation of dermatologic condition (psoriasis or eczema)
- Drug reaction (Penicillins, sulfa, etc)
- Cutaneous T-Cell Lymphoma (Mycosis Fungoides)

Clinical:
- Diffuse, uniformly red, warm skin on > 90% of body with scale
- Severe pain or itching
- Exfoliation
- Systemic symptoms (fever, chills, malaise) may be present
- Loss of fluids/electrolytes, ↑ perfusion of skin (may result in heart failure)

Diagnosis: Clinical

Management:
- Discontinue any potentially offending medications
- Supportive (fluids/electrolytes, support hemodynamics, monitor temp)
- Topical steroids/antihistamines for skin symptoms

BLISTERING DISEASE

Dermatology Medicine

Bullous Pemphigoid/Pemphigus Vulgaris

	Bullous Pemphigoid	Pemphigus Vulgaris
Gen	- Subepithelial bullous disorder of older adults - Autoantibody against basement membrane hemidesmosome protein (BP180/BP230, also known as BPAg)	- Intraepithelial bullous disorder with characteristic acantholysis - Autoantibody against intracellular keratinocyte adhesion molecules (desmoglein)
Clin	- Large (> 1 cm) tense bullae (Nikolsky sign [-]) - Trunks/extremities - Preceded by prodrome of itchy, erythematous plaques (similar to eczema)	- Flaccid blisters, which easily rupture, leading to painful erosions (Nikolsky sign [+]) - Mucosal involvement (most common is oral mucosa, which leave painful ulcers)
Dx	- Biopsy (direct immunofluorescence showing linear basement membrane Ig deposition) - Serology (ELISA for anti-BM Ig)	- Biopsy (direct immunofluorescence showing reticular intercellular Ig deposition) - Serology (for anti-desmoglein Ig)
Tx	- Acute: High potency topical steroids (systemic if can't do topical) - Chronic: Often requires steroid sparing agent long term (MTX, Mycophenolate or Azathioprine)	- Acute: Systemic corticosteroids +/- Rituximab - Chronic: Immunosuppressants (Azathioprine or Mycophenolate)

Dermatitis Herpetiformis

General: Autoimmune cutaneous eruption associated with Celiac's (gluten sensitivity)

Clinical:
- Pruritic skin eruption of papules and vesicles
- Excoriations and erosions from itching
- Extremities, buttocks, back, scalp involvement

Diagnosis: Biopsy (direct immunofluorescence showing IgA in the papillary dermis)
- Serology (Celiac serology also generally positive)

Management: Gluten free diet, Dapsone

SUN-RELATED SKIN DISEASE
Dermatology
Medicine, Pediatrics

Sunburn

General: Inflammatory skin reaction to exposure to excessive ultraviolet radiation. Repeated episodes increase risk for skin cancer. Also leads to:
- Photoaging (↑ wrinkles and skin discoloration)
- Senile purpura: Ecchymotic lesions on sun-damaged skin in older adults

Etiology:
- Natural sunlight
- Tanning beds or phototherapy

Clinical:
- Painful, erythematous skin within 24 hours of sun exposure
- Edema, blisters, and eventual skin sloughing all common

Management:
- Mild/Moderate: Cool compress, NSAIDs, aloe-vera or calamine
- Severe: Hospitalization for fluids and analgesia

Prevention:
- Wear protective clothing, avoid sun at peak hours
- Apply sunscreen (SPF ≥ 30) 30 minutes before going outside (reapply every 2 hours)

Photosensitivity/Photoallergic Reactions

Type	Features
Polymorphous Light Eruption	- Common rash (also known as sun-poisoning) that occurs with UV light exposure - Presents with pruritic papular rash in sun-exposed area within days of sun exposure
Phototoxicity	- Drug reaction, in which drug absorbs UV light in skin, and gives off energy/reactive species that damage surrounding tissue - Causes include tetracyclines, sulfa drugs, NSAIDs, and others - Presents similarly to sunburn, but reaction occurs more quickly and with greater severity than expected with typical sunburn
Photoallergic	- Delayed hypersensitivity with reaction to drug metabolites that are produced after sun exposure - Causes include topical agents (sunscreens, fragrances), other systemic drugs - Presents with itchy, eczematous eruptions

Other Causes of Sun-Related Skin Reactions:
- Solar urticaria (hives with sun exposure)
- Porphyria
- Autoimmune (SLE/Drug-Induced Lupus/Dermatomyositis)

MICROBIAL SKIN REACTIONS — Dermatology Medicine

	Clinical Presentation	Diagnosis/Management
Warts (Verruca vulgaris, others)	HPV 1-4. Subtypes: - Common wart (verruca vulgaris) - Flat wart (verruca plana) - Plantar wart (verruca plantaris) - Present as flesh colored hyperkeratotic lesion, can cause pain/discomfort	- Salicylic acid or cryotherapy
Molluscum Contagiosum	- Poxvirus. Transmitted skin to skin (highly contagious). - Can grow rapidly/large in immunosuppressed patients - Small papules (2 to 5 mm) with central umbilication, sparing palm/sole	- Cryotherapy, curettage, or podophyllin
Herpes Zoster (Shingles)	- Reactivation of VZV (must have had the virus previously), usually seen at ages > 50 y/o - Severe pain (neuritis) and vesicular rash in a dermatomal distribution Complications - Post-herpetic neuralgia - VZV ophthalmicus or oticus	- Acyclovir or Valacyclovir (if within 72 hours of symptoms or new lesions still appearing) * Only contagious to those without VZV in past or immunocompromised * Recurrent disease much more common in immunocompromised

FUNGAL SKIN DISEASE — Dermatology Medicine

	Clinical Presentation	Diagnosis/Management
Tinea versicolor	[See: Hypopigmentation]	
Candidal Intertrigo	- Burning red plaques in the skin folds with surrounding satellite macules - Inframammary fold, gluteal cleft, inguinal creases, under abdominal pannus	Dx: Clinical. KOH prep/fungal culture can confirm. Tx: Topical azoles or Nystatin
	Dermatophyte (tinea) infections - Caused by *Trichophyton*, *Microsporum*, and *Epidermophyton* - Diagnosis is generally clinical, but confirmation with KOH prep is recommended	
Tinea corporis [Ringworm]	- Risk: Skin-to-skin contact, infected animals, humidity - Presents as scaly, erythematous annular plaque, central clearing, pruritus	- Topical azoles or Terbinafine
Tinea capitis	- Scaly scalp patches with alopecia, pruritus - Wood's lamp fluoresces if microsporum	- Oral Griseofulvin, Terbinafine, or azole
Tinea unguium [Onychomycosis]	- Fungal nail infection, with thickened, discolored nails, subungual debris, and separation of nail plate from bed	- Oral Terbinafine (alt: azoles)
Tinea pedis [Athlete's foot]	- Interdigital, moccasin, and vesiculobullous subtypes - Redness, scaling in the foot and between toes causing pain/pruritus	- Topical azoles plus good hygiene
Tinea cruris [Jock Itch]	- Erythematous plaques in medial thigh, perineal areas	- Topical azoles or Terbinafine

PARASITIC SKIN DISEASE — Dermatology Medicine

	Clinical Presentation	Diagnosis/Management
Scabies	- *Sarcoptes scabiei* mite infection, spread by person-to-person contact - Mites tunnel into epidermis, lay eggs, and deposit feces, causing type IV hypersensitivity skin reaction - Pruritic erythematous rash with papules and burrows, excoriations - Most commonly on wrists/hands	Dx: Clinical. Scabies microscopic prep to confirm. Tx: Topical 5% Permethrin or oral Ivermectin
Pediculosis Capitis (Head lice)	- Common scalp infection in children - Can be asymptomatic or cause pruritus and excoriations	Dx: Visualize nits/adult lice Tx: Topical Permethrin (alt: Malathion, benzyl alcohol, topical Ivermectin) * No need to hold out of school, but examine household contacts
Pediculosis Pubis (Crabs)	- Sexually transmitted pubic lice infection - Presents as pubic itching	Dx: Visualize nits/adult lice Tx: Topical Permethrin
Cutaneous Larva Migrans	- Hookworm (*Ancylostoma*) infection, often acquired from walking barefoot on soil/sand - Erythematous migrating cutaneous tracks	Dx: Clinical appearance Tx: Oral Albendazole or Ivermectin
Bed Bugs	- Bugs that infest human dwellings - Presents with pruritic papules noticed upon waking	Dx: Detect bedbugs in sleeping area Tx: Professional pest eradication

BACTERIAL SKIN DISEASE

Dermatology — Medicine, Pediatrics

	Clinical Presentation	Diagnosis/Management
Impetigo	- Highly contagious, superficial skin infection from *Staph/Strep*, common in kids - Can be primary or secondary to minor skin trauma - Painful pustules, "honey" crusting - Bullae (in bullous impetigo) - Punched out ulcers (ecthyma)	- Limited: Topical antibiotics (Mupirocin) - Extensive: Dicloxacillin or Cephalexin
Erysipelas	- Infection of superficial dermis/lymphatics - Most common organism: *Streptococcus pyogenes* - Presents as acute onset well-demarcated raised erythematous rash, with systemic symptoms (fever/chill)	- *Strep* coverage (Oral Amoxicillin or Cephalexin. IV Cefazolin or Ceftriaxone)
Cellulitis	- Infection of deep dermis & subcutaneous fat - Most common: *Strep*, MSSA, MRSA - Presents with progressive skin erythema, edema, which is poorly demarcated - Can be nonpurulent (more commonly *Strep*) or purulent (MSSA/MRSA)	- *Strep*/MSSA: Cefazolin/Cephalexin - MRSA: PO TMP-SMX, Clindamycin. If admitted, IV Vancomycin.
Abscess	- Collection of pus within the dermis or subcutaneous space - Most common: MSSA/MRSA - Fluctuant, painful erythematous nodule - Possible purulent material/cellulitis	- I&D +/- antibiotics (TMP-SMX or Clindamycin)

*Note: For all skin infections, IV antibiotics are used for severe infections and those with systemic features. Oral antibiotics are appropriate for mild disease. Risk factors for MRSA dictate coverage (ie prior MRSA infection, purulent infection, infection resistant to empiric therapy)

BACTERIAL SKIN DISEASE
Dermatology — Medicine

Necrotizing Soft Tissue Infections

General: Includes necrotizing cellulitis, fasciitis, myositis. Subtypes:
- Necrotizing Fasciitis Type I: Polymicrobial
- Necrotizing Fasciitis Type II: Monomicrobial (group A *Streptococcus*)
- Necrotizing Myositis: Group A *Streptococcus*
- Necrotizing Cellulitis: *Clostridium perfringens* or polymicrobial

Risk: Traumatic wounds, immunosuppression, obesity, diabetes mellitus, cirrhosis

Clinical:
- Rapidly progressive soft tissue erythema and edema, with extreme pain
- Crepitus may be present (~50%)
- Tissue bullae and necrosis
- Systemic symptoms (fever, chills, etc)

Diagnosis: Primarily clinical: rapidly progressive infection, systemic signs, +/- crepitus
- CT (can reveal gas in soft tissue, which is highly specific)

Management:
- Surgical exploration/debridement PLUS
- Broad spectrum antibiotics: Vancomycin + Carbapenem or beta-lactam/lactamase inhibitor + Clindamycin (inhibits toxin production)

Staph Scalded Skin Syndrome/Toxic Shock Syndrome

	***Staph* Scalded Skin Syndrome**	**Toxic Shock Syndrome**
Gen	- *Staph* produced exfoliative toxin, which cleaves desmoglein-1 in the stratum granulosum - Seen commonly in infants or immunocompromised	- *Staph* or *Strep* produced TSST-1 "superantigen," causing massive T-cell response - Seen with tampon use, postpartum infections, and ENT surgery/sinusitis
Clin	- 24-48 hours of fever/skin tenderness followed by generalized erythematous rash w/ bullae formation and sloughing - Nikolsky's sign (+)	- Fever (> 102°F), hypotension. - Diffuse macular erythematous rash - Skin desquamation Organ Involvement: - Renal (AKI) - GI (vomit/diarrhea) - Liver (↑ AST/ALT) - Heme (thrombocytopenia) - MSK (myalgias, ↑ CK)
Dx	- Clinical - Culture all possible sources of infection (bullae are sterile)	- Clinical diagnosis (based on the presence of symptoms above plus organ system involvement)
Tx	- Supportive (fluids, skin care) - Antibiotics for MSSA or MRSA (Nafcillin or Vancomycin)	- Supportive (hemodynamic support) - Identification/treatment of cause (ie tampon, infection, etc) - Empiric antibiotics: Vanco + Clindamycin

| BACTERIAL SKIN DISEASE | Dermatology Medicine, Surgery |

Erythrasma

General: Superficial skin infection caused by *Corynebacterium minutissimum*. Seen frequently in those with diabetes mellitus, obesity.

Clinical:
- Interdigital: Scaly rash between toes
- Intertriginous: Dark erythematous to brown scaly plaques found in groin, inframammary, or axillae

Diagnosis: Clinical, plus Wood's lamp (Coral red fluorescence)

Management: Topical Clindamycin or Erythromycin. Oral antibiotics if widespread.

Hidradenitis Suppurativa

General: Chronic suppurative/inflammatory soft tissue process from follicular occlusion of the folliculopilosebaceous unit

Risk: Associated with diabetes, obesity, insulin resistance

Clinical:
- Severely painful/inflamed nodules
    - Most common in axilla, inguinal, inframammary, perineal areas
- Possible opening with purulent discharge
- Can be complicated by rope-like scarring, abscess or draining sinus tract formation, open comedones

Diagnosis: Clinical

Management:
- Behavioral (quit smoking, lose weight, avoid skin trauma)
- Antibiotics
    - Topical Clindamycin for mild disease
    - Oral Doxycycline or Clindamycin/Rifampin for severe disease
- Analgesia (NSAIDs) often required
- Limited surgical therapy
    - Surgical deroofing or intralesional steroids (to ↓ inflammation)
- Surgical Therapy: Wide excision of lesions

SOFT TISSUE ULCERS
Dermatology
Medicine, Surgery

Chronic Ulcers

Subtype	Clinical Features
Pressure	- Tissue damage from unrelieved pressure between soft tissue and bony prominence. Risk: Hospitalized patients, immobility. <table><tr><th>Stage</th><th>Findings</th></tr><tr><td>I</td><td>- Intact skin, but non-blanchable erythema</td></tr><tr><td>II</td><td>- Shallow ulcer with disrupted dermis</td></tr><tr><td>III</td><td>- Full thickness skin loss with possible visualization of subcutaneous fat</td></tr><tr><td>IV</td><td>- Full thickness skin loss with involvement of bone, joint, or tendon</td></tr><tr><td>Unstageable</td><td>- Full thickness tissue loss, with slough/eschar in ulcer</td></tr></table> - Management: Wound care, pain control, proper nutrition. Reposition patient at least every 2 hours.
Venous	- Ulcers that occur secondary to chronic venous insufficiency - Present as single or multiple shallow, exudative ulcers, most commonly over medial/lateral malleoli - Management: Compression stockings, elevate legs, diuretic
Arterial	- Ischemia from arterial obstruction, secondary to PAD or other arterial obstruction - Sharply demarcated ulcer at site furthest from vascular supply - Signs of arterial insufficiency (hairless legs, shiny skin, absent pulses) - Diagnosis: ABI/Doppler - Management: Stent/bypass graft
Diabetic	- Ulcers that occur due diabetic neuropathy (chronic trauma, abnormal vascular tone, etc) - Ulcers present on bony prominences (often on plantar surface of foot), appear punched out with irregular borders - Management: Mechanical offloading, wound care, debridement
Marjolin	- Ulcerating squamous cell carcinoma that occurs over an area of a chronic wound - Dx: Biopsy. Tx: Wide resection.

Other Ulcers

Ecthyma gangrenosum	- Occurs in immunocompromised patients with bacteremia (most commonly *Pseudomonas*). Due to vascular bacterial invasion causing ischemic necrosis. - Punched-out ulcer with crust, surrounded by violaceous margins
Pyoderma gangrenosum	- Inflammatory ulcer from abnormal neutrophil function - Risk: AI disease (IBD, inflammatory arthritis), malignancy - Acute, progressive, painful, purulent ulcer with irregular violaceous border

HAIR/HAIR FOLLICLE DISEASE — Dermatology Medicine

Hair Loss

Condition	Features
Androgenic Alopecia	- Selective loss of hair from the scalp due to genetic and hormonal factors (↑ DHT) - Temporal, anterior, and vertex commonly affected
Chemotherapy Alopecia	- Diffuse scalp hair loss from destruction of proliferating cells in the hair shaft
Alopecia areata	- Chronic autoimmune condition of relapsing episodes of hair loss - Smooth, discrete circular areas of hair loss - Tx: Topical/intralesional steroids, topical immunotherapy
Others (Discussed elsewhere)	- Trichotillomania - Tinea capitis

Folliculitis

General: Inflammation of the hair follicle, from infectious (bacterial/viral/fungal) or non-infectious cause

Etiology: Most commonly *Staph, Pseudomonas, Malassezia*

Clinical: Erythematous, follicular papules/pustules

Diagnosis: Clinical

Management: Topical antibiotics (Clindamycin/Mupirocin) or systemic antibiotics if severe

Specific Subtypes:

Hot-tub Folliculitis	- *Pseudomonas* folliculitis from dirty hot tub
Tinea Barbae	- "Barber's itch," is folliculitis of beard hair in adult men - *Trichophyton rubrum* most common culprit
Pseudofolliculitis Barbae	- Non-infectious folliculitis from shaving, with beard hair growth back into follicle
Keratosis Pilaris	- Common disorder of follicular keratinization - Papules on the back of extensor surfaces

VASCULAR SKIN TUMORS
Dermatology; Medicine, Pediatrics

	Clinical Presentation	Diagnosis/Management
Bacillary Angiomatosis	- Complication of *Bartonella* infection in HIV patients - Presents as friable red/purple nodule or papule	- Doxycycline/Erythromycin
Kaposi Sarcoma	- Abnormal vascular proliferation from HHV-8 infection - Commonly associated with HIV infection, but can occur without (commonly in Russian/Black patients) - Dark red or purple skin nodules or plaques - Can involve mouth/GI mucous membranes	Dx: Biopsy (vascular proliferation with lymphocytes) Tx: Can observe if asymptomatic. Symptomatic lesions can require local excision or chemotherapy.
Cherry Hemangioma	- Mature, adult hemangioma - Benign, unlikely to regress significantly	- Only excise if bothersome
Glomus Tumor	- Arises from the thermoregulatory glomus body - Painful red-blue tumor under fingernails	- Surgical excision
Pyogenic Granuloma	- Lobulated capillary hemangioma occurring with pregnancy or trauma - Rapidly growing, friable nodule. Risk for ulceration/bleeding.	- Surgical excision
Infantile Hemangioma	- Common childhood hemangioma - Erythematous nodules that rapidly grow for a few months after birth, then regress over time	- Monitor lesions - If disfigurement or symptomatic: Propranolol or laser/surgical excision

DERM MALIGNANCIES
Dermatology Medicine

Basal Cell Carcinoma

General: Neoplastic proliferation of basal layer of the epidermis. Can be locally destructive, but have low metastatic potential.

Risk: UV light, light skin

Clinical:
- Nodular: Pearly, waxy lesion, peripheral telangiectasia (most often in head/neck area). Frequent ulceration, bleeds.
- Superficial: Scaly plaques

Diagnosis: Biopsy (shave, punch or excisional). Nests of atypical basal epithelium.

Management: Excision (Surgical, electrodesiccation and curettage [ED&C], MOHS or topical therapy [Imiquimod or 5-FU]. 5 mm margins)
- MOHS for small (< 6 mm) head/neck lesions

Squamous Cell Carcinoma

General: Neoplastic proliferation of squamous cells in the skin. Actinic keratoses are precursor lesions. Higher potential than BCC for local recurrence or metastases.
- Keratoacanthoma: Well-differentiated SCC that grows rapidly over weeks and then resolves

Risk: UV light exposure, chronic wounds/inflammation/scars

Clinical: Erythematous plaques or nodules
- Scaling, crusting, ulceration, or increased pigment all possible

Diagnosis: Biopsy (shave, punch or excisional)

Management: Excision (Surgical, electrodesiccation and curettage [ED&C], MOHs, cryotherapy. 5-10 mm margins)

Melanocytic Nevi

General: Benign proliferation of melanocytes. Associated with UV light/fair skin.

Junctional	- Dark, macular lesions. Common in children. - From basal epidermis
Compound	- Darkly pigmented papules - From basal epidermis/upper dermis interface
Intradermal	- Skin colored to tan papules. Common in adults. - From dermis
Atypical (Dysplastic)	- Still benign, but have some high risk features consistent with melanoma. ↑ risk for development of melanoma.

Clinical: Varied appearance, but in general: < 6 mm, round/oval shape, regular border, even hyperpigmentation, homogenous surface

Diagnosis: Clinical. Biopsy if unsure.

Management: Observation. Excisional biopsy should be considered for lesions with atypical/concerning features OR changing over time.

DERM MALIGNANCIES

Dermatology Medicine

Melanoma

General: Malignant melanocytic neoplasm, with characteristic radial growth phase (lateral within epidermis) followed by nodular growth (deep into dermis)

Superficial Spreading	- Long radial growth phase. Good prognosis. - Generally a macule or very thin plaque
Lentigo Maligna	- Found on elderly chronically sun damaged skin - Proliferation of melanocytes along dermal/epidermal junction - Present as tan or brown macules, with slowly progressive growth
Acral Lentiginous	- Palmar, plantar, subungual location. More common if dark skinned.
Nodular	- Vertical growth phase melanomas. Poor prognosis. - Appear as darkly pigmented nodules

Risk: Sun/UV light exposure, fair skin, history of nevi, family history, xeroderma pigmentosum

Clinical: ABCDE (asymmetry, border irregularity, color variation, diameter [> 6mm], elevation)
- "Ugly Duckling Sign" (looks suspicious or different than other lesions)

Diagnosis: Clinical/dermoscopic features. Excisional biopsy (with 1-3 mm margin) for definitive diagnosis.

Management: Surgical Excision

Breslow Depth	Margins	Other Surgical Considerations:
In situ	0.5 cm	≥ 0.8 cm deep: Lymphatic mapping/sentinel LN biopsy
≤ 1 mm	1 cm	
1-2 mm	2 cm	
> 2 mm	2 cm	

Metastatic Disease:
- Resection if only a few sites involved/surgery is feasible
- Systemic therapy: Immunotherapy standard
    - Pembrolizumab and Nivolumab (Anti PD-1)
    - Ipilimumab (Anti CTLA-4)

Derm25

FEVERS
Infectious Disease Medicine

Overview of Temperature

General: Elevation in core body temperature, generally considered > 100.4°F or 38°C
- Temperature is controlled by the hypothalamus, which creates temperature "set point"
- Prostaglandin E2 formation can increase the "set point," leading to fever
- Acute fevers are most commonly due to infection

Management: COX inhibitors (Acetaminophen preferred, but ASA and other NSAIDs also have antipyretic effect)

Fever of Unknown Origin

General: Fever > 38.3°C (101°F), on multiple occasions over at least 3 weeks, without definitive diagnosis of underlying cause

Etiology:
- Infectious (TB, HIV, endocarditis, mononucleosis, parasitic infections)
- Malignancy (leukemia, lymphoma, multiple myeloma)
- Autoimmune (SLE, vasculitis, sarcoid, etc)

Workup:
- Blood cultures
- TB skin test or IGRA
- HIV serology
- Heterophile antibody test
- ANA, ESR/CRP, RF
- SPEP
- CT chest/abdomen

GRAM POSITIVE

Infectious Disease Medicine

	Clinical Presentation	Management/Antimicrobial Coverage
Staphylococcus		
Staphylococcus aureus	- Skin and soft tissue infections - Endocarditis - Septic arthritis/osteomyelitis - PNA (especially post influenza) - Toxin-mediated disorders (toxic shock, scalded skin, food poisoning)	Tx: - MSSA: Nafcillin, Oxacillin, beta-lactam/lactamase inh., cephalosporins - MRSA: Vancomycin (alt.: Linezolid, Daptomycin) for IV. TMP-SMX, Clindamycin, Doxycycline for PO.
Staphylococcus epidermidis	- Normal skin flora (most of the time if cultured it is a skin contaminant) - Can infect catheters, prosthesis	See *Staph aureus*, high risk for Methicillin resistance
Staphylococcus saprophyticus	- Cause of female UTI	
Streptococcus		
Streptococcus pyogenes	- Pyogenic: Pharyngitis, cellulitis, impetigo - Immunologic: Rheumatic heart disease/glomerulonephritis - Toxigenic: Toxic shock, scarlet fever	Tx: Susceptible to most beta-lactams (include Penicillin, cephalosporins)
Streptococcus agalactiae	- Infant pneumonia, meningitis, sepsis	
Streptococcus pneumoniae	- Meningitis, otitis media, pneumonia, sinusitis	Tx: Susceptible to most beta-lactams (not Penicillin, but beta-lactams/lactamase inhibitors, cephalosporins)
Streptococcus viridans	- *S. sanguinis* → Endocarditis - *S. mutans, S. mitis* → Dental Caries	
Enterococcus	- UTI, GI infections (diverticulitis, cholecystitis), subacute endocarditis	Tx: Susceptible to beta-lactams/lactamase inhibitors *Not susceptible to cephalosporins
Streptococcus bovis	- Subacute endocarditis (associated with colorectal cancer)	

GRAM POSITIVE   **Infectious Disease Medicine**

	Clinical Presentation	Management/Antimicrobial Coverage
Bacillus		
Bacillus anthracis	- Cutaneous: Painless ulcers with black eschar - Inhalation: Inhale spores → Fever, pulmonary hemorrhage, mediastinitis, shock, meningitis	- Systemic: Broad antibiotics, anthrax antitoxin, supportive care
Bacillus cereus	- Food poisoning ("reheated rice syndrome"): Vomit/Diarrhea	- Self-limited
Clostridium		
C. difficile	- Diarrhea [See: GI]	
C. perfringens	- Necrotizing cellulitis ("gas gangrene") - Food poisoning (spores ingested, can cause late onset GI symptoms)	
C. botulinum	- Produces toxin that inhibits presynaptic Ach release - Cause: Spores from environmental dust (infants), ingestion of pre-formed toxin in food (adults), rarely wound infection - Presents with descending flaccid paralysis/bilateral cranial palsy. Prodrome of abdominal pain, nausea, vomiting dry mouth, diplopia possible.	- Infants (< 1 y/o): Human-derived botulism Ig - Others (> 1 y/o): Equine-derived botulism antitoxin
C. tetani	- Produces exotoxin that blocks inhibitor NT release at spinal cord - Source: Wound infections (adult), umbilical stump (infants) - Clinical: Severe, generalized muscle contraction. Trismus, risus sardonicus, opisthotonos. Infants present with hypertonicity and failure to thrive.	Active Tetanus: Supportive care, tetanus Ig, Metronidazole, and benzodiazepines (for spasms) Prophylaxis (Vax=Td or TDap) | Vax	Minor/Clean Wound	Dirty/Severe Wound
≥ 3 Dose	Vax (if last dose > 10 yr)	Vax (if last vax > 5 yr)
< 3 Dose	Vax	Vax + Tet Ig	

ID3

GRAM POSITIVE — Infectious Disease Medicine

	Clinical Presentation	Management/Antimicrobial Coverage
Corynebacterium diphtheriae	- Causes diphtheria, which is rarely seen in US due to vaccines - Presents with pharyngitis, characteristic gray-white pseudomembranes - Toxin can disseminate and cause myocarditis, CNS damage, and renal injury	Tx: - Antibiotics: Penicillin or Erythromycin - Diphtheria antitoxin
Listeria monocytogenes	- Generally infects infants, elderly, or immunosuppressed Presents as: - Healthy: Self-limited, minor gastroenteritis - Immunosuppressed: Sepsis, invasive gastroenteritis - Pregnancy: Amnionitis, sepsis, abortion - Infants: Meningitis, granulomatosis infantiseptica (diffuse pyogenic granulomas)	Tx: Ampicillin or Penicillin G
Nocardia	- Infection occurs almost exclusively in immunocompromised Presents as: - Pneumonia (similar to TB) - CNS disease (brain abscess) - Cutaneous (skin infection, lymphangitis)	Tx: TMP-SMX
Actinomyces	- Bacteria that can cause cervicofacial invasion from dental infection or oromaxillofacial trauma. Pelvic actinomycosis from IUD. - Presents with mass, which progresses slowly into abscesses, draining sinus tracts (yellow sulfur granules), fistulae, and tissue fibrosis	Tx: Penicillin (or Ampicillin/Erythromycin)

ID4

GRAM NEGATIVE — Infectious Disease Medicine

	Clinical Presentation	Management/Antimicrobial Coverage
Neisseria meningitidis	- Cause of meningitis/meningoccemia [See: Neurology]	Tx: Penicillin or Ceftriaxone *PPX (close contacts): Rifampin, Ciprofloxacin, or Ceftriaxone
Neisseria gonorrhoeae	- Cause of gonorrhea urethritis/cervicitis, PID, septic arthritis, and neonatal conjunctivitis [See: STI]	Tx: Ceftriaxone/Azithromycin
Bordetella pertussis	- Cause of pertussis (whooping cough) Presents with: - Catarrhal: 1-2 weeks of flu like prodrome (cough/rhinitis) - Paroxysmal: 2-6 weeks. Severe cough with inspiratory whoop, post-tussive emesis. - Convalescent stage: Eventual resolution of symptoms	Dx: Culture or PCR for < 4 weeks of symptoms. Serology for > 4 weeks. Tx: Macrolides. Update Tdap. * Post-exposure ppx: Macrolide for close contacts
Legionella pneumophila	- Bacteria that thrives in and is transmitted from water - Pontiac fever: Mild flu-like syndrome of headache, fever, muscle aches that occurs with inhalation of *Legionella* endotoxin. Self-limited, no workup required. - Legionnaires disease: Atypical pneumonia, gastrointestinal symptoms, fever/myalgias, hyponatremia	Dx: Urine antigen and respiratory culture Tx: Azithromycin or Levofloxacin
Haemophilus influenzae	- Nontypable: Resp infection (otitis, PNA, sinusitis) - Encapsulated (Type B): Can cause meningitis, septic arthritis, pneumonia, and epiglottitis	Dx: Enlarged epiglottis on imaging or direct visualization Tx: Amox-Clav or cephalosporin usually sufficient *PPX: Rifampin (young, at risk household contacts of Type B)

GRAM NEGATIVE

Infectious Disease Medicine

		Clinical Presentation	Management/Antimicrobial Coverage
Escherichia coli	ETEC	- Causes watery diarrhea in children or travellers	- Self-limited. Fluids +/- antibiotics (Azithromycin or FQ).
	EHEC	- Invasive, bloody diarrhea in children - HUS	- Supportive care
	EPEC	- Cause of watery diarrhea in children in developing countries	- Supportive care
	EIEC	- Rare. Presents similar to *Shigella* with watery/bloody diarrhea.	- Supportive care
Salmonella spp		- Source: Infected poultry, milk, eggs, or pets (turtles) - Gastroenteritis (diarrhea, emesis, abdominal pain, fever) *Impossible to differentiate clinically from other causes of GE	Tx: - Supportive care (fluids/electrolytes) - Antibiotics (fluoroquinolone) if high risk (ie immunocompromised)
Salmonella typhi		Typhoid: - Obtained from ingesting contaminated food/water - Presents as abdominal pain, fever, HSM, possible GI bleeding - Bradycardia, pulse-temperature dissociation, and "rose-spots" (salmon colored macules) are classic findings - Dx: Blood/stool culture	Tx: Ceftriaxone or Ciprofloxacin PPX: Typhoid vax (either live oral or IM) for travellers to endemic areas
Shigella		- Common cause of bacterial diarrhea, transmitted person to person or through food - Presents with abdominal cramps, fever, and bloody diarrhea - Dx: Stool culture	Tx: Fluoroquinolone or macrolide
Campylobacter jejuni		- Common cause of acute enteritis (abdominal pain, diarrhea, sometimes bloody). Risk for GBS or reactive arthritis.	Tx: Supportive care, +/- antibiotics (fluoroquinolone or macrolide)
Yersinia enterocolitica		- Common cause of acute diarrhea illness (fever, abdominal pain, N/V, diarrhea). Can be confused with appendicitis.	Tx: Supportive care

GRAM NEGATIVE

Infectious Disease Medicine

	Clinical Presentation	Management/Antimicrobial Coverage
Klebsiella	- PNA (nosocomial, rarely community acquired) - GU infection	Tx: Cephalosporins, fluoroquinolone
Proteus	- GU infection, struvite stones	Tx: Ampicillin, TMP-SMX
Helicobacter pylori	- Peptic ulcer disease [See: GI]	
Vibrio cholera	- Acute secretory watery diarrhea ("rice water" diarrhea) - See in many third-world countries	Tx: - Aggressive fluids - Fluoroquinolone, macrolides, or tetracyclines
Vibrio vulnificus	- Lives in marine environments. Can be ingested (oysters) or due to wound infection. - Associated with ↑ Fe (ie hemochromatosis) - Can present with rapidly progressive cellulitis (necrotizing infection, bullous rash) and sepsis	Tx: - Tetracycline + Ceftriaxone - High mortality rate
Gardnerella	- Cause of bacterial vaginosis [See: GYN]	Tx: Metronidazole
Nosocomial		
Pseudomonas	- Feared, aggressive, water-loving nosocomial pathogen - Can cause sepsis, PNA, UTI, osteomyelitis (puncture wounds), otitis externa, skin infections (hot tub folliculitis, ecthyma gangrenosum, skin infections in burn victims)	Tx: Carbapenems, aminoglycosides, Cefepime, fluoroquinolones, Pip-Tazo
Burkholderia cepacia	- Opportunistic organism that can cause PNA in patients with underlying lung disease (CF) or immunocompromised	Tx: TMP/SMX, fluoroquinolone, cephalosporins
Acinetobacter baumannii	- Hospital acquired infections (most commonly PNA/bacteremia)	Tx: Often multidrug resistant; 4th gen cephalosporins, carbapenem, polymyxin, etc

ID7

Infectious Disease Medicine

GRAM NEGATIVE

	Clinical Presentation	Management/Antimicrobial Coverage
Zoonotic		
Yersinia pestis	- Cause of the plague. Transmitted by fleas, with rat reservoir. - Presents as fever, chills, malaise, myalgias - Swollen/painful lymph nodes ("bubo") - Eventual disseminated infection (sepsis, pneumonia)	Dx: Culture/serology Tx: Aminoglycosides, tetracyclines
Francisella tularensis	- Zoonotic infection from animal contact or tick vector - Tularemia presents nonspecifically within 1 week of contact - Fever, malaise, myalgias, GI symptoms all possible - Ulceroglandular: Ulcerative lesion at site of inoculation, with regional lymphadenopathy	Dx: Serology Tx: Aminoglycosides, tetracycline, fluoroquinolones
Brucella	- Brucellosis: Zoonotic infection from contact with infected animal fluid (cow, sheep, etc) or food products such as unpasteurized milk and cheese - Presents as insidious onset of fever, malaise, night sweats, myalgias, arthralgias - Specific organ system involvement possible (spondylitis, GU, pulmonary, hepatitis, endocarditis, meningitis/encephalitis)	Dx: Culture/serology Tx: Doxycycline/Rifampin
Pasteurella multocida	- Soft tissue infection after cat/dog bite, scratch, or lick - Rapid (within 24 hours) onset of inflammation	Tx: Amoxicillin-Clavulanate
Anaerobes		
Bacteroides fragilis	- Normal organism of the GI tract - Can be implicated in GI/GU/pulmonary abscesses, as well as dental infections and skin/soft tissue infections	Tx: Metronidazole, Clindamycin, or beta-lactam/lactamase inhibitors

ATYPICAL BACTERIA
Infectious Disease Medicine

	Clinical Presentation	Management/Antimicrobial Coverage
Chlamydia		
Chlamydia trachomatis	- Intracellular parasite - Serotype A-C: Trachoma (see ophthalmology) - Serotype D-K: Urethritis, cervicitis, PID (see STD section), neonatal conjunctivitis/PNA	
Chlamydophila psittaci	- Psittacosis: Atypical pneumonia. Obtained from inhalation of particles of bird feces.	Tx: Doxycycline/Macrolide
Chlamydophila pneumoniae	- Atypical pneumonia	Tx: Doxycycline/Macrolide
Rickettsia		
Rickettsia rickettsii	- Rocky Mountain Spotted Fever. Transmitted by dermacentor tick. Found in eastern US. - Presents initially with fever, chills, headache, myalgias, arthralgias. Eventual development of rash (starts at wrists and ankles, spreads inward [centrifugal])	Dx: Serology Tx: Doxycycline (alt: Chloramphenicol)
Rickettsia prowazekii	- Epidemic Typhus (rare, found in rural Africa/Asia/South America) - Transmitted by louse/flea - Acute onset fever, malaise, severe headache, followed later by maculo-papular rash and CNS involvement (confusion, lethargy) - Brill-Zinsser disease: Mild recurrence of symptoms later in life	Tx: Doxycycline (alt: Chloramphenicol)
Rickettsia typhi	- Endemic (murine) typhus. Rare in US, more in developing countries. - Transmitted by flea - Presents as acute, nonspecific flu-like illness, +/- rash	Tx: Doxycycline (alt: Chloramphenicol)

ATYPICAL BACTERIA

Infectious Disease Medicine

	Clinical Presentation	Management/Antimicrobial Coverage
Spirochetes		
Treponema pallidum	- [See: STD]	
Borrelia burgdorferi	- Lyme disease (ixodes tick vector, mouse reservoir) - Found in northeastern US - Presents early with erythema migrans, flu like symptoms - Stage 2: Carditis, AV block, facial nerve palsy, migratory myalgias/arthritis - Stage 3: Late disseminated, encephalopathies, chronic arthritis	Dx: ELISA, followed by confirmatory western blot Tx: Doxycycline (alt: Amoxicillin) - Ceftriaxone if CNS/cardiac involvement PPX: If tick bite < 36 hours, remove tick, no ppx If tick bite > 36 hours, remove tick, Doxycycline
Leptospira	- Tropical infection (in US → Hawaii) - Animal reservoir, excrete in urine, possibly into water/soil - Nonspecific illness (fever, severe myalgias, and headache) - Conjunctival suffusion - Possibly complicated by jaundice/renal failure ("Weil's disease")	Tx: Doxycycline or Azithromycin
Mycobacterium (non-TB)		
Mycobacterium leprae	- Causes Leprosy. Transmitted by respiratory droplets with infected humans, rarely armadillos. - Lepromatous: Diffuse hypopigmented, anesthetic skin lesions. Can have nodules, papules, plaques. Palpable nerves with neuropathy. Skin thickening (ie "lion facies") possible. - Tuberculoid: Few hypoesthetic, erythematous macules	Dx: Skin biopsy (with acid fast stain) Tx: Rifampin + Dapsone. In lepromatous: Add clofazimine.
Mycobacterium marinum	- Cause of skin/soft tissue infection in those exposed to fresh/salt water	Tx: Clarithromycin + Ethambutol/Rifampin
Mycobacterium avium complex	- Disseminated infection in immunocompromised patients [See: HIV]	

ATYPICAL BACTERIA — Infectious Disease Medicine

	Clinical Presentation	Management/Antimicrobial Coverage
Mycoplasma	- Atypical pneumonia. Young people/close proximity at risk. - Presents as: Pharyngitis, headache, malaise - Dry cough (diffuse interstitial infiltrate on CXR) - Possible cold-agglutinin (IgM)	Tx: Macrolides, respiratory fluoroquinolone
Ehrlichia chaffeensis	- Human monocytic ehrlichiosis (Vector: Lone-star tick) - Presents as: Nonspecific flu-like illness (fever, headache, myalgias) - Occasional rash - Leukopenia, thrombocytopenia, ↑ ALT/AST	Dx: Serology (ELISA/IFA) or PCR Tx: Doxycycline
Anaplasma phagocytophilum	- Human granulocytic anaplasmosis (Vector: Ixodes tick) - Presents as: Nonspecific flu-like illness (fever, HA, myalgias) - Leukopenia, thrombocytopenia, ↑ ALT/AST	Dx: Serology (ELISA/IFA) or PCR Tx: Doxycycline
Coxiella burnetii	- Q-Fever: Zoonotic infection, most commonly exposure to spores in farm animal bodily fluids - Presents as: High grade fever, fatigue, headaches, myalgias - Possible mild pneumonia, hepatitis. Rarely endocarditis.	Dx: Serology Tx: Doxycycline
Bartonella henselae	- Cat Scratch Disease (due to cat scratch or bite) - Presents with papule/nodule at site of inoculation, followed by erythematous painful lymphadenopathy, +/- fever	Dx: Clinical. Confirm with serology. Tx: Azithromycin

FUNGAL ORGANISMS — Infectious Disease Medicine

Cutaneous

	Clinical Presentation	Management/Antimicrobial Coverage
Sporothrix schenckii	- Note: *Tinea* infections (ie dermatophytes, *Malassezia*) covered in dermatology - Dimorphic fungi found in decaying plant matter - Presents with papule at site of inoculation, with ascending lymphangitis (lesions along lymphatic chain), and possible ulceration - Systemic disease (ie pneumonia, meningeal, sepsis) rare	Dx: Culture Tx: Itraconazole

Systemic

	Clinical Presentation	Management/Antimicrobial Coverage
Histoplasmosis	- Found in soil contaminated with bird/bat droppings - Midwestern/central US (Ohio and Mississippi River valleys) Clinical: (Note: Most are asymptomatic/clear organism) - Systemic symptoms (fevers, malaise, weight loss, etc) - Pulmonary (patchy/nodular infiltrates, with hilar LA) - Other: Arthralgias, skin nodules. Rarely disseminates. - Lab: Pancytopenia, ↑ AST/ALT, LDH	Dx: No specific test best. Culture, serology, and urine/serum antigen all contribute. Biopsy can show granulomas/yeast forms. Tx: - Mild: Itraconazole - Severe: Amphotericin B, followed by 1 year of Itraconazole
Blastomycosis	- Inhalation of conidia. Occurs in similar area to *Histoplasma*, but extends into upper midwest/great lakes. Clinical: (Can disseminate even if immunocompetent) - Pulm: Acute/chronic PNA (most common manifestation) - Derm: Verrucous lesions, violaceous nodules, skin ulcers - MSK: Osteomyelitis, osteolytic bone lesions	Dx: Visualization or culture (sputum, tissue, purulent material). Urine/serum antigen. Tx: - Mild: Itraconazole - Severe: Amphotericin B
Coccidioidomycosis	- Southwestern US (dust → Inhale spores) Clinical: (Often subclinical) - PNA (chest pain, cough) - Systemic symptoms (fever, night sweats, weight loss) - Arthralgias, erythema nodosum	Dx: Serology, culture Tx: Itraconazole (or Amphotericin if severe)

ID12

FUNGAL ORGANISMS

Infectious Disease Medicine

	General/Clinical	Management/Antimicrobial Coverage
Opportunistic		
Candida	- Can cause vaginitis, esophagitis, intertrigo, endocarditis, thrush - Can disseminate in immunocompromised patients	- See specific condition for treatment - In general, Nystatin for topical, azoles for others
Allergic Bronchopulmonary Aspergillosis	- Hypersensitivity in asthma/CF patient to *Aspergillus* colonization, which can lead to chronic inflammation/bronchiectasis - Presents as asthma with recurrent exacerbations, occasional coughing up of brown mucus plugs/bronchial obstruction	Dx: *Aspergillus* IgE/skin testing Tx: Acute flare: Corticosteroids + Voriconazole
Chronic Pulmonary Aspergillosis	- Risk: History of lung disease/damage (ie cavitary TB) - Presents with subacute onset weight loss, productive cough, hemoptysis, dyspnea, possible fever/night sweats	Dx: Imaging shows cavitary upper lobe lesions, possible fungus ball. (+) *Aspergillus* Ig. Tx: Surgically resect aspergilloma. Voriconazole.
Invasive Aspergillosis	- Pulmonary tissue infection with vascular invasion - Risk: Immunocompromised (ie HIV/immunosuppressant use) - Presents with fever, chest pain, dyspnea, hemoptysis - Imaging: Pulmonary nodules/infiltrates, + halo sign	Dx: Sputum stain/culture, biomarkers (beta-D-glucan, galactomannan). Tissue biopsy if uncertain. Tx: Voriconazole (+ Caspofungin if severe)
Cryptococcus	- Round yeast with thick capsule. Associated with pigeons. - Inhalation of fungus into lungs → Hematogenous spread may involve the brain and meninges - Clinical: Meningoencephalitis [See: HIV], PNA also possible	Dx: Lumbar Puncture (latex agglutination or Indian ink) Tx: Amphotericin B + Flucytosine (2 weeks) Oral Fluconazole (after)
Mucormycosis	- Risk: Diabetes (ketoacidosis), immunocompromised, neutropenia, deferoxamine - Presents as rapid, acute sinusitis, with necrotic invasion of surrounding structures (sinuses, palate, turbinates, skin) - Black necrotic eschar on skin and mucosa - CNS invasion: Frontal lobe abscess, cavernous sinus thrombosis	Dx: Tissue biopsy (histopathologic analysis) Tx: Surgical debridement, liposomal Amphotericin B

PROTOZOAL ORGANISMS

Infectious Disease Medicine

	General/Clinical	Management/Antimicrobial Coverage
Giardia lamblia	- Waterborne (esp hikers), foodborne, fecal-oral - Risks: Camping, traveling - Presents with bloating, flatulence, foul smelling, fatty diarrhea	Dx: Stool Antigen or PCR test (alt: stool microscopy) Tx: Metronidazole/Tinidazole +/- Nitazoxanide
Entamoeba histolytica	- Seen in contaminated food/water, especially in developing countries Presents as: - Mild diarrhea or severe bloody diarrhea/colitis - RUQ Abscess [See: GI]	Dx: Stool microscopy/antigen testing, Serology Tx: Metronidazole/Tinidazole. Paromomycin for intraluminal cysts.
Cryptosporidium	- Fecal-oral transmission (infected food/water) Presents as: - Asymptomatic or minor diarrhea in immunocompetent - Severe, chronic diarrhea in immunocompromised	Dx: Stool microscopy (and/or stool PCR) Tx: Nitazoxanide (for those with > 2 weeks of symptoms)
Trichomonas vaginalis	- Vaginitis [See: GYN]	
Naegleria fowleri	- Found in freshwater environments - Acute, rapidly fatal meningoencephalitis	Tx: Amphotericin B + Steroids
Acanthamoeba	- Chronic meningoencephalitis - Corneal eye infection (dirty contacts)	

ID14

PROTOZOAL ORGANISMS

Infectious Disease Medicine

	General/Clinical	Management/Antimicrobial Coverage
Toxoplasma gondii	- Transmitted by oocysts from the environment, cysts in infected meat, vertical transmission (mother to fetus) - Immunocompetent: Asymptomatic, mononucleosis-like illness, chorioretinitis - Congenital: TORCH infection - Immunosuppressed (esp HIV/AIDs): Encephalitis	Dx: Toxo Serology (IgM in active disease) Tx: Sulfadiazine + Pyrimethamine (+ Leucovorin) (TMP-SMX is alternative)
Trypanosoma brucei	- Transmitted by Tsetse fly - Human African Trypanosomiasis ("sleeping sickness") - Subtypes: Gambiense → Slow, chronic, Rhodesiense → Rapid - Early: Painful bite site (with possible chancre), flu-like symptoms (intermittent headache, fevers, malaise, and arthralgia) - Late: CNS (meningoencephalitis, somnolence, other neurologic issues)	Dx: Blood Smear (or identify organism in other tissue) Tx: Pentamidine/Suramin (early blood infection) and Melarsoprol (late CNS disease)
Trypanosoma cruzi	- Seen in South America. Transmitted by reduviid bug. Chagas Disease - Acute: Romana sign (periorbital swelling), nonspecific systemic symptoms - Chronic: Dilated cardiomyopathy, achalasia, progressive colonic dilatation	Dx: Acute: Blood Smear (trypomastigote) or PCR Tx: Benznidazole and Nifurtimox
Leishmania donovani	- Transmitted by sandfly Visceral (Kala-azar or old world) Subtype: - Spiking fevers, hepatosplenomegaly, pancytopenia Cutaneous Subtype: - Non-healing, crusty, non-painful skin ulcer	Dx: Histopathology (needle aspiration/tissue biopsy) Tx: Topical Paromomycin, liposomal Amphotericin B for visceral

PROTOZOAL INFECTIONS — Infectious Disease Medicine

Malaria

General: *Plasmodium* infection, transmitted by bite of Anopheles mosquito

Subtype	Features
P. falciparum	- Most common. sub-Saharan Africa, Haiti, Dominican - Severe symptoms, irregular fever pattern
P. vivax/ovale	- Next most common, Western Pacific and Americas - 48 hour cycle. Dormant form (hypnozoite) in liver.
P. malariae	- Rarer form, mostly found in sub-Saharan Africa - 72 hour cycle

Clinical:
- Paroxysmal fevers (timing depends on underlying organism)
- Systemic symptoms (malaise, headache, myalgias)
- GI (diarrhea, vomiting, abdominal pain, hepatosplenomegaly, jaundice)
- Can be complicated by hemolysis, hypoglycemia, acidosis, renal failure, noncardiogenic pulmonary edema or CNS disease (seizure/coma)

Diagnosis:
- Microscopy (thin/thick preps) are gold standard
- Rapid antigen testing in resource poor areas

Management:
If chloroquine resistant area:
- Artemisinin combination therapy (Artemether/Artesunate based regimen)
- Atovaquone-Proguanil
- Quinine + Doxycycline
- Mefloquine

If chloroquine sensitive area:
- Chloroquine or Hydroxychloroquine

Prophylaxis:
- Start 2 weeks before leaving and continue 4 weeks once back
- Regimen options: Doxycycline, Atovaquone/Proguanil, or Mefloquine
- Mosquito protection (sprays, netting)

Babesia

General: Spread by *Ixodes scapularis* (also lyme/anaplasma), in similar locations as those organisms

Clinical:
- Nonspecific flu-like illness (malaise, myalgias, fever, night sweats, headache)
- Hemolytic anemia, transaminitis, thrombocytopenia

Diagnosis: Blood smear (intraerythrocytic rings, "maltese cross") or blood PCR

Management: Atovaquone + Azithromycin

HELMINTH INFECTIONS

Infectious Disease Medicine

	General/Clinical	Management/Antimicrobial Coverage
Nematode (roundworms)		
Enterobius vermicularis (pinworm)	- Cycle: Fecal-oral (Adult worms → Lay eggs in perianal area → Itch and reintroduce via mouth) - Clinical: Asymptomatic OR anal pruritus	Dx: "Tape Test" (look for perianal eggs) Tx: Albendazole or Pyrantel pamoate
Trichuris (whipworm)	- Cycle: Ingest eggs, hatch larva, mature to adults in colon - Clinical: Asymptomatic often. Can cause diarrhea (+/- mucus or blood), and rectal prolapse if heavy worm burden.	Dx: Stool Microscopy (for ova/parasite) Tx: Albendazole
Ascaris lumbricoides (giant roundworm)	- Cycle: Ingest eggs into GI → Hatch, larva migrate to lungs → Cough up, swallow adult worms into GI - Clinical: Early infection → Nonspecific pulmonary symptoms (cough) Late Infection: GI symptoms (diarrhea, vomiting, abd pain), with possible SBO, hepatobiliary involvement, or malnutrition	Dx: Stool Microscopy (for ova/parasite) Tx: Albendazole or Pyrantel pamoate
Strongyloides stercoralis	- Cycle: Larvae in soil penetrate skin → Lung → Cough/swallow → GI → Mature to adult worms → Eggs in GI, which mature to larva and are secreted in feces - Clinical: Possible mild GI symptoms. Possible eosinophilia. - Immunocompromised: Hyperinfection (dissemination of larvae to lungs, liver, heart, CNS)	Dx: Stool Microscopy (for ova/parasite) Note: Often need serologic testing because larva burden low Tx: Ivermectin +/- Albendazole
Ancylostoma duodenale & Necator americanus (hookworms)	- Cycle: Larvae in soil penetrate skin → Lung → Cough/swallow → GI → Mature to adult worms → Eggs in GI, passed in stool - Clinical: Cutaneous larva migrans (see DERM), with eventual chronic GI symptoms. Chronic blood loss (iron/albumin) can lead to malnutrition.	Dx: Stool Microscopy (for ova/parasite) Tx: Albendazole

ID17

HELMINTH INFECTIONS

Infectious Disease Medicine

	General/Clinical	Management/Antimicrobial Coverage
Nematode (roundworms)		
Trichinella spiralis	- Cycle: Fecal-oral (undercooked meat, especially pork, wild meat) - Ingest cyst → Larvae released, invade SI, mature → Release larva that migrate and encyst in skeletal muscle - Clinical: Early GI symptoms (abd pain/diarrhea), followed by muscle stage (myositis/↑ CK), fever, periorbital edema, eosinophilia - Possible myocarditis, meningoencephalitis, pulmonary invasion	Dx: Serology. Biopsy is definitive but often unnecessary. Tx: Albendazole
Toxocara canis	- Cycle: Ingestion of eggs from soil/stool, with larvae hatching in GI, and systemic invasion - Visceral Larva Migrans: Pneumonitis, hepatitis with possible heart/CNS/muscle invasion - Ocular Larva Migrans: Unilateral ocular worm invasion	Dx: Serology Tx: Albendazole
Onchocerca volvulus	- Blackfly transmission (larva deposition in skin) - Clinical: Onchocerciasis, also known as "river blindness" Symptoms include: Ocular (keratitis/uveitis/chorioretinitis), derm (skin nodules/papules/plaques), systemic complaints	Dx: Skin-snip biopsy. Slit-lamp exam. Tx: Ivermectin
Wuchereria bancrofti	- Mosquito transmission (larva deposition with lymphatic invasion) - Clinical: Acutely causes lymphangitis, with chronic disease causing lymphedema ("Elephantiasis")	Dx: Antigen tests, blood smears Tx: Diethylcarbamazine
Loa loa	- Transmission: Deer/horse fly transmission - Clinical: Swelling in skin, conjuntivitis (from worm invasion)	Dx: Visualization in eye Tx: Diethylcarbamazine

HELMINTH INFECTIONS
Infectious Disease Medicine

	General/Clinical	Management/Antimicrobial Coverage
Cestodes (tapeworms)		
Taenia solium	- Cycle: Ingest eggs, which hatch larva that invade. Eggs often come from feces of asymptomatic carriers. Note: If larva ingested from raw meat, only mild GI infection occurs. Clinical: Cysticercosis (cysts throughout body, especially CNS) - Intraparenchymal: Seizures, headache, focal deficits - Intraventricular: Hydrocephalus, ↑ICP - Other: Spinal, ocular, intramuscular	Dx: - CT/MRI (depending on stage, calcified/edematous/enhancing brain lesions) - Serology Tx: Albendazole + Praziquantel + Glucocorticoids
Diphyllobothrium latum	- Fish tapeworm (transmitted from raw freshwater fish) - Nonspecific GI symptoms, vitamin B12 deficiency	Dx: Stool microscopy (for ova/parasite) Tx: Praziquantel
Echinococcus granulosus	- Ingestion of eggs in feces/soil (dogs are definitive hosts) - Clinical: Liver cysts [See: GI], lung cysts	Dx: Imaging (CT/US) and serology Tx: Albendazole +/- percutaneous intervention
Trematodes (flukes)		
Schistosoma	- Cycle: Snail host, cercariae (released into water) penetrate human skin Clinical: - Acute: "Swimmer's Itch" (itchy rash at penetration site) and Katayama fever (flu-like symptoms, fever, urticaria and angioedema, occurring within 2 months of initial infection) - Chronic: Liver fibrosis (and portal hypertension), GI infection, and GU (bladder inflammation, polyps, obstruction, cancer), renal (immune complex deposition, nephrotic syndrome)	Dx: Stool/urine microscopy (for ova/parasite), serology Tx: Praziquantel
Clonorchis sinensis (Chinese Liver Fluke)	- Can cause acute gastroenteritis/flu-like symptoms, but chronic infection can cause hepatobiliary disease (obstructive jaundice, pancreatitis, cholangitis, liver abscess)	Dx: Stool microscopy (ova/parasite) or bile aspirate Tx: Praziquantel

DNA VIRUS — Infectious Disease Medicine

	General/Clinical	Management/Antimicrobial Coverage
Parvovirus B19	- Small virus, respiratory spread, infects RBC precursors Clinical - In Utero: Hydrops fetalis - Adults: Flu-like, with polyarthralgias (resembles RA) - Kids: Erythema infectiosum (Fifth Disease): Low grade fever, followed by "slapped cheek," descending rash - Sickle/Thal: Aplastic crisis	Dx: B19 Serology (IgM) or PCR test Tx: Self-limited, supportive
Human Papilloma Virus (HPV)	- Types 1-4: Verruca vulgaris (Common Wart) - Types 6, 11: Anogenital warts (Condyloma acuminata), Laryngeal papillomatosis (respiratory tract tumors) - Types 16, 18, 31, 33: Anogenital cancers HPV makes E6 (inhibits P53) and E7 (inhibits Rb)	Dx: Either clinical or by cytology/serotyping Tx: See specific section
BK Polyomavirus	- Renal transplant: Tubulointerstitial nephritis	
JC Polyomavirus	- Progressive multifocal leukoencephalopathy [See: HIV]	
Adenovirus	- Common, seen in individuals in close proximity (ie military) Clinically can present as: - URTIs (rhinitis, sore throat, fever, conjunctivitis, tonsillitis) - Epidemic conjunctivitis (pink eye) - Diarrheal illness (infants/children) - Hemorrhagic cystitis	Dx: Viral antigen tests and culture exist, but are generally not needed
Pox Virus	- Smallpox - *Molluscum contagiosum*	

ID20

DNA VIRUS (HERPES) — Infectious Disease Medicine

	General/Clinical	Management/Antimicrobial Coverage
HSV-1	- "Herpes labialis," causes vesicular lesions - Primary herpes (gingivostomatitis/pharyngitis). Often presents with oral mucosal vesicular lesions (+/- ulceration), possible systemic symptoms. - Recurrent: Reactivation from sensory ganglion, with vesicle on lip Other Clinical Manifestations - Encephalitis - Herpetic Whitlow - Eczema herpeticum - Keratitis	Dx: Viral culture or PCR Tx: Acyclovir, Famciclovir, or Valacyclovir
HSV-2	- Genital Herpes [See: STD] - Neonatal Herpes [See: OB]	
Varicella-Zoster	Varicella (Chicken Pox) - Prodrome of fever, malaise, pharyngitis - Followed by generalized vesicular rash (red base with fluid filled vesicle on top) - Contagious 48 hours before rash starts until skin lesions have fully crusted - Complications: Bacterial superinfection (most commonly *Strep*), pneumonia, encephalitis/cerebellar ataxia Zoster (Shingles) [See: Derm]	Dx: Clinical Tx: Supportive care (antihistamines, NSAIDs). Acyclovir in those > 12 y/o. PPX: Varicella-Zoster vaccine, shingles vaccine

DNA VIRUS (HERPES) — Infectious Disease Medicine

		General/Clinical	Management/Antimicrobial Coverage
Epstein-Barr		Mononucleosis - Fever, pharyngitis, fatigue - Hepatosplenomegaly, posterior cervical lymphadenopathy - Generalized maculopapular rash (seen more commonly with amoxicillin administration) - Lab shows atypical lymphocytosis, elevated LFTs - Complications: GBS, meningoencephalitis, cranial nerve palsy - EBV associated with B-Cell lymphoma (Hodgkin's), Burkitt's lymphoma, nasopharyngeal carcinoma	Dx: Heterophile antibody test. Serology if unclear. Tx: Supportive * No athletics (3 weeks), no contact sports (4 weeks)
Cytomegalovirus		- Most individuals have had infection - Asymptomatic (in most) - CMV Mononucleosis (mono like syndrome, but without positive heterophile antibody test) - Immunosuppressed: Reactivation disease [See: HIV]. Can cause pneumonitis, retinitis, encephalitis, hepatitis, esophagitis. - Congenital infection [See: OB]	Dx: Serology/PCR (only required if presentation is heterophile negative mono OR immunocompromised) Tx: Severe infections treated with Ganciclovir, Cidofovir, or Foscarnet
	HHV 6/7	Roseola - High fevers for several days (seizures possible) - Followed by centrifugal maculopapular rash	Dx: Clinical Tx: Self-limited (NSAIDs for fever control)
	HHV 8	Kaposi Sarcoma [See: Derm]	

RNA VIRUS
Infectious Disease — Medicine

	General/Clinical	Management/Antimicrobial Coverage
Enteroviruses [Note: Most are cleared asymptomatically or with minor febrile illness. The following are rare syndromes associated with these viruses. Young children and immunocompromised patients are most at risk.]		
Entero	- Meningitis/encephalitis, viral pneumonia/bronchiolitis	Dx: If organism needs to be identified: RT-PCR
Echo	- Aseptic meningitis/encephalitis	Tx: Self-limited/supportive Care. IVIG or experimental antivirals for severe, life threatening infections.
Coxsackie A	**Hand-Foot-Mouth** - Common infection in kids - Fever, oral vesicles on the buccal mucosa/tongue, and small painful lesions on the hands/feet **Herpangina** - Fever, sore throat/odynophagia, vesicular lesions on tonsils and soft palate	
Coxsackie B	- Aseptic Meningitis - Myocarditis, pericarditis, or pleurodynia (fever + sharp pleuritic chest pain)	
Polio	- Most clear virus asymptomatically/minor febrile illness - Abortive Polio: Major viremia, with flu-like symptoms - Poliomyelitis: Only occurs in small fraction of those with viremia Destruction of anterior horn motor neurons. Presents with asymmetric flaccid proximal muscle weakness. Respiratory failure.	Dx: Clinical/CSF (PMN/lymphocyte pleocytosis). Confirmation via CSF PCR. Tx: Supportive PPX: Salk (IM) or Sabin (oral) vaccine
Rhinovirus	- Common cold (URTI)	
Norovirus	- Common cause of viral gastroenteritis	Dx: Clinical diagnosis. If definitive identification needed (ie for public health), ELISA/PCR available.
Rotavirus	- Common cause of viral gastroenteritis, especially in countries without rotavirus vaccine	Tx: Supportive (fluids/antiemetics if necessary). Note: Rotavirus can be fatal in young infants.

ID23

RNA VIRUS — Infectious Disease Medicine

		General/Clinical	Management/Antimicrobial Coverage
Toga Viruses	Arbo	- Mosquito transmitted. Eastern/Western Equine Encephalitis.	
	Chikungunya	- Aedes mosquito transmission. Endemic in Western Africa, but seen elsewhere (Central/South America, Caribbean). Chikungunya Fever: - High fever with severe, bilateral, symmetric polyarthralgia - Headache, myalgias, maculopapular rash all possible - Labs: ↑ AST/ALT, thrombocytopenia, leukopenia	Dx: RT-PCR or serology Tx: Supportive (fluid, NSAID pain control) *Some patients may develop chronic arthritis, requiring Methotrexate or glucocorticoids
	Rubivirus	Rubella ("German Measles") - Fever, lymphadenopathy, (cervical/postauricular), arthralgias - Maculopapular rash (starts on face and spreads inferiorly) - Severe congenital infection	Dx: Not needed, unless concern over congenital infection (serology) Tx: Supportive, PPX: MMR vax.
Flavi Viruses (all are mosquito transmitted)	Yellow Fever	- Initially causes flu-like symptoms, followed by ~48 hour remission - Followed by hepatic/renal failure, hemorrhage, shock	Dx: Serology or rtPCR Tx: Supportive care. High mortality rate. PPX: Vax.
	Dengue	Dengue Fever ("Breakbone") - High fever, severe myalgias/arthralgias, retro-orbital headache - Hepatomegaly/↑ LFTs, maculopapular rash possible findings - Hemorrhage (skin/mucosal bleeding) - Can lead to vascular leakage (shock, organ failure)	Dx: Clinical. Serology can confirm. Tx: Supportive care (Note: Acetaminophen okay, but no NSAIDs due to bleeding risk)
	Zika	- Found in Africa/Asia, now Americas. Mosquito and sexual transmission. - Causes febrile illness with flu-like symptoms and polyarthralgias/rash - Associated with fetal microcephaly, fetal loss	Dx: Serology or rtPCR Tx: Supportive
	West Nile Japanese/St.Louis	- All 3 are often asymptomatic, but can cause febrile flu-like symptoms, and CNS involvement (meningoencephalitis)	Dx: CSF serology/PCR (for CNS disease) Tx: Supportive

ID24

RNA VIRUS
Infectious Disease Medicine

	General/Clinical	Management/Antimicrobial Coverage
Coronavirus	- Common cause of URTIs - SARS/MERS Subtypes (flu-like symptoms, followed by period of respiratory failure)	
Influenza (Orthomyxo)	- Respiratory spread, cause of the common flu - Antigenic shift (epidemics) and antigenic drift (endemics)	Tx: Oseltamivir PPX: Flu vaccine. Consider Oseltamivir if high-risk and have flu exposure.
Ebola (Filo)	Ebola Virus Disease - Initial flu like syndrome, with vomiting/diarrhea (volume depletion) - Maculopapular rash, severe hemorrhage possible - Shock, multi-organ system failure (kidney/liver)	Dx: rtPCR Tx: Supportive care, proper precautions (isolation + contact/droplet)
Rabies (Rhabdo)	- Transmitted via infected animal bite (Bats/racoons/skunks in US, dogs in developing countries) - ~1-2 months after bite, presents with prodrome (flu-like symptoms, with possible pain/paresthesias at bite site) - CNS symptoms follow: Encephalitis (associated with hyperactivity, pharyngeal spasms, hypersalivation, hydrophobia), ascending flaccid paralysis - Coma, respiratory failure, and eventual death	Dx: Often clinical, but molecular tests available if confirmation needed Tx: Poor prognosis (can attempt experimental regimens) PPX: Rabies Vax/IVIG [See: EM] on bites for full algorithm
Retrovirus	- HIV [See: HIV] - HTLV-1/2: Associated with T-cell leukemia/lymphoma - HTLV-I-associated myelopathy (tropical spastic paraparesis) Presents with progressive muscle weakness, spasticity, hyperreflexia, and other upper motor neuron signs	Dx: ELISA serology, followed by western blot Tx: [See: Onc] for T-cell leukemia/lymphoma. Spastic paraparesis treated supportively +/- steroids

ID25

RNA VIRUS — Infectious Disease Medicine

Paramyxo

	General/Clinical	Management/Antimicrobial Coverage
Parainfluenza	- URTI/Lower respiratory infection (ie PNA) in adults - Croup (in children)	
RSV	- URTI/Lower respiratory infections - Bronchiolitis	
Metapneumovirus	- URTI, lower respiratory infections (bronchitis/pneumonia)	- Self-limited and usually goes unidentified
Mumps	- Respiratory/fomite spread - Decreased incidence due to vaccine, but vaccinated can still get disease - Clinical: Presents initially with fever/malaise/myalgias - Followed by parotid swelling - Complications: Orchitis/oophoritis, meningoencephalitis	Dx: Clinical (can consider serology/rt-PCR if uncertain) Tx: Supportive care PPX: MMR vaccine
Measles ("Rubeola")	- Highly contagious (respiratory/airborne spread) Clinical: - Prodrome: Fever, malaise, cough, conjunctivitis, coryza, Koplik spots (white lesions on the buccal mucosa) - Exanthem: Erythematous/brown maculopapular rash, starting at head and spreading down to body, and out (spares palms/soles) Complications: - Otitis media or PNA - Encephalitis - Encephalomyelitis - Subacute Sclerosing Panencephalitis	Dx: Serology or rtPCR Tx: Supportive care + Vitamin A PPX: MMR vaccine

ID26

HIV/AIDS
Infectious Disease Medicine

Overview of Human Immunodeficiency Virus

General:
- HIV: Retrovirus that infects immune cells (T-cells, macrophages), leading to progressive immunodeficiency
- AIDS: Acquired Immunodeficiency Syndrome, defined as:
  - CD4 cell count < 200 OR AIDs defining condition

Pathophysiology:
- Envelope Proteins: gp41 (enters host cells) and gp120 (docking)
- p17 (matrix protein), p21 (capsid protein)
- Reverse polymerase, integrase, protease
- Virus initially infects macrophages, with eventual spread to CD4 t-cells

Transmission:
- Transmission: Sexual, infected blood, or vertical at birth
  - Needlestick injury/shared needle: 20-60/10,000 exposures
  - Vaginal: 4-8/ 10,000 exposures
  - Anal: ~100/10,000 exposures
  - Vertical: ~30% (no meds). With medications, risk is < 2%.
- Increased risk if higher viral load, concurrent STIs, lack of circumcision

Clinical:

Stage	Clinical Features
Acute HIV	- Presents ~2-4 weeks after exposure - Presents with fever, lymphadenopathy, sore throat, HA, myalgias ("mono-like syndrome"). Painful mucocutaneous ulcers. - Macular rash, gastrointestinal symptoms (diarrhea) also possible * Viral load elevated, but antibody normal (no seroconversion yet)
Chronic HIV	- Asymptomatic for some period of years. May have persistent generalized lymphadenopathy. - Symptomatic ("pre-AIDs"): Occurs in some patients, but not all. Prior to AIDs level disease, patient may develop increased frequency of constitutional symptoms, infections (ie dermatologic, fungal). - Progressive decline in CD4 count
AIDS	- CD4 cell count < 200 OR - AIDS defining condition (most common listed below):

PCP Pneumonia	Candidiasis (esoph/pulm)	Cryptococcus
Chronic HSV	CMV (systemic or ocular)	Kaposi Sarcoma
Toxoplasmosis	Prog. Multifocal Leukoencep	HIV Wasting
MAI or TB Infection	Lymphoma (brain/Burkitt's)	Invasive Cervical Cancer
Chronic Cryptosporid.	Disseminated Histo/Coccidio	HIV Encephalopathy

HIV/AIDS
Infectious Disease Medicine

Diagnosis of HIV

Routine Screening/Diagnosis
- 4th Generation Immunoassay
    - Detects HIV p24 antigen and HIV antibodies
- HIV-1/2 Differentiation Immunoassay
    - Now preferred confirmatory test (over Western Blot)

Screening Indications
- One time screening between age 13-75
- Annual Screening: MSM (men sex with men), IV drug users, sex workers, sexual contact with high-risk partner
- Others: Routine prenatal screening, new STD, exposure to body fluids/blood

Acute HIV (testing given concern for symptoms consistent with acute HIV)
- 4th Generation Immunoassay
- HIV Viral Load (RNA): Should be ↑↑ in acute HIV

Management of HIV

Antiretroviral Therapy (ART)
- General Considerations
    - All with HIV should be treated with antivirals, regardless of CD4 count
    - Once initiated, ART is continued indefinitely

- Regimens
    - Treatment Naive (2 NRTIs + Integrase Inhibitor)
        - Emtricitabine + Tenofovir + Dolutegravir
        - Emtricitabine + Tenofovir + Bictegravir
        - Abacavir + Lamivudine + Dolutegravir
    - Adjust later based on mutation analysis

Pre-Exposure Prophylaxis
- Indications: HIV-uninfected patients at high risk to acquire HIV
- Regimen: Emtricitabine + Tenofovir, for as long as patient is determined to be at risk

Post-Exposure Prophylaxis
- Indications:
    - Needlestick or body fluid exposure in known HIV patient
        - Includes blood, semen, vaginal fluid
        - Does not include urine, saliva, sweat, etc
        - Exposure to non-intact skin or mucous membrane
    - Recent sexual exposure to known HIV carrier
    - High risk sexual activity
        - Condomless sex in high HIV prevalence area, condomless MSM, sex work
    - Recent IV drug use with needle sharing
- Regimens (similar to treatment naive above)
    - Emtricitabine + Tenofovir + Integrase Inhibitor
- Management:
    - 28 days of therapy
    - Test patient with 4th generation assay at start of PEP, 6 weeks, 4 months

HIV/AIDS — Infectious Disease Medicine

HIV Drugs

Drug	Mechanism	Side Effects/Management
NRTIs		
Abacavir Emtricitabine Lamivudine Tenofovir Zidovudine	- Competitive inhibitor of viral reverse transcriptase (incorporated into DNA, causing strand termination)	- Mitochondrial toxicity (neuropathy, pancreatitis) - Lipoatrophy (especially Zidovudine) - Hepatic steatosis - Renal insufficiency (Tenofovir) Abacavir Hypersensitivity - Associated with HLA-B*5701 - Fever, rash, GI problems, malaise
NNRTIs		
Efavirenz Etravirine Nevirapine Rilpivirine	- Binds reverse transcriptase at site outside active site, causing conformational change that ↓ enzymatic activity	- Efavirenz: Teratogenic, vivid dreams, other CNS symptoms (confusion), psychiatric changes (irritability, anxiety) - Mild hepatotoxicity across class
Integrase Inhibitor		
Bictegravir Dolutegravir Elvitegravir Raltegravir	- Inhibits enzyme that aids in viral DNA incorporation into host DNA	- Generally well tolerated - Levels boosted by CYP 3A4 inhibitors
Protease Inhibitor (PI)		
Atazanavir Darunavir Lopinavir	- Prevent viral maturation by inhibiting cleavage of key polyproteins to their active components	- Insulin resistance/hyperglycemia - Hyperlipidemia, lipodystrophy - Hepatotoxicity * Generally used with boosting agents
Fusion Inhibitor		
Maraviroc	- CCR5 entry inhibitor	- Both infrequently used, unless many other drugs failed
Enfuvirtide	- gp41 blocker	
Boosting Agents		
Cobicistat Ritonavir	- Cyp 3A4 Inhibitors, boosting the levels of protease inhibitors and Elvitegravir - Note: Ritonavir is a PI that has some antiviral efficacy, but is primarily used in low doses as booster	- Cobicistat: Mild renal insufficiency - Ritonavir: See PI class side effects

ID29

HIV/AIDS — Infectious Disease Medicine

Overview of HIV Complication Prophylaxis

Infection	Indication	Regimen
Tuberculosis	- Screen all HIV patients with IFN-γ or PPD	- Treat latent TB if present
Pneumocystis	- CD4 ≤ 200	- TMP-SMX - Alt: Atovaquone, Dapsone, or aerosolized Pentamidine
Toxoplasma	- CD4 ≤ 100 or - Positive Toxo IgG serology	- TMP-SMX - Alt: Dapsone + Pyrimethamine
MAC	- CD4 ≤ 50 and no ART - Not indicated if on ART	- Azithromycin
Coccidiomycosis	- CD4 ≤ 250 AND in AR/CA	- Fluconazole
Histoplasmosis	- CD4 ≤ 150 AND in highly endemic area (usually not needed in US)	- Itraconazole

Vaccinations in HIV

Vaccination	Indications
Live Vaccines (MMR/Zoster/Varicella)	- Contraindicated if CD4 ≤ 200 - Can give MMR/Zoster/Varicella vaccines if CD4 > 200 and patient has not previously received
Influenza, TDAP, HPV	- All have same indications as normal adult
Pneumonia	- PCV13 (one dose) - Followed in 8 weeks by PPSV23 - PPSV23 repeated in 5 years and at age 65
Hepatitis A	- If chronic liver disease or high risk (MSM, IV drugs)
Hepatitis B	- If not immune
Meningitis (ACWY)	- All HIV infected, regardless of age

HIV/AIDS — Infectious Disease Medicine

Mucocutaneous/Cutaneous HIV Complications

Disorder	Clinical Features
Oral Thrush	- Oropharyngeal Candidiasis: Most common HIV opportunistic infection. Most often seen with CD4 < 200. - Presents with white plaques on the buccal mucosa, palate, tongue - Tx: Topical Nystatin or Clotrimazole. Oral azoles if severe.
Oral Hairy Leukoplakia	- EBV-mediated disorder of tongue epithelium - White plaques on the side of tongue - Cannot be scraped off (unlike *Candida*) - Tx: Usually not necessary. Antivirals (Acyclovir) effective.
Bacillary Angiomatosis	- Bartonella infection, seen with CD4 < 100 - *B. Henselae* → Cats. *B. Quintana* → Lice exposure (ie homeless). - Presents with vascular cutaneous lesions (with varied appearance). Often red-purple nodules or papules. - Systemic symptoms (fevers/chills/malaise) - Dx: Biopsy (histopathology) - Tx: Doxycycline/Erythromycin. ART.
Kaposi Sarcoma	[See: Derm] - Tx: ART therapy usually leads to resolution (without requiring systemic chemotherapy)

Pneumocystis Pneumonia

General: Pulmonary opportunistic fungal infection with Pneumocystis jirovecii. Occurs almost exclusively in immunocompromised patients.

Clinical:
- Indolent onset fever, dry cough, dyspnea, hypoxemia
- Note: Usually slower onset in HIV, but acute fulminant resp failure in others
- ↑ LDH levels
- XR: Bilateral diffuse infiltrates

Diagnosis:
- Definitive: Organism identification in sputum or bronchoalveolar lavage
- However, often treated based purely on clinical presentation

Management:
- TMP-SMX
    - Alternatives: Pentamidine (IV), Atovaquone (oral), Clindamycin + Primaquine, Trimethoprim + Dapsone
- Corticosteroids if PO_2 < 70 or Aa Gradient > 35

Prophylaxis: (TMP-SMX)
- HIV with CD4 < 200
- Others: Immunosuppressant use (ie high dose steroids, Cyclophosphamide, etc), stem cell transplant/solid organ transplant, immunocompromised

HIV/AIDS — Infectious Disease Medicine

Gastrointestinal Infections

Esophagitis
Clinical: Presents with dysphagia/odynophagia
Diagnosis: Clinical, with confirmation via upper endoscopy in certain cases
Management: Treat empirically with Fluconazole
- If no improvement: Upper endoscopy indicated
- Acyclovir for HSV, Ganciclovir for CMV

Candidal	- White plaques, with likely oral thrush
HSV	- Round, herpetic ulcerations/vesicles
CMV	- Linear ulcerations

Diarrhea

Cryptosporidium *Isospora* *Microsporidium*	- Parasitic gastrointestinal pathogens, CD4 < 200 - Clinical: Low-grade fever, abdominal pain, weight loss, chronic watery diarrhea - Tx: Nitazoxanide (Cryptosporidium), TMP-SMX (Isospora), Albendazole (Microsporidium)
Mycobacterium avium complex	- CD4 count < 50, generally not on ART - Diarrhea is significant component of disseminated infection - Clinical: Fever, weight loss, night sweats, chronic diarrhea, abdominal pain, diffuse lymphadenopathy - Dx: Blood culture or lymph node biopsy - Tx: Clarithromycin + Ethambutol
Cytomegalovirus	- Reactivation of latent CMV infection, CD4 < 50 - Clinical: Systemic (fever/weight loss/malaise) - Abdominal pain/diarrhea (can be watery +/- blood) - Esophagitis - Must evaluate for CMV retinitis - Dx: Clinical symptoms + endoscopy (with both macroscopic and microscopic features of CMV) - Tx: Ganciclovir or Valganciclovir

HIV Nephropathy

General: Characterized by collapsing form of focal segmental glomerulosclerosis

Clinical: Proteinuria/nephrotic syndrome, with progressive renal insufficiency

Diagnosis: Renal biopsy (collapsing, focal areas of glomerulosclerosis, with dilated tubules and interstitial inflammation)

Management: ART. ACEi/ARB.

HIV/AIDS

Infectious Disease Medicine

Neurologic HIV Complications

Disorder	Clinical Features
Primary CNS Lymphoma	- Extranodal non-Hodgkin lymphoma originating from CNS - Associated with EBV - Can affect brain, eye, or meninges - Clinical: Focal neurologic deficits (depending on location of lesion), ↑ ICP, seizures all possible presentations - MRI w/ contrast: Single or multiple mass lesions - Dx: Brain biopsy (for definitive diagnosis) - Tx: Methotrexate, other chemotherapy/immunotherapy
Toxoplasmosis	- Common if CD4 count < 100 and not receiving PPX - Clinical: Presents with fever, headache, CNS symptoms (focal deficits, confusion, mental status change, etc) - +/- Extracerebral manifestations (pneumonitis/chorioretinitis) - MRI: Multiple ring-enhancing lesions - Dx: Clinical presentation + MRI + positive Toxo IgG - Tx: Sulfadiazine + Pyrimethamine (alt: Pyrimethamine & Clindamycin)
PML	- Progressive Multifocal Leukoencephalopathy. Due to JC Virus. - Demyelinating disease seen with HIV or certain immunosuppressant drugs - Clinical: Indolent and progressive mental status changes, ataxia, focal neurologic deficits, seizures - MRI: Multiple, asymmetric, non enhancing hypodense white matter lesions (no surrounding edema) - Dx: LP (CSF JC virus PCR). Brain biopsy is definitive but not often obtained. - Tx: ART, but poor prognosis
Cryptococcus	- Common cause of meningoencephalitis in HIV patients - Most common in CD4 count < 100 OR no ART therapy - Clinical: Systemic symptoms (fever/malaise) with headache, possible neck stiffness, vomiting, and photophobia - Dx: CSF (culture/Ag test/India Ink stain with encapsulated yeast) - Tx: Amphotericin B + Flucytosine induction, followed by 8 weeks of oral Fluconazole
HIV Dementia	- HIV-associated neurocognitive disorders. Occurs in advanced AIDs. - Clinical: Difficulty with attention, memory, concentration, and informational processing - Dx: Diagnosis of exclusion (no evidence for other etiology). May require MRI/LP to rule out other conditions. - Tx: ART

HIV/AIDS — Infectious Disease Medicine

Other HIV Complications

Disorder	Clinical Features
IRIS	- Immune Reconstitution Inflammatory Syndrome - Worsening of a preexisting infectious processes with initiation of ART - Clinical: Presents within 1-2 months of starting ART with exacerbations of one of the many opportunistic HIV infections - Management: Treat opportunistic infection, continue ART *If not on ART but have opportunistic infection, wait at least 2 weeks to initiate ART to avoid IRIS
HIV Wasting	- Rapid weight loss and tissue wasting with severe AIDs - Tx: Improves dramatically with ART
HIV-Associated Lipodystrophy Syndrome	- Multifaceted syndrome that can involve pure fat atrophy OR accumulation of fat - Fat atrophy: Preferential loss of subcutaneous fat, versus fat/muscle seen with HIV wasting - Most commonly associated with NRTI (Stavudine, Zidovudine) but seen with other antiretrovirals/HIV patients in general - Fat accumulation: Truncal fat accumulation (like Cushing's) - Not associated with any specific drug regimen - Both atrophy/accumulation can be associated with insulin resistance, hyperlipidemia
Disseminated Fungal Infection	- Disseminated candida - Histoplasmosis, Blastomycosis, Coccidioidomycosis

SEXUALLY TRANSMITTED INFECTIONS — Infectious Disease Medicine

Chlamydia

General: Sexually transmitted gram-negative intracellular bacterium, most common bacterial STI in the US

Risk: Sexual behavior (new partner, multiple partners), inconsistent condom use, history of STI, men who have sex with men

Clinical: Variety of potential presentations
- Asymptomatic (common, especially in men)
- Men
    - Urethritis (mucoid urethral discharge/dysuria)
    - Prostatitis, Epididymitis (rare)
- Women
    - Cervicitis
    - Pelvic Inflammatory Disease

Diagnosis: NAAT (vaginal swab or urine)
- Can also obtain NAAT from other sites, such as anal/pharyngeal

Management: Azithromycin (single dose 1000 mg)
Note: This is for simple urethritis or cervicitis. If advanced pathology (ie PID, epididymitis) is present, further antibiotics are indicated.

Gonorrhea

General: *Neisseria gonorrhoeae* infection, gram-negative diplococci, second most common cause of bacterial STI in the US

Risk: [See: Chlamydia]

Clinical:
- Asymptomatic (Often in both men/females)
- Men
    - Urethritis (mucoid urethral discharge/dysuria)
    - Epididymitis
- Women
    - Cervicitis (usually with urethritis)
    - Pelvic Inflammatory Disease
- Extragenital: Proctitis, pharyngitis, disseminated

Diagnosis: NAAT (vaginal swab or urine)
- Can also obtain NAAT from other sites, such as anal/pharyngeal
- Gram Stain: Gram-negative diplococci, PMNs

Management: Ceftriaxone + Azithromycin or Doxycycline

SEXUALLY TRANSMITTED INFECTIONS
Infectious Disease Medicine

Syphilis

General: Infection from the spirochete *Treponema pallidum*. Transmitted via sexual contact and vertically during pregnancy.
- Considered contagious during primary, secondary, and early latent disease

Clinical:

Primary	- Chancre: Papule, which ulcerates. Ulcer is nonexudative and painless. - Regional lymphadenopathy - Heals in a few weeks without therapy
Secondary	Weeks to months after chancre, presents with: - Constitutional symptoms (fever/malaise/other flu symptoms) - Diffuse lymphadenopathy (epitrochlear nodes are classic) - Rash: Maculopapular rash, pustules, white/gray plaques on mucous membranes and genitals (condyloma lata) - Alopecia
Tertiary	- Widely variable number of years after primary infection - Gummas (ulcers or granulomatous nodules) that occur on skin and bone - CV: Dilation of ascending aorta (aortic regurgitation/aneurysm) CNS: - Early Neurosyphilis: Meningitis (headache, neck stiffness, confusion), increased risk for thrombosis/stroke - Late Neurosyphilis: Focal paralysis, tabes dorsalis (posterior column degeneration, with sensory ataxia, sharp pains). Pupillary dysfunction (Argyll-Robertson pupil) a common sign of tabes dorsalis.
Latent	- Serologic evidence of syphilis without symptoms

Diagnosis:

Nontreponemal (RPR/VDRL)	- Increases with active disease, decreases after treatment - Frequent false positives, and false negative early in disease - False positive with: SLE, certain drugs/viral infections
Treponemal (FTS-Ab, TP-EIA)	- Persistently positive after infection - More specific than nontreponemal

- Screening: Use RPR/VDRL, followed by confirmatory FTS-Ab or TP-EIA
    - Note: Many are using reverse algorithm, starting with treponemal test as initial screen, followed by RPR/VDRL
- Lumbar Puncture (CSF-VDRL) to diagnose neurosyphilis

Management:
- IM Penicillin G (for primary, secondary, tertiary, and latent disease)
    - Alt: Doxycycline (best if Penicillin allergy)
- IV Penicillin G +/- Probenecid for neurosyphilis
- Jarisch Herxheimer: Worsening symptoms for ~24 hours after treatment

SEXUALLY TRANSMITTED INFECTIONS
Infectious Disease Medicine

Genital Herpes

General: Genital herpes is most commonly caused by HSV-2, but HSV-1 also possible

Clinical:
- Primary: Variable, but can have painful genital ulcers and systemic features
- Recurrent: Episodes of genital ulcers (less severe than initial episode)
  - Multiple vesicles on erythematous base is classic

Diagnosis:
- PCR/Culture (sample from unroofed lesion)
- Serology if no active lesions

Management:
- Primary infection: Acyclovir, Famciclovir and Valacyclovir
- Recurrent disease: Acyclovir, Famciclovir and Valacyclovir
  - Chronic acyclovir suppression if ≥ 6 episodes per year
  - Episodic antiviral therapy if < 6 episodes per year
- Note: No therapy requiring if episodes infrequent/not bothersome

Ulcerative Lesions DDx

Painful Ulcers	Painless Ulcers
Herpes	**Syphilis** (Chancre)
Chancroid - *Haemophilus ducreyi*. Rare in US. - Deep, painful exudative ulcer - Dx: Clinical (no good tests) - Tx: Azithromycin or Ceftriaxone	**Lymphogranuloma venereum** - Due to Chlamydia infection (L1-L3) - Small shallow ulcer clusters, followed by: - Severe, painful inguinal LA (buboes) - Anorectal disease (proctocolitis, anal mass) - Eventual fibrosis and strictures if untreated - Tx: Doxycycline/Azithromycin
	Granuloma Inguinale (donovanosis) - Due to *Klebsiella granulomatis* - Rare in US, more common in tropics - Nodules, which ulcerate, forming extensive ulcers with granulation tissue base - Tx: Azithromycin

Other STI

Disorder	Features
Pubic Lice (Crabs)	- *Phthirus pubis*. Transmitted sexually or via clothing/towel. - Presents with pruritus, diagnosed when bug visualized - Tx: Topical Permethrin
Anogenital Warts (*Condylomata acuminata*)	- HPV 6, 11 infection. Transmitted sexually. - Variable appearance (can be nodular or plaque like lesions that are white, erythematous, or skin colored) - Tx: Imiquimod, podophyllotoxin, cryotherapy, trichloroacetic acid, surgical (Note: May resolve on own, but takes months)

INFECTION PROHYLAXIS — Infectious Disease Medicine

Hospital Infection Prophylaxis

Precaution	Features	Indications
Standard	- Hand Hygiene - Proper gloves/gown/eye protection when exposed to body fluids	- All patients
Isolation		
Contact	- Gown/gloves	- MRSA, VRE - Drug resistant gram-negative - Viral (HSV, noro, VZV, RSV, entero, parainfluenza) - *C. Diff* - Scabies
Droplet	- Mask	- Virus: Influenza, Adeno, Parvo, Rubella, Mumps - Bacteria: Meningococcus, HiB, pertussis, diphtheria
Airborne	- Airborne isolation room (negative pressure, proper air filtering) - N95 Mask or Respirator (TB)	- Tuberculosis - Measles, Varicella - SARS, Ebola

Post-Exposure Prophylaxis

Organism	Regimen/Indications
N. meningitidis	- PPX for all close contacts (ideally within 24 hours) - Regimen: Ciprofloxacin, Ceftriaxone, Rifampin
HiB	- PPX for household contacts of invasive Type B infection that have not completed HiB vaccine OR are immunocompromised - Regimen: Rifampin
Pertussis	- Household/close contacts should receive PPX - Regimen: Macrolide
Hepatitis B	- Non-immune patient exposed to HepB or HepB unknown - Exposure: Percutaneous or mucosal exposure to body fluids - HBIG plus HepB Vax
Varicella	Post exposure to Varicella case: - VZV to healthy VZV-nonimmune children/adults - Varicella Ig to pregnant women, infants, and immunocompromised (ie not vaccine candidates)
Influenza	- Antivirals for close exposure to flu, in the following situations: Pregnancy, high-risk for complications, nursing home outbreaks

ANTIBIOTICS

Infectious Disease Medicine

	Mechanism	Indication	Side Effects/Management
Beta-Lactams			
Penicillin G (IM) Penicillin V (PO)	- Blocks peptidoglycan synthesis in cell wall	- Covers basic gram positive, spirochetes, and meningococcus	- Hypersensitivity reactions - Coombs (+) hemolytic anemia
Amoxicillin (PO) Ampicillin (IV)	- Same as Penicillin, but with penicillinase resistance	- Gram positive and some gram negative coverage	- Hypersensitivity reactions - Rash
Dicloxacillin Nafcillin		- MSSA coverage	- Hypersensitivity reactions
Piperacillin Ticarcillin	- Used with Tazobactam (β-lactamase inhibitor)	- *Pseudomonas* coverage	- Hypersensitivity reactions
Cephalosporins			
1st Generation Cefazolin Cefalexin	- Blocks peptidoglycan synthesis in cell wall - Less susceptible to (β-lactamase inhibitors)	- Basic gram positive and negative coverage	- Hypersensitivity reactions (some Penicillin cross-reactivity, but decreases in frequency in later generations) - Disulfiram-like reaction with EtOH (rare) - Hypoprothrombinemia (↑ bleeding risk)
2nd Generation Cefaclor Cefoxitin Cefuroxime		- Basic gram positive, extended gram negative coverage	
3rd Generation Ceftriaxone Ceftazidime Cefotaxime Cefdinir		- Extended gram negative coverage	
4th Generation Cefepime		- Extended gram negative coverage, plus pseudomonas	
5th Generation Ceftaroline Ceftolozane		- Ceftaroline has MRSA coverage - Ceftolozane has *Pseudomonas* coverage	

ID39

ANTIBIOTICS

Infectious Disease Medicine

	Mechanism	Indication	Side Effects/Management
Carbapenems Imipenem Meropenem Ertapenem	- β-Lactam: Blocks peptidoglycan synthesis in cell wall	- Broad gram positive, negative, and anaerobic coverage (including *Pseudomonas*)	- Seizures (Imipenem and Meropenem) - Hypersensitivity (some cross-reactivity with Penicillin)
Monobactams Aztreonam	- β-Lactam: Blocks peptidoglycan synthesis in cell wall	- Gram negative coverage	
Vancomycin	- Binds Dala/Dala precursors and inhibits further cell wall growth	- Gram positive coverage, including MRSA	- Nephrotoxicity/ototoxic (rare and uncommon) - Thrombophlebitis/injection site reactions - Red Man Syndrome (diffuse flushing with Vancomycin infusion, correct with antihistamines and slow infusions)
Aminoglycosides Gentamicin Neomycin Amikacin Tobramycin Streptomycin	- Inhibits 30s ribosome - Bactericidal	- Gram negative infections (including *Pseudomonas*)	- Nephrotoxicity - Ototoxicity - Neuromuscular blockade (exacerbates myasthenia gravis)
Tetracyclines Doxycycline Minocycline Tetracycline	- Inhibits 30s ribosome - Bacteriostatic	- Broad coverage, including atypicals, zoonotic, acne, and some MRSA coverage	- GI Distress - Photosensitivity - Teratogen: Discoloration of teeth, inhibition of bone growth

ANTIBIOTICS — Infectious Disease Medicine

	Mechanism	Indication	Side Effects/Management
Macrolide			
Azithromycin, Clarithromycin, Erythromycin	- Inhibits 50s ribosome - Bacteriostatic	- Basic gram positive and gram negative coverage, atypical infections	- ↑ GI motility - Arrhythmia (QT prolongation) - Cholestasis - CYP 450 inhibition
Fluoroquinolones			
Ciprofloxacin, Levofloxacin, Moxifloxacin	- Inhibits topoisomerase II (DNA gyrase) - Bactericidal	- Gram negative coverage, with some *Pseudomonas* activity	- Cramps/myalgias - Tendinopathy (especially older or those using steroids) - Cartilage damage in kids - CNS (insomnia, confusion, psychosis) - QT prolongation
Sulfonamides			
Sulfamethoxazole, Sulfisoxazole, Sulfadiazine, Dapsone	- Inhibit dihydropteroate synthase (part of DNA synthesis pathway)	- Gram positive and negative coverage - PCP treatment/PPX, toxoplasmosis - Dapsone: Leprosy	- Hemolysis if G6PD deficient - Pancytopenia (including megaloblastic anemia) - Nephrotoxicity (including interstitial nephritis) - Hyperkalemia (from ENAC channel inhibition)
Trimethoprim	- Inhibits bacterial dihydrofolate reductase		
Misc.			
Linezolid	- Inhibits 50s ribosome	- Gram positive coverage (including MRSA)	- Bone marrow suppression - Chemotherapy-associated peripheral neuropathy - Serotonin syndrome (has MAOI activity)
Clindamycin	- Inhibits 50s ribosome	- Gram positive and anaerobic coverage	- High risk of *C. Diff* infection

ANTIBIOTICS

Infectious Disease Medicine

	Mechanism	Indication	Side Effects/Management
Misc			
Daptomycin	- Lipopeptide that disrupts cell membrane of Gram (+) bacteria	- Gram positive coverage (including MRSA)	- Myopathy/rhabdomyolysis - Inactivated by pulmonary surfactant (don't use in PNA)
Metronidazole	- Forms free radical toxin that damages DNA	- Anaerobes - Some parasites (*Giardia, Entamoeba, Trichomonas*)	- Metallic taste
Nitrofurantoin	- Inhibits ribosome complex formation	- Used primarily for gram negative UTIs	- Rare interstitial pneumonitis and hepatotoxicity
Anti-tuberculosis			
Rifampin Rifabutin	- Inhibit RNA polymerase	- TB, leprosy, meningococcal ppx	- Minor hepatotoxicity - Red body fluids - CYP450 inhibition
Isoniazid	- ↓ mycolic acid synthesis	- TB	- Hepatotoxicity (usually minor transaminitis, but severe hepatitis possible) - Drug induced SLE - B6 deficiency (peripheral neuropathy, sideroblastic anemia)
Pyrazinamide	- Unknown MXN	- TB	- Hepatotoxicity - ↑ uric acid (gout flares)
Ethambutol	- Blocks arabinosyltransferase (part of mycobacterial cell wall)	- TB, MAI	- Optic neuropathy (red-green color blindness)

ID42

ANTIFUNGALS

Infectious Disease Medicine

	Mechanism	Indication	Side Effects/Management
Amphotericin B **Nystatin**	- Binds ergosterol, creating pores in cell membrane - Delivered in liposomes to decrease toxicity	- Nearly any serious fungal infection	- Nephrotoxicity - Electrolyte abnormalities (hypomag and hypokalemia) - "Shake and Bake": Fevers/chills/hypotension (infusion of medication, improves upon subsequent infusions) - Hepatotoxicity
Azoles Fluconazole Itraconazole Voriconazole Posaconazole Isavuconazole	- Inhibits ergosterol synthesis	- Cover basic fungal infections - Itraconazole covers endemic fungi - Voriconazole covers aspergillus	- Inhibits CYP 450 - Hepatotoxicity - Voriconazole: Vision changes, hallucinations, photosensitivity reaction
Echinocandins Caspofungin Micafungin	- Inhibit the synthesis of β-glucan in fungal cell wall	- All *Candida* species	- Flushing (with IV formulations)
Terbinafine	- Inhibits squalene epoxidase (part of ergosterol synthesis)	- Topical dermatophytes, including onychomycosis	- GI Disturbances (including abnormal taste) - Hepatotoxicity
Griseofulvin	- Disrupts microtubules, inhibiting fungal cell mitosis	- Topical dermatophytes	- CYP 450 inducer - Teratogen

	Yeast (Candida, Crypto)	Endemic Fungi (Histo/blasto/coccidio)	Molds (Aspergillus)	Molds (Mucor)
Amphotericin				
Fluconazole				
Itraconazole				
Voriconazole				
Micafungin				

ANTIVIRALS

Infectious Disease Medicine

	Mechanism	Indication	Side Effects/Management
Antivirals			
Oseltamivir Zanamivir	- Inhibit neuraminidase (prevent release of progeny virus)	- Influenza	- Nausea/vomiting - Psychiatric events
Acyclovir Famciclovir Valacyclovir	- Guanosine analog, inhibit viral DNA prolongation	- Herpes viruses (including HSV, VZV)	- Obstructive crystalline nephropathy (IV formulations given with fluids)
Ganciclovir Valganciclovir	- Guanosine analog, inhibits viral DNA kinase in CMV	- CMV	- Myelosuppression (leading to cytopenias) - Nephrotoxicity
Foscarnet	- Viral DNA/RNA polymerase inhibitor	- CMV/HSV (second line agent)	- Nephrotoxicity - Electrolyte abnormalities
Cidofovir	- Viral DNA polymerase inhibitor	- CMV retinitis - HSV (acyclovir resistant)	- Nephrotoxicity
Anti-helminth/louse			
Albendazole	- Inhibits microtubule assembly	- Variety of parasitic worm infections	- Hepatotoxicity
Pyrantel pamoate	- Neuromuscular blockade		
Diethylcarbamazine	- Inhibitor of arachidonic acid metabolism	- Filariasis, loiasis	
Ivermectin	- Increases parasitic cell membrane permeability	- Parasitic worm infections - Lice, scabies	- Neurotoxicity
Praziquantel	- Increases parasitic cell membrane permeability	- Parasitic worm infections (especially *Schistosoma*)	- GI disturbances
Permethrin	- Na channel blocker	- Anti-louse	- Skin irritation (at site of application)

NEUROLOGIC EXAMINATION

Neurology Medicine

Mental Status	- Attention (repeat back series of numbers)
	- Memory (remember 3 words after 5 minutes of distraction)
	- Language
	   - Repetition: Repeat complex phrases (no ifs, ands, or buts)
	   - Naming: Name objects
	   - Comprehension: Follow simple one-step commands
	   - Read/write
	- Visuospatial: Copy diamond or cube
	- Calculations: Serial sevens

Cranial Nerves	- CN II (Optic): Pupillary reaction, visual acuity (Snellen), visual fields, fundoscopy - CN III, IV, VI: Extraocular movements - CN V: Facial sensory, muscles of mastication - CN VII: Facial movement - CN IX: Uvula deviation, gag reflex - CN XI: "Shrugging" motor strength - CN XII: Tongue movements
Motor	- Muscle bulk/appearance - Strength testing (0/5 is no movement, 3/5 can overcome gravity, 5/5 is full strength)
Sensory	- Spinothalamics: Sharp/dull testing, temperature - Posterior column: Vibration testing (tuning fork), proprioception
Reflexes	- Achilles (S1/S2) - Patellar (L3/L4) - Biceps (C5/C6) - Triceps (C7/C8) - Babinski response (upper motor neuron sign) Grading: 2+ Normal (1+ is hyporeflexia, 3+ hyperreflexia, 4+ is clonus)
Coordination	- Finger-to-nose, heel-to-shin - Rapid alternating movements
Gait	- Romberg (stand in place with eyes closed) - Walk (check balance, speed, use of arms/legs) - Heel/toe walk (test of balance)

STROKE — Neurology / Medicine

Transient Ischemic Attack

General: Episode of transient neurologic dysfunction secondary to transient CNS ischemia that does not result in infarction

Etiology:
- Low Flow: From arterial stenosis (atherosclerosis)
- Embolic: Embolic thrombus, most commonly from heart
- Lacunar: Thrombosis over lipohyalinosis of small penetrating arteries

Clinical:
- Focal neurologic deficit, that spontaneously resolves within 24 hours
    - Often resolves quickly (low-flow in minutes, embolic in hours)

Diagnosis:
- MRI (preferred) or CT
- Source Localization:
    - Duplex US (or CTA/MRA)
    - Cardiac monitoring, ECHO

Management:
- Immediate outpatient workup for source of stroke
- Secondary prevention (weight loss, smoking cessation, ASA, Statin, etc)

Stroke Risk:
- Overall risk ~8% at 30 days and 10% at 90 days
- ABCD^2 score used in past (Age > 60, BP > 140/90, clinical features, duration > 60 min, diabetes) to predict stroke risk in next week
- High risk for stroke if MRI shows area of focal ischemia

STROKE

Neurology Medicine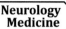

Ischemic Cerebrovascular Accident (CVA)

General: Inadequate brain oxygenation, leading to infarction of the brain parenchyma

Subtype	Etiology/Risk	Clinical Features
Thrombotic	- Atherosclerosis (often with history of TIA, HTN, HLD, DM) - Small vessel lipohyalinosis (responsible for lacunar infarct)	- Local thrombotic obstruction of artery - Fluctuating severity of symptoms initially, with periods of improvement
Embolic	- Atrial fibrillation - Endocarditis/valve disease - Septal defects (PFO/ASD)	- Thrombus thrown from outside CNS - Can have multiple infarcts in different vascular territories - Sudden onset of focal deficits - Maximal severity early on
Hypoperfusion	- Shock	- Global, nonspecific deficits

Diagnosis:
- Noncontrast CT (rule-out hemorrhage, occasionally see signs of ischemia)
    - Needed quickly to help determine tPA candidacy
- MRI (used later to help identify extent of ischemia and stroke subtype)
- Workup for stroke subtype:
    - Cardiac monitoring (for arrhythmia) and ECHO
    - Duplex US (or CTA/MRA) for evaluation vessels

Management:

Thrombolytic (IV Alteplase)	- Given for clear ischemia with measurable deficits - Must be given within 3-4.5 hours of symptoms - Exclusion Criteria: Hemorrhage, hx of intracranial lesion or stroke, stroke/head trauma within 3 months, recent intracranial surgery, BP > 185/110, current active bleeding, plt < 100k or INR > 1.7 - Relative Exclusion: Minor or improving neurologic deficits, recent major surgery/trauma/MI/GI bleed
BP Control	- ≤ 185/110 if tPA used, ≤ 220/120 if not - Labetalol, Nicardipine, and Clevidipine
Aspirin	- Aspirin (within 48 hours of stroke) *If tPA used, do not start ASA for at least 24 hours
Statin	- For all

Note: Mechanical thrombectomy utilized with increased frequency for proximal large artery obstruction

Secondary Prevention:
- Lifestyle modification
- Antiplatelet (Aspirin, Clopidogrel, or Aspirin-Dipyridamole)
- Continue with statin, HTN control, DM control, etc

STROKE

Neurology Medicine

Stroke Syndromes

Subtype	Clinical Features
Cortical	
Anterior Cerebral	- Contralateral motor/sensory deficit, with lower extremity predominance - Behavioral changes (abulia, dyspraxia, emotional change)
Middle Cerebral	- Contralateral motor/sensory deficit, with upper extremity and face predominance - Eye deviation towards side of infarction (frontal eye fields) - Homonymous hemianopsia - Aphasia (dominant) or neglect (non-dominant)
Posterior Cerebral	- Contralateral hemianopia with macular sparing - Possible sensory symptoms (from lateral thalamic infarct)
Brainstem	
Anterior Spinal	<u>Medial Medullary Syndrome</u> - Contralateral upper/lower limb paralysis - Ipsilateral hypoglossal (tongue deviates towards lesion) - Loss of proprioception (medial lemniscus)
Posterior Inferior Cerebellar (PICA)	<u>Wallenberg Syndrome</u> (Lateral Medullary) - Dysphagia/Hoarseness - ↓ Pain/temp from ipsilateral face/contralateral body - Ipsilateral Horner syndrome - Vertigo, nystagmus, ataxia, dysmetria
Anterior Inferior Cerebellar (AICA)	<u>Lateral Pontine Syndrome</u> - Ipsilateral facial paralysis (facial nucleus) - ↓ Pain/temp from ipsilateral face/contralateral body - ↓ Decreased lacrimation/salivation/taste from ant. tongue - Vertigo, nystagmus, ataxia, dysmetria
Basilar	- Medial pons, possible "Locked-In Syndrome" - Corticospinal: Unilateral or bilateral paresis - Bulbar: Unilateral or bilateral face weakness, dysarthria, dysphagia, limited jaw movement - Oculomotor: Horizontal gaze palsy, internuclear ophthalmoplegia
Lacunar	
Pure Motor	- Internal capsule (posterior limb) - Unilateral paralysis of face, arm, leg without sensory loss
Pure Sensory	- Thalamus (VPL/VPM) - Unilateral sensory deficit of face, arm, leg without motor loss
Ataxic Hemiparesis	- Internal capsule, basis pontis, or corona radiata - Unilateral weakness and limb ataxia
Dysarthria-Clumsy Hand	- Genu of internal capsule, basal pons - Unilateral face weakness, dysarthria, with hand weakness and clumsiness

STROKE
Neurology / Medicine

Intracerebral Hemorrhage

General: Parenchymal brain bleeds, second most common stroke (after ischemic)

Etiology:
- Hypertensive vasculopathy
    - Penetrating vessels develop pseudoaneurysms which rupture
- Cerebral amyloid angiopathy
- Vascular malformations
- Conversion from ischemic stroke

Clinical:
- Acute, progressive focal neurologic deficit (depending on location)
- Possible signs of increased ICP if large (HA, drowsiness, vomiting, seizures)

Diagnosis:
- Noncontrast CT (reveals bleed/hematoma)
- MRI (can aid in determining underlying cause)

Management:
- ICU level supportive care
- Stop antiplatelets/anticoagulants (and use reversal agents if available)
- BP Control (target MAP of 110, or 160/90)
    - Nicardipine, Labetalol, Enalapril
- ICP Control
    - Elevate head of bed, use sedation (ie Propofol)
    - If concern over ICP, can use invasive monitoring
    - Mannitol/hypertonic saline, hyperventilation, CSF drainage

< STROKE   Neurology Medicine >

Subarachnoid Hemorrhage

General: Bleeding into the subarachnoid space (between arachnoid/pia)

Etiology:
- Ruptured saccular aneurysms. Most common sites:
  (1) Anterior Communicating, (2) Posterior Communicating, (3) MCA
- Other Causes: Vascular malformations, arterial dissection, trauma

Clinical:
- Universally causes sudden, severe headache
- Nausea, vomiting, meningismus, loss of consciousness all possible

Diagnosis:
- Noncontrast CT
- LP (if CT negative, but suspicion high; xanthochromia is classic)
- Digital subtraction angiography (or CTA/MRA) to identify aneurysms

Management:
- Supportive ICU level care
- BP (< 160 systolic): Nicardipine, Labetalol, or Enalapril
- All get Nimodipine (improves outcomes)
- Aneurysm: Surgical Clipping or Endovascular Coil (↓ risk of rebleed)
- Seizure PPX (if seizure is part of presentation or high risk bleed)

Complications:
- Rebleeding (surgical intervention helps prevent)
- Vasospasm
  - No well-validated intervention, but hyperdynamic therapy is used
- Hydrocephalus (consider shunt placement)
- Hyponatremia (SIADH)

Unruptured Cerebral Aneurysm

General: Also called saccular ("berry") aneurysms. ↑ Risk for rupture and SAH.

Risk: Genetics (CT disease like Marfan/Ehlers Danlos, ADPKD), environmental (smoking, HTN)

Clinical: Generally asymptomatic unless ruptured. Large aneurysms can cause headache, visual loss or cranial nerve deficits.

Diagnosis: CTA or MRA

Management:
- Controversial. Generally, small aneurysms observed/monitored, and large symptomatic aneurysms can be intervened upon endovascularly.

| STROKE | Neurology Medicine |

Venous Sinus Thrombosis

General: Thrombosis of cerebral veins or dural sinuses, leading to backup of blood, with eventual CNS dysfunction

Etiology: Prothrombotic states (Genetic thrombophilia, OCP, pregnancy, malignancy)

Clinical: Highly variable presentation, with variable timing of onset
- Headache
- Other signs of increased ICP (vomiting, papilledema, and visual problems)
- Focal neurologic deficits in some
- Seizures

Diagnosis: MR venography + Brain MRI

Management:
- Anticoagulation (LMWH or IV Heparin)
  - Long term Warfarin (or DOAC)
- Other acute management: ICP management, seizure ppx (if seizures)

Cavernous Sinus Thrombosis

General: Infection and thrombosis of the cavernous sinus, which multiple cranial nerves run through (CN III, IV, V1, V2, VI). Organisms commonly implicated include MRSA/MSSA, or *Strep pneumoniae*/viridans.

Etiology:
- Certain sinus infections
- Facial infections (from areas around eyes/nose, which drain via ophthalmic veins)
- Dental infections

Clinical:
- Early signs: Headache, fever, periorbital edema (can be acute or slow and progressive)
- Lateral gaze palsy (CN VI)
- CN III (oculomotor) deficits (mydriasis, eyelid drooping, diplopia)
- Changes in sensation in the V1/V2 dermatomes

Diagnosis: CT or MRI with contrast

Management:
- Antibiotics (generally Vancomycin + 3rd/4th generation cephalosporin)
- Surgical drainage in severe cases

SUBDURAL/EPIDURAL BLEEDS
Neurology — Medicine, Surgery

Subdural Hematoma

General: Bleed into potential space between dura and the arachnoid membranes, due to rupture of bridging veins (drain brain to dural sinus). Rarely due to arterial bleed.

Etiology:
- Trauma (ie MVA, assault, falls in elderly)
    - ↑ Risk: Elderly (cortical atrophy), previous TBI, EtOH abuse

Clinical:
- Acute: Increased ICP (HA, vomit), anisocoria, CN palsies, coma
- Chronic: Progressive headaches, neurologic impairment, somnolence

Diagnosis:
- Contrast CT (crescentic hyperdense lesion, possible midline shift)
- MRI (higher sensitivity)

Management: Acute Subdural

Operative	- Indicated if signs of herniation/severely ↑ ICP, clot thickness ≥ 10 mm or midline shift ≥ 5 mm, clinically deteriorating - Surgical craniotomy (or alternative decompressive method)
Nonoperative	- Serial CT scans - ICP management (head elevation, hyperventilation, and Mannitol)

Chronic Subdural: Surgery if clinically severe/progressive neurologic decline, OR clot thickness ≥ 10 mm or midline shift ≥ 5 mm

Epidural Hematoma

General: Bleeding into potential space between dura/skull, most commonly from sphenoid damage/rupture of middle meningeal artery

Etiology: Trauma

Clinical:
- Altered consciousness, confusion, drowsiness
- Headache, vomiting, seizures
- Possible loss of consciousness, followed by "lucid interval" (transient recovery), and subsequent deterioration

Diagnosis: Noncontrast CT. MRI can be used if diagnosis unclear.

Management:
- Urgent/emergent surgical hematoma evacuation
- If asymptomatic, can consider serial CT monitoring/nonoperative care

INTRACRANIAL HYPERTENSION
Neurology / Medicine

Overview of ICP

General: Intracranial pressure is normally ≤ 15 mmHg, intracranial hypertension defined as ≥ 20
- CPP = MAP - ICP

Etiology:
- Cerebral edema (ie post trauma)
- Intracranial mass lesion or bleed (tumor, hematoma, hemorrhage)
- Hydrocephalus/increased CSF production/decreased CSF absorption

Clinical:
- Headache
- Papilledema, CN VI palsy
- Cushing's triad: Bradycardia, respiratory depression, and hypertension
- Herniation syndromes (see below)

Management:
- ICP monitoring (intraventricular/intraparenchymal)
- Interventions
    - Treat underlying condition
    - Head elevation, hyperventilation, Mannitol
    - Sedation (ie Propofol), which reduces brain metabolic demand
    - BP control (maintain CPP > 60 mmHg)
    - Fever control (Acetaminophen)

Herniation

Syndrome	Clinical Manifestations
Transtentorial (Uncal)	- Ipsilateral hemiparesis (compression of contralateral crus cerebri against the tentorial edge [Kernohan notch], "false-localizing sign") - Contralateral homonymous hemianopia (compression of PCA) - Mydriasis and down/out gaze (compression of CN III) - Eventual central herniation/death
Transtentorial (central)	- Thalamus and temporal lobe herniation through tentorium cerebelli, rupturing branches of the basilar artery feeding the pons ("Duret Hemorrhage") - Fatal CV/respiratory depression
Tonsillar	- Respiratory depression/CV instability/death (cerebral tonsils herniate through the foramen magnum, compressing midbrain)
Subfalcine	- ACA infarction (cingulate gyrus under falx cerebri)

TRAUMATIC BRAIN INJURY

Neurology, Medicine, Surgery

Overview of Traumatic Brain Injury (TBI)

General: TBI is a heterogenous term that includes brain trauma of a variety of mechanisms and varying severity. Often occurs from the direct impact, rapid acceleration/deceleration, or penetrating trauma. Injuries include:
- Brain contusions
- Diffuse axonal injury (due to shearing mechanism)
    - Especially poor prognosis (present with coma/increased ICP)
    - Imaging shows blurring of gray/white junction
- Hemorrhages (subdural, epidural, intracranial)

Subtypes:

GCS 13-15	Mild TBI (concussion). See below.
GCS 9-12	Moderate TBI
GCS < 8	Severe TBI

Mild TBI (Concussion)

General: Mild brain injury from blunt force or acceleration/deceleration injury

Clinical:
- Possible loss of consciousness at time of event
- Confusion and amnesia (for events just before and after trauma)
- Headaches, dizziness, or imbalance
- Disorientation, poor concentration, inability to maintain attention
- Delayed reaction/verbal expression
- No focal neurologic deficits

Diagnosis:
- Clinical (see above)
    - Can use clinical scoring tool like SAC or SCAT5
- CT (with contrast) in select patients

Adult CT Indications	Child CT Indications (2-18 y/o)
- GCS < 15 - Focal neuro deficits - Skull fracture - Seizure - Anticoagulant use - > 60 y/o - Multiple vomiting episodes - Severe mechanism of injury	- GCS < 15 - Focal neuro deficits - Skull fracture - Prolonged loss of consciousness - Seizure - Can observe OR CT the following: Headache, vomiting, severe MOI, loss of consciousness

Follow up with CTA/MRA if vascular injury suspected

Management:
- 24 hours of monitoring (for worsening symptoms)
    - CT for worsening symptoms
- Graduated return to play for sports (ie do not return until asymptomatic and off medication for symptoms)
- Cognitive rest (ie from work) until symptoms resolve

COMPLICATIONS OF HEAD TRAUMA
Neurology / Medicine, Surgery

Carotid/Vertebral Artery Dissection

General: Separation of arterial wall layers, leading to creation of false lumen

Etiology:
- Minor trauma (sports, sex, yoga, chiropractic manipulations)
- Underlying CT/vascular disorder (ie Marfans, Ehlers-Danlos, fibromuscular dysplasia)

Clinical:
- Local neck pain or headache
- TIA/CVA symptoms
    - Carotid: Anterior circulation stroke symptoms (ie MCA, ACA, etc)
    - Vertebral: Posterior circulation stroke symptoms (ie brainstem, cerebellar, visual)
- Horner syndrome
- Audible bruit

Diagnosis: MRA/CTA

Management:
- Aspirin or anticoagulation
- tPA (used if ischemic stroke symptoms and meets criteria)
- Endovascular stents if symptoms recurrent strokes persist on med therapy

Skull Fractures

Subtype	Clinical	Management
Linear	- Simple, linear fracture through full thickness of calvarium - Generally not clinically significant, but can rarely cause bleeding	Dx: CT Tx: No intervention required if patient has no underlying brain injury/bleed
Depressed	- Segment of skull driven below the plane of adjacent skull - Almost all have some degree of TBI - Risk for infection, bleed, seizures - Can have "step off" on physical exam	Dx: CT Tx: Tetanus/Abx prophylaxis, +/- surgical repair
Basilar	- Fracture of bone forming base of skull (ie sphenoid, occipital, cribriform plate, petrous temporal) - High risk for bleeds and dural tears (causing CSF leaks) **Clinical:** - Battle Sign: Bleed behind ear/mastoid - Periorbital ecchymosis ("raccoon eye") - Clear/blood tinged rhinorrhea or otorrhea (concern for CSF leak) - Hemotympanum	Dx: CT - CSF Leak: "Halo-sign" or beta-2 transferrin level Tx: Surgery (for bleeds), others simply admitted for observation

HYPOKINETIC MOVEMENT DISORDERS

Neurology Medicine

Parkinson's

General/Clinical

- Loss of dopamine containing neurons in the substantia nigra in the midbrain, causing reduced excitatory input to the motor cortex
- Risk: ↑ Age. Smoking is protective.

Clinical: (Cardinal 4 symptoms numbered)
(1) Bradykinesia (slow movements)
(2) Tremor (pill-rolling rest tremor, improves with movement)
(3) Rigidity (increased resistance to passive movement)
(4) Postural instability (impaired postural reflex, manifested as imbalance)
- Masked facial expression, hypophonia
- Gait: Shuffling, short-steps, "freezing"
- Neuropsychiatric or cognitive dysfunction

Management

Dx: Purely clinical diagnosis (Criteria are complex, but essentially bradykinesia + tremor or rigidity, without any evidence of an alternative diagnosis)

Tx:
- Levodopa-Carbidopa
  - First line therapy
- Dopamine agonists (ie Ropinirole, Pramipexole)
  - Used as adjunctive agents in advanced disease
- MAO-B Inhibitors (Selegiline, Rasagiline)
  - Adjunctive agents
- Anticholinergics (Trihexyphenidyl and Benztropine)
  - Treats tremor, generally used in early disease
- COMT Inhibitors (Tolcapone and Entacapone), occasionally used as adjunct in advanced disease
- Amantadine: Mild effects, useful in early disease

Parkinson's Plus

General/Clinical

- Overarching term for multiple diseases (olivopontocerebellar atrophy, Shy-Drager, and striatonigral degeneration), which all have Parkinsonian features plus other symptoms

Management

Dx: Clinical. Some improve on Levodopa/Carbidopa but a lack of improvement would indicate MSA over Parkinson's.

Multiple Systems Atrophy

General/Clinical

Clinical
- Parkinsonian features (bradykinesia, rigidity, tremor)
- Autonomic dysfunction (ED, orthostatic hypotension)
- Cerebellar dysfunction (ataxia)

Management

Tx: Levodopa (see if response). Otherwise all care is purely supportive, no other effective treatments.

HYPOKINETIC MOVEMENT DISORDERS

Neurology Medicine

	General/Clinical	Management
Parkinson's Plus (con't)		
Progressive Supranuclear Palsy	- Tau-positive neurodegenerative disease, resulting in rapidly progressive Parkinsonism and other features Clinical: - Parkinsonian features (postural instability causing falls) - Supranuclear ophthalmoplegia (vertical gaze palsy) - Others: Cognitive dysfunction, dysarthria, dysphagia	Dx: Clinical. MRI findings can be supportive (mid-brain atrophy, "Hummingbird" sign) Tx: Supportive. No effective therapies. Poor response to Levodopa.
Corticobasal Degeneration	- Progressive tau-positive neurodegenerative disease Clinical: - Initially presents with focal akinesia, dystonia, myoclonus, or apraxia (ie of one limb) - Can progress to diffuse parkinsonian features - Progressive cognitive dysfunction/behavioral changes - CT/MRI shows asymmetric frontal cortical atrophy	Dx: Clinical. Poor response to Levodopa. Tx: No effective therapies
Other "Parkinson Plus" (covered elsewhere) - Lewy body dementia - Pick's disease		
Bradykinesia in Children (can rarely get early-onset Parkinson's, early-onset Huntington's, or Wilson disease)		
PKAN	- AR mutation in pantothenate kinase 2, causing iron accumulation in CNS with progressive neurologic dysfunction starting in first decade of life Clinical: - Parkinsonism - Dystonia or choreoathetosis - Retinopathy, cognitive decline	Dx: Clinical. MRI can support ("eye of the tiger" sign in globus pallidus) Tx: Supportive. Levodopa may help in some cases.

HYPERKINETIC MOVEMENT DISORDERS

Neurology Medicine

Tremors

	General/Clinical	Management
Resting Tremor	- Usually due to Parkinson's disease - "Pill-rolling" tremor, disappears with movement (4-6 hz freq)	Tx: [See: Parkinson's]
Physiologic Tremor	- Normal low-amplitude, high-frequency (10-12 hz) - Normally subclinical, but can become apparent in high adrenergic states (ie anxiety, use of certain medications, etc)	Tx: Manage underlying exacerbating factor
Essential Tremor	- AD, familial tremor - Action tremor; most commonly of hands/forearms (6-12 hz)	Tx: Propranolol (alt: Primidone, moderate EtOH)
Intention Tremor	- Almost always occurs in association with some underlying neurologic disease (ie stroke, MS) - Tremor occurs with goal-directed movements, worsening as hand gets close to target	
Functional Tremor	- Psychogenic tremor with varying presentation (ie frequency and characteristics), but disappears with distraction	
Myoclonus	- Clinical: Quick, rapid involuntary movements. Multiple underlying causes. - Physiologic (jerks associated with sleep) - Essential (idiopathic, can be acquired or hereditary) - Epilepsy (associated with seizures)	Tx: Antiepileptics (ie Levetiracetam or Valproate) or benzodiazepines
Fasciculations	- Clinical: Brief, spontaneous contraction involving small group of muscle fibers (appears as flicker under skin) - Can be sign of motor neuron disease (ie ALS), but often benign	
Tardive Dyskinesia	- Writhing movements of the mouth, face and limbs - Secondary to chronic antipsychotic medication use	Tx: Discontinue antipsychotic med, but often irreversible

HYPERKINETIC MOVEMENT DISORDERS

Neurology Medicine

Chorea

General: Movement disorder characterized by involuntary quick, random, and irregular movements. Several disorders are on the choreiform spectrum:

Chorea	- Quick, involuntary, unpredictable contractions - Most commonly affect distal limbs, but also face and trunk
Athetosis	- Slow, writhing, "snake-like" movements
Ballism	- Large amplitude (ie flinging/kicking) movements of proximal muscles - Hemiballism (unilateral) most common, usually due to lesions involving the subthalamic nucleus

Etiology:
- Hereditary (Huntington, other rare syndromes)
- Secondary (certain infections, autoimmune disease, drugs)
    - Sydenham's Chorea with rheumatic heart disease
- Idiopathic

Huntington Chorea

General: Progressive neurodegenerative disorder. AD CAG nucleotide repeat in the huntingtin gene on chromosome 4. Causes loss of GABA-producing neurons in the striatum.

Clinical:
- Gradual and progressive onset of symptoms between 30-50 years of age
- Chorea
- Progressive motor function decline
- Psychiatric: Irritability, depression, or psychotic symptoms
- Progressive cognitive decline
- MRI: Can show caudal atrophy (in late-stage disease)

Diagnosis:
- Clinical/family history
- Confirmatory genetic testing

Management:
- Supportive, multidisciplinary care
- Chorea: Tetrabenazine (alt: antipsychotics)
- Behavioral symptoms (ie psychosis): Atypical antipsychotics

HYPERKINETIC MOVEMENT DISORDERS — Neurology Medicine

Dystonia

General: Sustained, prolonged muscle contractions, causing repetitive abnormal, often stereotypical movements. Can be focal or diffuse, and it can be isolated or occur in association with another movement disorder/neurodegenerative disorder.

Adult Onset Focal Dystonia:

Cervical	- Spasmodic torticollis: Horizontal turning of neck with lateral tilt
Blepharospasm	- Involuntary blinking and spasms of involuntary eye closure
Spasmodic Dysphonia	- Laryngeal muscle involvement, resulting in abnormal phonation (voice cracks/strained voice)
Oromandibular/ Lingual	- Involuntary jaw clenching, chewing, opening, etc - Possible tongue protrusion
Task Specific	- Writer's cramp - Musician's dystonia

Management:
- Trial of Levodopa (see if responsive)
- Other drugs: Trihexyphenidyl, Tetrabenazine
- Botulinum toxin injection

Stiff Person Syndrome

General: Progressive, full body stiffness. Anti-GAD antibodies in CSF (decreases available GABA, resulting in uninhibited muscle contraction).

Clinical:
- Progressive axial muscle spasms, stiffness, and rigidity
- Spasmodic episodes, impaired ambulation

Diagnosis: Clinical, plus EMG (continuous motor activity, improves with diazepam)

Management: Benzodiazepines or Baclofen

Restless Leg Syndrome

General: Idiopathic disorder characterized by uncomfortable urge to move legs

Etiology: Idiopathic, but associated with decreased central iron stores (↓ ferritin)

Clinical:
- Uncomfortable urge to move legs during periods of inactivity (ie at night)
- Felt in lower legs, varied sensation (restless, cramping, electric)
- Transient relief with movement

Diagnosis: Clinical (but work up for low iron with ferritin levels)

Management:
- Iron replacement (for low or borderline low ferritin)
- Nonpharmacologic therapy (massage, heat, exercise, etc)
- Avoid exacerbating agents (ie anti-dopaminergic agents, antihistamines)
- Pharm: Pramipexole, Ropinirole (alt: Gabapentin/Pregabalin)

GAIT/CEREBELLAR DYSFUNCTION

Neurology Medicine

Abnormal Gaits

Subtype	Clinical Features	Etiologies
Hemiplegic	- Drags affected leg in semicircle (circumduction)	- Stroke
Neuropathic	- "Steppage Gait." Patient with foot drop lifts leg high to avoid tripping over it.	- Motor neuropathy (ie L5 nerve disease OR motor neuron disease like ALS)
Myopathic	- Hip drop on contralateral side due to weak gluteal muscles on ipsilateral side - "Trendelenburg sign"	- Myopathy (ie muscular dystrophy)
Cerebellar	- Staggering, wide-based gait with ataxia	- Cerebellar disease (stroke or degeneration) - EtOH intoxication
Parkinsonian	- Stooped, head forward posture - Walks with shuffling, short steps - Decreased arm swing	- Parkinson's - Movement disorders
Sensory	- Lack of proprioception, so slams foot to help localize/feel	- Peripheral sensory neuropathy, dorsal column degeneration
Vestibular	- Unsteady, falling over - Complain of associated features such as vertigo	- Any cause of vertigo
Frontal	- Gait apraxia, difficulty starting to walk - Freezing, "magnetic" gait - En bloc turns. Falls backwards.	- Dementia - Normal pressure hydrocephalus

Clinical Manifestations of Cerebellar Dysfunction

General: Cerebellum functions to modulate movement, especially aiding with coordination and balance

Lesion	Abnormality
Lateral Cerebellum	- Ipsilateral limb dysmetria (test with finger/nose, heel/shin) - Ipsilateral dysdiadochokinesia (test with rapid alternating movements) - Intention tremor
Medial Cerebellum	- Truncal ataxia (wide-based cerebellar gait)
Flocculonodular	- Vertigo - Nystagmus

CEREBELLAR DISORDERS

Neurology
Medicine, Pediatrics

	General/Clinical	Management
Genetic		
Spinocerebellar Ataxia	- Wide variety of genetic mutations responsible. Mutations can be inherited (most commonly AD) or sporadic. - Clinical: Cerebellar ataxia, with other symptoms depending on specific mutation	Tx: No effective therapies
Friedreich's Ataxia	- AR GAA-trinucleotide expansion (frataxin gene). Most common inherited cerebellar ataxia. Part of spinocerebellar ataxia family. Clinical: - Cerebellar atrophy (limb and gait ataxia) - Degeneration of multiple spinal cord tracts (motor weakness, loss of DTR, loss of sensation/proprioception, dysarthria) - Cardiomyopathy - Other: Diabetes mellitus, kyphoscoliosis, hammer toes	Dx: Clinical. Confirm with genetic testing. Tx: No specific disease altering therapy. Supportive, multidisciplinary care.
Toxin Mediated		
EtOH Cerebellar Degeneration	- Degeneration of cerebellar vermis from chronic alcohol abuse - Clinical: Poorly coordinated, wide-based gait	Dx: Clinical Tx: EtOH cessation, nutritional supplementation
Inflammatory Cerebellar Disease		
Acute Cerebellar Ataxia (Post-infectious Cerebellitis)	- Occurs weeks after certain viral/bacterial infections or rarely post vaccination. Seen in young children. - Autoimmune white matter demyelination of the cerebellum - Clinical: Acute, rapid onset of gait disturbance, ataxia, etc	Dx: Clinical (must rule out meningitis with LP. CSF analysis usually normal or mild lymphocytosis) Tx: Self-Limited. Most fully recover.

CENTRAL DEMYELINATING DISEASE
Neurology Medicine

Multiple Sclerosis

General: CNS inflammatory demyelinating disease, believed to be due to autoreactive lymphocytes. Typical clinical courses below:
- Relapsing-Remitting: Episodes followed by full recovery
- Primary Progressive: Progressive accumulation of disability (temporary improvements or partial recoveries possible, but overall worsens)
- Secondary Progressive: Initial relapse-remit, then progressive disease

Risk: Female, aged 20-40, far from equator (↓ vitamin D)

Clinical:
- White Matter CNS lesions, separated by space and time
    - Optic neuritis (blurry vision, painful eye movements)
    - Internuclear ophthalmoplegia (nystagmus of abducting eye contralateral to lesion)
    - Transverse myelitis (spinal cord lesions causing sensory or motor deficits)
    - CNS white matter lesions
- Cerebellar disease (ataxia, intention tremor, dysarthria)
- Bladder Incontinence
    - Urge incontinence initially (from detrusor overactivity)
    - Eventually can develop overflow incontinence
- Autonomic dysfunction (ED, constipation)
- Fatigue, depression, neuropathic pain, cognitive decline
- Classic Signs
    - Uhthoff's: Symptoms worse with heat (axons conduct worse)
    - Lhermitte: Electric sensation with neck flexion
    - Charcot's Triad (Scanning speech, intention tremor, nystagmus)

Diagnosis: Combination of clinical symptoms and MRI lesions
- MRI: New and old white matter lesions in multiple typical CNS areas
    - New lesions tend to enhance with contrast
    - Dawson's fingers from corpus callosum (classic sign)
- Other supportive tests:
    - LP (CSF shows oligoclonal IgG bands). Used if above is equivocal.
    - Visual Evoked Potentials: Latency of P100 peak

Management:

Acute Exacerbation	- IV High-dose Methylprednisolone
Relapse-Remit	- Options include Glatiramer, IFN-β (both safe, less efficacious), Natalizumab (more side effects, but better effect) - If refractory to first line agents: Alemtuzumab, Fingolimod, Teriflunomide, Cyclophosphamide all options - Vitamin D for all
Primary Progressive	- Ocrelizumab

CENTRAL DEMYELINATING DISEASE
Neurology Medicine

Acute Disseminated Encephalomyelitis (ADEM)

General: Postinfectious, autoimmune demyelinating disorder. More common in kids than adults.

Etiology: Post infection or vaccination

Clinical:
- Multiple focal neurologic deficits (can present with motor, sensory, or cranial nerve defects)
- Encephalopathy

Diagnosis:
- MRI: Multifocal, asymmetric, white matter lesions
- LP: Increased protein, lymphocytosis

Management: IV Methylprednisolone +/- IVIG

Neuromyelitis Optica

General: Inflammatory CNS disorder, due to autoantibodies against aquaporin-4

Clinical:
- Acute episodes of optic neuritis PLUS
  - Transverse myelitis
  - Brainstem syndromes (Area postrema; intractable hiccups, emesis)

Diagnosis: MRI plus AQP-4 antibody test

Management:
- Acute: IV Methylprednisolone
- Chronic: Azathioprine, Rituximab, or others

Progressive Multifocal Leukoencephalopathy

General: JC virus infection of CNS oligodendrocytes → White matter demyelination

Risk:
- HIV
- Natalizumab
- Hematologic malignancies, inflammatory disorders

Clinical: Progressive, subacute focal neurologic deficits (ie encephalopathy, motor dysfunction, sensory issues, ataxia, visual issues)

Diagnosis:
- MRI: Multifocal, asymmetric white matter lesions
- LP (CSF shows JC virus IgG)
- Brain biopsy (definitive, but rarely used due to side effects)

Management: Supportive. No effective therapy.
- Treat underlying disorder (ie start ART)

PERIPHERAL DEMYELINATING DISEASE
Neurology Medicine

Guillain Barre/AIDP

General: Acute immune-mediated peripheral neuropathy, believed due to molecular mimicry, causing immune-mediated damage to peripheral nerves. Variants include:
- Acute inflammatory demyelinating polyneuropathy (AIDP)
    - Most common, with typical presentation (see clinical)
- Acute motor axonal neuropathy (like typical AIDP, but no sensory symptom)
- Acute motor and sensory axonal neuropathy (more sensory involvement)
- Miller Fisher syndrome (ophthalmoplegia, ataxia, areflexia)

Etiology: Associated with certain infections (*Campylobacter jejuni*, EBV, CMV, HIV, HSV), and rarely post immunization

Clinical:
- Rapidly ascending extremity weakness/paralysis/loss of DTR
- Can involve respiratory, facial, and bulbar muscles
- Autonomic dysfunction (arrhythmias, tachycardia, postural hypotension)
- Paresthesias

Diagnosis: Clinical diagnosis, supported by following labs
- LP (CSF analysis shows ↑ protein, but normal cell count, called "Albuminocytologic Dissociation")

Management:
- Supportive care (hemodynamic monitoring, respiratory support)
    - Monitor FVC and maximum inspiratory pressure
    - Low pulmonary function tests → Invasive ventilation indicated
- Plasma Exchange or IVIG
- Corticosteroids not effective

Chronic Inflammatory Demyelinating Polyneuropathy (CIDP)

General: Acquired disorder of chronic demyelination of the peripheral nervous system

Clinical:
- Progressive or relapsing/remitting peripheral neuropathy
    - Motor usually more pronounced than sensory deficits
    - Hyporeflexia or areflexia

Diagnosis: Clinical, plus the following diagnostic evidence
- Electrodiagnostic (↓ conduction velocities, supporting demyelination)
- Nerve biopsy
- LP (CSF analysis shows ↑ protein, but normal cell count)

Management:
- IVIG, plasma exchange, or glucocorticoids
- Other immunosuppressants if multiple relapses/refractory to first-line

SPINAL CORD LESIONS

Neurology Medicine

Spinal Cord Syndromes

Syndrome	Clinical Findings
Brown Sequard (Hemisection)	- Ipsilateral hemiparesis - Ipsilateral dorsal column signs (vibration/proprioception) - Contralateral pain and touch (from spinothalamic which crosses two levels above the loss of sensation)
Central Cord	- Loss of pain/temperature at the level of the lesion - Weakness (more pronounced in UE compared to LE) - Occurs with syringomyelia, certain tumors, trauma
Ventral Cord	- Loss pain/temperature, motor weakness
Dorsal Cord	- Loss of proprioception, vibration, fine touch
Transection	- Loss of all sensation and motor function - Bladder dysfunction

Spinal Cord Disorders

Disorder	Clinical Findings
Syringomyelia	- Fluid filled dilation of the spinal cord, most commonly in cervical or thoracic spine - Associated with Chiari I malformation, but also infection, tumor, inflammation, or trauma - Causes central cord syndrome ("cape-like" loss of pain/temp)
Subacute Combined Degeneration	- Associated with B12 deficiency - Leads to degeneration of dorsal cord and corticospinal tracts
Transverse Myelitis	- Associated with MS, and other autoimmune conditions - White matter lesion, usually 1-2 segments, in thoracic cord
Spinal Cord Infarctions	- Most commonly anterior spinal infarct (ventral cord syndrome)
Compressive Lesions	- Epidural abscess or hematoma - Neoplasms - Cervical spondylotic myelopathy
Tabes Dorsalis	- Advanced neurosyphilis (now rare with antibiotics) - Posterior column disease (sensory ataxia and sharp pains) - Argyll-Robertson pupils (does not respond to light, but does contract with accommodation)

NEUROMUSCULAR DISEASE
Neurology
Medicine, Pediatrics

Amyotrophic Lateral Sclerosis

General: Motor neuron degeneration, with combined lower motor neuron atrophy, and subsequent degeneration of the upper motor corticospinal tracts

Etiology:
- Sporadic (90%): Increased risk with ↑ age, family history, and smoking
- Hereditary (10%): Many genes. SOD 1 (superoxide dismutase type 1) is common subtype.

Clinical:
- Most commonly presents asymmetric limb weakness, with other UMN and LMN signs. Bulbar (dysphagia, dysarthria) symptoms also possible.
- Upper Motor Signs: Muscle weakness, spasticity, hyperreflexia
- Lower Motor Signs: Muscle weakness, fasciculations, atrophy
- Progressive cognitive impairment
- Progressive worsening of disease, with prognosis of ~3-5 years on average

Diagnosis: Clinical diagnosis (combination of UMN/LMN signs, without evidence of an alternative diagnosis, plus the following)
- EMG: Reveals evidence of acute/chronic denervation
- MRI: Typically normal

Management:
- Disease Modifying Therapy:
    - Riluzole (only drug to show improved survival)
    - Edaravone (slow neurodegeneration in some)
- Other management is symptom based (ie PEG tube for dysphagia, PPV for respiratory compromise, antispasmodics, mucolytics, etc)

Spinal Muscular Atrophy

General: Inherited degeneration of the anterior horn cells that results in muscular atrophy. Presents in kids. Due to AR SMA gene mutation.

Clinical:
- Diffuse symmetric proximal muscle weakness (UE greater than LE)
    - Often flaccid, unable to sit upright, "Frog-leg" posture
- Weak cry, difficulty sucking/swallowing
- Hyporeflexia/areflexia

Diagnosis: Genetic testing

Management:
- Supportive care (respiratory, nutritional, etc)
- Nusinersen (intrathecal injection of antisense DNA that increases SMN gene expression)

NEUROMUSCULAR DISEASE

Neurology, Medicine, Pediatrics

Muscular Dystrophy

	General/Clinical	Management
Duchenne (DMD)	- X-linked dystrophin mutation (frameshift mutation) Clinical: (onset < 5 years old) - Proximal muscle weakness (with ↑ CK, aldolase). Starts with lower extremity (ie hip-girdle), then progresses. - Cardiomyopathy - Scoliosis, bone fractures - Calf pseudohypertrophy, Gowers' sign	Dx: Genetic testing confirms. Muscle biopsy (with dystrophin stain) used in equivocal cases. Tx: - Prednisone for motor function - Multidisciplinary supportive care (physical therapy, nutritional, monitoring of cardiac/respiratory function)
Becker (BMD)	- X-linked dystrophin mutation (non-frameshift mutation) - Clinical: Similar presentation to DMD, but later onset (ie 10-15 years old), with milder disease course	- DMD: Poor prognosis (most die in 10-20's from respiratory failure or cardiomyopathy) - BMD: Improved prognosis compared to DMD
Myotonic	- AD inheritance of DMPK gene CTG trinucleotide repeat Clinical: (Presents in late teens/young adults) - Muscle weakness (skeletal and respiratory muscle) - Myotonia - Arrhythmias, balding, cataracts	Dx: Genetic testing Tx: No disease modifying therapies available. Supportive care only.
Limb-Girdle	- Group of AR or AD muscular dystrophy - Clinical: Weakness in the pelvic girdle and/or shoulder girdle - Bulbar/ocular muscle weakness typically mild or absent	Dx: Genetic testing. Biopsy if uncertain. Tx: Multidisciplinary supportive care
Facioscapulo-humeral	- AD (but frequently sporadic) mutation in DUX4 gene - Clinical: Onset generally as young adult. Asymmetric muscle weakness of face, scapula, upper arms, lower abdomen.	Dx: Genetic testing (alt: muscle biopsy, EMG) Tx: Multidisciplinary supportive care

NEUROMUSCULAR DISEASE

Neurology Medicine

Myasthenia Gravis

General: Autoimmune dysfunction of the neuromuscular junction, due to autoantibody formation against acetylcholine receptor

Clinical:
- Skeletal muscle weakness (worse with repeated activity)
    - Initially transient symptoms, eventually more frequent/severe
    - Preserved reflexes/sensory function
    - Can test clinically with bedside ice-pack test OR Edrophonium (Tensilon) infusion test. Both should improve muscle strength.
- Ocular symptoms (most common initial): Ptosis, diplopia
- Bulbar symptoms: Fatigue with chewing, dysphagia, and dysarthria
- Neck extensors and UE/LE also involved
- Exacerbated by certain drugs (Hydroxychloroquine, fluoroquinolone, aminoglycoside, beta-blockers)
- Myasthenic crisis: Respiratory distress due to resp muscle fatigue
- Thymoma (seen ~15% of MG cases, rule out with CT chest)

Diagnosis:
- Lab: AChR-Ab (alt: MuSK) autoantibodies (confirms diagnosis in someone with clinical symptoms, but not always present [seronegative disease])
- Electrophysiologic tests
    - Repetitive nerve stimulation (progressive decline in compound muscle action potential)

Management:

Acute Exacerbation	- Plasmapheresis/exchange and IVIG - Monitor vital capacity and maximum inspiratory pressure (if low, may require invasive ventilation)
Chronic	- Acetylcholinesterase inhibitors (Pyridostigmine) is first line - Most require chronic immunotherapy (ie glucocorticoids, Azathioprine, Mycophenolate, Cyclosporine) - Thymectomy: Indicated in those with thymoma, all patients < 60 y/o with MG

Lambert-Eaton Syndrome

General: NMJ disorder: Autoantibody against presynaptic voltage-gated Ca channels

Etiology: Most commonly associated with small-cell lung cancer

Clinical:
- Progressive, symmetric proximal muscle weakness (improves with activity)
- Autonomic (ED, dry mouth) and decreased reflexes
- Can develop ocular features, but not typically the presenting complaint

Diagnosis: VGCC antibody titers. Increase in compound muscle action potential (CMAP) with exercise or repetitive nerve stimulation.

Management: Pyridostigmine (alt: 3,4-diaminopyridine, Guanidine)
- IVIG/Prednisone if refractory

VENTRICULAR PATHOLOGY

Neurology Medicine

	General/Clinical	Management
Hydrocephalus	- Excessive CSF in the ventricles with subsequent dilatation and increased ICP Causes: - Obstructive (ie non-communicating): Neoplasm or cystic lesion, congenital obstruction of aqueduct/foramen of Monro (including genetic aqueductal stenosis, or malformation like Dandy-Walker) - Communicating (poor absorption from arachnoid): From intraventricular hemorrhage, scarring from meningoencephalitis, Chiari 2 or Dandy-Walker malformations Clinical: - ↑ ICP (headache, vomiting, papilledema, etc) - Irritability, behavioral changes, altered mental status - Focal deficits can develop if severe - In children: Increased head-circumference	Dx: CT/MRI (ventriculomegaly) Tx: Surgical correction in symptomatic patients (CSF shunt or endoscopic third ventriculostomy)
Normal-Pressure Hydrocephalus	- Enlarged ventricles but normal opening pressure on LP. Due to impaired CSF absorption. Clinical: - Cognitive impairment - Gait ataxia - Urinary incontinence	Dx: MRI (ventriculomegaly out of proportion with sulcal/cortical atrophy). Lumbar puncture (check pressure, improvement of symptoms after tap). Tx: Ventricular shunting
Hydrocephalus Ex-vacuo	- Cortical atrophy with enlarged ventricles (see in older people or those with dementia)	

Neuro26

DEMENTIA

Neurology Medicine

Neurocognitive Disorder

Disorder	Findings/Criteria
Normal Aging	- Slight but steady decreases in fluid intelligence (processing new information, problem solving, working memory, etc) - Word finding difficulties (expressive aphasia) - Sleep changes (advanced sleep-wake cycle)
Mild Neurocognitive Disorder	- Deficit in at least one cognitive domain that cannot be attributed to normal aging - Unlike dementia, function is primarily intact
Major Neurocognitive Disorder (Dementia)	- Significant decline in one or more cognitive domains (executive, learning/memory, language, attention, motor, social) - Requires assistance in IADL's or ADL's - Not caused by delirium or medical condition - MMSE is generally < 24/30

Differential Diagnosis for Dementia

<u>Delirium</u> (Waxing and waning cognitive changes, not chronic)
<u>Infections</u>
    - HIV dementia
    - Neurosyphilis
<u>Metabolic</u>
    - Hypothyroidism
    - B12 Deficiency
    - Thiamine deficiency (Wernicke's)
<u>Drugs</u>
    - EtOH abuse
    - Other drug abuse
<u>Pseudodementia</u> (depression)
<u>Chronic Traumatic Encephalopathy</u>

IADL/ADL

IADL	ADL
- Shopping - Cooking - Managing finances, meds - Telephone	- Bathing - Dressing - Feeding - Toileting - Transferring - Continence
- Higher-level activities that one must perform to remain independent - Often can receive aid from outside to remain independent	- Basic self-care activities that must be performed to stay self-sufficient

DEMENTIA — Neurology Medicine

		General/Clinical	Diagnosis/Management
Alzheimer's (AD)		- Most common cause of dementia. Almost exclusively presents > 65 y/o. - Early onset (< 60): Rare. Can be idiopathic or associated with genes: Presenilin 1,2, or APP (amyloid precursor protein) - Involves β-amyloid plaques and tau neurofibrillary tangles - Risk: ↑ Age, females, family history of dementia, APOE4 allele Clinical: - Generally starts with memory impairment - Progressive to other domains (ie executive, language, and visuospatial) - Neuropsychiatric/behavioral, motor symptoms late in disease	Dx: Clinical. MRI can show cortical/hippocampal atrophy Tx: Cholinesterase inhibitor (Donepezil, Galantamine, and Rivastigmine), Memantine in severe disease
Frontotemporal "Pick's Disease"		- Cause of early onset dementia (ie 50s-60s). Multiple subtypes based on the types of symptoms primarily involved. Pathophys: Involves tau, TDP-43. Clinical: - Behavioral Subtype: Disinhibition, loss of sympathy, increased apathy, compulsive behaviors, hyperorality (binge eating, putting things in mouth) - Aphasia Subtype: Progressive language disturbance (ie aphasia), with cognition intact	Dx: Clinical. MRI can show unilateral or bilateral frontal and temporal atrophy Tx: No disease modifying therapy. Treat psychiatric symptoms (SSRI, antipsychotics, etc).
Lewy Body		- 2nd MCC dementia. Seen > 65 y/o. Path shows cortical Lewy-Body formation. Clinical: Dementia (progressive cognitive decline) - Extreme cognitive fluctuations - Visual hallucinations, REM sleep-behavior disorder. - Parkinsonism develops after other symptoms	Dx: Clinical. MRI can show cortical atrophy (w/o significant hippocampal disease) Tx: Cholinesterase inhibitors, low-dose antipsychotics, Levodopa (for parkinsonism)
Vascular		- Due to combo of large/small artery infarcts & chronic vascular injury Clinical: (Often presents in stepwise fashion) - Executive dysfunction (memory mostly preserved, vs AD) - Focal cortical deficits (aphasia, neglect, etc) - Focal subcortical deficits (motor, gait, etc) - History of stroke	Dx: Clinical. MRI can show focal white matter lesions, with cortical and or subcortical infarcts Tx: Treat underlying vascular disease. Trial of cholinesterase inhibitor.

PRION DISEASE
Neurology Medicine

General: Neurodegenerative disease due to prions, which are abnormally conformed proteins. Once exposed, the abnormal protein induces conformational change in the host's normal PrP, which then forms a chain reaction, aggregates, and causes cell death.

Etiology: Most commonly spontaneous mutation, but can also be acquired or familial

Management: No effective therapies. Universally fatal.

Subtype	Features
Creutzfeldt-Jakob	- Pathophys: Spongiform change and accumulation of abnormal PrP Clinical - Rapidly progressive cognitive deterioration - Behavioral changes (depression, apathy, mood changes) - Myoclonus (startle) - Extrapyramidal signs (ataxia, nystagmus) or corticospinal (motor dysfunction) Diagnosis - MRI: Abnormal signal in putamen/caudate - EEG: Periodic, triphasic sharp "spike" wave complexes - CSF: 14-3-3 protein - Brain biopsy (definitive but rarely performed)
Bovine Spongiform Encephalopathy	- "Mad Cow Disease." Variant of Creutzfeldt-Jakob caused by ingestion of infected meat products.
Kuru	- Neurodegenerative prion disease seen in certain tribes in Papua New Guinea that practice cannibalism
Fatal Familial Insomnia	- Neurodegenerative disease from inherited or acquired PrP mutation - Presents with progressive mental status change, behavioral change, and insomnia

ALTERED MENTAL STATUS

Neurology / Medicine

Encephalopathy Overview

General: Defined as acute period of altered consciousness characterized by cognitive or perceptual dysfunction. Due to a medical condition and not underlying dementia.

Etiology:

CNS	- Seizures, encephalitis, meningitis
Organ Failure	- Cardiac failure/ACS - Hepatic encephalopathy - Pulmonary (hypoxemia/hypercarbia) - Renal (uremia)
Metabolic	- Electrolyte disturbances (K, Ca, Na) - Endocrine (ie thyroid, adrenal, etc) - Hypoglycemia, hyperglycemia
Infection	- Any, including UTI's (MCC in elderly)
Drugs	- Opiates, Benzodiazepines
Toxins	- EtOH, ethylene glycol, methanol, cyanide, carbon monoxide, other heroin, hallucinogens, drugs of abuse - Drug withdrawal
Nutritional	- B1 (Wernicke), B12 deficiency

Clinical:
- Acute deterioration in mental status (over hours to days)
- Fluctuating level of awareness. Frequently disoriented.
- Visual hallucinations (frequently present)
- Subtypes
    - Hyperactive: Agitation, mood lability, uncooperative
    - Hypoactive: Decreased psychomotor activity (drowsy/lethargic), slow, blunted responses.
    - Mixed (features of both)

Diagnosis:
- MMSE generally < 24/30
- Workup should include labs (electrolytes, glucose, CBC, urinalysis/culture)
    - Drug levels, tox screen, LFTs, ABG in appropriate circumstances
    - Vitamin B12, thiamine
- Neuroimaging/LP not required

Management:
- Treat underlying cause
- Protocols to prevent delirium
    - Orientation protocols (clocks, dates visible, etc)
    - Avoid physical restraints (use one-to-one sitter if necessary)
    - Avoid polypharmacy (especially benzos)
    - Frequent reorientation from familiar persons
    - Nonpharmacologic sleep aids
- Severe agitation or psychosis: Haloperidol or atypical antipsychotic

ALTERED MENTAL STATUS

Neurology Medicine

Coma

General: A state of unarousable unresponsiveness

Etiology: Variety of causes, including metabolic, drug/toxic, infections, and CNS lesions

Glasgow Coma Scale:

	Eye	Motor	Verbal
1	Does not open eyes	None	No verbal
2	Opens to pain	Decerebrate posture	Incomprehensible
3	Opens to voice	Decorticate posture	Inappropriate words
4	Opens spontaneously	Withdraws from pain	Confused
5		Localizes pain	Appropriate, oriented
6		Moves w/ command	

Diagnosis: Requires wide range of labs, neuroimaging (CT head), EEG, possible LP

Persistent Vegetative State

General: State of wakefulness without awareness (of environment, stimuli, etc). No response to visual, auditory, painful stimuli. Preserved reflexes/autonomic function.

Etiology: Can occur after severe anoxic brain injury

Brain Death

General: Irreversible loss of cortical and brainstem function. Legally equivalent to cardiopulmonary death in US.

Diagnosis: Algorithm below. If the patient does not meet the criteria for the following tests, ancillary tests (CTA/MRA, EEG, evoked potentials) may be performed.

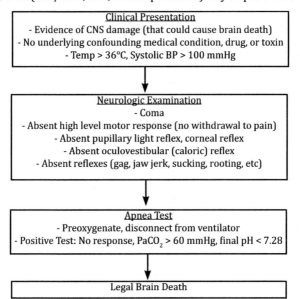

HEADACHE — Neurology Medicine

	General/Clinical	Diagnosis/Management
Tension	- Most common HA subtype. Due to heightened CNS pain pathways. - Precipitants: Mental tension and stress Clinical: - Generalized, usually bilateral aching headache of mild-to-moderate intensity - Often with tender muscles (post cervical, temporal, frontal, posterior neck muscles) - No other issues/normal neurologic examination - Can occur infrequently or be chronic (ie >15 days per month)	Dx: Clinical Tx: NSAIDs (Ibuprofen, Naproxen) first-line therapy. Caffeine can be added. If in-hospital: can try Ketorolac or Metoclopramide +/- Diphenhydramine PPX: TCA (Amitriptyline) only drug with established prophylactic evidence. Biofeedback or other therapies can also be helpful.
Migraine	- Pathophys: Cortical spreading depression with trigeminal activation - Risk: Female, family history - Triggers: Fasting, stress, menstruation, weather change, EtOH/wine Clinical: Episodic, passing through multiple phases - Prodrome: Depression, irritability, neck stiffness, tiredness - Aura: Visual (flashing lights, blurry/hazy lines in vision), sensory (paresthesias), or auditory (tinnitus) - HA: Generally unilateral, throbbing, pulsatile. Nausea, vomiting and photophobia are common.	Dx: Clinical. Neuroimaging not necessary unless atypical presentation/want to rule out other pathology. Tx: High-dose NSAIDs, triptans, IV Metoclopramide +/- Diphenhydramine. Glucocorticoids can be added if frequent exacerbations. PPX: General measures (good sleep/diet, regular exercise). Pharm (indicated if migraines impact QoL). See next page for options.
Cluster	- Rare. Seen primarily in men. Thought to be due to overactivation of trigeminal/hypothalamic pathway. Clinical: Severe, unilateral periorbital/temporal pain - Autonomic phenomena (rhinorrhea, congestion, ptosis, miosis, lacrimation, facial flushing, conjunctival injection) - Episodes are short (~15 min to 2 hours), and can occur multiple times per day, usually daily over a period of weeks with complete remission between "cluster" periods	Dx: Clinical. Head imaging to rule out other dangerous causes of headache. Tx: Inhaled O_2, Sumatriptan. PPX: Verapamil or Prednisone

HEADACHE

Neurology Medicine

Migraine PPX

General: Indicated in anyone that has impaired quality of life from migraines. All have equal efficacy, so pick based on possible treatment of comorbid conditions.

Agent	Comorbid Conditions Treated
Beta-blocker (Propranolol, Timolol)	- HTN, other heart diseases
Amitriptyline and Venlafaxine	- Depression, mood disorder, insomnia (Ami)
Valproate and Topiramate	- Epilepsy
Verapamil	- HTN, rate control

Differential Diagnosis for Headaches

"VOMIT"
- Vascular (subarachnoid hemorrhage, subdural hematoma, epidural hematoma, intraparenchymal hemorrhage, temporal arteritis)
- Other (malignant HTN, pseudotumor cerebri, post lumbar puncture)
- Meds (nitrates, chronic analgesic abuse)
- Infection (meningitis, encephalitis, cerebral abscess, sinusitis)
- Tumor

Red Flag Symptoms: Sudden onset, "worst ever," new onset without previous episode, increasing in severity and frequency over time, worse after lying down, mental status change, focal neurologic deficits, trauma, fever, stiff neck

Other Causes of Headache:

Medicine Rebound	- Due to excessive (> 3x per week) amounts of acute symptomatic medication use for chronic headaches - Tx: Abruptly stop medication
Paroxysmal Hemicrania	- Presents as 5-30 minute unilateral excruciating headaches in trigeminal distribution - Episodes happen multiple times throughout the day, occurring a couple of times per year with remission between - Tx: Indomethacin usually effective
Idiopathic Intracranial Hypertension (pseudotumor)	- Elevated pressure in the subarachnoid, possibly due to poor arachnoid reabsorption - Risk: Obese women of childbearing age, retinoids, Tetracycline - Clinical: Headaches, worse in mornings, associated with nausea, tinnitus (pulsatile) - Transient visual obscurations, papilledema, 6th nerve palsy - Dx: MRI (rule out causes of ↑ ICP). LP (elevated CSF pressure). - Tx: Acetazolamide (alt: Topiramate). LP/steroids can help acutely. If visual loss (despite therapy): Optic nerve sheath fenestration or CSF Shunt
Low Pressure	- Occurs post LP or rupture of arachnoid cyst - Orthostatic headache (better laying down, worse sitting up)

SYNCOPE
Neurology / Medicine

Overview and Approach to Syncope

General: Transient loss of consciousness due to inadequate cerebral blood flow

Etiology: See next page for differential diagnosis
- Important non-syncopal mimics of syncope: Seizures/pseudoseizures, sleep issues, mechanical falls (with subsequent LOC from head trauma)

Clinical:
- Transient loss of consciousness (usually for ~10 seconds)
- Can result in fall (ie loss of postural tone) or accident if driving
- Specific prodromal features specific to syncopal etiology (see next page)

Workup:
- History/physical is key
- Labs
- ECG
- ECHO if concerned for structural abnormality

Management: Risk stratification
- Low risk (ie clear vasovagal syncope, no red flags): Discharge home
- High risk (syncope during exercise, palpitations, abnormal ECG findings [VTach, sinus bradycardia, prolonged QT, heart block, bifascicular block])
  - Requires admission for further evaluation

SYNCOPE

Neurology Medicine

	General/Clinical	Management
Neurocardiogenic		
Vasovagal	- Increased parasympathetic outflow, resulting in transient bradycardia and hypotension - Triggers: Emotional stress, pain, fear, heat, prolonged standing - Clinical: Presents with prodrome of nausea, diaphoresis, pallor, nausea and overall feeling of unwellness, followed by syncope	Dx: Usually clinical. Tilt-table testing reserved for special circumstances. Tx: Reassurance. When prodromal symptoms, try counterpressure maneuvers or laying down.
Situational	- Syncope with one of the following situations: Cough/sneeze, urination, postprandial, swallowing, defecation - Carotid Sinus Syncope: Specific situational subtype from hypersensitive carotid sinus to stimulation. Significant drop in BP/HR with carotid massage.	Tx: Reassurance. Pacing may be requiring for carotid sinus syncope.
Orthostatic	- Can be primary autonomic failure, or secondary to chronic disease (ie diabetes), medication, or volume depletion - Clinical: Lightheadedness, dizziness upon standing, with syncopal episode upon standing or prolonged standing.	Tx: Fluids
Cardiogenic (arrhythmias)	- Includes bradycardia (sinus, heart-block, sick sinus) or ventricular arrhythmias (long QT, underlying heart disease, etc) - Clinical: Syncope often sudden (without prodrome) or with prodromal palpitations	Dx/Tx: ECG, cardiac monitoring, and inpatient workup essential
Cardiogenic (structural)	- Causes: Aortic stenosis, hypertrophic CM - Clinical: Generally presents during exertion	Dx: ECHO in addition to normal workup
Other	- Pulmonary embolism, subarachnoid hemorrhage	

VERTIGO

Neurology Medicine

	General/Clinical	Management
Vertigo (OVERVIEW)	- Transient feeling of spinning and dizziness (appears as if surrounding is spinning) - Can be peripheral (vestibular canal/CN VIII problem) or central (cerebellum or brainstem lesion)	Dx: Head thrust test (can help differentiate central from peripheral vertigo) Tx: Acute episodes can be treated with antihistamines, antiemetics, and benzodiazepines
Differential Diagnosis		
Benign Paroxysmal Positional Vertigo	- Due to canalithiasis (calcium debris) in semicircular canal - Clinical: Recurrent episodes of vertigo (< 1 min), often triggered by head movements	Dx: Dix-Hallpike maneuver (causes nystagmus) Tx: Particle repositioning (Epley) maneuver
Vestibular Neuritis (Labyrinthitis)	- Acute viral or postinflammatory CN VIII disorder - Clinical: Acute, single, episode of vertigo that is persistent and lasts for several days. Possibly associated with or following viral symptoms. Nausea, vomiting, and gait unsteadiness present.	Dx: Clinical Tx: Symptomatic care (antiemetics, antihistamines like meclizine), Corticosteroids.
Meniere's	- Due to increased endolymph/pressure Clinical - Episodic vertigo (often episodes last > 0.5 hours) - Hearing loss - Tinnitus/ear fullness	Dx: Clinical Tx: - Acute: Antihistamine (Meclizine) or Anticholinergic (Scopolamine), antiemetics - Chronic: Limit salt intake, caffeine, EtOH, diuretics (ie HCTZ). Surgical interventions (destructive procedure or endolymphatic sac surgery).
Migraine	- Migraine symptoms (ie HA, aura, etc) PLUS vertigo during episodes	Dx: Clinical Tx: Treat as migraine
Stroke	- Stroke in brainstem (vestibular nuclei) or cerebellum	

SEIZURES

Neurology
Medicine, Pediatrics

Overview of Seizures

General: Episode of abnormal activity caused by excessive, synchronous electrical activity in the cerebral cortex

Etiology:

Infants (< 6 M)	- Most commonly secondary to acute process (hypoxic-ischemic encephalopathy, intraventricular or other CNS hemorrhage, metabolic disturbances [hypoglycemia, hypocalcemia], CNS infection) - Rarely neonatal onset epilepsy syndrome
Children	- Febrile (usually 6 months to 5 y/o) - Epilepsy (variety of genetic and idiopathic subtypes)
Adults	- Stroke (ischemic/hemorrhagic, subarachnoid hemorrhage), subdural hematoma, anoxic brain injury - Infection (abscess, meningitis, encephalitis) - Brain mass or vascular malformation - Alcohol/Drug withdrawal - Drug intoxication - Electrolyte disturbances (HypoNa, HyperNa, HypoCa, Hypoglycemia) - Epilepsy (usually presents in childhood, but rare subtypes can present later in adulthood)

Clinical:
- Occur spontaneously and randomly
- First sign can be vocalization (cry): Pharyngeal muscles tighten
- Can maintain awareness (simple) or be without awareness (complex)
- Can have motor, sensory, and/or autonomic features
    - Tonic: ↑ tone
    - Atonic: Loss of tone, can drop if standing
    - Myoclonic: Muscle jerks
- Transient perioral cyanosis (most commonly in children)
- Tongue biting, incontinence, and self-injury are all classic signs
- Postictal state: May appear confused or disoriented after episode
- Todd's paralysis: Rare, focal weakness/paralysis post seizure, resolves over hours
- Status Epilepticus: > 5 minutes of continuous seizure activity or cluster of seizures without normal recovery in between

Diagnosis: Clinical diagnosis. Full workup to characterize seizure includes:
- MRI
- EEG

Neuro37

SEIZURES
Neurology
Medicine, Pediatrics

Management of Seizure

Active Seizure	- Most are self-limited (~ 2 minutes) - First aid: Protect bystanders, loosen tight clothing, nothing in mouth, place on side to avoid aspiration - Actively seizing: Can give benzo (ie IV Lorazepam, IM Midazolam, others)
Status epilepticus	- ABCs - IV Lorazepam - Fosphenytoin (or Phenytoin, Valproate, Levetiracetam) - Refractory: IV Midazolam, Propofol, or Pentobarbital

Chronic Prevention	- Pharm indicated if recurrent, unprovoked seizures
	- Drug choice is complex, without clear evidence of superiority of any specific drug. Side effects large consideration with selection.
	
	- Broad Spectrum Agents (for both generalized and focal):
	  - Levetiracetam, Lamotrigine, Topiramate, Valproate
	- Narrow Spectrum Agents (focal seizures)
	  - Carbamazepine, Oxcarbazepine, Phenytoin
	  - Ethosuximide (narrow spectrum, but for absence specifically)
	
	- Refractory cases: Epilepsy surgery, vagus nerve stimulation, ketogenic diet all possible options
	- Period of seizure free (generally 6-12 months) required before resume driving

Epilepsy Syndromes

Childhood Absence Epilepsy	- Syndrome of chronic, recurring absence seizures - Occurs in kids ~5-10 years old
Juvenile Myoclonic Epilepsy	- Presents in young teens - Myoclonic jerks, full tonic-clonic seizures, absence seizures - Occur early morning, after waking up
Benign Rolandic Epilepsy	- Occurs between 6-10 years old, often remitting after a few years - Focal seizures are characteristic, often starting in face and spreading to other body areas
Lennox-Gastaut	- Presents in children between 3-5 years old - Multiple seizure subtypes (tonic, atonic, myotonic, and atypical absence seizures) - Impaired development, intellectual disability

SEIZURES
Neurology — Medicine, Pediatrics

	General/Clinical	Management
Focal Seizures	- Originates from one hemisphere Clinical: - Motor Features: Movements/jerks in one part of body - Sensory Features: Paresthesias, auditory/visual symptoms	
Generalized Seizures (Previously Grand-mal)	- Originates focally, but spreads and involves both hemispheres Clinical: - Motor Features: Diffuse movements/jerks throughout body. Sensory, autonomic features also possible.	
Absence Seizures	- Common type of seizure in children - Presents with episodes of "spacing out", < 20 seconds, can recur multiple times per day - Automatisms (eyelid flickers, tongue smacking, etc), tone usually intact	Dx: EEG (3 Hz spike and wave pattern), provoked by hyperventilation Tx: Ethosuximide (alt: Valproate)
Febrile Seizures	- Occur between 6 months and 5 years old - Generally occur with viral or bacterial infection - Generalized tonic-clonic activity most common - Must not have prior history of epilepsy, or possible metabolic/infectious etiology Note: Children with febrile seizures are at risk for recurrent febrile seizures and have a ↑ risk for epilepsy	Dx: Clinical diagnosis. MRI, EEG, LP only required if atypical features (suspicion for meningitis, other serious pathology) Tx: IV Lorazepam if seizing for > 5 min. If back to baseline after, can reassure and send home. No evidence for antipyretics or antiepileptic medications.
Psychogenic Nonepileptic Seizures	- Clinically present like epileptic seizures, but no focal CNS changes are found on workup - Variety of subtle features can provide hints that episode is not true epileptic seizure (movements more variable, changing in type and magnitude over course of seizure, often more writhing, thrashing)	Dx: EEG (patient seizes, but no abnormal EEG activity) Tx: Patient/family education. Psychotherapy (CBT) and treat underlying psych disorders.

NEUROPATHY/NEUROPATHIC PAIN

Neurology Medicine

Overview

	Features	Etiology
Neuropathy		
Mononeuropathy	- Peripheral insult to one nerve, most commonly due to compression	- Carpal tunnel - Cubital tunnel - Meralgia paresthetica - Peroneal n. compression
Mononeuritis multiplex	- Multiple, single nerve abnormalities	- Vasculitis
Polyneuropathy	- Diffuse peripheral nerve disease	- Diabetes mellitus - GBS - EtOH, chemotherapy, heavy metals - Infections (HIV) - B12 deficiency
Radiculopathy	- Compression of nerve root, causing motor weakness, sensory loss, and/or episodic lancinating pains	- Disc herniation - Osteoarthritis - Spinal stenosis
Myelopathy	- Spinal cord compression causing neurologic dysfunction	- Trauma - Spinal stenosis

Management:
- Management for underlying condition is essential
- Pharm (for neuropathic pain)
    - Gabapentin/Pregabalin
    - TCA (Amitriptyline)
    - Topical Capsaicin or Lidocaine

Complex Regional Pain Syndrome

General: Previously named reflex sympathetic dystrophy. Disorder of extremity with pain and other neurologic abnormalities, that is disproportionate to any reported trauma or underlying pathology. Pathophysiology unknown, but thought to involve neurogenic inflammation and abnormal changes in CNS pain pathways.

Clinical: Limb pain, sensory/motor impairments, autonomic symptoms, atrophy
- Examples: Burning skin, muscle spasms, vasospasm, skin/nail changes, edema

Diagnosis: Clinical

Management:
- Patient education, PT/OT
- Pharm: NSAIDs, TCA, Gabapentin, topical Lidocaine
- Surgical interventions (nerve block, trigger point injections) lack evidence
- PPX: Vitamin C (after distal limb surgery/fracture)

NEUROPATHY

Neurology / Medicine

	General/Clinical	Management
Trigeminal Neuralgia	- Caused by compression of CN V nerve root (ie by artery, vein, tumor), or can be secondary to another condition (Herpes-Zoster, or demyelination seen with MS) - Clinical: Sudden, quick, severe, unilateral, paroxysmal episodes of shock-like pain in the distribution of CN V	Tx: Carbamazepine (alt: Oxcarbazepine)
Facial Nerve Palsy	- Paralysis of facial muscles due to CN VII lesion - Bell's Palsy (idiopathic facial palsy): Usually caused by reactivation of HSV or VZV - Non-idiopathic causes: Lyme disease, congenital, otitis media, HIV - Clinical: Acute onset unilateral facial paralysis. Associated with decreased lacrimation, hyperacusis, loss of taste sensation on the anterior $2/3$ tongue.	Tx: Self-limited (resolves within weeks to months). Prednisone. Treat infection if suspected (HSV with Valacyclovir, Lyme with antibiotics).
Ramsay Hunt (Herpes Zoster Oticus)	- Reactivation of VZV in multiple cranial nerves - Clinical: Triad of unilateral facial paralysis, vesicles in ear/ear canal, and ear pain	Tx: Typical VZV antiviral management
Post Herpetic Neuralgia	- Pain left in distribution of VZV reactivation (shingles)	Tx: Gabapentin, Pregabalin, TCA, or topical Capsaicin.
Drug-Induced Neuropathy	- Common agents: Vincristine/Vinblastine, Cisplatin, Paclitaxel - Clinical: Sensory neuropathy (stocking-glove distribution), rare motor involvement	

CNS INFECTIONS
Neurology
Medicine, Pediatrics

Etiology and Presentation of Meningitis

General: Inflammatory disease of the leptomeninges. Infectious agent often spreads via hematogenous spread, contiguous spread (sinusitis, otitis media, trauma, surgery), or retrograde transport up nerves.

Etiology	Organism
Bacterial Meningitis	
Neonates	- Group B *Streptococci*, gram-negatives (*E. Coli*), *Listeria*
Children	- *Neisseria meningitidis*, pneumococcus, *H. influenzae*
Adults	- *S. pneumoniae, N. meningitidis, H. influenza* - *Listeria* in elderly
Immunocomp.	- *Listeria*, gram-negative (*E. Coli*), pneumococcus
Trauma/Surg	- MRSA, *Staph epidermidis*, gram negatives
Aseptic	- Enterovirus (coxsackie, echo), HIV, HSV, mumps, VZV, West-Nile - Syphilis, Lyme
Other	- Tuberculosis, fungal (*Cryptococcus, Coccidioides*)

Clinical:
- Fever, nuchal rigidity, headache
- Lethargy, but intact sensorium (vs encephalitis)
- Other signs:
    - Seizure, focal deficits (occur in some)
    - Maculopapular rash (with meningococcus)
    - Kernig sign: Inability to extend knees with patient supine and hips flexed
    - Brudzinski sign: Leg flexion elicited by passive flexion of neck

Diagnosis: Lumbar puncture (CSF findings are diagnostic). Blood cultures should also be obtained.

Subtype	WBC	Diff	Protein	Gluc	Gram Stain
Normal	< 5	--	15-60	50-75 (66% serum)	--
Bacterial	> 1000	> 80% PMN	↑↑	↓	(+)
Viral (Aseptic)	5-500	> 50% L	↑	↔	--
Fungal	20-2000	> 50% L	↑	↔	--
TB	20-2000	> 80% L	↑	↓	(+) in some

- CT (Needed before LP?)
    - Previously performed to rule out ↑ ICP in fear of herniation
    - Usually not required. Only indicated if: History of mass lesion or stroke, new onset of seizure, papilledema, focal neurologic deficit, abnormal consciousness, or immunocompromised (ie HIV)

CNS INFECTIONS
Neurology
Medicine, Pediatrics

Management of Meningitis

General Principles:
- Empiric antibiotic therapy: Start immediately after LP is performed
  - Adjust once culture/sensitivity are resulted
- Steroids: Indicated in some (see below)
  - Has been shown to reduce complications in certain groups
- Contact PPX: For meningococcus (Rifampin or Ceftriaxone)

Type	Group	Antibiotic/Drug Regimen
Bacterial	Neonate (< 1 month)	- Ampicillin + Gentamicin +/- Cefotaxime
	Children (> 1 month)	- Vancomycin + Ceftriaxone (or Cefotaxime) - Dexamethasone (for HiB, controversial w/ *S. Pneumo*)
	Adults	- Vancomycin + Ceftriaxone (or Cefotaxime) - Add Ampicillin if > 50 y/o - Dexamethasone (if pneumococcus)
	Immunocomp	- Vancomycin + Ampicillin + Cefepime or Meropenem
	- Trauma - Surgery - Health-Care Acquired	- Vancomycin + Cefepime or Meropenem
Aseptic		- Observe - Consider Acyclovir if HSV suspected

Complications:
- Hearing loss (evaluate all children after for hearing loss)
- Seizures
- Intellectual disability
- Hydrocephalus

CNS INFECTIONS

Neurology Medicine

Encephalitis

General: Diffuse inflammation of the brain parenchyma

Etiology	Specific Findings
HSV-1	- Red cells in CSF - Temporal lesions/hemorrhage
West Nile	- Often associated with ascending flaccid paralysis - Must have appropriate location/timing of year
Mumps	- Associated with parotitis, lack of vax status
Other	- St Louis encephalitis virus - Eastern/Western equine encephalitis virus - California encephalitis viruses - EBV - HIV - Rabies

Clinical:
- Altered mental status (confused, agitated, or unresponsive)
- Seizures
- Focal deficits (cranial palsies, motor/sensory deficit)
- Meningismus and headache (in those with meningoencephalitis)

Diagnosis:
- LP (CSF cell count/gluc/protein, PCR for HSV, serology for west nile, others)
    - WBC < 250 (usually lymphocytes)
    - Protein mildly increased, glucose normal
- MRI (rule out mass, abscess, etc)

Management:
- Empiric acyclovir (for possible HSV)
- ICP management if appears elevated

CNS INFECTIONS
Neurology / Medicine

Brain Abscess

General: Focal collection of pus within the brain parenchyma. Usually due to contiguous spread (sinusitis, otitis, mastoiditis) or hematogenous spread (bacteremia).

Etiology:
- *Strep* viridans, other *Strep*
- *Staph aureus*, other *Staph*
- Gram negatives, anaerobes

Clinical:
- Headache, fever
- Focal neurologic deficits (cranial nerve defects, hemiparesis)
- Papilledema

Diagnosis:
- MRI (or CT): Ring-enhancing brain lesion
- LP (avoid due to increased risk of herniation)
- CT- guided aspiration

Management:
- Aspiration or surgical drainage
- Empiric antibiotics (Vancomycin + Ceftriaxone + Metronidazole)
- Glucocorticoids

CNS MALIGNANCIES

Neurology Medicine

Brain Malignancy

Etiology:
- Primary (see cancer subtypes on next two pages)
- Secondary (mets most commonly from lung, melanoma, breast cancer)
  - Most common cause of brain cancer in adults

Clinical:
- Can be asymptomatic or symptomatic
- Symptoms can progressive rapidly over weeks or slowly over time
- Headache (Early morning classic but rarely found)
  - Can be worse bending over/with valsalva (if ICP ↑)
- Focal neurologic deficits (weakness, sensory, aphasia, etc based on location)
- ↑ ICP (headache, vomiting, papilledema)
- Seizures

Diagnosis: MRI with contrast (best for visualization compared to CT)

Management: Specific therapies depend on tumor type (see next page)

Paraneoplastic Syndromes of CNS

Disorder	Features
Paraneoplastic Encephalomyelitis	- Autoantibody formation against CNS antigens. Can cause encephalitis, myelitis, or combination of both. - Common antigens include Hu (SCLC), Ma-2 (testicular), and CMPR-5 (SCLC, thymoma) - Clinical presentation varies based on location. Neuropsychiatric defects common (impaired cognition, psychosis, memory loss, etc).
Anti-NMDA Receptor Encephalitis	- Subtype of above, often associated with teratomas, but can also be idiopathic autoimmune condition - Clinical: Psychiatric disturbance, memory deficits, seizures, dyskinesias, autonomic instability, language dysfunction - Dx: CSF finding of anti-NMDA IgG - Tx: Corticosteroids, IVIG, tumor resection
Opsoclonus-Myoclonus Ataxia Syndrome	- "Dancing eyes, dancing feet" - Occurs most commonly with neuroblastoma (in children) and SCLC (adults), but can be idiopathic or occur with other tumor - Clinical: Ataxia, myoclonus, opsoclonus (multi-directional rapid eye movements)
Paraneoplastic Cerebellar Degeneration	- Associated with SCLC, Hodgkin lymphoma, breast cancer - Antibodies against Hu, Yo, Tr antigens in Purkinje cells - Clinical: Gait instability, dizziness, nausea, vomiting

CNS MALIGNANCIES

Neurology / Medicine

	General/Clinical	Management
Metastasis	- Most common brain malignancy in adults - Clinical: Focal deficits, cognitive dysfunction, and headache all possible. Must work up for brain mets in any cancer patient presenting with neurologic symptoms.	Dx: MRI (multifocal lesions, most commonly occur at gray-white junction) Tx: Single lesion (surgical removal, stereotactic radiosurgery), or multiple lesions (whole brain radiation). Glucocorticoids (reduce edema/ICP).
Glioblastoma Multiforme	- High grade glioma, with poor prognosis - Clinical features: Develop rapidly over days to weeks	Dx: MRI (classic butterfly appearance with central necrosis). Histologic confirmation (with surgery). Tx: Surgical resection. Neoadjuvant radiation therapy and Temozolomide.
Meningioma	- Derived from meninges and located along dura - Risk: Radiation, NF2 - Clinical: Often asymptomatic, but can cause focal findings where compression occurs, seizures	Dx: MRI (extra-axial, dural based mass, with tail) Tx: Surgical resection. Radiation therapy (if not resectable or high risk for recurrence based on histo).
Vestibular Schwannoma	- Also known as acoustic neuroma, Schwann cell tumors derived from CN VIII, occuring at cerebellopontine angle - Clinical: Presents with loss of hearing, tinnitus, and vertigo. Can compress other cranial nerves (ie CN V, VII).	Dx: MRI Tx: Surgical resection or radiation therapy
Oligodendroglioma	- Rare, slow growing glioma - Associated with IDH mutation, deletion of chromosome 1p and 19q - Clinical: Slow, progressive symptoms over years	Dx: MRI. Histologic confirmation. Tx: Surgical resection, radiation, chemo

CNS MALIGNANCIES

Neurology
Medicine, Pediatrics

	General/Clinical	Management
Pilocytic Astrocytoma	- Well-differentiated, low grade, glioma - Posterior fossa tumor, with cystic +/- solid components	Dx: MRI. Confirm with histology. Tx: Surgical resection (can achieve cure due to well circumscribed nature)
Medulloblastoma	- Most common childhood brain tumor - Clinical: Cerebellar dysfunction, ↑ ICP (headache, vomiting, altered mental status, papilledema) - Can metastasize inferiorly to spinal leptomeninges	Tx: Surgery + Chemoradiation
Ependymoma	- Glial tumor of ependymal lining of ventricles	Tx: Surgery + Radiation
Craniopharyngioma	- Most common childhood supratentorial tumor, but also seen in adults - Tumor derived from ectodermal remnants of Rathke's pouch - Clinical: Headache, visual symptoms (bitemporal hemianopsia), endocrine changes (hyperprolactinemia, diabetes insipidus, or panhypopituitarism)	Dx: MRI (calcified, solid or cystic masses in the suprasellar area) Tx: Surgical resection +/- radiation therapy
Pinealoma	- Germ cell tumor arising from pineal gland - Presents with ↑ ICP and hydrocephalus - Parinaud syndrome: Vertical gaze palsy, eyelid retraction, diplopia, pupils do not react to light - Can produce β-hCG (causing precocious puberty)	Tx: Radiation therapy
Brain Stem Glioma	- Can be low grade (focal brainstem glioma) or high-grade (diffuse intrinsic pontine glioma, which has poor prognosis)	Tx: Surgery + Chemoradiation

Neuro48

AUDITORY PATHOLOGY

Neurology Medicine

Etiology of Hearing Loss

	Conductive	Sensorineural
Path	- Caused by lesions in the outer or middle ear, which interfere with mechanical conduction	- Due to lesions in the cochlea or CN VIII (inner ear)
Clin	- Worse with low frequency	- Worse with high frequency OR intensity - Poor sound discrimination - Possible tinnitus
Cause	External Ear - External otitis - Cerumen - Exostoses (bony outgrowths in auditory canal) Middle Ear - Otitis media - Cholesteatoma - Otosclerosis - Tympanic membrane perforation	Inner Ear - Hereditary/congenital hearing loss - Presbycusis - Noise-induced hearing loss - Ototoxic drugs - Meniere - Acoustic neuroma - Multiple sclerosis - CVA - Complication of CNS infection (ie meningitis, neurosyphilis) - Sudden sensorineural hearing loss

Evaluation of Hearing Loss

(1) Clinical Evaluation
   - Whispered voice test, or tone-emitting otoscopes
   - External auditory canal exam (rule out cerumen, external otitis, etc)
   - Rinne/Weber Test (differentiates conductive vs sensorineural hearing loss)

	Rinne	Weber
Normal	Air > Bone	Equal both ears
Conductive	Bone > Air in affected ear	Lateralizes to affected ear
Sensorineural	Air > Bone	Lateralized to unaffected ear
Mixed	Bone > Air in affected ear	Lateralized to unaffected ear

(2) Audiologic testing (for all that do not have obvious cause of hearing loss)
(3) MRI (or CT) for asymmetric disease

HEARING LOSS — Neurology Medicine

	General/Clinical	Management
Conductive		
Cerumen Impaction	- Ear wax can accumulate and obstruct, due to cerumen overproduction or tortuous/narrow ear canal	Tx: Mineral oil or hydrogen peroxide, irrigation, mechanical removal (only remove if patient symptomatic)
Cholesteatoma	- Growth of desquamated squamous epithelium debris in the middle ear - Can be primary (from negative pressure retraction pocket) or secondary (perforation from trauma or chronic inflammation) - Present with hearing loss and ear drainage. Possible pearly mass behind tympanic membrane.	Dx: Clinical. MRI/CT can aid in ruling out cranial involvement. Tx: Surgical (tympanomastoidectomy)
Otosclerosis	- Bony overgrowth of the stapes, resulting in mechanical failure of sound conduction in the inner ear	Tx: Hearing aids or surgical correction (stapedectomy plus prosthesis)
Sensorineural		
Presbycusis	- Age-related hearing loss (from generalized damage to cochlea or other inner ear structures) - Presents with gradual, progressive symmetric hearing loss, difficulty with high pitches and voice discrimination	Tx: Hearing aids
Noise-Induced	- Chronic exposure to sounds > 85 dB	
Ototoxicity	- Aminoglycosides and Cisplatin most commonly implicated - Aspirin, Quinine, Chloroquine, loop diuretics other causes	
Sudden Sensorineural Hearing Loss	- Acute, unilateral, hearing loss, due to idiopathic, autoimmune, or viral etiology	Dx: MRI, Audiology used to rule out other disorders. Tx: Steroids. Generally regain hearing in a week.

OPHTHALMOLOGY

Eyelid Pathology

	General/Clinical	Management
Hordeolum (stye)	- Small abscess of the eyelid (most commonly *Staph aureus*) - Presents as small, painful, erythematous swelling, either externally at eyelid margin, or internally on conjunctiva	Dx: Clinical Tx: Self-limited. Warm compress. I&D if persistent.
Chalazion	- Chronic granulomatous infection of meibomian gland - Presents as painless, localized eyelid nodule or swelling on inner eyelid (less painful, red, and angry compared to styes)	Dx: Clinical Tx: Self-limited. Persistent lesions: I&D or steroid injection.
Xanthelasma	- Cholesterol-filled yellow plaques associated with hypercholesterolemia	Dx: Cholesterol panel Tx: Intervention not required
Dacryocystitis	- Infection of lacrimal sac from nasolacrimal duct obstruction - Pain, erythema, swelling over the medial canthus	Dx: Clinical Tx: Oral antibiotics
Dacryostenosis	- Obstructed lacrimal duct. Common congenital abnormality in children. - Presents with chronic, excessive tearing, debris in eyelids. Possible swelling in medial eye.	Dx: Clinical Tx: Self-limited in most cases. Can perform lacrimal sac massage. Surgical probing for refractory cases.
Blepharitis	- Inflammation of the eyelids, most commonly occurring near eyelid margin - Present with erythematous, swollen, itchy eyelids. Possible associated symptoms include blurry vision, excessive tearing, gritty sensation, flaking/scaling.	Dx: Clinical Tx: Eyelid massage, warm compress, and washing. Topical antibiotics for severe or refractory cases.

OPHTHALMOLOGY

	General/Clinical	Management
Conjunctival Disorders		
Conjunctivitis		
Bacterial	- Erythema, thick mucoid discharge, most often unilateral. Eye often stuck shut in morning (common conjunctivitis feature). - *Staph aureus*, pneumococcus, *H. influenzae*, most common	- Erythromycin ointment or Trimethoprim/Polymyxin drops
Viral	- Erythema, mucoid/serous discharge, itching/burning/gritty sensation, most often bilateral - Can occur as part of viral syndrome (ie URI). Adenovirus most common.	- Self-limited. Fake tears, antihistamines.
Allergic	- Bilateral erythema, watery discharge, and itching - History of atopy (ie atopic dermatitis, asthma, etc)	- Avoid allergens. Cool compress/fake tears. - Acute: Topical antihistamine/vasoconstrictor (ie Naphazoline/Pheniramine) - Chronic: Antihistamine/Mast cell stabilizer (Olopatadine, Azelastine)
Trachoma	- MCC blindness in world. Infection with *Chlamydia trachomatis*. - Active trachoma causes mild conjunctival inflammation - Repeated episodes can lead to cicatricial disease, in which chronic eyelid inflammation and scarring turns lids inwards (entropion), ingrown eyelashes (trichiasis), and eventual blindness	Dx: Clinical. Culture/PCR for chlamydia if unsure. Tx: Antibiotics (Azithromycin, Tetracycline). Surgery for trichiasis.
Subconjunctival Hemorrhage	- Can be idiopathic or occur with trauma/eye contact - Presents as focal collection of blood between conjunctiva and sclera	Tx: Self-limited (resolve in a few weeks)
Dry Eye	- Also referred to as keratoconjunctivitis sicca - Decreased tear production or excessive tear evaporation - Presents with chronic dry eye, irritation, burning	Tx: Artificial tears

OPHTHALMOLOGY

Sclera Disorders

	General/Clinical	Management
Scleritis	- Acute inflammation of the sclera. Potentially blinding. - Often associated with RA or vasculitis (ie Wegener's) - Presents with ocular redness, severe pain (worse with eye movements), eye watering, possible visual impairment	Dx: Clinical/slit-lamp examination Tx: NSAIDs. Prednisone + Rituximab for severe cases.
Episcleritis	- Inflammation of the episclera. Benign and self-limited. - Usually idiopathic, can be associated with rheumatologic condition - Presents with focal erythema/injection, vasodilation of the episcleral vessels, possible irritation, but no visual loss	Tx: Self-limited. Topical lubricants.

Lens Disorders

	General/Clinical	Management
Cataracts (adult)	- Opacification of the lens (present in 50% over 75) - Risk: ↑ Age, smoking, EtOH, light exposure, diabetes, steroids - Presents with decreasing visual acuity (especially in the dark, with glare around bright lights) - Myopic shift: Increased refractive power of the lens, causing nearsightedness	Dx: Clinical (slit-lamp exam) Tx: Surgical extraction/artificial lens replacement
Presbyopia	- Loss of normal accommodating power of lens, occurring with ↑ age - Presents with difficulty reading close, fine print	Tx: Reading glasses
Refractive Errors	- Myopia (nearsightedness) - Hyperopia (farsightedness) - Astigmatism (abnormal corneal shape)	Dx: Snellen chart (worse than 20/25) Tx: Glasses, contact lenses, or refractive surgery (Lasik)

OPHTHALMOLOGY

Corneal Disorders

	General/Clinical	Management
Corneal Abrasion	- Corneal insult from direct trauma, foreign bodies, contact lens - Presents with severe eye pain (CN V) - Foreign body sensation in eye, irritation - Photophobia, refusal to open eye	Dx: Fluorescein examination. Rule out retained foreign body with careful exam under eyelid. Tx: Usually improve within 2-3 days. Topical antibiotic prophylaxis (Erythromycin, Ciprofloxacin), Oral or topical NSAIDs for analgesia.
Keratitis	- Inflammation of the cornea, with bacterial, viral, fungal causes - Often associated with contact lens use (especially with bad hygiene, overuse of single-use lens, etc). Also dry eyes, topical corticosteroid use. - Presents with corneal infiltrate +/- mucopurulent discharge - Red eye, photophobia, foreign body sensation	Dx: Penlight exam (infiltrate appears like small white spot, stains (+) with fluorescein) Tx: See specific etiology below
Bacterial Keratitis	- *Staph aureus, Pseudomonas* most commonly	Tx: Topical antibiotics
Viral Keratitis	- Most commonly HSV - Corneal lesion is classically described as dendritic (forms from initial vesicular lesions)	Tx: Oral or topical antivirals
Amebic Keratitis	- *Acanthamoeba* infection almost always associated with poor contact lens hygiene - Can rapidly lead to vision loss if not treated	Tx: Topical antiparasitic agents (Polyhexamethylene Biguanide, Hexamidine, etc)

< OPHTHALMOLOGY | Neurology Medicine >

Glaucoma (Chronic)

General: Increased IOP leading to damage to optic neuropathy and irreversible vision loss (peripheral vision, followed by central)

	Open Angle	Closed Angle
Path	- ↑ Aqueous humor production or ↓ outflow	- Narrowing of the anterior chamber angle, ↓ aqueous humor outflow
Risk	- ↑ Age, family history, black	- Primary: ↑ Age, family history, hyperopia - Secondary: Fibrosis, inflammation, mass, or neovascularization
Clin	- Asymptomatic - Progressive peripheral visual field loss with eventual "tunnel vision," followed by central vision loss	- Can present with acute blockage (see below) OR chronic, asymptomatic process (like open angle) with progressive peripheral visual field loss
Dx	- Fundus examination (cupping) - Tonometry. ↑ IOP (> 25 mmHg) is consistent with glaucoma, but not diagnostic - Gonioscopy (diagnostic for closed-angle, allows for visualization of angle)	
Tx	- First line therapy: Pharm and surgery equal efficacy **Pharm** - Prostaglandins (Latanoprost, Bimatoprost), beta-blockers (Timolol) - Others (less frequently): CA inhibitors, alpha-agonists, cholinergic agonists **Surgery:** Trabeculoplasty	- Surgery: Laser peripheral iridotomy is definitive treatment Note: Treat/remove underlying cause if secondary to another process

Drug	Class/Mechanism	Side Effects
Timolol	β-blocker	- Generally well-tolerated
Bimatoprost Latanoprost	Prostaglandins	- Heterochromia, ↑ eyelash length - Conjunctival hyperemia
Acetazolamide	Carbonic Anhydrase Inh.	
Pilocarpine Physostigmine	Cholinomimetics	- Miosis (if chronic use)
Epinephrine Brimonidine	α-agonist	- Ocular hyperemia, blurred vision, discomfort - Mydriasis

Acute Angle Closure Glaucoma

Clinical:
- Decreased visual acuity, abnormal halo around light
- Headache/severe eye pain, possibly associated with nausea and vomiting
- Conjunctival erythema, dilated pupils

Management:
- Emergent therapy/ophtho referral
- Topical beta-blocker (Timolol), alpha-agonist (Brimonidine, Apraclonidine), miotic agents (Pilocarpine)
- Acetazolamide or Mannitol

<OPHTHALMOLOGY | Neurology Medicine>

Sudden Visual Loss

	General/Clinical	Management
Central Retinal Artery Occlusion	- Similar etiology to CVA (atherosclerosis, embolic, etc) - Presents with acute, painless single sided visual loss - Poor prognosis, often leads to permanent visual loss	Dx: Clinical plus fundoscopy (pale retina whitening with cherry red spot) Tx: Ocular massage, anterior chamber paracentesis, reduce intraocular pressure
Central Retinal Vein Occlusion	- Thrombotic occlusion of retinal veins, with resulting ischemia - Risks: Coagulopathy, hyperviscosity, atherosclerosis - Presents with acute/subacute progressive loss of visual acuity (less sudden than arterial). Can be asymptomatic.	Dx: Fundoscopy (Disc swelling, venous dilation, hemorrhages, cotton wool spots) Tx: Observation. anti-VEGF injections for macular edema, laser treatment for neovascularization.
Retinal Detachment	- Separation of the neurosensory retina from the retinal pigment epithelium, leading to ischemia and vision loss - Often evolves from underlying posterior vitreous detachment or retinal tears - Risk: Eye trauma, diabetes mellitus, myopia - Presents with floaters/flashes of light, which can progress to peripheral vision loss ("curtain over visual field")	Dx: Fundoscopy (retinal breaks/abnormalities, grey elevated retina, pigmented cells in vitreous) Tx: Laser retinopexy or cryoretinopexy
Vitreous Hemorrhage	- Leakage of blood into vitreous humor of the eye - Associated with retinal tears, trauma and child abuse - Presents with impaired vision, floaters, and light flashes	Dx: Fundoscopy (retina obscured by floating cells in vitreous) Tx: Elevated head, allow hemorrhage to settle. Treat underlying cause (ie tear, detachment).

OPHTHALMOLOGY

Retinal Disorders

	General/Clinical	Management
Diabetic Retinopathy	- Associated with DM1 and DM2 Classification - Nonproliferative: Microaneurysms, hemorrhages, exudates, and cotton wool spots - Proliferative: Neovascularization (can lead to vitreous hemorrhage and/or retinal detachment) - Generally asymptomatic until late stage	Dx: Fundoscopy (screen diabetics yearly) Tx: - Glycemic control (Hgb A1C < 7%), BP control - Proliferative: Photocoagulation or anti-VEGF
Hypertensive Retinopathy	- Refers to retinal changes directly associated with chronic HTN - Arterial wall thickening, AV nicking, flame hemorrhage, exudate, cotton-wool spots, optic disc edema/papilledema	Dx: Fundoscopy Tx: Manage underlying hypertension
Macular Degeneration	- Most common cause of blindness in developed countries Classification - Dry: Atrophy and degeneration of the central retina, drusen deposition - Wet: Leakage of serous fluid/blood with neovascularization - Risk: ↑ Age, smoking, EtOH use, family history - Presents with central vision loss, scotomas, metamorphopsia	Dx: Fundoscopy (areas of retinal atrophy, depigmentation, drusen). Edema, hemorrhage, and neovascularization in wet MD. Tx: - Dry: Supportive. eye vitamins, quit smoking - Wet: anti-VEGF injections
CMV Retinitis	- Reactivation of latent CMV, with full thickness inflammation of the retina - Common disease in AIDS with CD4 < 50 - Presents with loss of central vision, scotoma/floaters	Dx: Fundoscopy (fluffy retinal lesions, hemorrhage) Tx: Ganciclovir (either oral or intravitreal), proper ART therapy
Retinitis Pigmentosa	- Inherited progressive retinal degeneration - Presents with night blindness, peripheral visual field loss - Ophthalmoscopy: Pigment deposits, pale optic nerve	Dx: Clinical, plus advanced retina testing

< OPHTHALMOLOGY   Neurology / Medicine >

Uveitis

General: Intraocular inflammation

Etiology: Systemic inflammatory condition, viral (HSV, VZV), parasite (toxoplasmosis)

	Anterior	Posterior
Path	Anterior chamber inflammation, including: - Iritis - Iridocyclitis	Inflammation posterior to lens, including: - Vitritis - Pars planitis - Chorioretinitis
Clin	- Red eye, pain, photophobia, possible decreasing visual acuity	- Presents with decreased visual acuity, painless
Dx	- Clinical (history + slit lamp) - Leukocyte/protein accumulation in anterior chamber	- Clinical (history + slit lamp) - Chorioretinal inflammation, leukocytes in vitreous humor
Tx	- Topical glucocorticoids	- Intraocular glucocorticoids

Associated Conditions:
- Sympathetic Ophthalmia: Anterior uveitis that occurs ~ 1 year after penetrating trauma to other eye (believed due to systemic antigen exposure/AI response)

- Acute Retinal Necrosis: Reactivation of HSV, HZV or other virus seen in severe immunocompromised states. Presents with prodrome of keratoconjunctivitis, then progresses to bilateral necrotizing retinitis. Clinical diagnosis (ophthalmoscopy shows retinal/vitreal inflammation, retinal vascular arteriolitis). Treat with Acyclovir/Valacyclovir.

Endophthalmitis

General: Infection within eye, including vitreous/aqueous humor

Etiology: Post-surgery, penetrating eye trauma, keratitis

Clinical: Presents with eye pain, decreased visual acuity, conjunctival injection, hypopyon (WBCs in anterior chamber)

Management: Vitrectomy. Intravitreal antibiotics.

OPHTHALMOLOGY

Misc. Eye Disorders

	General/Clinical	Management
Globe Rupture	- Can be caused by blunt trauma or penetrating trauma - Presents with eye deformity and volume loss. Possible findings include eccentric pupil, pupillary defects, decreased visual acuity.	Dx: Clinical. CT is used to better characterize. Tx: Prophylactic antibiotics, tetanus. Avoid increasing eye pressure (no pressure on eye). Primary surgical closure is definitive.
Optic Neuritis	- Acute inflammatory demyelination of optic nerve - Associated with MS, NMO, etc - Presents with monocular vision loss. Possible color desaturation or pupillary defect. - Possible optic nerve inflammation or atrophy on exam	Dx: MRI Tx: High-dose steroids

OPHTHALMOLOGY — Neurology Medicine

Eye Movement Disorders

Lesion	Features
CN III	- Parasympathetic (external nerve fibers): Subject to compression. Causes pupillary dilation with abnormal light reflex. - Motor (internal nerve fibers): Damaged from vascular disease (ie diabetes mellitus). Causes down/out gaze, ptosis, diplopia.
CN IV	- Innervates superior oblique muscle - Presents as vertical/oblique diplopia, worse with downward gaze. Patients often head tilt toward side of lesion. Worsening misalignment (eye moves upward) with adduction of eye.
CN VI	- Impaired abduction on side of lesion
Internuclear Ophthalmoplegia	- Lesion in medial longitudinal fasciculus (normally coordinates CN VI/CN III movements) - Lesions cause conjugate horizontal gaze palsy - Example (right MLF): With leftward gaze, left eye abducts with nystagmus, right eye has impaired adduction (does not move past midline)
Frontal Eye Field Lesions	- Lesions in the frontal eye field result in eyes deviated towards the side of the lesion

OPHTHALMOLOGY — Neurology / Pediatrics

Pediatric Eye Disorders

	General/Clinical	Management
Cataracts	- Can be idiopathic, or associated with trauma, glucocorticoid use, or congenital infections/disorders - Presents with asymmetric red reflex, leukocoria, photophobia, decreased visual acuity	Dx: Clinical (slit-lamp exam) Tx: Surgical extraction/artificial lens replacement
Dacryostenosis	- Due to congenital nasolacrimal duct obstruction - Presents with persistent tearing and discharge	Dx: Clinical Tx: Lacrimal sac massage, observation (self-limited)
Amblyopia ("Lazy Eye")	- Decreased visual acuity from abnormal visual development, due to strabismus, refractive errors, or other structural eye issues	Dx: Routine screening < 5 y/o (fixation testing for preverbal, visual acuity if verbal) Tx: Treat underlying condition. Encourage use of lazy eye (patch/Atropine drops for other eye).
Strabismus	- Abnormal ocular alignment - Primary (idiopathic) or secondary to acquired ocular or CNS diseases - Definitions: Esotropia (nasal), exotropia (temporal), hypertropia (upward), and hypotropia (downward) - Presents with asymmetry of red or corneal light reflexes, possible head tilt, abnormal cover-uncover test - Amblyopia can develop if not treated	Tx: < 4 months: Watchful waiting - Occlusion therapy (patch good eye) OR penalization therapy (cycloplegic drops in good eye) - Eyeglasses (to correct refractive errors) - Surgery if refractory
Retinopathy of Prematurity	- Overproliferation of retinal blood vessels from excess O_2 exposure (seen in premature, low birth weight babies) - Common cause of childhood blindness	Dx: Retinal examination Tx: Monitor mild disease, laser coagulation and VEGF inhibitors for severe disease
Retinoblastoma	- Most common childhood ocular malignancy - Can be heritable (germline RB1 mutation) or sporadic - Presents with leukocoria, strabismus	Dx: Retinal exam, plus ocular US/MRI Tx: Laser or cryotherapy, +/- local/systemic chemotherapy

CONGENITAL NEUROLOGIC DEFECTS
Neurology — Medicine, Pediatrics

Disorder	Features
Neural Tube Defects Risk Factors: Folate deficiency/antagonists, neuroleptic drugs (Valproate, Phenytoin)	
Spina bifida occulta	- Failure of fusion of the vertebral bodies, without herniation of spinal cord - Can range from being asymptomatic to causing neurologic dysfunction, including weakness and autonomic symptoms - Can have skin abnormalities (ie dimple, tuft of hair) overlying lesion - Tx: Surgery if any neurologic dysfunction
Meningocele	- Meninges (but no neural tissue) herniate through bony defect. Rare. - Usually asymptomatic - Surgically repair, with good prognosis
Meningomyelocele	- Meninges and neural tissue herniate through bony defect - Often associated with severe neurologic deficits (paralysis below the level of lesion, bladder dysfunction), Chiari II malformation, hydrocephalus, other defects in neuronal migration - ↑ AFP on prenatal screening, confirmed with US - Surgically repair (emergently)
Anencephaly	- Malformation of anterior neural tube, resulting in abnormal forebrain, open calvarium - ↑ AFP on prenatal screening, confirmed with US - Not compatible with life
Holoprosencephaly	- Failure of separation of the left and right hemispheres - Often associated with other midline defects, such as cleft lip, midface cleft and cyclopia - Severe defects not compatible with life
Encephalocele	- Skull/dural defect, with herniation of meninges +/- brain - Can be surgically corrected
Posterior Fossa Malformations	
Chiari I	- Ectopic, downwardly displaced cerebellar tonsillar - Manifests with headaches, ataxia (especially with cough, valsalva), during childhood
Chiari II	- Herniation of cerebellar vermis through foramen magnum - Associated with myelomeningocele - Causes hydrocephalus and hind brain dysfunction (paralysis below the level of the lesion)
Dandy-Walker	- Agenesis of cerebellar vermis with cystic enlargement of 4th ventricle - Associated with non-communicating hydrocephalus, spina bifida

NEUROCUTANEOUS DISORDERS

Neurology · Medicine, Pediatrics

	General	Clinical	Management
Neurofibromatosis (von Recklinghausen)	- AD NF1 mutation on chromosome 17	- Café-au-lait macules - Axillary freckling - Lisch nodules (iris hamartomas) - Neurofibromas - Other: Optic glioma, long bone dysplasia, pheochromocytoma	Dx: Clinical + Genetic testing Tx: Careful medical supervision with treatment of complications
Neurofibromatosis 2	- AD NF2 mutation on chromosome 22 (Merlin tumor suppressor gene)	- Bilateral acoustic schwannomas - Tumors (meningiomas, spinal tumors) - Neuropathy, cataracts, skin lesions	
Tuberous Sclerosis	- AD TSC1/2 gene mutations, most often sporadic	- Derm: Ash-leaf spots (hypopigmented patches), Shagreen patches (thick orange peel skin), Angiofibromas - CNS: Glioneuronal hamartomas ("Tubers") and subependymal nodules, epilepsy, intellectual disability - CV: Cardiac rhabdomyoma - Renal: Angiomyolipoma	Dx: Clinical + Genetic testing Tx: Antiepileptics, screening brain MRI
Sturge Weber	- Sporadic mosaic mutations in GNAQ gene	- Port wine stain (facial capillary malformation) - Ipsilateral leptomeningeal cavernous angioma (can cause seizures) - Glaucoma, heterochromia of iris, vascular malformations in the eye - Intellectual disability	Dx: Clinical, plus MRI with contrast to determine extent of CNS disease Tx: Medically manage complications

CEREBRAL PALSY

Neurology / Pediatrics

General: Abnormal fetal CNS development, resulting in nonprogressive and permanent motor dysfunction

Risk: Prematurity, low birth weight, congenital abnormalities, multiple gestation, IUGR, placental pathology, intrauterine infection, perinatal hypoxic-ischemic injury

Clinical:

Subtype	Risk	Clinical Features
Spastic Diplegia	- Preterm - PVL	- Lower extremities usually affected - Spasticity, UMN signs, muscle contractures
Spastic Hemiplegia	- Neonate stroke - Congenital CNS maldevelopment	- Unilateral arm/leg involvement - Spasticity, UMN signs, muscle contractures
Spastic Quadriplegia	- SGA/Preterm - Variety of global brain abnormalities	- Entire body - Spasticity, UMN signs, muscle contractures
Dyskinesia (athetoid)	- Kernicterus - Hypoxemic-ischemic	- Hypotonia, reduced purposeful movements - Development of involuntary movements - Choreiform, athetoid, and dystonic movements all possible
Ataxic	- Cerebellar hypoplasia	- Hypotonia, poor coordination, ataxia

Common comorbids: Intellectual disability, epilepsy, behavioral disorder, visual/hearing defects, orthopedic problems (hip subluxation, scoliosis)

Diagnosis: Clinical (combination of symptoms, plus characteristic MRI findings)

Management:
- Physical/occupational/speech therapy
- Spasticity: Botulinum toxin, antispasmodics (ie Baclofen), surgical (selective dorsal rhizotomy)
- Preventative: Magnesium (in moms at risk of premature birth), delayed cord clamping, proper neonatal supportive care

NEURO PHARM — Neurology Medicine

	Mechanism	Indication	Side Effects/Management
GABA Targeting Antiepileptics			
Barbiturates Phenobarbital Pentobarbital Thiopental	- GABA potentiator (↑ duration of action)	- Seizures (Acute, Status) - Anesthesia - Alcohol withdrawal	- Respiratory and CNS depression - CYP 450 Induction
Benzodiazepines Diazepam Lorazepam Midazolam Chlordiazepoxide Alprazolam	- GABA potentiator (↑ frequency of opening)	- Seizures (Acute, Status) - Alcohol withdrawal - Anxiety - Spasticity - Insomnia	- Respiratory and CNS depression - Tolerance over time (limits usefulness chronically) - Dependence/withdrawal - Overdose can be reversed with Flumazenil
Tiagabine	- ↑ GABA concentration and activity	- Narrow-spectrum antiepileptic	
Vigabatrin			- Visual field loss
Ca²⁺ Channel Blocking Antiepileptics			
Ethosuximide	- Blocks T-type Ca²⁺ channels	- Absence seizure	- GI Upset - Drowsiness
Na⁺ Channel Blocking Antiepileptics			
Phenytoin Fosphenytoin	- Blocks Na⁺ channels	- Status epilepticus - Narrow-spectrum antiepileptic	- Gingival hypertrophy - ↑ body hair - Rash/SJS/DRESS (HLA-B*1502, most commonly Asian) - Neuro: Confusion, blurry vision, ataxia with long term use - ↓ Folate/megaloblastic anemia - Teratogen/fetal hydantoin syndrome - CYP450 induction/↓ vitamin D/osteopenia

NEURO PHARM

Neurology Pharm

	Mechanism	Indication	Side Effects/Management
Na⁺ Channel Blocking Antiepileptics (continued)			
Carbamazepine Oxcarbazepine	- Blocks Na⁺ channels	- Narrow-spectrum antiepileptic	- Hyponatremia/SIADH - Myelosuppression - Hepatotoxicity - Sedation/ataxia/diplopia - SJS (HLA-B*1502, most commonly Asian) - CYP450 Induction
Lacosamide	- Blocks Na⁺ channels	- Narrow-spectrum antiepileptic	- Well-tolerated
Lamotrigine	- Blocks Na⁺ channels	- Broad-spectrum antiepileptic	- SJS
Misc. Antiepileptics Drugs			
Gabapentin	- GABA analog, but acts mainly inhibiting Ca²⁺ channels	- Narrow-spectrum antiepileptic - Neuropathic pain - Used off label for EtOH use disorder, fibromyalgia, hot flashes, etc	- Sedation - Dizziness, ataxia, weight gain - Toxicity worse with worsening renal failure
Levetiracetam	- Unclear mechanism	- Broad-spectrum antiepileptic	- Well-tolerated (possible fatigue/somnolence/depression)
Topiramate	- Blocks Na⁺ channels, ↑ GABA activity, blocks NMDA receptors	- Broad-spectrum antiepileptic	- Weight loss - Impaired cognition/mood issues/somnolence - Inhibits carbonic anhydrase (metabolic acidosis, nephrolithiasis)
Valproate	- Blocks Na⁺ channels, ↑ GABA concentration	- Broad-spectrum antiepileptic	- GI Disturbances - Weight gain/metabolic syndrome - Thrombocytopenia - Hepatotoxicity - Teratogen

NEURO PHARM — Neurology Pharm

Anti-Parkinson Drugs

	Mechanism	Indication	Side Effects/Management
Levodopa-Carbidopa	- L-Dopa crosses BBB, converted to dopamine in CNS - Carbidopa inhibits peripheral breakdown of L-Dopa	- Parkinson's disease	- Dopaminergic stimulation: Confusion, hallucinations, psychosis, orthostatic hypotension, nausea - "Wearing-Off Effect": Motor fluctuations, dyskinesias that develop years after beginning levodopa (unclear if drug related, or part of natural progression of disease)
Pramipexole Raniperole	- Dopamine agonist	- Parkinson's disease - Restless leg syndrome	- Similar dopaminergic stimulation side effects as Levodopa
Entacapone Tolcapone	- COMT Inhibitors (prevents peripheral L-Dopa breakdown)	- Parkinson's disease (L-dopa adjunct only, no effect on own)	- Similar dopaminergic stimulation side effects as Levodopa
Selegiline	- MAO-B Inhibitors (prevents dopamine breakdown)	- Parkinson's disease (only modest efficacy)	- Similar dopaminergic stimulation side effects as Levodopa - Rare risk for serotonin syndrome
Amantadine	- ↑ synaptic dopamine availability	- Parkinson's disease (mainly used early in mild disease)	- Livedo reticularis - Lower extremity edema
Benztropine Trihexyphenidyl	- Anticholinergic agents	- Parkinson's disease (mainly tremor)	- Typical anticholinergic side effects (confusion, dry mouth, urinary retention, blurry vision, etc)

ALS Drugs

	Mechanism	Indication	Side Effects/Management
Riluzole	- ↓ glutamate-induced excitotoxicity	- ALS	

Huntington Drugs

	Mechanism	Indication	Side Effects/Management
Tetrabenazine	- Inhibits dopamine packaging into vesicles	- Huntington (for chorea)	- Akathisia, parkinsonism

NEURO PHARM

Neurology Medicine

	Mechanism	Indication	Side Effects/Management
Dementia			
Memantine	- NMDA antagonist	- Dementia	
Donepezil Galantamine Rivastigmine	- Acetylcholinesterase inhibitor		- Nausea, vomiting, diarrhea
Misc Neurologic Agents			
Sumatriptan	- 5-HT1B/1D agonist	- Migraine abortant	- Coronary vasospasm and myocardial ischemia - Paresthesias
Dantrolene	- Binds RY-R, ↓ Ca release from SR in skeletal muscle	- Malignant hyperthermia	
Baclofen	- GABA-B agonist at spinal cord	- Muscle relaxant	- Drowsiness, dizziness - Withdrawal syndrome (similar to benzo/alcohol)
Zolpidem Zaleplon Eszopiclone	- Acts on BZ1 subtype GABA receptor	- Insomnia	- Headaches - ↓ cognitive functioning (possibly lasting into next day) - Tolerance/dependence over time (though less risk compared to benzos)

ADULT PREVENTATIVE CARE — Primary Care/Emergency Medicine

	Male	Female
Screening (Note: The following are for average risk adults unless noted. For high-risk conditions, refer to specific sections for screening intervals)		
HTN	- Optimal screening not known, but typically performed every visit	
HLD	- 1x screen between 17-21 - Lipid screens once > 35 (> 25 for high risk individuals)	- 1x screen between 17-21 - Lipid screens once > 45 (> 35 for high risk individuals)
DM	- Screen those with HTN, HLD, or 40-70 y/o and BMI > 25	
Osteoporosis	- DEXA screen in clinical signs of low bone density, fracture history, or fracture risk factors	- DEXA scan all > 65, < 65 if risk factors (ie elevated FRAX) - q5 years if T-score > -1
Colon Ca	- 50-75 y/o - Methodology and risk determines interval [See: GI]	
Prostate Ca	- PSA screening (> 50 y/o) is an individual decision (discuss pros/cons with patient)	
Lung Ca	- Annual low dose CT scan - Indications: 55-74 y/o, 30 pack-year history, and either current smoker or quit within last 15 years	
Breast Ca		- Mammography, starting at age 40-50 (societies vary on age), with q2 yr repeat testing
Cervical Ca		- 21-29 y/o: Pap smear (q3 yr) - > 30 y/o: Pap smear (q3 yr) OR Pap + HPV (q5 yr)
STD	- Chlamydia/Gonorrhea (all sexually active women < 25 and all male and females > 25 with risk factors) - HIV: One time between 13-75 years old. Annual screening for high risk individuals.	
Hep B	- Screening reserved for high risk individuals (risks include IV drug use, high risk sexual activity, MSM, inmates, history of liver disease, close contact of Hep B patient, individuals born in endemic areas)	
Hep C	- One time screen for those born between 1945 and 1965	
Abd Aortic Aneurysm	- One time between 65-75 in smokers OR first-degree family history of AAA	
Other Preventative Care		
Aspirin (daily low dose)	- Highly controversial, but overall evidence lacking for use of aspirin for primary prevention of cardiovascular events given elevated bleeding risk - Should be considered in those with significantly elevated cardiovascular risk scores	

ADULT PREVENTATIVE CARE — Primary Care/Emergency Medicine

Vaccine	General Indications	Special Considerations
Influenza	- All patients, yearly	
Tdap/Td	- Booster q10 years (at least 1x should be Tdap)	
Varicella	- All (without documented evidence of immunity)	- Contraindicated for pregnant women and severe immunodeficiency
Zoster	- All > 50 y/o - Note: Historically, only live vax (ZVL) was available, but now new recombinant vax (RZV) is available and preferred (but 2 dose series required)	- ZVL (Contraindicated for pregnant women and adults with severe immunodeficiency)
HPV	- Recommended all < 26 y/o	- Now approved up until age 45

PCV13
PPSV23
	> 65: PCV13 1x (if no prior dose)
	    PPSV23 (1 year after PCV 13, and repeat dose 5 years later)
	
	19-64: PPSV23 1x if at intermediate risk (smokers, chronic heart disease, COPD, DM, alcohol abuse, or chronic liver disease)
	    Note: Revaccinate at age 65 (assuming > 5 years since first dose)
	
	19-64: PCV13 and PPSV23 if high risk (asplenia, immunocompromised, CSF leak, cochlear implant, advanced CKD)
	    Note: PCV13 first, followed by PPSV23 8 weeks later
	    Revaccinate PPSV 5 years later + once > 65 years old	

Men-ACWY Men-B	- 11-18 y/o (recommended for all) - 16-23 y/o (suggested for all)	- Used outside age range for those at increased risk, including: travel to endemic area, military, microbiologist working with meningococcus, asplenia, complement deficiency, eculizumab use, or recent epidemic in area of living
Hep A	Patients that want protection (personal preference)	- High risk individuals (travel to endemic area, MSM, IV drug use, chronic liver disease, etc)
Hep B	Patients that want protection (personal preference)	- High risk individuals (liver disease, mucosal/percutaneous exposure risk, HIV, sexual exposure risk, etc)

True Contraindications: Previous anaphylactic reaction, anaphylaxis to egg (for egg prepared live vaccines, like MMR, yellow fever), immunocompromised/pregnant (no live vaccine), household of immunocompromised (no oral polio)

False Contraindications: Mild illness, convalescent phase of an illness, recent exposure to communicable disease, breastfeeding, current antibiotic use

SMOKING — Primary Care/Emergency Medicine

Smoking

General: Smoking is the leading preventable cause of mortality. Increases risk for:
- Cardiovascular Disease (#1 reversible risk factor)
  - Atherosclerosis (CAD, stroke)
- Pulm (COPD)
- Malignancy (lung, esophageal, pancreatic, genitourinary)
- Peptic ulcer disease
- Osteoporosis
- OB-GYN (placental insufficiency)

Clinical:
- Nicotine Withdrawal
  - Increased appetite/weight gain
  - Irritability, anxiety, or depression
  - Insomnia
  - Poor concentration, restlessness

Smoking Cessation: Behavioral intervention + pharm is first line

Drug	Mechanism	Side Effects/Contraindications
Varenicline	- Partial agonist of α4β2 (of nicotinic Ach receptor)	- Nausea - Sleep disturbance (insomnia, atypical dreams) * No issue with increased suicidality
Nicotine Replacement	- Long acting patch + short acting gum/lozenge	- Irritation at site of drug - Headache, nausea possible
Bupropion	- ↑ NE and D release	- Increases seizure risk - Headache, dry mouth, insomnia common

Hospitalized Patients:
- Nicotine replacement (usually patch + short term breakthrough)

OBESITY

Primary Care/Emergency Medicine

Obesity

Class	BMI Range
Underweight	< 18.5 kg/m²
Normal weight	≥ 18.5 to 24.9 kg/m²
Overweight	≥ 25.0 to 29.9 kg/m²
Obese	≥ 30 kg/m²
Severely obese	≥ 40 kg/m²

Increases Risk For:
- Type II DM, metabolic syndrome
- CAD
- HTN, HLD
- OSA

Evaluation:
- BMI should be calculated at each visit
- Waist circumference
    - ≥ 40" in men and ≥ 35" in women → ↑ Cardiometabolic risk
- Should screen for obesity related comorbid conditions

Management:
- Behavior Modification and Counseling (first line)
    - Diet (most important) and exercise
- Pharmacotherapy (if BMI > 30 and failed behavior modification)

Drug	Mechanism	Side Effects
Orlistat	- Inhibits fat absorption through lipase inhibition	- GI (flatulence, cramps, steatorrhea)
Liraglutide	- GLP-1 analog, often used in diabetics	- Nausea, vomiting - ↑ risk pancreatitis
Lorcaserin	- Serotonin 2C-R agonist	
Phentermine-Topiramate	- Stimulant (↑ NE)	- Dry mouth, constipation - Avoid in those with cardiovascular disease
Bupropion-Naltrexone	- ↑ NE/D (unclear how naltrexone modulates/if it is effective)	- Avoid in those with cardiovascular disease

- Bariatric Surgery
    - Indicated if BMI > 40 or > 35 + comorbidity

GERIATRICS — Primary Care/Emergency Medicine

Normal Aging

System	Normal Findings
CNS	- Minor forgetfulness, word finding difficulty, and memory loss - Functional loss not normal - Decreased brain weight, enlarged ventricles/sulci - Impaired vision and hearing
Pulmonary	- ↓ Alveolar surface area (increased dead space) - Decreased lung compliance
Renal	- ↓ Creatinine clearance
Heme	- ↓ Bone marrow reserves (increased risk for cytopenias) - ↑ Risk for clotting
MSK	- Decreased muscle, increased fat - Increased fracture risk
Sleep	- ↓ REM latency and total REM - Decreased total sleep - Advanced sleep cycle - Increased frequency of nocturnal awakenings

VITAMINS/MINERALS — Primary Care/Emergency Medicine

Vitamin	Overdose	Deficiency
A	- Caused by excessive supplements or dietary source (liver of certain wild animals) - Acute: Nausea/vomiting, vertigo, blurry vision - Chronic: Alopecia, dry skin, hepatic toxicity, arthralgias, pseudotumor - Severe teratogen	- Xerophthalmia (dry conjunctiva, keratomalacia, Bitot spots [abnormal areas of corneal keratinization]) - Night blindness (nyctalopia) - Abnormal bone development - Derm (hyperkeratosis)
D	- Due to inappropriate use of vitamin D supplements - Symptoms are that of hypercalcemia (confusion, polyuria, polydipsia, nausea, vomiting, weakness)	- Rickets (children) - Osteomalacia (adults)
E	- Can increase bleeding risk	- Hemolytic anemia - Acanthocytosis - Neuromuscular (spinocerebellar tract demyelination, manifesting with ataxia, weakness)
K	- Not known	- Increased bleeding risk (manifests as easy bruisability, mucosal bleeding, melena, hematuria, etc)

| VITAMINS/MINERALS | Primary Care/Emergency Medicine |

Vitamin	Deficiency
B1 (Thiamine)	Risk: Alcoholism Clinical: Beriberi: Rare. Wet (high output heart failure). Dry (peripheral neuropathy). Wernicke-Korsakoff - Wernicke: Triad of confusion, ophthalmoplegia, and ataxia - Korsakoff: Irreversible memory loss
B2 (Riboflavin)	Risk: Rare Clinical: Stomatitis, glossitis, cheilosis, corneal vascularization
B3 (Niacin)	Risk: Developing countries (corn dependent), carcinoid tumors, isoniazid toxicity, Hartnup syndrome Clinical: Pellagra - Dermatitis (blistering rash in sun-exposed skin) - Diarrhea - Dementia (MS change, depression, poor concentration, etc)
B6 (Pyridoxine)	Risk: Isoniazid (inactivates B6) Clinical: Stomatitis, glossitis, cheilosis, CNS (confusion, depression), peripheral neuropathy, anemia *Can cause toxicity with massive intake (neuropathy)
B7 (Biotin)	Risk: Rare. Occurs with large consumption of raw egg whites. Clinical: Dermatitis, alopecia, conjunctivitis, altered mental status
B9 (Folate) B12	[See: Heme/Onc]
C	"Scurvy" - Hemorrhages/hemarthrosis/skin petechiae (bone and gums) - Gingivitis - Poor wound healing - Periosteal hemorrhage - Corkscrew hairs

< VITAMINS/MINERALS >   < Primary Care/Emergency Medicine >

Mineral Deficiency

Mineral	Deficiency
Chromium	- Decreased sensitivity to insulin
Copper	- Brittle hair - Skin depigmentation - Osteoporosis - Sideroblastic anemia - Peripheral neuropathy
Selenium	- Cardiomyopathy - Muscle dysfunction - Immune dysfunction
Zinc	- Alopecia - Impaired wound healing - Rash (pustules in perioral region) - Dysgeusia, anosmia - Hypogonadism * Can be caused by Acrodermatitis enteropathica (AR genetic disorder, causing decrease in Zn gut absorption)

Severe Malnutrition

Marasmus	- Complete energy (protein + nonprotein) deficient state - Very thin, from loss of protein/body fat
Kwashiorkor	- Pure protein deficient state (seen in parts of world where people live off starches) - Generalized edema, abdominal distension, skin hypo/hyperpigmentation, and thin/sparse hair

TOXICOLOGY			Primary Care/Emergency Medicine, Pediatrics
	General	**Clinical**	**Management**
Carbon Monoxide	- Binds hemoglobin, left-shifting oxyhemoglobin curve - Risk: Smoke, fuel-burning devices with poor ventilation, poorly functioning furnace	- Mild: Headache, nausea, dizziness, malaise - Severe: Altered mental status, seizure, coma, cardiac ischemia Dx: ABG with co-oximetry	- 100% O_2 - Mechanical ventilation/hyperbaric O_2 if severe
Methemoglobinemia	- Exposure to oxidizing substance (turns Fe^{2+} to Fe^{3+}), which has poor affinity for O_2 - Risks: Dapsone, topical anesthetics, NO, other sulfa/nitrite drugs	- Cyanosis, dark blood - Nonspecific symptoms (HA, dyspnea, fatigue, etc) Dx: Co-oximetry	- IV Methylene blue
Cyanide	- Inhibits electron transport chain Risk: - Fires - Industrial exposure - Iatrogenic (ie nitroprusside)	- Flushing ("cherry red") - CV: Arrhythmia, bradycardia/hypotension - Pulm: Respiratory depression - CNS: Confusion, coma, seizure - Lactic acidosis *Bright red blood/lacks cyanosis (high oxyhemoglobin concentration)	- Supportive care - Decontamination (depending on type of exposure) - Hydroxocobalamin + Sodium thiosulfate - Nitrites are alternative therapy
Organophosphates	- Cholinesterase inhibitors - Risk: Insecticides, "nerve gas" (ie Sarin). Exposure can be cutaneous, ingestion, inhalation.	Excessive cholinergic activity: - Bradycardia, miosis - Lacrimation, salivation - Bronchospasm, excess secretions - Diarrhea/vomiting	- Atropine, Pralidoxime - Intubation, 100% O_2 * Avoid Succinylcholine

TOXICOLOGY

Primary Care/Emergency Medicine, Pediatrics

	General	Clinical	Management
Arsenic	- Binds to sulfhydryl groups, affecting cellular respiration - Risk: Pesticides, pressure treated wood, contaminated well water	- Acute: GI (watery diarrhea, vomiting, pain), garlic breath, QT prolongation - Chronic: Hypo/hyperpigmentation of skin, hyperkeratosis, sensory/motor neuropathy, ↑ Ca risk (skin/bladder)	- Supportive - Decontamination - BAL chelation
Iron	- Damages via free radicals and lipid peroxidation - Risk: Ingestion of iron supplements	- GI: Pain, bleeding, hematemesis/melena - Hypotensive shock/metabolic acidosis - Radiopaque pills on XR - After initial episode: GI obstruction, hepatic toxicity	- IV Deferoxamine - Gastric lavage/bowel irrigation (if pills on xray)
Salicylate	- COX inhibitor, increases respiratory drive, interferes with cell metabolism - Risk: ASA overdose	- Tinnitus, vomiting, dizziness, altered mental status - Mixed respiratory alkalosis/metabolic acidosis	- Sodium bicarbonate - Supportive care
Ricin	- Ribosome inhibitor - Found in castor beans, potential agent of terror	- Inhalation → Respiratory distress/pulm edema - Ingestion → GI bleeding/inflammation	- Supportive - Decontamination (skin, or GI via charcoal/lavage)
Seafood Toxins			
Tetrodotoxin	- Pufferfish - Binds Na channels	- Nausea, diarrhea, paraesthesia, paralysis	- Supportive
Ciguatoxin	- Reef fish (barracuda, snapper) - Opens Na channels	- Cholinergic poisoning symptoms (nausea, vomiting, abdominal pain, paresthesia, etc)	- Supportive
Histamine (scombroid)	- Dark meat fish (tuna, mahi-mahi) - Bacterial histidine decarboxylase forms histamine	- Anaphylaxis like symptoms - Burning, flushing, erythema, diarrhea	- Diphenhydramine - Epi/Albuterol for anaphylaxis-like symptoms

PC/EM10

TOXICOLOGY
Primary Care/Emergency Medicine, Pediatrics

Acetaminophen Overdose

General: Metabolized to NAPQI by CYP system, forms toxic free radicals, damaging DNA, proteins, and lipid membranes

Risk: Overdose usually > 150 mg/kg for kids or > 7.5 g in adults

Clinical: Acute hepatic failure (AST and ALT > 1000, ↑ INR/PT)
- Hypovolemia, jaundice, renal failure all possible

Diagnosis: Serum Acetaminophen concentration

Management:
- If within 4 hours: Activated charcoal
- N-acetylcysteine (either IV or oral protocols available). Indicated if:
    - Acetaminophen level > 10 ug/mL at any point in time
    - Above line on Rumack-Matthew Nomogram
    - Evidence of liver injury
    - High-risk liver condition

Alcohol Toxicity

Type	Source	Clinical	Management
Ethanol	- EtOH beverages	- CNS depression/inebriation	- Supportive
Isopropyl	- Rubbing Alcohol - Antifreeze - Solvent	- CNS depression - Ketonemia (Acetone) with normal AG	- Supportive
Methanol	- Moonshine - Solvents	- Metabolized to formic acid - CNS depression - Visual changes (scotoma, blurry vision) due to retinal toxicity - AG metabolic acidosis	- Fomepizole - Sodium bicarb - Hemodialysis (if end organ damage, high alcohol levels)
Ethylene Glycol	- Antifreeze	- Renal: AKI, oxalate stones - CNS depression - AG metabolic acidosis	

*Note: All the above present with elevated osmolar gap, but only methanol and ethylene glycol cause significant elevation in the anion gap

INGESTIONS
Primary Care/Emergency Medicine, Pediatrics

Caustic Esophageal Injury

General: Ingestion of alkali or acidic material, causing mucosal damage
- Alkali (ie ammonia, NaOH): Liquefactive necrosis, usually more damage to esophagus, buffered by stomach
- Acid: Coagulation necrosis. Causing pain immediately in oropharynx, often limiting ingestion. Causes more gastric damage.

Clinical: Varied. Can cause oropharyngeal, chest, or abdominal pain, dysphagia, odynophagia, vomiting.

Diagnosis: Upper GI endoscopy within 24 hours to determine extent of injury
- Contraindicated if signs of hemodynamic instability/surgical complication

Management:
- Supportive care
- Contraindicated: Emetics, NG tubes, neutralizing agents, NG lavage/charcoal
- Surgery if complicated by peritonitis, mediastinitis, etc

Complications:
- Strictures, perforation, ↑ cancer risk

Foreign Body Ingestion

General: Objects most commonly become stuck in esophagus/stomach. Often asymptomatic, unless complete obstruction (causes dysphagia, impaired swallowing of secretions, etc).

Object	Features	Management
Coins	- Most often in stomach and pass without problem	- Most pass spontaneously - Remove if in esophagus > 24 hr
Flat Battery	- Can conduct electricity across esophagus, causing necrosis	- Urgent removal (if in esophagus)
Sharps/Bones	- High perforation risk	- Urgent removal
Magnets	- Multiple magnets can attract across bowel layers, causing necrosis, obstruction, etc	- Urgent removal (if multiple)
Food Impaction	- Often in adults with esophageal strictures	- Emergent removal if complete obstruction (otherwise within 24 hr)

Diagnosis: Multiple view plain XR

Management: Flexible endoscope is preferred method for removal. In general, if not a high risk object, can observe for 24 hours for spontaneous passage into lower GI tract, then follow with serial radiographs
- Note: Any signs of obstruction or complications is indication for removal
- If any object is stuck in esophagus for > 24 hours, removal is indicated
- Once any object passes beyond proximal duodenum, follow with serial radiographs and monitor for any symptoms of complications

HEAT ILLNESS — Primary Care/Emergency Medicine

General: Group of disorders caused by the failure of thermoregulation, most commonly in extreme heat/humidity

Risk: Exercise during hot/humid weather, dehydration, poor physical fitness

Disorder	Features	Management
Heat Cramp	- Exercise-induced muscle cramps	- Rehydrate, stretch
Heat Syncope	- Syncope associated with physical activity in high temperature areas	- Cool, rehydrate
Heat Exhaustion	- Inadequate cardiac output secondary to heat, which results in inability to continue exercising - Temperature usually > 101°F - No neurologic dysfunction or end organ damage	- Remove from play, remove excess clothing - Cool patient (cold water or evaporative therapy) - Rehydration
Heat Injury	- Temp > 104°F with end-organ damage (but no CNS dysfunction) - Often complicated by DIC, ARDS, organ failures	- Remove from play, remove excess clothing - Cool patient (cold water or evaporative therapy) - Rehydration - Hospital level supportive care
Exertional Heat Stroke	- Temp > 104°F, CNS dysfunction, and end-organ damage	- Rapid cooling (ice-water immersion) - Fluid and electrolyte repletion - Supportive care for organ dysfunction
Non-exertional Heat Stroke	- Temp >> 104°F, CNS dysfunction, and end-organ damage - Seen in elderly, with chronic medical conditions that can impair thermoregulation	- Supportive (ABC's, intubation if necessary) - Rapid cooling (evaporative)

COLD — Primary Care/Emergency Medicine

Hypothermia

General: Core temperature < 35° C

Risk: Outdoor extreme cold, water submersion, EtOH abuse, sepsis, hypothyroidism, elderly

Class	Temp (C)	Clinical Findings
Mild	32-35°	- Shivering, tachycardia, tachypnea, ataxia, dysarthria
Moderate	28-32°	- CNS depression, bradycardia, hypoventilation, loss of shivering reflex
Severe	< 28°	- Hemodynamic instability, severe CNS depression (ie coma), ventricular arrhythmias/asystole

Management:

Class	Management
Mild	- Supportive care (ABC's, intubate if necessary) - Warmed IV crystalloid - Remove wet clothing, passive external warming (ie blankets)
Moderate	- Above, plus: Active external warming (warm blankets, heating pads)
Severe	- Above, plus: Active internal warming if refractory to above options (warmed pleural/peritoneal fluids)

Frostbite

General: Freezing and subsequent necrosis of tissue. Frequently occurs in distal extremities, ears, nose, and other parts of face. Other types of cold injury include:
- Frostnip: Completely reversible paresthesias due to cold exposure
- Pernio (chilblains): Painful, erythematous lesions from repetitive damp cold exposure
- Trench foot: Seen from consistent exposure of feet to wet/cold conditions. Results erythematous, painful, edematous foot.

Risk: Cold wind exposure, or conductive loss through cold water/metal

Clinical:
- Coldness, paresthesias
- Superficial pallor with hard/waxy texture
- Eventual development of bullae, eschar formation

Diagnosis: Clinical. Bone scan (Tc-99) can help determine extent of injury/prognosis.

Management:
- External rewarming (warm water), analgesia, wound care
- tPA/Heparin (due to frequent clotting in affected tissues)
- IV Iloprost for severe injury

DROWNING/LIGHTNING — Primary Care/Emergency Medicine

Drowning

General: Aspiration of water, causing pulmonary edema/laryngospasm, pulmonary edema, with eventual hypoxemia

Management:
- Immediate: Rescue breaths, followed by CPR (if breaths fail)
- Airway: Often requires supplemental O_2/intubation
- Supportive care (manage hypothermia, end organ damage, etc)

Electrical Injuries

General: Electrical current through tissues, causing various degrees of thermal injury

Etiology:
- Electrical (work related in adults, accidental in children)
- Lightning (DC current. Extremely high voltage. Severe, frequently fatal.)
- Stun guns/tasers (may cause minor superficial injury, but severe organ injury is rare)
    - No medical care necessary if < 15 sec of stun gun discharge

Clinical: If severe, findings include
- Burns (severity of internal burns may not be apparent on the skin)
- Cardiac (arrhythmias, asystole [DC] and ventricular fibrillation [AC])
- CNS: Altered mental status, neuropathy, autonomic failure, etc
- Renal: Rhabdomyolysis
- MSK: Bone necrosis, dislocations, compartment syndrome

Management:
- CPR (if necessary), trauma evaluation, etc
- Supportive care
- Burn management

BITES

Primary Care/Emergency Medicine

Type	Features	Management
Spider		
Black Widow	- Muscle pains/spasms - Localized diaphoresis - Abdominal pain, autonomic hyperactivity	- Wound care, tetanus, analgesia - Benzodiazepines - Antivenom if severe
Brown Recluse	- Bite site develops erythema, with possible necrosis/ulceration over next few days	- Wound care, tetanus, analgesia - Debridement if severe
Snake		
Coral	- "Red on yellow, kill a fellow" - Neurotoxin causes muscle weakness/paralysis (anti-ACH at NMJ) - Possible respiratory failure	- Antivenom - Atropine + Neostigmine - Intubation (if necessary)
Crotalinae	- Rattlesnake, copperhead, or water moccasin - Causes local tissue damage/edema - Can be complicated by rhabdo, coagulopathy	- FabAV
Other		
Scorpion	- Pain, swelling at sting site - Certain subtypes cause autonomic or neuromuscular toxicity	- Wound care, tetanus, analgesia - Antivenom for neurologic

BITES — Primary Care/Emergency Medicine

Mammal Bites

Type	Organism
Human	- Organisms: *Staph, Strep, Eikenella*. Usually polymicrobial.
Cat/Dog	- *Pasteurella, Staph, Strep*, anaerobes

Diagnosis: Wound culture only if appears infected

Management:
- Wound care, irrigation, debridement if necessary
- Closure
    - Primary Intention: If uninfected, < 12 hours, not on hands/feet
    - Secondary Intention: All others
- Antibiotics (Amoxicillin-Clavulanate, etc)
    - Indicated if infected
    - Prophylactic: If high risk, especially cat bites
- Tetanus PPX
- Rabies PPX (see below)

Rabies

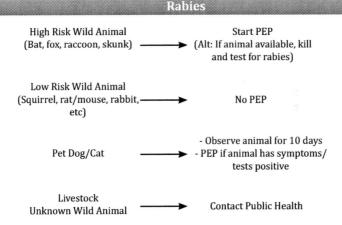

High Risk Wild Animal (Bat, fox, raccoon, skunk) → Start PEP (Alt: If animal available, kill and test for rabies)

Low Risk Wild Animal (Squirrel, rat/mouse, rabbit, etc) → No PEP

Pet Dog/Cat → - Observe animal for 10 days
- PEP if animal has symptoms/tests positive

Livestock / Unknown Wild Animal → Contact Public Health

PC/EM17

MENTAL STATUS EXAMINATION — Psychiatry

General: Mental status examination is the core "physical exam" in psychiatry, with the components in the figure below

Component	Examples
Appearance	- Well-groomed, poorly-groomed - Physical build, appeared age, etc - Any other changes in physical appearance (ie scars, etc)
Behavior	- Eye contact - Attitude (ie level of cooperativity)
Speech	- Rate - Rhythm - Articulation
Mood	- Mood based on the patient's words (ie "happy")
Affect	- Observer's assessment of the patient's mood - Common descriptions include euphoric, dysphoric, neutral - Range of emotions described flat, blunted, constricted, or full
Thought Process	- Description of the patient's pattern of thoughts - Common descriptors include logical/linear, circumstantial, tangential, flight of ideas
Thought Content	- Types of thoughts the patient is having
Hallucinations	- Assessment of sensory perceptions that occur without actual stimulus - Illusions: Abnormal perception of actual stimulus
Suicidal/Homicidal Ideation	- Assessment of patients risk toward self and others - Always assess for actual plan
Cognition	- Assessment of patient's orientation, memory, concentration, consciousness, etc
Insight	- Patient's awareness of their own problem
Judgment	- Patient's ability to approach their problems in an appropriate manner

PSYCHIATRY BASICS

Defense Mechanisms

Type	Features	Example
Immature		
Acting Out	- Expressing feelings through inappropriate actions	- Temper tantrums
Denial	- Rejecting reality	- Reject new diagnosis
Projection	- Internal feelings displaced onto another person	- Individual who is angry states that the other person has angry feelings
Regression	- Going back to earlier modes of dealing with the world	- Bedwetting
Psychotic		
Displacement	- Transferring unwanted feelings to another person or object	- Mother yells at her child, because her husband yelled at her
Isolation of Affect	- Separation of feelings from stressful life event	- Description of death without any emotion
Intellectualization	- Overuse of facts/logic to avoid negative feelings	- Focus on statistics after life threatening diagnosis
Rationalization	- Avoid self-blame by coming up with other logical reasons for an action	- Blames another person after getting fired
Reaction Formation	- Actions in opposition of feelings	- Mother overprotective of a child that she did not desire
Repression	- Involuntary withholding of feeling from consciousness	- Person does not remember episode of sexual abuse
Splitting	- Alternation between belief that others are all good or all bad	- Person says that all the nurses here are great but all doctors are bad
Undoing	- Action or words designed to cancel some disapproved thoughts, impulses, or acts	- Think about physically hurting someone, but act nicely instead
Mature		
Altruism	- Alleviating negative feelings through charity	
Humor	- Appreciating the nature of an anxiety provoking situation	
Sublimation	- Transferring unwanted feelings into more appropriate activity	
Suppression	- Intentionally withholding an idea or feeling from conscious	

PSYCHOTIC/DELUSIONAL DISORDER — Psychiatry

Disorder	Overview	DSM-5 and Clinical Features	Management
Schizophrenia	Pathophysiology: - Excess dopamine - Hypofunction of NMDA-R - MRI: Enlarged ventricles, decreased cortical size Risk: - Presents between 15-50 (men earlier, poorer prognosis) - Family history - "Downward Drift" - High suicide risk	* ≥ 2 of the following, with at least 1 being #1-3 (1) Delusions (2) Hallucinations (3) Disorganized speech (4) Disorganized/catatonic behavior (5) Negative symptoms (flat affect, apathy, anhedonia) Brief Psychotic (< 1 month) - Rare. Associated with borderline personality - Triggered by extreme stressor Schizophreniform (1-6 months) Schizophrenia (> 6 months)	Antipsychotics - Typical and atypical have equal efficacy, but atypical preferred due to side effect profile - Clozapine reserved for refractory Psychotherapy - Family Therapy (want decreased home stress) - Behavioral/Group Therapy
Schizoaffective		- Meet criteria for major depressive or manic episode with concurrent psychotic symptoms - Psychotic symptoms for ≥ 2 weeks in the absence of mood symptoms	- Antipsychotics (2nd generation preferred) - Treat mood disorder (SSRI for depression, mood stabilizer if manic)
Psychotic Disorder Due to Medical Condition	- Etiologies include dementia, Parkinson's, CVA, encephalitis, and other neurologic/endocrine abnormalities	- Hallucinations or delusions - Evidence of a non-psychiatric cause	- Treat underlying
Substance-Induced Psychotic Disorder	- Corticosteroids, antiepileptic, anticholinergics, others - Drug use or withdrawal	- Hallucinations or delusions - Evidence of medication or substance - Not better explained by psychotic disorder	- Withdraw substance

PSYCHOTIC/DELUSIONAL DISORDERS — Psychiatry

Delusional Disorder

General: Presence of delusion without functional impact or other psychotic features. Often have poor insight into their own condition.

Subtypes of Delusions:
- Erotomanic: Belief that other person is in love with the patient
- Grandiose: Delusions of having great talent
- Somatic: Delusion of physical abnormality
- Persecutory: Delusion of being persecuted
- Jealous: Delusion of lack of faith
- Folie a deux (Shared delusion disorder)
    - Two people share delusion (started by one, imposed on the other)
    - Should interview separately

DSM-5:
* ≥ 1 delusion for at least 1 month
- Functionality is NOT significantly impaired, delusions not obviously bizarre
- Psychotic symptoms (ie consistent with schizophrenia) not present

Management:
- Establish patient rapport (patients often reject that they have condition)
- Antipsychotic therapy
- CBT

Clinical Features of Psychosis

Positive Symptoms:
- Hallucinations, delusions, bizarre behavior, disorganized speech
- Ideas of reference (draw conclusions from every day sensory experiences)
- Generally respond to antipsychotics

Negative Symptoms:
- Flat or blunted affect, anhedonia, apathy, alogia (poverty of speech), and lack of interest in socialization
- More often resistant to pharmacologic treatment

Cognitive Symptoms:
- Impairments in attention, executive function, and working memory
- Neologisms (newly coined words that only have meaning to patient)
- Eye tracking defects

Phases:
- Prodromal: Decline in functioning that precedes the first psychotic episode
    - Often becomes socially withdrawn with atypical behavior
- Psychotic: Hallucinations, delusions, and disordered thoughts

MOOD DISORDERS — Psychiatry

Manic Episode

DSM-5: At least 3 of the following
1) Distractible
2) Insomnia
3) Grandiosity
4) Flight of ideas
5) Activity/Agitation
6) Speech (pressured)
7) Thoughtlessness

Mania	Hypomania
≥ 7 days - Severe functional impairment - Possible psychotic features	≥ 4 days - No marked functional impairment - No psychotic features

Bipolar Disorder

Condition	DSM-5 Definition
Bipolar I	- Mania (at least one episode) +/- hypomania or depressive episodes
Bipolar II	- Hypomania + ≥ 1 major depressive episodes
Cyclothymic	≥ 2 years with periods of hypomania and depressive symptoms - No episodes qualify as mania or major depressive episodes

Management:

Situation	Intervention
Acute Mania	- Mild: Antipsychotic (atypical) - Severe: Mood stabilizer (Lithium, Valproate) PLUS antipsychotic - Refractory: Change drugs. ECT if failure to respond to > 4-5 different meds
Acute Bipolar Depression	- Mood stabilizer (Quetiapine, Lurasidone, Lamotrigine, Lithium, Valproate, or Olanzapine + Fluoxetine)
Chronic Bipolar	- Mood Stabilizer (Lithium first line, with alternatives: Valproate, Quetiapine, or Lamotrigine) - Refractory: Lithium or Valproate PLUS antipsychotic - Patients typically require lifelong treatment
Pregnancy	- Acute Mania: Use typical antipsychotics. ECT also safe option. - Maintenance: Lamotrigine, atypical antipsychotics

MOOD DISORDERS — Psychiatry

Major Depressive Episode

DSM-5: 5 of the following for at least a two week period
1) Depressed mood most of the time
2) Anhedonia (Loss of interest in pleasurable activities)
3) Change in appetite or weight
4) Feelings of worthlessness or guilt
5) Sleep changes (Insomnia or hypersomnia)
6) Diminished concentration
7) Psychomotor agitation or retardation
8) Fatigue or loss of energy
9) Recurrent thoughts of death or suicide

Major Depressive Disorder

Pathophysiologic Changes:
- Decreased CSF 5-HIAA
- Elevated cortisol
- Multifactorial genetic inheritance

Condition	DSM-5 Criteria
Major Depressive Disorder	- ≥ 1 major depressive episode - No mania

Persistent Depressive Disorder (Dysthymia)	- Depressed mood for at least two years
	- ≥ 2 of the following
	   (1) Hopelessness
	   (2) Decreased appetite
	   (3) Sleep problems
	   (4) Low energy
	   (5) Low concentration
	   (6) Low self-esteem

Specifiers:

Atypical	- Mood reactivity - Hypersomnia - Hyperphagia/weight gain (due to increased appetite) - Leaden paralysis - Hypersensitivity to interpersonal rejection
Melancholic	- Anhedonia, dysphoric affect, loss of sleep/appetite
Catatonic	- See next page
Psychotic	- Major episodes contain hallucinations and delusions (that are not present outside the episode) - Themes tend to be consistent with mood
Anxious	- High levels of anxiety
Seasonal	- Symptoms start during one season, remit during another

MOOD DISORDERS — Psychiatry

Management of Depression

- Hospitalization (if potential harm to self)
- Ideal treatment of depression is the combination of psychotherapy plus pharm

- Pharmacotherapy
    - SSRI (first line)
    - SNRI, atypical agents generally second line
    - MAOi, TCA, others are alternatives, but rarely used
    - Atypical Antipsychotics: Can be used as adjunctive agents/to treat psychotic features
- Psychotherapy:
    - Cognitive-behavioral therapy
    - Interpersonal psychotherapy

- Initiating and Adjusting Pharm Therapy
    - Must give around 4-6 weeks to assess for efficacy of drug
    - If patient still symptomatic, either increase dose or try different drug
    - Phases:
        - Acute: Remission is induced (minimum 1.5-2 months in duration)
        - Continuation Phase: Remission is preserved and relapse prevented (usually 5-10 months)
        - Maintenance Phase: Susceptible patients are protected against recurrence or relapse (many require indefinite therapy)

- Refractory (Patient that fails at least two drug monotherapy trials)
    - Augment with atypical antipsychotic, Lithium, or thyroid hormone
    - Electroconvulsive Therapy (for severe, refractory cases)

Electroconvulsive Therapy

Procedure:
- Anesthetic (Methohexital, Etomidate, etc) plus Succinylcholine, Atropine
- Generalized seizure is induced via electricity across the brain
- Repeated ~6-10 times over a few weeks

Side Effects:
- Retrograde and anterograde amnesia (usually resolve within 6 months)
- Note: Lithium/Benzos contraindicated (lower seizure threshold)

Indications:
- Severe, refractory depression, catatonia, or mania
- Emergent correction required (won't eat, imminent suicide risk)

Contraindications:
- No absolute contraindication
- Increased risk in those with:
    - Recent MI or CV risk
    - Recent stroke/aneurysm or space occupying brain mass

MOOD DISORDERS — Psychiatry

Suicide

Risk Factors:
- Sex (male 3x more completion, but women make more attempts)
- Age (older)
- Depression
- Prior attempt
- EtOH/Substance abuse
- Rational thought loss (psychosis)
- Social support
- Organized thought
- No significant other
- Sickness

Management:

Highest Risk (ideation/intent/plan)	- Hospitalize with constant observation - Ensure safety
High Risk (ideation, w/o plan)	- Close follow-up, use social supports to monitor patient - Treat underlying psychiatric conditions - Reduce access to firearms/other means of suicide

Catatonia

General: State of immobility and abnormal stuporous behavior, associated with mood disorders and schizophrenia (but also underlying medical conditions)

Clinical:
- Immobility or excessive activity
- Stupor, mutism
- Negativism (resistant to instructions)
- Catalepsy (remains in fixed position for prolonged time)
- Posturing or waxy flexibility (resistant to movement)
- Echolalia, echopraxia

Management:
- Benzodiazepines (first line)
- ECT for refractory cases

Grief

Typical Grief	< 6 months - Shock, numbness, distress, crying, sleep issues, decreased appetite, poor concentration, weight loss, survivor guilt - Hallucinations of loved one
Complex Grief	> 6 months - Loss of function - Emotional dysregulation, preoccupation with death
Major Depression	- Meets criteria for major depressive episode - No breakthrough happiness, self-loathing, or suicidal ideation are all signs

ANXIETY DISORDERS — Psychiatry

Panic Disorder

General: Spontaneous episodes of intense fear and other symptoms

Clinical: Panic attacks characterized by the following symptoms (lasting minutes to hours)
- Dyspnea, chest pain, palpitations, diaphoresis
- Paresthesias (hyperventilation)
- Abdominal pain/nausea
- Dizziness, derealization, depersonalization, fear of dying

DSM-5:
- Recurrent unexpected panic attacks without trigger
- ≥ 1 attacks followed by > 1 month of continuous worry about experiencing subsequent attacks (+/- behavior change to avoid potential triggers)

Management:
- Acute Episode: Benzodiazepine
- Chronic: SSRI, CBT

Agoraphobia

General: Intense fear of public places, where escape may be difficult

DSM-5:
Intense fear/anxiety about > 2 situations for ≥ 6 months (due to concern of escape or inability to obtain help)
- Fear of triggering situation out of proportion to actual danger posed
- Situations often include both open spaces (ie bridges) and confined spaces (ie public transportation, stores, crowds)
- Causes significant functional impairment

Management:
- Cognitive-behavioral therapy
- SSRI

Specific Phobia/Social Anxiety Disorder

General: Irrational fear and anxiety of a specific feared object or situation
- Specific: An intense fear of a specific object or situation
- Social: Fear of scrutiny by others or of acting in an embarrassing way

DSM-5: > 6 months with the following features:
- Persistent excessive fear elicited by a specific situation or object
- Exposure to the situation triggers an immediate fear response
- Situation or object is avoided
- Functional impairment

Management:

Specific Phobia	- Cognitive-behavioral therapy
Social Phobia	- Cognitive-behavioral therapy - SSRI - PRN beta-blockers for performance anxiety/public speaking

ANXIETY DISORDERS — Psychiatry

Generalized Anxiety Disorder

General: Persistent, excessive anxiety regarding many facets of daily life

DSM-5:
- Excessive anxiety/worry about various daily events for > 6 months
- Associated with ≥ 3 of the following:
    - Restlessness, impaired concentration, irritability, muscle tension, insomnia, fatigue

Management:
- CBT
- SSRI (can augment with buspirone)
- Benzos have been used, but dependence limits their utility

Obsessive Compulsive Disorder

General: Presence of distressful and impairing obsessions and compulsions
- Obsessions: Recurrent intrusive, anxiety producing thoughts
- Compulsions: Repetitive behaviors aimed to alleviate stressor
- Common Patterns:
    - Contamination/cleaning
    - Doubt or harm/checking multiple times to avoid danger
    - Can be dark (ie obsessed over child being harmed, patient stabs self to relieve these thoughts)
- Ego-dystonic

DSM-5:
- Experiencing obsessions and or compulsions (definition above)
- Time consuming (> 1 hr/day) OR cause significant distress/dysfunction

Management:
- CBT (exposure and response therapy)
- SSRI
    - Alternative: Venlafaxine, Clomipramine
    - Augment with atypical antipsychotics

ANXIETY DISORDERS — Psychiatry

Post-Traumatic Stress Disorder

General: Multiple symptoms after exposure to one or more traumatic events

DSM-5:
- Exposure to death, threatened death, serious injury, or sexual violence
- Plus > 1 month of the following symptoms
    - Persistently re-experienced event (ie flashbacks, nightmares, etc)
    - Avoidance of trauma-related stimuli
    - At least two negative cognitions/mood changes: Negative feelings of self/others/world, self-blame, anhedonia, etc
    - At least two symptoms of arousal and reactivity: Hypervigilance, exaggerated startle, irritability/angry outbursts, impaired concentration, insomnia

Management:
- Pharmacotherapy:
    - SSRI or SNRI (Venlafaxine)
    - Prazosin (for nightmares, sleep disruption)
    - Augmentation with atypical antipsychotics if severe
- Psychotherapy:
    - CBT (containing eye movement desensitization and reprocessing)

Acute Stress Disorder:
- < 1 month of symptoms that occur within one month of a traumatic event
- Tx: Mobilize social supports, brief CBT, treat symptoms (insomnia/anxiety)

Adjustment Disorder

General: Behavioral or emotional symptoms develop after a stressful life event

DSM-5: Emotional or behavioral symptoms within 3 months in response to an identifiable stressful life event:
- Marked distress in excess of what would be expected after such an event
- Impairment in daily functioning
- Symptoms resolve within 6 months after stressor has ended
- Does not meet criteria for other mental disorder (including normal grief)

Management: Psychotherapy

ANXIETY DISORDERS — Psychiatry

Disorder	DSM-5 and Clinical Features	Management
Selective Mutism	- Situational mutism, often seen in children - > 1 month of consistent failure to speak in select social situations - Able to speak in other situations, and no underlying communication disorder	- CBT/Family Therapy
Body Dysmorphic Disorder	- Preoccupation with perceived defects or flaws in physical appearance - Not observable/minimal defect to other observers	- CBT/SSRI
Excoriation Disorder	- Recurrent skin picking resulting in lesions - Repeated attempts to reduce skin picking - Repetitive behaviors in response to concerns	- CBT/SSRI - Atypical Antipsychotics
Trichotillomania	- Recurrent episodes of pulling out hair, resulting in hair loss - Usually involves the head or eyebrows/lashes, but can involve any hair - Not due to another medical condition (ie alopecia) or psych disorder	- CBT > SSRI
Hoarding Disorder	- Persistent inability to discard possessions, regardless of value - Accumulation of possessions that fill living areas and affect use	- CBT
Gambling Disorder	- Persistent and recurrent problematic gambling for at least a year - Issues seen include preoccupation, need to gamble for pleasure, jeopardizing relationships, lying about gambling, etc	- Support Group - CBT

PERSONALITY DISORDERS — Psychiatry

Personality Disorder (Overview)

General: Pervasive, maladaptive personality change that cause significant functional impairment
- Usually have lack of insight
- Ego-syntonic
- Increased risk for other disorders

DSM-5:
- Enduring pattern of behavior that deviates from person's culture
- The pattern is pervasive, inflexible, and has an onset no later than adolescence or early adulthood

Cluster A ⟶ Eccentric, peculiar withdrawn
- Associated with psychotic disorders

Cluster B ⟶ Emotional, dramatic, inconsistent
- Associated with mood disorders

Cluster C ⟶ Avoidant, dependent, obsessive-compulsive
- Associated with anxiety

Management:
- Generally very difficult to treat
- Patients often do not realize they need help
- Psychotherapy is cornerstone of care
- Comorbid psychiatric illnesses should be treated

PERSONALITY DISORDERS

Psychiatry

Personality	Overview	DSM-5 and Specific Clinical Features	Management
Cluster A			
Paranoid	- Pervasive distrust and suspiciousness of others	- Distrust of others, with ≥ 4 of the following: Suspicion of exploitation or deception, preoccupation with doubts of loyalty, reluctance to confide in others, interpretation of benign remarks as threatening, persistence of grudges, etc	- Individual Psychotherapy (not group) - Antipsychotics (if psychotic)
Schizoid	- Lifelong pattern of social withdrawal - Eccentric and reclusive	- Voluntary social withdrawal and restricted emotions - ≥ 4 of the following: Chooses solitary activity, no desire for relationship, little interest in sexual activity, few friends, lack of emotion	- Generally lack insight for therapy
Schizotypal	- Eccentric behavior and peculiar thought patterns - Magical thinking (ie belief in superstition, telepathy, bizarre fantasies, etc)	- Eccentric behavior, perceptual distortions, and discomfort with relationships - ≥ 5 of the following: Ideas of reference, magical thinking, illusions, suspiciousness, restricted affect, odd appearance/behavior, odd beliefs, few friends, social anxiety	- Psychotherapy - Antipsychotics (if required)
Cluster B			
Antisocial	- Exploitive of others, lacks empathy/compassion - Violates the law - Begins in childhood as conduct disorder	- Pattern of disregard for and violation of the rights of others + history of conduct disorder - ≥ 3 of the following: Fails to conform to social norms, deceitfulness/lies for personal gain, impulsivity, irritability/aggressiveness, lacks remorse, irresponsible, reckless	- Low utility for psychotherapy or pharmacotherapy

Psych14

PERSONALITY DISORDERS — Psychiatry

Personality	Overview	DSM-5 and Specific Clinical Features	Management
Borderline "unstable, hx of abuse"	- Unstable moods, behaviors, interpersonal relationships - Splitting is characteristic - Associated with childhood physical, emotional, sexual abuse - High rate of psychotic episodes	- Pervasive pattern of impulsivity and unstable relationship - ≥ 5 of the following: Unstable relationships, unstable self-image, unstable mood, SI/ self-mutilation, anger, paranoid ideation, impulsivity (sexually/spending/substance use)	- Dialectical behavior therapy (CBT plus mindfulness skills) - Pharm: Mood stabilizers, antipsychotics, SSRI
Histrionic "attention + sex" "hysterically sexual"	- Attention seeking behavior and emotionally labile	- ≥ 5 of the following: Provocative behavior, exaggerated emotion, easily influenced, perceives intimacy, wants to be center of attention, uses appearance for attention	- Psychotherapy
Narcissistic	- Pattern of grandiosity, need for admiration, and lack of empathy	- ≥ 5 of the following: Exaggerated sense of importance, requires admiration, entitled, takes advantage of others, lacks empathy, arrogant, envious, belief they are special	- Psychotherapy
Cluster C			
Avoidant	- Social inhibition, hypersensitivity, and feelings of inadequacy	- ≥ 4 of the following: Avoids interpersonal contact, cautious, unwilling to interact, afraid of criticism/rejection, feels socially inept	- Psychotherapy
Dependent	- Excessive need to be taken care of that leads to submissive and clinging behavior	- ≥ 5 of the following: Feels helpless alone, seeks relationships, fear of being alone, seeks support from others, needs other to assume their responsibilities	- Psychotherapy
Obsessive-Compulsive	- Preoccupation with orderliness, control, and perfectionism - Unlike OCD, ego-syntonic	- ≥ 4 of the following: Perfectionism, excessive devotion to work, rigid/stubborn, preoccupied with detail	- Psychotherapy

DISSOCIATIVE DISORDERS — Psychiatry

Dissociative Amnesia

General: Inability to remember important personal information
- Usually post-traumatic event or extreme stressors
- Procedural memory preserved
- Rarely generalizes to complete memory loss

DSM-5:
- Inability to recall important autobiographical information, usually due to traumatic or stressful event
- Often with dissociative fugue: Wandering from home, without knowledge of autobiographical information

Management:
- Generally self-limited
- Psychotherapy is cornerstone

Depersonalization/Derealization Disorder

General: Detachment from one's self or surroundings
- Depersonalization: "Out of body experience"
- Derealization: "In dream or movie"

DSM-5:
- Recurrent experience of either depersonalization or derealization
- Reality testing remains intact during episode

Management:
- Psychotherapy (CBT, psychodynamic, etc)

Dissociative Identity Disorder (Multiple Personality)

General: Presence of more than one distinct personality state
- Often occurs in victims of significant and chronic/childhood trauma

DSM-5:
- Disruption of identity manifested as two or more distinct personality states
- Extensive memory lapses in autobiographical information, daily occurrences, and or traumatic events

Management: Psychotherapy

SOMATIC AND FACTITIOUS — Psychiatry

Somatic Symptom Disorder

General: Chronic perseveration over subjective symptom

DSM-5: > 6 months
- ≥ 1 somatic symptoms causing distress/functional impairment
- Excessive thoughts, feelings, behaviors related to the somatic symptoms

Management:
- Regular visits with single primary care physician
    - Minimize unnecessary medical workups and treatments
    - Address psychological issues slowly (patients likely to resist)

Conversion Disorder

General: Neurological symptoms without underlying neurologic condition
- Onset often in adolescence or early adulthood
- Neurologic conditions include: Weakness/paralysis, non-epileptic seizure, visual, or speech problems
- Often calm and unconcerned (la belle indifference)

DSM-5:
- ≥ 1 symptoms of altered voluntary motor or sensory function
- Incompatibility between the symptom and recognized neurological or medical conditions

Management:
- 1st Line: Education, with self-help techniques and family education
- 2nd Line: CBT
- Often spontaneously recover, but remission rate is high

Illness Anxiety Disorder

General: Excessive concern about having medical condition
- Previously called hypochondriasis

DSM-5: > 6 months of:
- Preoccupation with having or acquiring a serious illness
- Somatic symptoms none or minimal
- High level of anxiety about health
- Performs excessive health-related behaviors

Management:
- Regularly scheduled visits (establish good relationship with PCP)
- CBT

Psych17

SOMATIC AND FACTITIOUS — Psychiatry

Factitious Disorder

General: Intentionally falsify medical or psych symptoms to assume the role of a sick patient. Previously called Munchausen.
- Risk Populations:
    - Healthcare workers
    - Associated with personality disorders
- Common Scenario
    - Medical: Fever, infection, hypoglycemia, seizures
    - Psych: Hallucinations, depression

DSM-5: Falsification of physical or psych symptoms OR induction of injury or disease
- Absence of obvious external rewards

Management:
- Collect collateral information from medical providers and family
- Collaborate with PCP and treatment team to avoid unnecessary procedure
- Patients may require confrontation

Malingering

General: Intentional reporting of physical or psychological symptoms in order to achieve personal gain (ie obtain narcotics, avoid police, receive monetary reward)

DSM-5: Not a medical condition

IMPULSE CONTROL DISORDERS

Psychiatry

Disorder	Clinical Features	Management
Intermittent Explosive Disorder	- Recurrent behavioral outbursts, characterized by verbal and/or physical aggression - Either weekly for > 3 months OR outbursts result in physical damage to people or property	- CBT + SSRI (first line) - Anticonvulsants (ie Phenytoin) used in refractory cases
Kleptomania	- Failure to resist urge to steal objects, despite having no personal or monetary need - Objects often discarded or returned - High rate of comorbid bulimia, and other anxiety/mood disorders	- CBT - Pharm (SSRI) has potential benefit
Pyromania	- At least two episodes of deliberate fire setting - Tension before act, with gratification after watching - Excessive fascination with fires	- Often remits on own - CBT/SSRI can be used

EATING DISORDERS — Psychiatry

	Overview	DSM-5 and Other Clinical Features	Management
Anorexia Nervosa	- Low body weight, with limited caloric intake and preoccupation with weight - Can be restricting (weight limitation from ↓ caloric intake/excessive exercise) OR binge-purge subtypes	- DSM-5: Restriction of energy intake relative to requirements, leading to significant low weight - Fear of gaining weight or becoming fat - Disturbed body image/concern with weight Physical Findings/Complications: - CV: Cardiomyopathy, arrhythmia - Endocrine: Amenorrhea, hypothyroid, hypopituitary, osteoporosis - Fluid/electrolyte abnormalities (hypotension) - Lanugo hair, alopecia	- Nutritional replenishment - CBT - Pharm: Not standard therapy, but can modulate with olanzapine - Hospitalization (Indications include dehydration, hemodynamic instability, arrhythmia, very low weight/refusal to eat) * Monitor for refeeding syndrome
Bulimia Nervosa	- Eating disorder characterized by binge eating/purging Methods of Purge: - Laxative - Ipecac - Induced vomiting - Diuretics - Fasting/excessive exercise	- DSM-5: Recurrent episodes of binge eating, with compensatory purging behaviors (at least once per week for 3 months) - Perception of self excessively influenced by physical appearance Physical Findings/Complications - Parotid enlargement, dental erosions/caries - Hand calluses ("Russell's sign") - Mallory-Weiss tear/acid reflux - Hypokalemia, hypochloremia, metabolic alkalosis	- CBT + SSRI
Binge Eating Disorder	- Periods of overeating without sense of control over eating	- Recurrent episodes of binge eating (at least once per week for 3 months) ≥ 3 of the following: Rapid eating, eating until too full, eating when not hungry, eating alone, feeling disgusting/gross after eating	- Psychotherapy (CBT) - If overweight: Behavioral modification for weight loss

SEXUAL/SEXUALITY DISORDERS — Psychiatry

Gender Dysphoria

General: Distress accompanying incongruence between patient's expressed gender and assigned gender. Definitions below;
- Gender: What a person identifies with
- Sex: Biologic sex
- Transsexualism: Desire to live as the opposite sex
- Transvestism: Wearing clothes of the opposite sex

DSM-5: > 2 of the following:
- Difference between experienced gender and primary/secondary sex characteristics
- Strong desire to be other gender
- Strong desire to be treated as other gender
- Strong desire for primary/secondary sex characteristics of the other gender
- Strong belief one has typical feelings/reactions of the other gender

Management:
- Child/Adolescents: Provide education, support, and mental health referral
    - Treat comorbid psych conditions
- Onset of Puberty: If still unsure of gender, provide pubertal suppression
    - GnRH agonists are preferred (alt: anti-estrogen/anti-androgen)
- Gender-affirming hormones
    - Androgens or Estrogen + Spironolactone
- Surgical sex reassignment
    - Indicated after 1 year of living in gender role + hormonal therapy

Paraphilias

General: Sexual arousal to atypical situations, fantasies, individuals, or acts. DSM recognizes the following subtypes:

Pedophilia	- Sexual interest in children (generally < 13 y/o, while individual is > 5 years older)
Transvestic	- Sexual arousal from cross dressing
Fetishistic	- Sexual arousal from use of non-living objects or non-genital body parts (ie feet)
Sexual Masochism	- Arousal from being beaten, bound, humiliated, etc
Sexual Sadism	- Arousal from physical or psychological suffering of another
Exhibitionism	- Arousal from exposure of one's genitals to others
Voyeuristic	- Arousal from observing an unsuspecting individual
Frotteuristic	- Arousal rubbing against/touching nonconsenting person

DSM-5:
- > 6 months of engaging in unusual sexual activities or preoccupation with unusual sexual urges
- Occurs either with nonconsenting person and/or causes loss of functioning

Management:
- Psychotherapy, support groups

SEXUAL/SEXUALITY DISORDERS — Psychiatry

Psychologic Sexual Dysfunction

General: Sexual dysfunction include a variety of problems with sexual response, which can be due to either medical or psychological etiology

DSM-5:
- Significant clinical distress from a sexual dysfunction, which cannot be better explained by another mental or medical disorder
- Subtypes Include:

Disorder	Definition (for all: > 6 months of the following symptoms)
Men	
Premature Ejaculation	Recurrent ejaculation during sex within one minute
Erectile Dysfunction	Difficulty in getting or maintaining an erection
Delayed Ejaculation	Marked delay in or absence of orgasm
Women	
Sexual Interest/ Arousal Disorder	Absence or deficiency of sexual thoughts, desire
Female Orgasmic Disorder	Marked delay in or absence of orgasm

Management:
- Psychotherapy
    - Sex therapy
    - CBT
- Pharm/Mechanical
    - SSRI (if premature ejaculation)
    - Hormone replacement
    - Phosphodiesterase inhibitors
    - Vacuum devices, rings, etc

Normal Aging:
- Desire does not usually change as people age
- Men require more direct stimulation of the genitals and more time to achieve orgasm
- Women experience vaginal dryness and thinning

SLEEP DISORDERS — Psychiatry

Overview of Sleep Disorders

Awake (eyes open)	Beta	
Awake (eyes closed)	Alpha	
Non-REM N1	Theta	Light sleep
Non-REM N2	Spindles/K-complex	Deeper sleep
Non-REM N3	Delta	Deepest non-REM sleep
REM	Beta	

Sleep disorders can be placed in the following classes:
- Insomnia
- Sleep-related breathing disorders
- Central disorders of hypersomnolence (ie narcolepsy)
- Circadian rhythm sleep-wake disorders
- Parasomnias (ie unusual sleep related behaviors)
- Sleep-related movement disorders

Nonpharmacologic Sleep Advice:
- Sleep Hygiene (avoid caffeine/EtOH around bedtime, avoid naps, exercise regularly, try relaxing activities near bedtime)
- Relaxation (progressive muscle relaxation, guided imagery, meditation)
- Stimulus Control (go to sleep when you feel sleepy, try for 10 minutes max, use bed only for sleep, regular schedule, avoid naps)
- Sleep restriction

Insomnia

General: Difficulty initiating or maintaining sleep. Can be:
- Primary (idiopathic)
- Secondary (adverse med effect, symptoms of concurrent psych disorder, or related to medical disorder)

Can also be defined as:
- Acute (< 3 months): Most often related to stressor
- Chronic (> 3 months, see DSM criteria below)

DSM-5: > 3 days a week for > 3 months of:
- Difficulty initiating or maintaining sleep, or waking up too early
- Adequate opportunity/chance for sleep
- Functionally impairing, often causing daytime symptoms (hypersomnolence)

Management:
- Sleep Hygiene
- CBT (therapy >>> medication)
- Pharm (for refractory cases)
    - Sleep Onset Insomnia: Zaleplon/Zolpidem (short acting)
    - Sleep Maintenance Insomnia: Eszopiclone, other long acting benzo
    - Trazodone commonly used off label

SLEEP DISORDERS — Psychiatry

	Overview	Clinical Features	Management
Obstructive Sleep Apnea	- Intermittent oropharyngeal airflow obstruction (20-30 seconds of hypoxemia, which awakens patient) Risks: - Obesity - Structural (tonsils, uvula) - Increased neck circumference - Family history - Alcohol	Clinical symptoms include: Snoring, daytime somnolence, nighttime desats Diagnosis: Polysomnography - > 5 episodes of apnea or hypopnea in 1 hour (in symptomatic patient) is diagnostic - > 15 episodes diagnostic if not symptomatic	- Behavioral modification (weight loss/exercise) Mild-to-moderate - PEEP therapy - Oral appliance (alternative) Severe - CPAP is preferred - Uvulopalatopharyngoplasty - Tracheostomy (refractory)
Central Sleep Apnea	- Repetitive decrease in airflow and ventilatory effort during sleep - Primary: Idiopathic - Secondary: CHF, stroke, medical conditions, drugs, Cheyne-stokes (periodic crescendo-decrescendo breathing pattern)	Clinical: Daytime somnolence, insomnia, signs of nocturnal hypoxia (eg morning headaches) Diagnosis: Polysomnography - > 5 apneic episodes per hour	- Noninvasive PAP therapy - Supplemental O_2
Obesity Hypoventilation Syndrome	- Alveolar hypoventilation secondary to obesity (BMI > 30)	- Clinical: Hypersomnolence plus witnessed hypopnea. Presents similarly to OSA (because it is frequently comorbid). - Diagnosis: Chemistries (elevated bicarbonate) plus ABG (CO_2 > 45 mmHg) * Should perform polysomnography to rule out OSA	- Noninvasive PAP therapy - Tracheostomy (if refractory)

SLEEP DISORDERS — Psychiatry

Narcolepsy

General: Inherited disorder of REM dysregulation, resulting in hypersomnolence

Clinical:
- Daytime hypersomnolence
- Cataplexy (loss of muscle tone with emotional stimulus)
- Sleep paralysis
- Hypnagogic hallucinations (going to sleep)
- Hypnopompic hallucinations (awakening)

DSM-5: Irrepressible need to sleep or daytime lapses into sleep occurring for ≥ 3 months PLUS either
(1) Low CSF hypocretin-1 concentration or
(2) Cataplexy and decreased sleep/REM latency on polysomnogram

Management:
- Education/behavioral modification (sleep hygiene, scheduled naps, avoid car accidents)
- Daytime Sleepiness: Modafinil or other stimulants
- Cataplexy: Venlafaxine, Fluoxetine, or Sodium oxybate at night

Circadian Sleep-Wake Disorders

Disorder	Description	Management
Delayed	- Delayed onset of sleep, delayed wake time	- Morning bright light - Nighttime melatonin
Advanced	- Early sleep onset, early wake time	- Nighttime bright light
Non-24-Hr	- Circadian rhythm off 24 hour cycle - Results in wakefulness at times during night, drive for sleep during day	- Phototherapy - Melatonin
Irregular	- Failure to consolidate periods of sleep and wakefulness (ie 4 hours of sleep, 4 hours wake, etc)	- Phototherapy - Melatonin
Jet Lag	- Excess daily sleep time due to poor sleep/misaligned circadian rhythm - > 2 time zones	- Self-limited - Melatonin
Shift Work	- Sleep-wake difficulties due to shifts off of the light-dark cycle	- Change schedule - Sleep hygiene/melatonin

Diagnosis:
- Sleep diaries
- Actigraphy (sensor tracking movement during sleep)

SLEEP DISORDERS — Psychiatry

		Overview	Clinical Features	Management
Parasomnias	Sleepwalking (Somnambulism)	- Ambulation and other acts, with underlying purpose, occurring during slow wave sleep - Risks: Stress, irregular sleep, fatigue	- Sitting up, walking around, eating, and other acts during sleep - Open eyes, blank stare, glassy look - Difficulty arousing, may become agitated	- Lifestyle modification - Low dose Clonazepam
	Sleep Terror	- Awakening from sleep from sudden terror, occurring during slow wave sleep	- Screaming, agitation, and fear, with event - Autonomic symptoms (flushing, sweating) - Usually little recall of event - Difficult to arouse	- Lifestyle modification - Low dose Clonazepam
	Nightmare Disorder	- Dysphoric dreams occurring during REM sleep	- Repeated episodes of extended, extremely dysphoric, and well-remembered dreams - Cause significant distress/functional impairment	- Often self-limited - Lifestyle modification - Psychotherapy - Prazosin
	REM Sleep Behavior Disorder	- Dream movements that occur after the loss of REM atonia - High association with movement disorders (ie Parkinson's)	- Dream enactment (sleep talking, yelling, walking, punching, etc) - Generally remember dream - Dx: Polysomnography (see loss of REM atonia, dream enactment)	- Make sleep environment safe - Pharm therapy with melatonin or Clonazepam
Sleep Movement Disorder	Periodic Limb Movement Disorder	- Involuntary myoclonic limb movements occurring during sleep	- > 15 periodic limb movements /hr of sleep - Significant sleep disturbance or functional impairment - Dx: Polysomnography	Similar to RLS: - Pramipexole/Ropinirole - Gabapentin

CHILD PSYCHIATRY

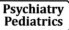
Psychiatry
Pediatrics

Intellectual Disability

General: Severely impaired cognitive and adaptive/social functioning (replaces mental retardation)

Etiology:
- About 50% are idiopathic
- Fragile X (most common inherited), Down's (most common genetic)
- Infections, metabolic derangements, hypothyroidism, etc

DSM-5:
- Significant limitations in both adaptive and intellectual function
- Onset during developmental period
- Deficits affect multiple domains: Conceptual, practical, and social
- IQ > 2 SD below mean

Severity	~IQ	Description
Mild	50-70	- Can often live/function if provided some support
Moderate	35-50	- Requires high amounts of supervision
Severe	20-35	- Not independent, needs help with self-care
Profound	< 20	- Needs nursing care throughout life

Management:
- Multidisciplinary support (behavioral intervention, educational assistance, family counseling, physical/occupational/speech therapy)

Other Developmental/Learning Disorders

Diagnosis	Features
Global Developmental Delay	- Failure to meet expected developmental milestones in several areas (ie motor, social, communication, etc)
Specific Learning Disorder	- Delayed development in a particular academic domain (ie reading, writing, arithmetic)
Language Disorder	- Difficulty learning and using language due - Reduced vocabulary, limited sentence structure
Fluency Disorder (stuttering)	- Dysfluency and speech motor production issues
Speech-Sound Disorder	- Difficulty producing articulate, intelligible speech

Psych27

CHILD PSYCHIATRY

Autism Spectrum Disorder

General: Disorder of impaired social communication/interaction and restrictive repetitive behaviors/interests

Etiology: Multifactorial. High comorbid rate with ID. Also associated with genetic disorders (Fragile X, Down's, Rett's).

DSM-5:
- Problems with social interaction and communication (ie lack of interest in peers, poor eye contact, impaired social interactions)
- Restricted, repetitive patterns of behavior, interests, and activities (ie peculiar interest, adherence to rituals, repetitive movements)
- Symptoms not accounted for by ID, learning disorder, deafness (rule out with audiology)

Management:
- Early Intervention
- Multidisciplinary (special education, behavior therapy, speech/language/occupational therapy)

Attention Deficit Hyperactivity Disorder

General: Characterized by inattention, hyperactivity, impulsivity. Subtypes:
- Inattentive
- Hyperactive
- Features of both

DSM-5: Symptoms > 6 months and present in at least two settings, onset before age 12
- At least 6 inattentive symptoms and or 6 hyperactive symptoms

Inattentive	Hyperactive
- Difficulty sustaining attention	- Difficulty remaining seated
- Does not appear to listen	- Fidgets/squirms
- Difficulty organizing	- Runs about or climbs excessively
- Loses things	- Talks excessively
- Easily distracted	- Blurts out answers
- Careless mistakes	- Interrupts others
- Struggles following instructions	- Difficulty taking turns

Management:
- Combination of pharmacologic plus educational/behavioral interventions
- Nonpharm:
- Behavior modification, educational intervention
- Pharm
- Stimulants: Methylphenidate, Dextroamphetamine
- Atomoxetine
- Alpha-2 Agonists (Clonidine, Guanfacine)

CHILD PSYCHIATRY

Psychiatry Pediatrics

Tic Disorders

General: Tics are repetitive, stereotyped movements or vocalizations, that are generally spontaneous and difficult to repress

Risk: Behavioral disorders, ADHD, and OCD are frequently comorbid with Tourette's

Clinical:

Syndrome	DSM-5 Criteria
Persistent Chronic Motor Tic Disorder	- ≥ 1 motor tic (repetitive, stereotyped movement) - Occurs for at least 1 year
Persistent Chronic Vocal Tic Disorder	- ≥ 1 vocal tic (repetitive, stereotyped vocalization) - Occurs for at least 1 year
Tourette Syndrome	- Multiple motor and vocal tics - Occurs for at least 1 year

Management:
- Therapy (psychoeducation, habit reversal therapy)
- Pharm (indicated if tics are bothersome)
    - Tetrabenazine
    - Fluphenazine, Risperidone (Haloperidol/Pimozide in the past)
    - Guanfacine/Clonidine (especially if also suffering from ADHD)

Disruptive Mood Dysregulation Disorder

General: New disorder to DSM-5. Described as chronic severe persistent irritability occurring in childhood and adolescence.

DSM-5: > 12 months of the following symptoms
- Severe recurrent verbal and/or physical outbursts (> 3x /week)
- Occur in at least 2 settings
- Persistently irritable or angry mood most
    (*differentiates from intermittent explosive)
- No mania (ie no bipolar disorder), or underlying substance/medical issue

Management:
- Psychotherapy (CBT)
- Pharm (none have great evidence yet)
    - Atypical antipsychotics
    - Antidepressants

CHILD PSYCHIATRY

Psychiatry
Pediatrics

Separation Anxiety Disorder

General: Excessive anxiety due to separation from parents

DSM-5:
- Excessive and developmentally inappropriate fear/anxiety regarding separation from attachment figures
- ≥ 4 weeks in children/adolescents and ≥ 6 months in adult
- ≥ 3 of the following:
    - Separation leads to extreme distress
    - Constant worry about harm
    - Reluctance to leave home
    - Reluctance to be alone
    - Reluctance to sleep alone
    - Complaints of physical symptoms when separated
    - Nightmares of separation

Management:
- Psychotherapy (CBT, family therapy, school therapy)

Oppositional Defiant Disorder

General: Maladaptive pattern of irritability/anger, defiance, or vindictiveness

DSM-5: Least four symptoms present for ≥ 6 months
- Anger/Irritability: Touchy, loses temper, easily annoyed, often angry
- Vindictiveness: Multiple spiteful acts in the past
- Defiant Behavior: Breaks rules, argues with authority figures, annoys others

Management:
- Therapy (behavior modification)
- Parent management training

Conduct Disorder

General: Serious disruptive behaviors, which violate the rights of other humans and animals, generally without guilt

DSM-5: Recurrent (at least 3 over the last year) acts that violate rights of others or societal norms. Examples below:
- Aggression to humans/animals (bullies, fights, physically harms animals/other people, rape)
- Property destruction
- Theft (steals items, breaks into home/car, lies to get goods)
- Serious rule violation (runs away from home, breaks curfew)

Management:
- Psychotherapy (behavior modification)
- Parent management training

CHILD PSYCHIATRY

Psychiatry
Pediatrics

Elimination Disorder

General: Developmentally inappropriate elimination of urine or feces
- Incontinence normal at young age (feces until 4 and urine until 5 y/o)
- Can be primary (idiopathic, continence never achieved) or secondary (continence achieved, then later lost, usually due to stressor)

DSM-5:
Enuresis
- Recurrent urination into clothes or bed-wetting
- ≥ 5 years old
- 2×/week for ≥ 3 consecutive months

Encopresis
- Recurrent defecation into inappropriate places
- ≥ 4 years old
- 1×/month for ≥ 3 consecutive months

Management:
- Psychoeducation (high spontaneous remission rate for both conditions)

Enuresis
- Bladder training (limit caffeine, nighttime fluid intake, scheduled voids)
- Urine alarm
- Pharm if refractory (Desmopressin or Imipramine)

Encopresis
- Behavioral Program (bowel retraining)
- If constipation, initial "clean out", followed by stool softeners/ high fiber diet

SUBSTANCE ABUSE — Psychiatry

	Overview	Intoxication	Withdrawal

EtOH	- Activates GABA receptors	**Clinical:**
		- ↓ fine motor, impaired judgement/coordination, poor balance, lethargy, coma, respiratory distress/death
		
		Management:
		- Supportive care (ABC's, lytes)
		- Thiamine, folate
		- GI Evacuation (only if significant EtOH intake in last hour)
			Clinical:
			- Mild Withdrawal (6-24 hr): Anxiety, tremors, diaphoresis, palpitations, insomnia
			- Seizures (24-48 hr)
			- Alcoholic Hallucinosis (24-48 hr): Visual, auditory, or tactile hallucinations, but orientation is normal and vital signs stable
			- Delirium Tremens (48-96 hr): Confusion, hallucinations, hypertension/fever
			
			Management:
			- Benzodiazepines (CIWA scale) or Phenobarbital
			  - Normal Liver → Chlordiazepoxide, Diazepam
			  - Bad Liver → Lorazepam
			- Thiamine, folate, vitamins ("Banana bag")

Benzodiazepine	- Potentiate GABA channels	**Clinical:** (Similar to EtOH) - Drowsiness, confusion, slurred speech - Incoordination, ataxia - Respiratory/CNS depression **Management:** - Supportive Care (ABC's, lytes, O$_2$) - Flumazenil/GI Evacuation in some	**Clinical:** - Similar to EtOH (hallucinations, tremors, anxiety, tremors, and seizures) **Management:** - Long acting benzo (requires gradual tapering over months)

SUBSTANCE ABUSE — Psychiatry

Alcohol Use Disorder

General: Recurrent drinking that causes functional impairment

Risk: Multifactorial, but high genetic basis

DSM-5: Recurrent drinking, resulting in failed obligations, hazardous situations, social problems, tolerance, history of withdrawal, inability to cut back, alcohol cravings, etc

Clinical Complications:
- GI: Gastritis, hepatitis, cirrhosis, pancreatitis
- Cardiac: Dilated cardiomyopathy, hypertension
- CNS: Neuropathy, cerebellar degeneration
    - Wernicke's
        - Thiamine deficiency
        - Nystagmus, ataxia, ophthalmoplegia, confusion
        - Precipitated by glucose administration in alcoholics
    - Korsakoff
        - Amnestic disorder, often irreversible, with confabulation
- Malignancy: ↑ risk esophageal, oropharyngeal cancers

Management:
- Support Groups (Alcoholics Anonymous)

Pharm
- Naltrexone (Opioid receptor blocker)
    - Decreases desire/craving and "high" associated with alcohol
    - Can be initiated without complete alcohol abstinence
    - Cannot be used with severe hepatitis (mild liver disease is okay)
- Acamprosate (Glutamate transmission modulator)
    - Should be started post-detoxification for relapse prevention
    - Can be used in patients with liver disease, but not in severe renal disease

Other options: Baclofen, Disulfiram, Topiramate, Gabapentin, SSRI, Ondansetron
- Disulfiram (inhibits aldehyde dehydrogenase)
    - Causes adverse reaction to EtOH (flushing, headache, vomiting, palpitations, dyspnea)
    - Used less frequently now

Screening:
- CAGE (Cut Down, Annoyed, Guilt, Eye opener)
- Validated tool (AUDIT, MAST)

SUBSTANCE ABUSE — Psychiatry

	Overview	Intoxication	Withdrawal
Cocaine	- 5-HT, Dopamine, Epi, Norepi reuptake inhibitor	Clinical: - Euphoria, heightened self esteem, hypertension/tachycardia, dilated pupils - Paranoia/hallucinations - Can cause dangerous symptoms like respiratory depression, seizures, MI, or arrhythmias Management: - Reassurance/supportive care - ACS/MI: Aspirin, benzo, stenting	- Abrupt abstinence not life threatening (symptoms usually last ~1 week) - Can experience depression, anxiety, anhedonia, cocaine craving, and increased sleep
Amphetamines	- Block reuptake and facilitate release of Dopamine and Norepi	Clinical: - Euphoria, dilated pupils, tachycardia, diaphoresis - Hyperthermia, dehydration, rhabdomyolysis - Can develop psychosis Management: - Supportive. Restraints/antipsychotics for agitation/hallucination.	- Dysphoria, hypersomnolence, fatigue

SUBSTANCE ABUSE — Psychiatry

	Overview	Intoxication	Withdrawal

Opioids	- Stimulate mu, kappa, delta opiate receptors	Clinical:
		- Drowsiness, nausea, vomit, slurred speech, constricted pupils
		- Hypothermia, seizures, respiratory depression if severe
		
		Management:
		- ABC/Ventilation, naloxone
			Clinical:
			- Dysphoria, insomnia, lacrimation, rhinorrhea, yawning, weakness, sweating
			- Nausea, fever, abdominal cramps, arthralgia, myalgia
			
			Management:
			- Clonidine (Alternative: Methadone as inpatient, especially if severe)
			- Symptomatic Management (COWS scale)
			  - NSAIDs
			  - Dicyclomine for cramps
			  - Loperamide (diarrhea)
			  - Promethazine (nausea)

Marijuana	- CB receptor activator (THC is active substance in cannabis)	Clinical: - Euphoria, anxiety, impaired coordination - Perceptual disturbance or psychosis - Conjunctival injection, dry mouth, increased appetite - Tachycardia, fluctuations in blood pressure Management: - Purely supportive - Benzos if agitation	Clinical: - Only occurs after heavy/prolonged use - Irritability, anger, depressed mood, insomnia Management: - Generally self-limited. Relaxation techniques and sleep hygiene may be helpful. - Dronabinol or Gabapentin for severe symptoms

Psych35

SUBSTANCE ABUSE — Psychiatry

Substance	Clinical Features
MDMA	- Amphetamine (increases D/NE/E in synapse) - Mild hallucinogenic properties - Clinical: Increased sociability, sexual desire, HTN, tachycardia, hyperthermia - Complications: Serotonin syndrome, hyponatremia
LSD	- Activates D, 5-HT, NE, hallucinogenic - Clinical: Perceptual distortion (visual, auditory), depersonalization, anxiety, paranoia, psychosis

PCP	- NMDA antagonist
	- Clinical: Agitation, depersonalization, hallucinations, impaired judgement, memory impairment, aggression
	- Nystagmus (rotary, horizontal, vertical), ataxia, dysarthria, hypertension, tachycardia, muscle rigidity
	- Overdose: Seizures, delirium, coma, death
	- Management:
	    - Monitor (dark quiet room, restraints only if necessary)
	    - Benzos/Haloperidol (if needed)

Psilocybin	- 5-HT2 stimulating hallucinogenic - Found in certain mushrooms
Mescaline	- 5-HT2 stimulating hallucinogenic - Found in peyote
Inhalants	- Inhaled CNS depressant drugs - Types include toluene (solvents, paint thinners), glue, nitrous, and amyl nitrite (poppers)
Caffeine	- cAMP antagonist > 250 mg: Anxiety, insomnia, muscle twitching, rambling, diuresis > 1 g: Tinnitus, severe agitation, visual light flashes

PSYCHOTHERAPY — Psychiatry

General: Interpersonal therapy that attempts to alleviate psychological symptoms

Subtypes	Features
Cognitive-Behavioral Therapy	- Helps the patient identify and correct maladaptive beliefs - Utilizes cognitive/behavioral techniques (ie education, relaxation, stress management, coping skills, etc)
Psychodynamic	- Developing insight on patient's past experiences and relationships that may affect unconscious thought patterns
Interpersonal	- Emphasizes current relationships and the connection with depressive feelings
Supportive	- Conversational therapy that focuses upon current problematic relationships and maladaptive patterns of behavior - Promotes coping skills and improved self-esteem
Dialectical	- Promotes mindfulness, emotional regulation, in addition to other CBT type techniques - Designed for borderline personality patients
Motivational Interviewing	- Technique utilized to encourage patients to change maladaptive behaviors

Format: Most commonly individual therapy, but can be performed with couples, families, or in groups

Specific Technique	Features
Systematic Desensitization	- Relaxation techniques while being exposed to increasing doses of an anxiety-provoking stimulus
Flooding	- Confronted with an anxiety-provoking stimulus and not allowed to withdraw until they feel calm and in control
Aversion	- Negative response (ie shock) when specific behavior occurs
Biofeedback	- Monitor physiologic data as patients try to control their physiologic state (ie HR/BP) - Used in patients with anxiety, chronic pain, hypertension, migraines

PSYCHOPHARMACOTHERAPY — Psychiatry

	Mechanism	Indication	Side Effects/Management Concerns
SSRI Fluoxetine Sertraline Paroxetine Citalopram Escitalopram Fluvoxamine	- Inhibitor of 5-HT reuptake at synapse	- Depression/GAD/Panic Disorder - OCD (Fluvoxamine) - Bulimia - PTSD - Premenstrual Dysphoric Disorder - Premature Ejaculation	- All (usually subside): Headache, insomnia, vivid dreams, anorexia, GI (nausea, diarrhea), mania, platelet dysfunction - Sexual Dysfunction: Anorgasmia, decreased libido (does not subside, ~40% occurrence) - Lower dose, change med, or add Bupropion or Sildenafil - Rare/Life Threatening: Seizures (rare), SIADH, serotonin syndrome - Discontinuation Syndrome: Fatigue, HA, myalgias, paresthesias for rapidly stopping SSRI (except fluoxetine, which has long half life)
SNRI Venlafaxine Desvenlafaxine Duloxetine Milnacipran Levomilnacipran	- Inhibitor of 5-HT and Norepi reuptake	- Depression, GAD - PTSD, panic disorder, OCD - Neuropathic pain/fibromyalgia	- Side effects similar to SSRIs (PLUS noradrenergic symptoms like diaphoresis/dizziness) - BP can increase at higher doses

Psych38

PSYCHOPHARMACOTHERAPY — Psychiatry

	Mechanism	Indication	Side Effects/Management Concerns
TCA **Tertiary Amine** Amitriptyline Imipramine Clomipramine Doxepin **Secondary Amine** Desipramine Nortriptyline	- Inhibitor of 5-HT and Norepi reuptake - Highly Anticholinergic	- Amitriptyline: Chronic pain, migraines, insomnia - Imipramine: Enuresis - Clomipramine: OCD - Doxepin: Chronic pain	- Cardiotoxicity (prolonged QT, wide QRS) - Seizures/Coma - AntiHIS: Sedation, weight gain - AntiADR: Orthostasis, dizziness - AntiMUSC: Dry mouth, constipation, urinary retention, blurry vision - Anti-5-HT: Erectile dysfunction *TCA Overdose* - Presents with encephalopathy, anticholinergic symptoms, seizures, cardiac issues (QRS prolongation, heart block, risk for VTach/VFib) - Tx: $NaHCO_3$ (for > 100 ms QRS interval) - Benzo for seizures
MAO-I Tranylcypromine Phenelzine Isocarboxazid Selegiline	- Nonselective MAO A/B irreversible inhibitors	- Refractory/atypical depression	*Serotonin Syndrome* - Must wait weeks before switching from SSRI OR switching to MAO - Watch for SSRI, TCAs, St John's Wort, Meperidine, Dextromethorphan *Hypertensive Crisis* - Precipitated by tyramine rich foods (red wine, cheese, chicken liver, fava beans, cured meats) - HA, diaphoresis, photophobia, autonomic instability - Tx: Nifedipine or Phentolamine

PSYCHOPHARMACOTHERAPY — Psychiatry

	Mechanism	Indication	Side Effects/Management
Atypical Antidepressants			
Bupropion	- Increased Dopamine and Norepinephrine	- Depression - Smoking cessation	- Tachycardia, insomnia, anxiety, headache - Decreased seizure threshold (Contraindicated: Epilepsy, eating disorder) - No sexual side effects
Mirtazapine	- α2 antagonist (increases NE/5-HT release) - 5-HT, H1 antagonist	- Depression	- Sedation - Weight gain - Dry mouth, other anticholinergic effects
Trazodone Nefazodone	- Inhibitor of 5-HT2, α1 adrenergic, and H1	- Depression - Insomnia	- Sedation - Dizziness, orthostatic hypotension - Priapism (Tx: Epi injection into corpus) - Nefazodone → Black box warning for liver failure
Stimulants			
Amphetamines Methylphenidate	- Increases catecholamines in synaptic cleft	- ADHD	- Decreased appetite, weight loss - Possible growth delay (reversible with stopping) - Insomnia - Irritability/mood change - BP elevation - Exacerbation of tics - Decreased seizure threshold
Atomoxetine	- Inhibits norepi synaptic uptake	- ADHD	- Less abuse potential and side effects, but less effective

Psych40

PSYCHOPHARMACOTHERAPY — Psychiatry

	Mechanism	Indication	Side Effects/Management
Antipsychotics (first generation)			
Low Chlorpromazine Thioridazine *Mid* Perphenazine *High* Haloperidol Fluphenazine Pimozide	- D2 Receptor Blocker	- Schizophrenia - Bipolar	- Anti-H → Sedation, weight gain - Anti-α → Orthostatic hypotension - Anti-M → Dry mouth, tachycardia, urine retention - QT prolongation - Increased Prolactin (tuberoinfundibular) - Decreased libido, galactorrhea, gynecomastia - Extrapyramidal symptoms - Chlorpromazine → Blue gray skin deposition, photosensitivity, jaundice - Thioridazine → Pigmented retinopathy
Antipsychotics (second generation, or atypical)			
Clozapine Risperidone Quetiapine Olanzapine Ziprasidone Aripiprazole *Newest:* Paliperidone Iloperidone Lurasidone	- D2, 5-HT Receptor Blocker (Note: Aripiprazole is a partial D2 agonist)	- Schizophrenia - Bipolar - Borderline personality - Tic disorders	- Metabolic syndrome (monitor with weight, waist, BP, glucose, lipids) - AntiHis, Antiα, Anti-M (see above) - QT prolongation - Elderly: Increased risk of mortality - Clozapine: Agranulocytosis (must monitor WBC for 6 months weekly, next 6 months bi-weekly, then monthly). Stop if neutrophils < 1500. Can also cause seizures, myocarditis. - Quetiapine: Sedation, cataracts - Risperidone: Ends up in breast milk

PSYCHOPHARMACOTHERAPY — Psychiatry

Extrapyramidal Symptoms

	Features	Management
Dystonia	- Involuntary muscular contraction - Specific examples include oculogyric crisis, torticollis, opisthotonus	- Diphenhydramine - Benztropine
Dyskinesia (Parkinsonism)	- Impaired ability to perform normal movements	- Benztropine - Amantadine
Akathisia	- Restlessness	- Reduce dose - Benzo, beta-blockade, or benztropine
Tardive Dyskinesia	- Writhing movements of mouth and tongue, choreoathetoid movements of extremities - Believed due to D2 upregulation and hypersensitivity - Often irreversible	- D/C medication - Clozapine (if med is needed)

Neuroleptic Malignant Syndrome and Serotonin Syndrome

	NMS	Serotonin Syndrome
Gen	- Occurs in those using antipsychotics (especially first generation)	- Precipitated by the use of multiple serotonergic meds (MAO-I, SNRIs, TCAs, SSRIs, triptans, Meperidine, Dextromethorphan, St. John's wort)
Clin	- Encephalopathy - Fever (often > 40°C) - Muscle contractions - Autonomic instability (tachycardia, arrhythmias, tachypnea, diaphoresis) - Elevated CK, leukocytosis	- Neuromuscular activity (clonus, hypertonia, hyperreflexia, tremors) - Autonomic Instability (tachycardia, arrhythmias, tachypnea, diaphoresis) - Agitation/Confusion
Tx	- Stop neuroleptics - Supportive (fluids, cooling) - Dantrolene/Bromocriptine	- Stop offending medications - Supportive care - Benzos for agitation/spasms - Cyproheptadine

PSYCHOPHARMACOTHERAPY — Psychiatry

	Mechanism	Indication	Side Effects/Management
Mood Stabilizers			
Lithium	- Unknown	- Bipolar disorder - Augmentation of antidepressant	- Acute Side Effects: GI (nausea, diarrhea), tremor (give propranolol), ataxia, weakness - Chronic Side Effects: Nephrogenic DI, hypothyroidism, hyperparathyroidism, teratogen (Ebstein's), benign leukocytosis Toxic Levels - Precipitated by: Illness/dehydration, NSAIDs, ACE-I, diuretics, Metronidazole, Tetracycline - Altered mentation, tremors, convulsions, delirium - Tx: Hemodialysis if lithium level > 5 or > 2.5 with severe symptoms Contraindications: Severe renal or CV disease Management - Prior to start: ECG, chemistries (Cr/BUN), CBC, TSH, pregnancy test, urinalysis - Blood levels at 5 days, then every 2-3 days until therapeutic (after that every 6-12 months) - Monitor Cr/TSH q3-6 months
Carbamazepine Lamotrigine Valproate	[See: Neuro]		

NEONATOLOGY

Primary Care Pediatrics

Delivery Room Care

- Dry infant, clear airway secretions, provide warmth. Stimulate the infant.
- Apgar score (at minutes 1, 5. Helps to assess neonatal status, does not predict prognosis or mortality)

	Sign	0	1	2
A	Appearance	All blue	Blue extremities	All pink
P	Pulse	Absent	< 100 bpm	> 100 bpm
G	Grimace	Absence	Weak grimace	Cough/cry
A	Activity	Limp	Some flexion	Fully active
R	Respiratory	Absent	Weak cry	Good cry

- APGAR > 7: Good status. Do not require any resuscitation. Give to mom for skin-to-skin contact and early breastfeeding.

Neonatal Resuscitation

Situation	Intervention (in order of escalation of care)
HR < 100 bpm	(1) Positive pressure ventilation (intubation if prolonged/inadequate) (2) Chest compressions (if no improvement despite ventilation) (3) Epinephrine (if no response to compressions)
Labored Breathing Cyanosis	- Supplemental O_2 with O_2 monitoring

Newborn Nursery

Eye Care	- Erythromycin ophthalmic ointment Note: Serves as PPX for gonococcal conjunctivitis (not chlamydia)
Vitamin K	- Single IM dose - Prevents vitamin K deficiency bleeding
Hepatitis B Vax	- First vaccine within 24 hours of delivery (regardless of maternal status)
Umbilical Cord	- Sterile clamp/cutting, with "dry cord care" (keep clean/dry) - Umbilical Granuloma: Friable, moist, pink pedunculated lesion that can occur at umbilical stump. - Tx: Silver nitrate
Feeding	- 8-12 feeds per day. Helps prevent hypoglycemia. Note: Up to 10% weight loss is typical in first few days after birth, but should be regained by 14 days

NEONATOLOGY		Primary Care Pediatrics

Newborn Nursery

Screening	- O_2 Saturation (to monitor for congenital heart disease) - Genetic Panel: "Blood spot" testing, which is sent to identify a variety of inherited disorders - Hearing screening
Monitoring	- Glucose - Bilirubin
Circumcision	- Elective procedure that is controversial. Generally believed that benefits > risks, but information should be provided to family to make informed decision. - Benefits: ↓ Risk of penile cancer, UTI, foreskin retractile disorders. ↓ transmission of HIV/HPV/HSV. - Risks: Bleeding, infection, glans injury (extremely rare), fistula formation, excess skin removal, etc.

Breastfeeding

	Benefits
Infant	- Improved immunity (decreased risk of acute illnesses, such as sepsis, respiratory disease, gastroenteritis, UTI, and gastroenteritis) - Improvement of GI function/maturity - Possible long term benefits (cancer, obesity, etc)
Maternal	- Reduced rates of breast and ovarian cancer - Maternal-infant bonding - Accelerated recovery from childbirth - Quicker return to prepartum weight - Improved child spacing (from suppression of normal cycle) - Reduced expense

Contraindications:
Maternal
- Active herpetic breast lesions
- HIV or HTLV infection
- Current chemotherapy or radiation therapy
- Abuse of street drugs or alcohol

Infant
- Galactosemia

[See: OB] for maternal complications of breastfeeding.

NEONATOLOGY

Primary Care Pediatrics

Prematurity

General: Birth at < 37 gestational weeks. Associated with increased risk for multiple complications (see below).
- Corrected Gestational Age
    - Chronologic age minus number of weeks born before 40 weeks
    - Useful until age of 2 years old, when preemies should be caught up

Complications:

Immediate	Long-Term
- Systemic (Hypothermia, hypoglycemia, hypotension, hypocalcemia) - Respiratory (RDS, apnea of prematurity, bronchopulmonary dysplasia) - GI (gastroesophageal reflux, NEC) - CNS (intraventricular hemorrhage) - Retinopathy of prematurity - ↑ Infection/sepsis risk - Hyperbilirubinemia	- Overall increased mortality, morbidity (↑ hospitalizations) - Neurodevelopmental delay - Growth impairment - Impaired respiratory function

Postterm

General: Birth at > 42 gestational weeks. Associated with the below complications:

Immediate	Long-Term
- Meconium aspiration syndrome - Polycythemia - Neonatal asphyxia - Dysmaturity syndrome - Overall ↑ neonatal morbidity/mortality	- N/A

Weight

General:
- Small for Gestational Age (< 10 percentile) or 2500 g
- Large for Gestational Age (> 90 percentile) or 4000 g

Risk:
- SGA: IUGR, genetics
- LGA: Diabetes mellitus (both gestational and preexisting), excessive weight gain, fetal sex (male), ↑ gestational age

Complications:

Small for Gestational Age	Large for Gestational Age
- Hypothermia, hypoglycemia - Polycythemia	- Hypothermia - Birth injuries common (clavicle fracture, brachial plexus injury, facial nerve palsy, shoulder dystocia)

NEONATOLOGY
Primary Care Pediatrics

Indirect Hyperbilirubinemia

General: Almost all newborns have elevated levels of indirect bilirubin, and severely ↑ levels (> 25 mg/dL) put at risk for bilirubin-induced neurologic dysfunction (BIND)

Etiology	General	Clinical/Timing
Physiologic	- High bilirubin production, low hepatic UDPGT, low levels of bile metabolizing intestinal flora	- Within days of birth
Hemolysis	- ABO incompatibility - Anti-Rh disease	- Within 24 hours of birth
Breast Milk Jaundice	- High β-glucuronidase in breast milk	- Starts ~3-5 days, peaks at 2 weeks - Jaundice, but normal otherwise without issues feeding
Breastfeeding Jaundice	- Failure of lactation, resulting in ↑ enterohepatic circulation	- Around 1 week - Poor feeding - Often have signs of dehydration
Others	- Crigler-Najjar - Congenital hypothyroidism - Galactosemia - Chronic disorders of hemolysis (ie spherocytosis) - Sepsis - Increased RBC load from birth trauma	

Clinical:
- Jaundice (yellow discoloration of conjunctiva/extremities)
    - If below level of umbilicus, exact level should be checked
    - Note: Any jaundice within 24 hours is pathologic

Diagnosis: Can measure with blood test or transcutaneous bilirubinometer
- Defined as > 95th percentile on the hourly Bhutani nomogram

Management:
- Phototherapy (for any with hyperbilirubinemia based on nomogram)
- Exchange transfusion (for any with signs of neurologic dysfunction)
- IVIG (for isoimmune hemolytic disease)

… NEONATOLOGY — Primary Care Pediatrics

Direct Hyperbilirubinemia

General: Elevations of direct bilirubin are always pathologic in neonates

Etiology:
- Biliary atresia
- Choledocal cysts
- Hepatitis
- Genetic/inherited metabolic conditions

BIND/Kernicterus

Bilirubin-induced neurologic dysfunction (BIND): Acute neurologic deficits from hyperbilirubinemia
- Lethargy, hypotonia initially
- Progresses to coma, seizures, hypertonia (opisthotonos/retrocollis) if not treated

Kernicterus: Long term sequelae of CNS bilirubin deposition
- Cerebral palsy
- Hearing loss
- Gaze defects
- Dental enamel hypoplasia/dysplasia

NEONATOLOGY — Primary Care Pediatrics

Birth Trauma

Disorder	Clinical Findings
Cephalohematoma	- Subperiosteal collection of blood, causing head mass - Usually self-limited, resolve over next few months
Caput Succedaneum	- Swelling of the scalp above the periosteum - Presents as irregular swelling that crosses suture lines - Usually self-limited, resolves over few days
Subgaleal Hemorrhage	- Blood accumulation between periosteum of the skull and the aponeurosis (usually due to dural venous sinus injury) - High risk for massive blood loss in this space - Presents with shifting, fluctuant, skull mass, plus eventual hemodynamic instability
Clavicle Fracture	- Most common fracture associated with birth - Can present with immobility of affected arm, crepitus, and edema - Dx: XR - Tx: Reassurance, NSAID analgesia, long sleeved garment, pin arm to chest
Others	- Intracranial hemorrhage (subdural, epidural, etc) - Fracture (humeral, femur, etc) all fairly rare - Nasal septal dislocation - Brachial plexus injury

Other Musculoskeletal

Neonatal Torticollis	- Postural deformity of the neck, characterized by lateral neck flexion and neck rotation. Can be due to hypertonic sternocleidomastoid muscle. - Associated with multiple gestation, breech, oligohydramnios - Risk for developing craniofacial abnormalities or plagiocephaly, as well as other musculoskeletal abnormalities - Dx: Clinical - Tx: Positioning changes, physical therapy. Surgery if refractory.
Positional Plagiocephaly	- Head asymmetry from pressure on head from prolonged sleeping position - Tx: Change positioning

NEONATOLOGY — Primary Care Pediatrics

Respiratory Failure

	General	Clinical	Management
Neonatal Respiratory Distress Syndrome	- Diffuse atelectasis from insufficient quantity of surfactant - Risk: Prematurity, maternal diabetes	- Severe respiratory distress and cyanosis - CXR (diffuse ground glass, low lung volumes, air bronchograms)	- Supplemental O_2 (+ CPAP or intubation) as needed - Surfactant - PPX: [See: OBGYN]
Transient Tachypnea of Newborn	- Mild pulmonary edema from failed alveolar fluid clearance at birth - Risk: Prematurity, C-section, maternal diabetes	- Tachypnea starting at birth, and improving within days - CXR shows bilateral perihilar linear streaks	- Supportive - Supplemental O_2 (+ CPAP or intubation) as needed
Persistent Pulmonary Hypertension	- Right-to-left shunt from persistently elevated pulmonary pressures post birth - Risk: Meconium aspiration, perinatal asphyxia	- Tachypnea and cyanosis - CXR (clear lungs, possible ↓ pulmonary vasculature)	- Supportive care - 100% O_2 (helps to ↑ PVR) - If severe: IV NO, Sildenafil, or ECMO
Meconium Aspiration	- Aspiration of meconium-stained amniotic fluid	- Diagnosis of exclusion - Respiratory distress, tachypnea, cyanosis. Trachea may have meconium. - CXR (patchy densities and areas of hyperinflation)	- Avoid suctioning/intubation immediately after birth - Supplemental O_2, supportive care - Antibiotics
Apnea of Prematurity	- Periods of apnea in premature neonate from immaturely developed respiratory drive or airway obstruction	- Cessation of breathing > 20 seconds OR - Shorter period of apnea that causes hypoxemia or bradycardia	- Supportive care - CPAP therapy - Methylxanthine (caffeine)

NEONATOLOGY
Primary Care Pediatrics

Newborn Skin Rashes

Condition	Features	Management
Congenital Melanocytic Nevus	- Large benign moles - Low rate of malignant transformation, but should be monitored closely	- Monitor - Biopsy if suspicious
Congenital Dermal Melanocytosis	- Also known as "Mongolian Spot" - Hyperpigmented, congenital blue-grey patches over low back/butt of infants - Benign, fades spontaneously over first few years of life	- Monitor, document well
Nevus Sebaceous	- Overgrown epidermis/hair follicles - Presents with smooth, yellow, hairless patch, oval in shape - Scalp most common location	- Monitor, usually benign
Aplasia Cutis Congenita	- Congenital lesion of abnormal skin development - Presents with erosion/ulcerative lesion - Scalp most common, but can occur anywhere	- Wound care or surgical closure
Nevus Simplex	- "Stork Bite." Common neonatal finding. - Benign vascular proliferation found on glabella, neck, eyelid - Presents as blanchable, pink-red patches	- Fades within years
Nevus Flammeus	- "Port wine stain" vascular malformation - Associated with Sturge-Weber (if in V1 formation)	- Grows with child
Erythema Toxicum Neonatorum	- Scattered erythematous papules, pustules throughout the body	- No treatment - Resolves within days
Neonatal Acne	- Inflammatory papules/pustules on face	- No treatment - Resolves within days
Seborrheic Dermatitis	- Yellow, erythematous, greasy plaques, on scalp ("cradle cap"), face, body	- Topical steroids
Miliaria	- Blockage of sweat ducts, causing small papules and vesicles on head/upper torso	- Resolves with cooling/avoiding excess clothes
Neonatal HSV	- Clusters of vesicles on skin and mucous membranes - CNS, organ system involvement possible	- Acyclovir

NEONATOLOGY — Primary Care Pediatrics

Germinal Matrix Hemorrhage/Intraventricular Hemorrhage

General: Germinal matrix hemorrhage due to vascular fragility in premature babies

Risk: Prematurity, low birth weight, respiratory distress/neonatal resuscitation

Clinical: Can be clinically silent, or result in altered level of consciousness, hypotonia, decreased activity, seizures, coma, or other neurologic deficits

Diagnosis: Cranial US

Management:
- Purely supportive (maintain proper hemodynamic status, correct fluid/electrolytes, proper nutrition, etc)
- Monitor for complications with serial US

Complications:
- Ventricular dilation
    - May result in ↑ ICP and further neurologic damage
    - Tx: Serial lumbar punctures or ventricular drain

Neonatal Conjunctivitis (ophthalmia neonatorum)

Type	Clinical	Management
Gonococcal	- Within 2-5 days of birth - Severe exudates/swelling of eyelids - Corneal edema/ulceration - Dx: Gram stain/culture	- IM Ceftriaxone - Eye irrigation
Chlamydial	- Presents at 5-14 days post birth - Watery/ mucopurulent eye discharge	- PO Erythromycin
Chemical	- Conjunctivitis from ointments used for bacterial conjunctivitis PPX - Commonly due to silver nitrate (no longer used in US), but can also be due to others	- Self-limited - Lubricant eye drops
HSV	- Presents at 5-14 days - Unilateral serous discharge	- Acyclovir

| NEONATOLOGY | Primary Care Pediatrics |

Hypoglycemia

General: Blood sugar < 50-60 mg/dL

Risk: Preterm infant, fetal growth restriction, large babies/maternal diabetes

Clinical:
- Often asymptomatic
- Can manifest as jitteriness, irritability, poor tone, lethargy, poor suck/feed, seizures

Management:
- Oral feedings (if asymptomatic/not severe)
- Parenteral glucose (if symptomatic/severe)

Polycythemia

General: Hematocrit > 65%

Risk: Delayed cord clamping, twin-to-twin transfusion, maternal diabetes

Clinical:
- Often asymptomatic
- Possible lethargy, poor feeding, etc
- Hyperviscosity symptoms
- Associated with hypoglycemia

Management:
- IV Hydration/Glucose
- Partial fluid exchange: Reserved for severe or progressive symptoms

Neonatal Sepsis

General: Systemic signs of infection plus isolation of a bacteria from blood. Most commonly due to Group B *Strep*.

Risk: Chorioamnionitis, prematurity, prolonged rupture of membranes

Clinical:
- Fever, respiratory distress, tachycardia
- Poor feeding, lethargy, irritability

Diagnosis: Blood, urine and CSF cultures

Management:
- Empiric antibiotics (Ampicillin and Gentamicin)
    - Vanco can be substituted in if concern for MRSA

PEDIATRIC VACCINATIONS

Primary Care Pediatrics

	0M	1M	2M	4M	6M	9M	12M	15M	18M	2Y	2.5Y	3Y	4Y	5Y	7-10Y	11-12Y	13-18Y
Hep B	#1	#2			#3												
DTaP			#1	#2	#3			#4					#5				
Hib			#1	#2	#3		#4										
PCV13			#1	#2	#3		#4										
IPV			#1	#2	#3								#4				
Rota			#1	#2	*3												
MMR							#1						#2				
Varicella							#1						#2				
Hep A							#1		#2								
Influenza							Yearly Vaccination (2 doses at first ever)										
MenACWY																#1	#2 (@16)
MenB																	*: 2 Dose Series
HPV																	#: 2 Dose Series
Tdap																#1	

#= Normal recommended vax.   *= Special Circumstances

Contraindications (do not give vaccine in future)	Precautions (defer vaccines until the condition is improved)
- Anaphylaxis after prior administration - Severe immunodeficiency (heme/solid tumor, chemo, HIV, congenital immunodeficiency, etc) → No live vaccines - Pregnancy → No live vaccines - Encephalopathy within 7 days (any pertussis-containing vax) - Intussusception, SCID (Rota vax)	- Moderate or severe acute illness, +/- fever - DTaP: Temp > 40.5°C within 48 hr, seizures within 3 days, or inconsolable crying > 3 hr within 48 hr of vaccine - MMR/VZV: IVIG within year prior to administration (may prevent proper immune response to vaccine)

Peds11

DEVELOPMENTAL MILESTONES

Primary Care Pediatrics

	Motor	Fine Motor	Communication/Social	Cognitive
2 M	- Lifts head	- Holds hands together	- Social smile	- Recognizes parent
4 M	- Rolls	- Grasps rattle	- Laughs, soothed by parents	- Directs head to voice
6 M	- Sits without support	- Transfers objects	- Babbles, stranger anxiety	- Feeds self
9 M	- Pulls to stand - Creeps/crawls	- Immature pincer - Bangs two cubes	- Says mama/dada - Waves bye	- Object permanence - Separation anxiety
12 M	- Stands/begins to walk	- Fine pincer - Throws objects	- Follows one step command with gesture	- Points
15 M	- Stoops and recovers	- Scribbles	- 3-5 word vocab	- Turns page
18 M	- Runs - Creeps down stairs	- 3 cube tower	- 10-25 word vocab - Imitates sounds	- Removes clothes
2 Y	- Throws a ball - Kicks ball	- Copies line	- 2 word combos - 50 word vocab, 50% intelligible	- Sorts objects - Matches objects to picture
3 Y	- Rides tricycle - Goes up stairs alt feet	- Copies circle - Line of cubes	- 3 word sentences - 75% intelligible, parallel play	- Knows own gender/age
4 Y	- Hops	- Copies square/cross	- 100% intelligible	- Knows 4 colors
5 Y	- Skips	- Copies triangle	- Defines simple words	- Dresses self

DEVELOPMENTAL MILESTONES

Primary Care Pediatrics

Primitive Reflexes

	Description	Disappears by
Hand grasp	- Reflex grasp of object placed in palm	3M
Sucking	- When roof of mouth is touched	4M
Moro	- Abduction/extension of arms after startle	4M
Rooting	- Turn head toward side of cheek stimulus	6M
Galant	- Stroke spine, causing baby to laterally flex torso towards side of stimulus	9M
Plantar	- Dorsiflexion of foot and flexion of toes with plantar stimulation	12M

SCREENING

Primary Care Pediatrics

Test	Timing/Frequency	Details
H/H (Fe Def Anemia)	- 1 y/o - Repeated if risk factors	
Developmental Screen	- 9M, 18M, 24/30M	- Variety of questionnaires, such as Parents Evaluation of Developmental Status
Autism Screen	- 18, 24 M	- MCHAT-RF
Hearing	- Start at 4 y/o	
Vision	- Start at 3 y/o	- Test for strabismus - Test for visual acuity (as soon as child old enough to perform test)
TB Risk Assessment	- 6M, 12M, then annually	- Only use PPD/other screen if risk factors presents
Lead	- Blood Screen: 1Y, 2Y - Risk Assessment: 6, 9, 12, 18, 24 M	- Screening should be adjusted to location (CDC recommendations)
Lipid	- Once 9-11 y/o - Once 17-21 y/o	
Drug/Alcohol	- Annually starting at 11Y	- CRAFFT Screen
Depression	- Annually starting at 12Y	
STD	- Chlamydia/Gonorrhea: Annually screen sexually active females < 25 y/o - HIV: One time screen (between 15-65 y/o)	

ANTICIPATORY GUIDANCE — Primary Care Pediatrics

Topic	Advice
Weight	- Infants can lose up to 10% of weight in first few days of life, but should regain birth weight by 2 weeks old - Infants double birth weight by 4M and triple birth weight by 1Y - Infants gain ~20-30g per day - Gain about 2 kg (4-5 lbs)/yr after this
Height	- Height increases 50% by 1Y, doubles by 4Y, triples by 13Y - Height growth velocity varies, but is ~2-4 inches/year between 1Y and 10Y, progressively slowing as pubertal growth spurt approaches
Diet	- Feed infants every 2-3 hours (8-12 times/day), ~15 min per breast - Supplement vitamin D if breastfeeding - Energy requirement 100 kcal/kg/day (which should be more if premature or low birth weight) - Introduce iron fortified cereals ~6 months and slowly add other solid foods - Switch to whole milk (~12 months) - Encourage healthy food choices, avoiding sweets - Limit juice to < 5 oz due to risk of dental caries
Dental	- Teeth erupt around 6 months and onwards - See dentist within 6 months of first tooth eruption - Ensure proper fluoride (usually tap water sufficient, but depends on area) - Should start brushing teeth once they emerge
Bowel Movements	- Over first week, stool transitions from meconium, to yellow/seedy, and eventually more brown - 4/day during the first week, 2/day by 1Y, and 1/day by 4Y
Urine	- For first week, # of wet diapers should be about the age of child in days - After first week, ≥ 4 wet diapers/day - Can start toilet training around 18M, usually successful by 3-4 y/o
Sleeping	- Initially sleep at 3-4 hour stretches for 18-20 hours per day - As child gets older, they sleep less overall and for longer stretches - Many sleep through night by 6M - 1-2 naps/day normal in years 1-4
Car Seats	< 2 Y: Rear-facing car seat (in rear) 2-4 Y: Forward facing car seat (in rear) 4-8 Y: Belt-positioning booster seat (until reach 4'9" tall) < 13 Y: Should ride in rear seats

ANTICIPATORY GUIDANCE — Primary Care Pediatrics

Safety	(Infant) - Sleep on back - Hot water heater < 120°F - Avoid objects that can be aspirated - No walkers - Weapons and pet safety - Sunscreen (1 yr) - Childproof house (3 yr) - Helmets - Street safety - Stranger danger - Water safety/swimming lessons

Misc. Infant/Toddler Problems

Diaper Rash	- Irritant contact dermatitis from constant contact with diaper - Involves anywhere, but spares skin folds (if hits folds, concern for *Candida*) - Tx: Topical barrier ointments (Petrolatum, Zinc oxide), topical steroids if severe
Breath Holding Spells	- Involuntary, harmless breath holding events - Toddler can become cyanotic or pallid (pale/limp) - Reassurance
Temper Tantrum	- Angry outbursts from fatigue or frustration - Decrease as child gets older
School Phobia	- Vague physical complaints only prior to school

ANTICIPATORY GUIDANCE
Primary Care Pediatrics

Adolescents: Puberty

Puberty (Females)
- Girls start puberty between 8 and 13 years of age
    - Breast buds appear (age 10-11 years)
    - Pubic hair appears (age 10-11 years)
    - Growth spurt (age 12 years)
    - Menarche (age 12-13 years)
    - Attainment of adult height (age 15 years)

Tanner	Breast	Pubic Hair
1	Elevation of papilla	None
2	Breast bud (elevation of breast/papilla)	Sparse hair along labia
3	Further growth in breast/papilla	Darker hair grows along labia
4	Projection of breast/papilla (secondary mound)	Coarse, curly hair covering symphysis pubis
5	Normal adult contour	Adult hair extends to medial thigh

Puberty (Males)
- Boys start puberty between 10 and 15 years of age
    - Growth of testicles (age 12 years)
    - Pubic hair appears (age 12 years)
    - Growth of penis, scrotum (age 13-14 years)
    - First ejaculations (age 13-14 years)
    - Growth spurt (age 14 years)
    - Attainment of adult height (age 17 years)

Tanner	Phallus	Pubic Hair
1	Prepubertal testes	None
2	Testes start to enlarge	Sparse, long
3	Testes continue to enlarge Penis length increases	Some dark, coarse, curly hair
4	Penis length/width further increases	Dark coarse curly hair of symphysis pubis
5	Adult sized testes/penis	Dark coarse curly hair extending to medial thigh

ANTICIPATORY GUIDANCE — Primary Care Pediatrics

Adolescents: Guidance/Screening

Early Adolescence (10-13 y/o)	- Starts to desire independence from family - Preoccupation with pubertal changes - Risk taking behaviors
Middle Adolescence (13-18 y/o)	- Conflicts with family - Preoccupation with physical appearance/presentation - Peer-group involvement, begins romantic relationships
Late Adolescence (18-21 y/o)	- Development of self separate from parents - Comfortable with body image

Screening (also see the screening/vaccination charts)

Social Hx	HEADSSS (Home, Education, Activities, Drugs, Sex, Suicide, Safety)
Drugs/EtOH	CRAFT - Have you ever ridden in a CAR driven by someone (including yourself) who was "high" or had been using alcohol or drugs? - Do you ever use alcohol or drugs to RELAX, feel better about yourself, or fit in? - Do you ever use alcohol/drugs while you are by yourself, ALONE? - Do you ever FORGET things you did while using alcohol or drugs? - Have you gotten into TROUBLE while you were using alcohol or drugs?
Confidentiality	- Important to create rapport with adolescents, and should keep all discussions confidential from parents - Includes: Pregnancy, birth control, mental health, drugs/EtOH - Excludes: Abuse (sexual/physical), suicidal/homicidal

GROWTH DISTURBANCES
Primary Care Pediatrics

Failure to Thrive

General: Abnormal weight gain in first 2 years of life. No definitive definition, but considered when weight < 2 percentile, weight falls more than 2 lines on growth curve, or weight gain is less than linear growth velocity.

	Organic	Non-organic
Definition	- Acute/chronic medical disorder - Usually have signs/symptoms associated with this disorder	- No underlying disease or disorder - Due to malnutrition for caregiver neglect, stress, or lack of parenting skills
Etiologies	- Cystic fibrosis - Congenital heart defects - Chronic vomiting (from GI disorder like bowel obstruction or GER) - HIV - CNS (cerebral palsy, hydrocephalus)	- Poverty - Poor feeding techniques - Inadequate breast milk or formula

Diagnosis: Clinical diagnosis based on definition provided above. Thorough H/P and workup required to determine underlying cause.

Management:
- Interdisciplinary care (nutritionist, OT, speech therapy, social worker, etc)
- Nutritional catch-up: Calculate daily energy requirement, provide enough calories to overcome this level
    - High calorie formulas for infants, high calorie additions for those eating solid foods
- Hospitalization for severe cases

GROWTH DISTURBANCES

Primary Care Pediatrics

Differential for Microcephaly

General: Occipitofrontal circumference < 2 SD below mean for age

Etiology:

Congenital	Acquired
- TORCH infections - Teratogen exposure (ie EtOH) - Trisomy 13, 18, 21	- Late pregnancy infections - Meningitis - Ischemic brain insults - Metabolic (hypothyroid)

Clinical:
- Associated with small brain size
- Often occurs with intellectual disability, developmental delay, cerebral palsy

Differential for Macrocephaly

General: Occipitofrontal circumference > 2 SD below mean for age

Etiology:
- Increased Brain Size: Anatomic or familial megalencephaly
- Increased CSF: Hydrocephalus
- Hemorrhage
- Mass lesions

Clinical:
- Work up if single measurement > 2 SD OR
- Crosses multiple lines on the head circumference growth curve

Diagnosis: Evaluate with MRI (or CT)

Management: Treat underlying condition

SIDS/CHILD ABUSE

Primary Care Pediatrics

Sudden Infant Death Syndrome (SIDS)

General: Sudden death of infant < 1 y/o, with no clear underlying cause after thorough autopsy and evaluation. Pathophysiology unknown. Most common cause of death between 1M and 1Y.

Risk Factor	Prevention
- Smoking (in household) during/after pregnancy	- Smoke avoidance
- Prone/side sleep position	- Supine sleeping
- Soft sleep surface with loose bedding	- Firm surface, without extra blankets/ pillows
- Bed sharing	- Avoid bed sharing
Other: - Maternal age < 20 - Prematurity	Other: - Use pacifier

Clinical: Often no signs, but can have evidence of terminal event like bloody froth in mouth, clenched fists

Child Abuse

General: Physical injury inflicted on a child by a caretaker

Clinical:
- Bruises (in pre-mobile infant, located on butt/back, in pattern of striking object)
- Oral injuries
- Burns (if well-demarcated, appear due to immersion injury)
- Fractures (multiple fractures in different healing stages, most commonly ribs/sternum fx, metaphyseal corner fx, bilateral long bone fx, skull fx)
- Head trauma
    - Retinal hemorrhages
    - Skull fractures
    - Bulging fontanelles
    - Encephalopathy
- Suspect if: Inconsistent stories from caregiver, story is out of proportion with injury, vague history, story not consistent with age of child

Diagnosis:
- Skeletal survey
- Dry CT (if head trauma suspected)

Management:
- Remove from caregiver's care
- Contact appropriate authorities
- Manage patient's injuries

Peds21

COLIC/PEDIATRIC CONSTIPATION
Primary Care Pediatrics

Colic

General: Crying for no clear reason, lasting for ≥ 3 hr/day and occuring on ≥ 3 days/week, in healthy infant < 3 months old

Clinical:
- Paroxysmal episodes of crying
- Compared to normal crying, colic is higher pitched, louder, and involves clenched fists and facial flushing
- Normal physical examination/developmental history

Management:
- Most often improves as child gets older
- Provide parental support
- Soothing techniques (pacifier, rocking baby, rubbing tummy)
- Feeding techniques (fix underfeeding/overfeeding, inadequate burping)

Differential:

Normal Crying	- Intermittent, < 2 hr/day - Generally consolable with soothing methods

Pediatric Constipation

General: Common primary care presentation in preschool-aged children

Risk: Excess cow's milk, newly introduced solid foods, toilet training, school entry

Clinical:
- Painful, firm/small bowel movements
- Refusal to defecate, with eventual encopresis possible
- Can be complicated by anal fissure, hemorrhoid, or UTI

Management:
- Increase fiber intake, increase water intake, minimize cow's milk to < 24 oz
- Laxatives (ie polyethylene glycol or lactulose)
- Suppositories/enemas if necessary

Growing Pains

General: Pain that wakes child at night, not associated with MSK disease

Clinical: Bilateral pain in thighs or calves that occurs at night, resolves in morning

Management:
- Education/reassurance
- Stretching, massage, heat, analgesics

CHROMOSOMAL ABNORMALITIES

Genetics — Pediatrics

	General/Clinical	Management
Trisomy 13 (Patau)	- Dysmorphic features: Microphthalmia, microcephaly, cleft lip/palate, cutis aplasia, polydactyly - Holoprosencephaly, severe intellectual deficits - Cardiovascular defects (ASD/VSD/PDA) - Umbilical hernia, omphalocele	Dx: Karyotype (alt: FISH) Tx: None. Most die within days to weeks after birth.
Trisomy 18 (Edward's)	- Dysmorphia: Micrognathia, low-set ears, prominent occiput - Clenched fists with overlapping fingers - Cardiovascular defects (VSD, PDA) - Renal (horseshoe kidney) - GI (Meckel's diverticulum and malrotation)	Dx: Karyotype (alt: FISH) Tx: None. Most die within 1 yr (those that survive have severe intellectual defects).
Trisomy 21 (Down's)	- 95% meiotic nondisjunction, 4% Robertsonian translocation (14-21) - Intellectual disability, slowed growth (both length/weight) - Facies (Upslanting palpebral fissures, small ears, flattened midface, epicanthal folds) - Hypotonia, redundant nuchal skin, reduced startle - Brushfield spots, protruding tongue, single palmar crease, gap between first two toes - CV: Complete AV septal defect, ASD, VSD - GI: Duodenal atresia, imperforate anus, esophageal atresia, Hirschsprung, Celiac's - Endo: Congenital hypothyroidism, shore stature, obesity, T1DM - Heme: ↑ Risk ALL/AML - CNS: Early onset dementia (Alzheimer's subtype) - Atlantoaxial instability	Dx: Karyotype (lymphocyte). 2nd Line: FISH. Tx: - Monitor for complications (ie screen patient with CBC, TSH, ECHO, hearing/ophtho tests, cervical MRI, etc) - Life expectancy reduced

CHROMOSOMAL ABNORMALITIES

Genetics — Pediatrics

	General/Clinical	Management

Turner (XO)	- Partial or full loss of X chromosome (from paternal nondisjunction, mosaicism, or partial X)
	- Short stature, shield chest, widely spaced nipples, webbed neck, cubitus valgus, cystic hygroma/lymphedema
	- Primary hypogonadism (amenorrhea, lack of pubertal development)
	- Cardiovascular
	  - Bicuspid valve, aortic coarctation, other arch/septal abnormalities
	  - High risk for aortic dissection, especially during pregnancy
	- Osteoporosis
	- Endocrine (obesity, insulin resistance, hypothyroidism)
	- Risk for gonadoblastoma (if Y chromosome present)
	- Generally infertile, but can become pregnant with IVF/donor eggs
		Dx: Karyotype
		
		Tx:
		- GH replacement during childhood
		- E2 replace starting around 11-12 (to initiate puberty)
		- Screen for common complications (ie ECHO and monitoring for cardiovascular disease)

Klinefelter (47 XXY)	- Due to nondisjunction of sex chromosomes - Small, firm testes with abnormal leydig cells/seminiferous tubules - Subnormal sperm count/infertility (↑ FSH/LH) - Gynecomastia, female hair distribution - Eunuchoid body shape, abnormally tall with long arms/legs - Psychosocially abnormal	Dx: Karyotype
XXX	- Generally normal, with increased likelihood of being tall, and average IQ less than normal	Dx: Karyotype
XYY	- Tall stature, mild intellectual disability, developmental delays	Dx: Karyotype

GENETICS

	General/Clinical	Management
Fragile X	- FMR1 (CGG repeats → ↑ FMR methylation → ↓ gene expression) - Long/narrow face, prominent forehead, large ears, macroorchidism - Moderate intellectual disability (most common inherited form of ID) - Behavioral abnormalities (ADHD, stereotyped movements, etc) - Associated with hypermobile joints, GERD, MVP - Girls can be asymptomatic or have mild retardation/behavioral issues	Dx: Genetic testing Tx: Multidisciplinary management of behavioral and cognitive problems
Rett's	- XD disease females in the MECP gene - Normal initial development, followed by progressive loss of speech and motor skills starting around 1-2 y/o - Stereotypical hand movements, seizures, autism all possible	Dx: Clinical features/DNA analysis Tx: Multidisciplinary supportive care
Lesch-Nyhan	- XR HGPRT enzyme deficiency (defective purine metabolism) - Onset @ 6 months of hypotonia, persistent vomiting - Develop intellectual disability, choreoathetosis, spasticity, compulsive self injury, other behavioral abnormalities - Uric acid deposition (gouty arthritis, tophi, obstructive nephropathy)	Dx: Clinical, plus genetic testing Tx: Allopurinol

GENETICS

Genetics Pediatrics

	General/Clinical	Management
Ehlers-Danlos	- AR or AD defects in collagen synthesis - Depending on subtype, some combination of skin hyperextensibility, joint hypermobility, joint dislocations, scoliosis, translucent/hyperextensible skin, poor wound healing, easy bruising, vascular dissection/dilatation - Type I/II (classic, MSK/skin symptoms) - Type III (mostly MSK) - Type IV (high risk for vascular problems, MSK normal)	Dx: Clinical + genetic testing Tx: Supportive care/monitor for complications
Marfan's	- AD defect in fibrillin-1 - Cardiovascular: Aortic dissection/regurgitation/dilatation, MVP - Ectopic lens - MSK: Joint hypermobility, arachnodactyly, long arms/legs, pectus deformity, kyphosis/scoliosis - Pulm: Lung bullae/spontaneous PTX	Dx: Clinical (aortic dilatation/ectopic lens) plus genetic mutation Tx: - Aortic dilatation: Monitor with ECHO, add beta-blocker/ARB, surgery if severely enlarged
Menkes	- XR defect in ATP7A, leading to severe copper deficiency - Brittle kinky hair, growth retardation, hypotonia, epilepsy, progressive neurodegeneration	Tx: Administer Cu
Osteogenesis Imperfecta	- AD defect in COL1A gene - Bone Abnormalities: Can range from mild (premature osteoporosis/bone loss) to severe (multiple fractures from minimal/no trauma) - Other features: Blue sclera, short stature, scoliosis, hearing loss, opalescent teeth, easy bruising - Multiple subtypes. Type I (mild), Type II (severe/fetal demise), types III-VI (moderate symptoms)	Dx: Clinical + genetic testing Tx: - Multidisciplinary care - Monitor for complications - Bisphosphonates for most

GENETICS

Genetics Pediatrics

	General/Clinical	Management
Xeroderma Pigmentosum	- AR abnormality in repair of pyrimidine dimers from UV light - Risk for SCC, BCC, and melanoma starting in childhood - Keratitis, hypo/hyperpigmentation, opacification of the cornea	Dx: Clinical, plus genetic testing Tx: Avoid sunlight exposure
Primary Ciliary Dyskinesia (Kartagener)	- AR defect in dynein arms, resulting in abnormal ciliary movement - Chronic rhinosinusitis, cough - Recurrent otitis media - Infertility: Immotile sperm, dysfunctional fallopian tubes - Situs inversus - Screening test: Low nasal NO	Dx: Electron microscopy (showing ciliary dysfunction) Tx: Chest physiotherapy, surgical intervention for advanced disease
McCune Albright	- Sporadic, postzygotic mutation in GNAS gene (inappropriate G-protein signaling, resulting in excess cAMP). Always mosaic. - Fibrous dysplasia of bone - Endocrinopathies (hyperthyroid, GH secretion, hypercortisolism, etc) - Multiple café-au lait spots - Precocious puberty	Dx: Clinical (genetics if uncertain) Tx: Aromatase inhibitors (Letrozole) to prevent precocious puberty, management of other endocrine/bone disease that occurs
Noonan Syndrome	- Heterogenous AD disorder due to a variety of defects in Ras-MAPk - Classically presents with short stature and congenital heart defects (pulmonic stenosis) - Many features similar to Turner's (short webbed neck, low set ears, shield chest, etc)	Dx: Clinical, plus genetic testing Tx: Fairly good prognosis, often have good ability function

GENETICS

Genetics Pediatrics

	General/Clinical	Management
Prader-Willi	- Deletions on paternal 15q11-13, or maternal uniparental disomy - Hypotonia (earliest sign during infancy) - Obesity, hyperphagia, binge eating - Intellectual disability, hypogonadism/microphallus, short stature	Dx: Genetic testing Tx: GH therapy, attempt to prevent weight gain
Angelman	- Deletions of maternal 15q11-13, or paternal uniparental disomy - Severe intellectual disability - Ataxia, seizures - Frequent smiling/laughing behavior, with hand flapping	Dx: Genetic testing Tx: Interdisciplinary care, management of complications (ie seizures)
Cri-du-chat	- 5p microdeletion - High pitched cry/mewing, hypotonia, microcephaly, intellectual disability, facial dysmorphia, cardiac defects (VSD)	Dx: Genetic analysis
Williams	- 7q microdeletion (includes elastin gene) - Elfin facies (wide mouth, small jaw, long philtrum, thick vermillion border of the lips) - Intellectual disability, but good verbal skills/extreme friendliness - Supravalvular aortic stenosis, renal artery stenosis - Hypercalcemia	Dx: Genetic analysis
DiGeorge Syndrome	- 22q11 microdeletion, causing 3rd/4th branchial arch defects - Thymus/parathyroid hypoplasia (↑ infection risk, hypocalcemia) - Conotruncal cardiac defects - Facial dysmorphia (cleft lip/palate)	Dx: Clinical (↓ T-cells, cardiac disease, etc) or genetic testing Tx: - Thymic transplantation or HCT - Treat hypocalcemia, cardiac disease

GENETICS

Glycogen Storage Disease (all AR)

	General/Clinical	Management
Type I von Gierke	- Glucose-6-Phosphatase Deficiency - Hypoglycemia (months after birth) and lactic acidosis - Hyperuricemia and hypertriglyceridemia - Thin upper extremities, doll like face, hepatosplenomegaly	Dx: Genetic testing Tx: Maintain glucose levels with regular snacks/cornstarch
Type II Pompe	- Lysosomal acid alpha-1,4-glucosidase deficiency - Cardiomyopathy, hypotonia, death during infancy - Can present later with limb-girdle weakness and respiratory failure	Dx: Genetic testing Tx: Enzyme replacement therapy
Type III Cori	- 1,6 Glucosidase (glycogen debrancher) deficiency - Hypoglycemia, hepatomegaly, hypotonia, failure to thrive - Muscle weakness - Normal lactate (vs type I) - Limit dextrans accumulation	Dx: Genetic testing Tx: Avoid hypoglycemia, supportive
Type V McArdle	- Glycogen phosphorylase deficiency - Painful muscle cramps, myoglobinuria, exercise intolerance, presenting in early adolescence - Normal blood glucose and lactate - Second wind phenomenon (due to increased muscular blood flow)	Dx: Genetic testing Tx: Pre-exercise carbohydrate loading

GENETICS

Genetics Pediatrics

	General/Clinical	Management
Carbohydrate Intolerance Disorders		
Essential Fructosuria	- AR Fructokinase deficiency - Benign condition with fructose found in blood and urine	Dx: (+) urinary reducing sugar test Tx: Benign, none required
Fructose Intolerance	- AR Aldolase B deficiency (Fructose 1-P accumulates in cells, using up intracellular phosphate), resulting in inhibition of glycogenolysis and gluconeogenesis - Presents as hypoglycemia, liver failure/jaundice, vomiting, failure to thrive - Often appear normal, until new fructose-containing foods introduced to diet	Dx: (+) urinary reducing sugar test, confirm with genetics Tx: Dietary modification (avoid fructose/sucrose)
Galactokinase Deficiency	- AR Galactokinase deficiency - Causes development of infantile cataracts	Tx: Treat cataracts, dietary modification
Classic Galactosemia	- AR defect in galactose-1-P uridylytransferase deficiency - Presents with infantile cataracts, hepatomegaly/jaundice, failure to thrive, intellectual disability, increased risk for infection/sepsis	Dx: Enzyme activity assay, confirmatory genetics Tx: Dietary modification (avoid galactose)
Urea Cycle Disorders		
Ornithine Transcarbamylase Deficiency	- XR defect in key urea cycle enzyme - After protein ingested, infant develops vomiting, lethargy, poor feeding - ↑ Orotic acid, ornithine, ↓ citrulline	Dx: Clinical, with confirmatory genetic testing Tx: Low protein diet, sodium benzoate

GENETICS

Genetics Pediatrics

	General/Clinical	Management
Amino Acid Disorders		
Phenylketonuria	- AR phenylalanine hydroxylase deficiency (rarely from BH4 deficiency which is an essential cofactor) - Intellectual disability, epilepsy, ataxia - Fair complexion, eczema, "mousy" body odor - Maternal PKU: If not controlled during pregnancy, infant will suffer from intellectual disability, growth disturbance, development delay	Dx: Elevated phenylalanine concentration, confirm with genetic testing Tx: Dietary restriction of phenylalanine, can consider BH4 in mild cases Note: If controlled/recognized early, patients have good prognosis *New enzyme replacement therapy available
Maple Syrup Urine	- AR defect in branched-chain ketoacid break down - Within days of birth, develop vomiting, poor feeding, irritability/lethargy, ketonuria - Later develop intellectual disability, growth retardation	Dx: ↑ plasma/urine branched AA (leucine, isoleucine, and valine), can confirm with genetics Tx: Dietary (restrict branched-chain AA), give thiamine
Alkaptonuria	- AR defect in homogentisic acid dioxygenase (part of the degradation pathway of tyrosine) - Ochronosis: Black pigment deposition in connective tissues - Urine turns black after long exposure to air - Black cartilage (ie ear), sclera. Can develop arthropathies.	Dx: ↑ HGA in urine/plasma Tx: None
Homocystinuria	- AR deficiency in cystathionine synthase or methionine synthase - Marfanoid body habitus, ectopic lens (downward dislocation) - Intellectual disability - Thrombosis/atherosclerosis	Dx: Urine/blood homocysteine levels Tx: - Mild: B6 supplementation (+ B9/B12) - Antiplatelets/anticoagulation

GENETICS

Genetics Pediatrics

	General/Clinical	Management
Mitochondrial Disorders (maternally inherited mitochondrial DNA conditions)		
MELAS	- Mitochondrial encephalomyopathy with lactic acidosis and stroke-like episodes (results in hemiparesis, hemianopia, etc)	Dx: Mitochondrial DNA testing Tx: Supportive
MERRF	- Myoclonic epilepsy with ragged red fibers - Myoclonus, followed by development of epilepsy, myopathy, ataxia	
Peroxisomal Disorders		
Zellweger Spectrum	- Includes Zellweger, infantile refsum, and neonatal adrenoleukodystrophy, which are all disorders of abnormal peroxisome biogenesis, with resulting accumulation of very-long chain fatty acids - Causes abnormal CNS development, hypomyelination	- Patients rarely survive past 1 y/o
Fatty Acid Disorders		
Oxidation Disorders	- Defects in fatty acid oxidation, including AR medium-chain acyl-CoA dehydrogenase deficiency, AR very-long-chain acyl-CoA dehydrogenase deficiency - Presents during infancy or early childhood, with hypoketotic hypoglycemia (especially after fasting) increased ammonia (decreased urea cycle function) - Vomiting, lethargy, seizures, hepatomegaly, and myopathy	Dx: Can confirm with genetic testing Tx: - Fat-restricted diets - Avoidance of prolonged fasts
Carnitine Deficiency	- Variety of AR mutations in carnitine transport - Toxic accumulation of LCFA in the blood - Causes acute encephalopathy, severe hypoketotic hypoglycemia, hyperammonemia, arrhythmias	Tx: - Fat-restricted diets - Avoidance of prolonged fasts - Carnitine supplementation

GENETICS

Sphingolipidoses

	Enzyme Deficient [Substrate accumulates]	Clinical Features	Management/Prognosis
Fabry	XR Alpha Galactosidase A (Globotriaosylceramide)	- Slowly progressive painful neuropathy, anhidrosis, angiokeratomas, restrictive cardiomyopathy, CKD	- Enzyme replacement therapy - Lives into adulthood
Gaucher	AR Glucocerebrosidase (Glucocerebroside)	- Hepatosplenomegaly, pancytopenia - Bone: Osteoporosis, aseptic necrosis, bone pain	- Enzyme replacement therapy - Can live into adulthood
Niemann-Pick	AR Sphingomyelinase (Sphingomyelin)	- Progressive neurodegeneration, loss of motor milestones, hypotonia, "cherry-red" macula - Hepatosplenomegaly, areflexia	- Progressive death within few years
Tay-Sachs	AR Hexosaminidase A (GM2 ganglioside)	- Progressive neurodegeneration, loss of motor milestones, hypotonia, "cherry-red" macula - Hyperreflexia	- Progressive death within few years
Krabbe	AR Galactocerebrosidase (Galactocerebroside)	- Presents ~6M old, with progressive weakness, developmental delay, areflexia, optic atrophy	- Progressive death within few years
Metachromatic Leukodystrophy	AR Arylsulfatase (Cerebroside sulfate)	- Presents ~2 years old, with progressive demyelination, CNS dysfunction, weakness	- Progressive death within early childhood

Mucopolysaccharidoses

	Enzyme Deficient	Clinical Features	Management/Prognosis
Hurler	AR Iduronidase (Heparan sulfate)	- Coarse facies (" gargoylism"), short stature, HSM, intellectual disability, OSA/airway obstruction - Dysostosis multiplex, frequent respiratory infections - Corneal clouding (Hurler only) - Behavioral issues, like ADHD (Hunter only)	- Supportive care only - Live on average to ~10 y/o
Hunter	XR Iduronate sulfatase (Heparan sulfate)		

Mucolipidosis

	Enzyme Deficient	Clinical Features	Management/Prognosis
I-Cell Disease	Failure of delivery of key enzymes to lysosomes	- Growth failure, motor delay/hypotonia, coarse facies - Corneal clouding, dysostosis multiplex	- High plasma lysosomal enzymes - Supportive care

GENETICS

Genetics Pediatrics

	General/Clinical	Management
Hereditary Hemorrhagic Telangiectasia	- AD condition (endoglin, ALK-1, or SMAD4) - Epistaxis - Mucocutaneous telangiectasia - Mucosal bleeding, leading to anemia - AV Malformation (pulmonary can result in paradoxical strokes, polycythemia, shunting, etc) - Venous thrombosis	Dx: Clinical. Consider confirmatory genetic test. Tx: - Screen for AVM, consider embolization - Treat anemia - Treat mucosal bleeding, consider medical/surgical interventions if recurrent
Li-Fraumeni	- Germline p53 predisposition for cancer - Breast cancer, sarcomas, brain tumors, and adrenocortical carcinomas	- MRI screening for breast cancer - Colon cancer screening - Consider whole body MRI screens

GENETICS

Genetics Pediatrics

Genetic Associations

VACTERL	- Vertebral defects - Anal atresia - Cardiac anomalies - TracheoEsophageal fistula - Renal (+ GU) defects - Limb defects (ie radial hypoplasia, syndactyly and polydactyly)
CHARGE	- Colobomas: Absence/defect of ocular tissue - Heart (tetralogy of fallot) - Atresia (choanal) - Retarded growth/cognitive development - Genital anomalies - Ear anomalies

Other Genetic Syndromes

Cornelia de Lange	- Very short stature, small birth weight, and failure to thrive - Single "bushy" eyebrow, micrognathia, microcephaly - Mental retardation, behavioral abnormalities (ie autism) - A variety of CV, GI, hearing and visual impairments
Silver Russell	- Short stature - Limb asymmetry - Triangle face, small downturned mouth - Excess sweating as infant
Pierre Robin	- Retrognathia - Cleft lip/palate - Backward displacement of tongue (causes airway obstruction)

APPROACH TO FEVERS

Infectious Disease – Pediatrics

Fever without Source: An acute febrile (rectal temp >100.4°F) illness in which the etiology of fever is not apparent after H/P

Age	DDx/General Considerations	Workup	Management
< 7 days old	[See: Neonatal Sepsis]		
Infant (7-28 days)	- High risk for IBI*, including UTI, bacteremia/sepsis, and meningitis (risk decreases with older ages) - Viruses (ie RSV, influenza, parainfluenza, enterovirus) - HSV	- Full workup (CBC w/ diff, blood cx, urine cx/urinalysis) - Lumbar puncture with CSF studies	- Hospitalize all - Empiric antibiotics (Ampicillin + Gentamicin or Cefotaxime) - Add Acyclovir (if HSV suspicion)
Infant (28-60 D)	*Infant Bacterial Infection (IBI): Includes meningitis, bone and joint infections, soft tissue, pneumonia, UTI, sepsis/bacteremia, enteritis	- Full workup (CBC w/ diff, blood cx, urine cx/urinalysis) +/- Lumbar puncture w/ CSF (only if high risk: see below)	- Hospitalize patients with high risk features on initial workup - Empiric antibiotics if admitted (Cefotaxime/Ceftriaxone +/- Ampicillin)
Infant (60-90 D)		- Urine cx/Urinalysis - Full workup only if significant underlying comorbidities	- (+) UA: Empiric abx for UTI - (-) UA: Close outpatient followup
Children (3-36 M)		- Toxic appearing, T ≥ 102°F: Full workup, hospitalization, empiric abx (Cefotaxime +/- Vancomycin) - Nontoxic, T ≤ 102°F: No workup, but consider UA in boys < 6-12M and females < 24M. Outpatient monitoring with careful follow up.	

Organisms: Group B Strep, *E. Coli, Listeria, S. pneumoniae, H. influenzae, N. meningitidis, S. aureus, Pseudomonas, Enterococcus*

Risk Stratification: Low risk for IBI if laboratory workup reveals the following
- WBC > 5K and < 15 K, bands < 1.5K, normal urinalysis, normal CSF (if LP performed)

- Note: If history of fever at home, but afebrile now, can safely discharge (assuming child looks well, H/P normal, no antipyretics used)

APPROACH TO FEVERS

Infectious Disease Pediatrics

Fever of Unknown Origin

General: Fever (> 101°F) that persists ≥ 8 days, with no clear diagnosis

Etiology:
- Infectious disease (atypical viral presentations, bacterial/fungal infections)
- Connective tissue disease (Juvenile idiopathic arthritis, SLE, Kawasaki, etc)
- Neoplasms (leukemia, lymphoma, etc)

Clinical:
- Most often unusual/nonspecific presentation of common infectious disease

Diagnosis:
- Workup includes detailed H/P, CBC, ESR/CRP, blood cx, urine cx/urinalysis, chest radiograph, tuberculosis/HIV screening

Management: Avoid empiric antibiotics, but can consider antipyretics (ie NSAIDs)

Cervical Lymphadenitis

General: Enlarged, inflamed, tender lymph node in the neck

Etiology:
- Bilateral: Viral URI, GAS pharyngitis, HSV, EBV
- Unilateral: *S. aureus* and GAS

Clinical:
- > 2 cm, tender lymph node or nodes
- Possible overlying skin erythema/cellulitis

Diagnosis: Clinical diagnosis. Consider workup in those with moderate/severe symptoms (blood cultures, cx of draining lesion, throat culture, or needle aspiration).

Management:
- Bilateral: Most commonly self-limited (but do workup if severe sx)
- Unilateral: Workup, empiric abx therapy (ie Amoxicillin-Clavulanate)

Cat Scratch Disease

General: Regional lymphadenopathy, from *Bartonella henselae* infection. Most often spread from kittens, other animals, and rarely fleas.

Clinical:
- Papule at scratch area
- Regional lymphadenopathy, fever

Diagnosis: Clinical. Serology (for confirmation).

Management: Azithromycin

PRE-OPERATIVE EVALUATION

General Surgery
Surgery

System	Evaluation
Cardiovascular	- After coronary stenting, delay elective surgeries for 1 month after bare metal stent and 1 year after drug eluting stent - Postpone surgery if unstable angina or MI within 60 days - Stabilize CHF prior to surgery - ECG: Not necessary in healthy patients, but obtain if CAD, arrhythmia, PVD, or other cardiac disease history - Use preoperative risk stratifying tools. If high risk, with poor functional capacity (< 4 METs), then obtain stress test. Otherwise, proceed to surgery.
Pulmonary	- Smoking: Ideally quit > 4-8 weeks prior to surgery (reduced post-operative complication rates) - Optimize COPD/asthma/OSA prior to surgery - Consider PFTs in someone with unexplained exercise intolerance
Renal	- Creatinine > 2 mg/dl associated with increased surgery risk
Liver	- Child Pugh Class A/B or MELD < 15: Surgery acceptable - High surgery risk for Class C or MELD > 15
Hematology	- Hgb > 7 - Platelets > 50K - INR < 1.5 Anticoagulation: - Hold warfarin for 4-5 days prior to surgery (or until INR < 1.5) - LMWH: Can use to bridge. Last dose should be at least 24 hours prior to surgery, and 50% of normal dose.
Infectious Disease	- Cancel elective surgery if current acute infection

Medications
- Drugs to Continue:
    - Statins, beta-blockers
    - Insulin (but consider reduced dose the day of surgery)
- Drugs to Hold:
    - ACEi/ARB, diuretics (morning of surgery)
    - NSAIDs (1 week prior to surgery)
    - Antiplatelets (balance risk of continuation with risk of holding)
        - Stop ASA within 5-10 days and Clopidogrel within 7
    - OCPs (hold in surgery with high risk for thrombotic events)
    - Oral hypoglycemic agents

POST-OPERATIVE FEVER

General Surgery — Surgery

DDx	General	Diagnosis	Management/PPX
Immediate (< 24 hours)			
Malignant Hyperthermia	- AD RYR1 mutation: Hypersensitivity to succinylcholine	- Clinical (Presents with acute muscle rigidity, rhabdo, hypercapnia, tachycardia, hyperkalemia, hyperthermia)	- 100% O_2, Dantrolene, cool off - PPX: Careful family history
Blood Product Reaction	- Acute febrile reaction to blood product		- Stop blood product
Acute (1-7 days)			
Idiopathic	- Benign, transient fever within first few days after surgery - Often attributed to atelectasis (but no longer believed to cause fever)		- Monitor
Nosocomial Infection (UTI, PNA, catheter)		- Urinalysis, CXR, check catheters, etc	- Appropriate antibiotics
Surgical Site Infection	- Early SSI usually presents outside of first week, but group A Strep and *Clostridium perfringens* can be earlier	- Clinical	- Antibiotics - Surgical debridement/cleaning
Other	- PE/DVT - MI		
Subacute (7-28 days)			
Soft Tissue Infection	See next page		
C. Difficile Colitis	- Severe diarrhea	- Stool toxin ELISA	- Vancomycin +/- Metronidazole
Febrile Drug Reaction	- Antibiotics, PPIs, Heparin, etc		- Withdraw drug

Surg2

POST-OPERATIVE COMPLICATIONS — General Surgery / Surgery

Surgical Wound Complications

Surgical Site Infection	- Presents with localized erythema, warmth, edema and pain - Possibly associated with purulent drainage, separation of wound, fever, leukocytosis - Tx: Surgical (open/drain/irrigate/debride). Antibiotics.
Fascial Dehiscence	- Fascial disruption, most commonly due to abdominal wall tension overcoming strength of sutures - Risk: Inadequate closure/technique, or host factors like infection, malnutrition, diabetes, etc - Tx: Abdominal binders, surgical exploration/repair
Evisceration	- Dehiscence with visceral protrusion through wound - Tx: Surgical emergency
Hematoma	- Failure of primary hemostasis, resulting in collection of blood near site of incision - Increased risk for surgical site infection - Tx: Drainage of large collections

Fistula

General: Abnormal connection between two organs. Enteric fistulas are communications between bowel lumen and skin or another organ.

Risk:
- Postoperative (ie abdominal surgery, vascular surgery)
- Crohn's disease, malignancy, PUD, malignancy, infections
- "FETID" (foreign body, epithelialization, tumor, irradiation/inflamed/IBD, distal obstruction)

Clinical: Variable based on the connection
- Skin drainage
- Diarrhea
- Fecaluria

Diagnosis:
- Either clinical (for obvious ones) OR
- CT abdomen (if suspected)

Management:
- Initially supportive (treat infection, control drainage, etc)
- Surgical repair
    - Some enterocutaneous fistulas can heal spontaneously, so short trial of supportive care is appropriate prior to surgery

POST-OPERATIVE COMPLICATIONS — General Surgery

Abdominal Distension/Constipation

Ileus	- Typical for lack of flatus or feces in first 1-2 days after surgery - Risk: Worse with use of opioids, long/more intensive surgery - Presents with absent bowel sounds, mild obstructive symptoms (ie distension), and constant dull pain - KUB XR shows diffuse bowel dilatation - Tx: Purely supportive (fluids, out of bed, etc)
Obstruction	- Suspicion grows for SBO (vs ileus) with lack of flatus/feces on days 4-5 - KUB XR can reveal proximal bowel dilatation, with decompressed bowel distally - Dx: CT can confirm location - Tx: NG decompression, pain control, consider surgical correction
Ogilvie	- Functional ileus of the colon - Seen in elderly, chronically ill patients - XR/CT shows diffuse large bowel dilatation (vs LBO, which shows a transition area at the site of obstruction) - Tx: Supportive care, consider Neostigmine

Other Post-Op Complications

Complication	Etiology/Causes
Post-Op Bleeding	- Surgical bleeding - Medications (antiplatelets, anticoagulation) - Chronic liver/kidney disease - DIC
Perioperative Myocardial Infarct	- Dx and treat as if normal STEMI/NSTEMI
Decreased Urine Output	> 0.5 mL/kg/hr is normal - Obstructive (bladder, scan, relieve obstruction) - Renal failure (can try small fluid bolus to see if prerenal)
Hypoxemia	- Atelectasis (common soon after surgery) - Aspiration - PE, PNA, ARDS

EMERGENCIES/FRACTURES
Orthopedics Surgery

Compartment Syndrome

General: Increased pressure within a compartment bound by fascial membranes, resulting in compromised vascular flow and tissue ischemia

Risk: Trauma (ie fractures, penetrating, or blunt), ischemia/reperfusion (ie vascular injury or arterial insufficiency), prolonged limb compression, IV drugs

Clinical:
- Progressive, tense, swollen extremity compartment
- Pain with passive motion of extremity
- Paresthesias
- Motor symptoms or pulselessness (late findings, poor prognosis)

Diagnosis:
- Compartment pressure measurement
    - < 8 mmHg is normal. Symptoms develop at > 20-30 mmHg.
    - Δ Pressure < 30 mmHg (diastolic BP - compartment pressure)

Management:
- Remove all dressings, keep limb at body level
- Emergent fasciotomy

Fracture Basics

Open Fracture	- Defined as fracture with direct communication externally - Clinically diagnosed (grossly obvious) - Tx: Antibiotics, tetanus PPX, surgery (aggressive irrigation and debridement)
Closed Fracture	- Bone fracture without external communication - Can be traumatic or pathologic (weak bone from osteoporosis, metastasis, etc) Displacement - Can be nondisplaced OR - Displaced (ie sideways/translated, angulated, rotated, etc) Fragments - Complete: Bone fully broken into separate pieces - Incomplete: Crack in bone, but still partially joined - Comminuted: Bone is broken into several pieces Fracture Pattern - Linear: Parallel to long bone axis - Transverse: Perpendicular to long bone axis - Oblique: Diagonal to long bone axis - Spiral: One part of bone is twisted - Compression: Bony collapse (usually vertebrae) - Impacted: Fx from bone fragments being driven into each other - Avulsion: Fragment of bone ripped from main bone

FRACTURES

Orthopedics Surgery

Fracture Diagnosis/Management

Diagnosis: Plain XR imaging is almost always first step and sufficient for diagnosis

Management:
- Closed, non-displaced fractures: Treated conservatively with analgesia, ice, and immobilization (splinting, sling, etc)
- Displaced fractures: Require either open or closed reduction prior to immobilization

Stress Fractures

General: Small bone fracture from repeated stress from overuse. Common sites include tibial (most common), foot, ankle, femur.

Risk: Sudden increased in intensity of physical activity, low fitness, low bone density, female, irregular menstruation, prior stress fractures

Clinical:
- Insidious onset of pain, associated with recent increase in activity
- Focal tenderness to palpation over bone

Diagnosis:
- XR (insensitive/often negative)
- MRI (highly sensitive, but only used if definitive diagnosis is required)

Management:
- Reduced weight bearing, splinting/boot for protection
- Rest, ice, analgesia
- Gradual return to activity

Rib Fractures

Risk: Blunt chest trauma, severe coughing, pathologic fractures (usually bony mets)

Clinical: Localized pain in the chest wall, which is tender with palpation

Diagnosis: CXR (PA/lateral)

Management:
- Analgesia
    - NSAIDs, opioids. intercostal nerve blocks
    - Adequate relief required to prevent atelectasis/pneumonia
        - Also incentive spirometry
- ≥ 3 rib fractures or rib fractures in high risk patients (ie elderly) likely require hospitalization for monitoring/prevention of complications

FRACTURES

Orthopedics Surgery

Upper Extremity Fractures

Clavicle	- Most commonly middle third (~70%) with ~25% in the distal third - Usually caused by trauma (fall on shoulder, MVA, etc) - Tx: Sling, analgesia for minimally displaced fx. Surgical intervention if displaced.
Proximal Humerus	- Often caused by falls - Tx: Conservative (sling). Surgical (if in many pieces).
Mid-Humeral Shaft	- Uncommon. From serious trauma. High risk for neurovascular compromise (especially radial nerve). - Tx: Surgery/splinting (in most cases)
Distal Radius	- Often referred to as Colles (with dorsal displacement of distal radius) or Smith (with palmar displacement of distal radius) - Common. Risk: Elderly with fall on outstretched hand. - Tx: Splinting (nondisplaced), closed reduction/splint (displaced)
Monteggia	- Midshaft ulna fracture, with dislocation of radial head
Galeazzi	- Radial midshaft fracture, with instability of radioulnar joint
Scaphoid	- Tenuous, retrograde blood supply. High risk for avascular necrosis, especially with proximal scaphoid. - Fall on outstretched arm with wrist in dorsiflexion - Pain is localized to radial wrist, with focal pain in the anatomic snuff box - Dx: XR. Often negative initially, so if high suspicion, immobilize and repeat imaging in a week. (alt: MRI) - Tx: Surgery (if displaced, or proximal 1/5 of scaphoid). Cast immobilization for others.
Metacarpal Neck	- "Boxer's" fractures (5th MC) - Mechanism: Striking object with clenched fist or hand trauma - Tx: Reduction and splinting in most cases

FRACTURES

Orthopedics Surgery

Lower Extremity Fractures

Pelvic	- Can occur with minor trauma in elderly or major trauma in healthy adults - Traumatic hip fractures have high risk for injury complications, such as GU, vascular, or spinal
Hip	- Common elderly injury, associated with ↑ morbidity/mortality - Presents after fall, with shortened leg and external hip rotation Classified as: - Intracapsular (femoral neck/head): High risk for complications (ie avascular necrosis, due to tenuous blood supply) - Extracapsular (intertrochanteric): Less risk for complication (good blood supply), but high risk for bleeding - Tx: Arthroplasty or open reduction w/ internal fixation. Must prophylaxe for DVT.
Femur	- Related to severe trauma - Risk for fat embolism - Tx: Adults (surgical nailing). Kids (casting).
Patellar	- Blunt knee trauma - Tx: Simple → Immobilization. Displaced or complex → Surgical.
Tibia/ Fibula Shaft	- High speed trauma or sports injury - Often involve both tibia and fibula, requiring ortho consult - Isolated fibula (non-weight bearing bone) can be treated nonoperatively in most cases
Ankle	- Most commonly unimalleolar, but can be bimalleolar - Similar mechanism to ankle sprains, but severe, focal bone tenderness and inability to bear weight

PEDIATRIC ORTHOPEDICS

Orthopedics, Pediatrics, Surgery

	General/Clinical	Management
Developmental Dysplasia of Hip	- Abnormal development of acetabulum/femoral head, with resulting instability of the hip joint - Risk factors: Breech, family hx, females Clinical - Ortolani (abduction/elevation) - Barlow (adduction) - The above maneuvers result in jerks or clunks - Leg length discrepancy, asymmetric inguinal folds	Dx: Clinical, with imaging confirmation (US if < 4 M, XR > 4 M) Tx: - < 6 M: Abduction splint (Pavlik harness) - > 6 M: Often require reduction (either open or closed) - Monitor for long term complications (OA, avascular necrosis)
Slipped Capital Femoral Epiphysis (SCFE)	- Posterior displacement of capital femoral epiphysis from the femoral neck through the growth plate - Commonly affects 10-15 year-olds, overweight, males - Presents as groin (or occasionally knee) pain with limp - Limited internal rotation	Dx: XR (ice cream falling off cone) Tx: Surgical femoral head pinning
Legg-Calves-Perthes	- Avascular necrosis of idiopathic origin - Peak age ~5-7 - Presents with insidious onset hip pain, worse with activity, and limp (note the subacute, often > 1M onset, vs other causes)	Dx: XR (often insensitive/normal early). MRI is highly sensitive). Tx: Splinting, with surgery if refractory. Usually resolves on own, but can lead to OA/other complications
Other Hip Pain	- Septic arthritis - Transient synovitis	

PEDIATRIC ORTHOPEDICS
Orthopedics — Pediatrics, Surgery

Back

Scoliosis	- Excessive lateral curvature of the spine - Common in young adolescents (usually idiopathic) - Dx: Inspection, Adams forward bend test, measurement of angle of trunk rotation, XR imaging - Tx: Monitoring, bracing, or surgery (depending on severity of the curvature)

Knee

Osgood-Schlatter	- Overuse injury with strain and avulsion of the secondary ossification center of the tibial tubercle - Seen in running/jumping athletes - Presents with pain over tibial tubercle, which is exacerbated with contraction of quad muscles. Pain generally insidious in onset. - Dx: Clinical - Tx: Conservative (RICE), physical therapy

Foot

Metatarsus Adductus	- Congenital medial deviation of forefoot and neutral position of hindfood, so the toes point inward - Often bilateral. Common cause of "pigeon toes" at < 1 y/o. - Tx: Reassurance
Club Foot (Talipes equinovarus)	- Pathologic congenital foot deformity, with medial deviation of forefoot, combined with foot supination (plantar surfaces facing inward), ankle plantar flexion, and cavus (high arch) - Tx: Manipulation/casting, followed by achilles tenotomy, and bracing to maintain shape. Surgery for refractory cases.

Misc Benign

Genu Varum	- Bow legged. Normal before 2-3 years old, after which time child progresses to valgus. - If older than 3, concern for pathologic variant (ie Rickets, skeletal dysplasias, or Blount disease [disturbance of medial tibial growth plate])
Genu Valgum	- Knock knees. Normal variant between 4-7 years old.
Flat Feet	- Totally normal in children, as pedal arch is developing in first 8 years of life - However, if foot does not have full range of motion, then needs referral to orthopedics

TRAUMA OVERVIEW

Trauma Surgery

Initial Evaluation in Trauma

Airway	- Airway is generally normal if patient is conscious and speaking with normal voice Indications for intubation: (1) GCS < 8 (2) Compromised airway (3) Failure of oxygenation/ventilation (4) Anticipation of rapid deterioration - Cricothyroidotomy reserved for failed intubation and serious need for airway
Breathing	- Check breath sounds and look for symmetric chest wall motion
Circulation	- Evaluation of hemodynamic status (for shock). Check pulses. - Need to establish IV access (preferably two 16 gauge peripheral IVs, but if unable to obtain can attempt intraosseous placement or central line) - If signs of shock/hypovolemia, provide boluses of crystalloid fluids. Can consider going straight to type O blood and activate massive transfusion protocol of 1:1:1 blood products if severe bleeding. - Immediate intervention for severe bleeding (ie tourniquet placement for severe extremity bleeding, pelvic binder for hip fracture with possible bleed, and thoracotomy if suspicion for severe aortic injury)
Disability	- Focused neurologic examination - GCS evaluation - Pupil assessment, extremity sensation/strength assessment
Exposure	- "Primary Survey": Examine the patient entirely for any other wounds or injuries

Shock (in trauma)

Hypovolemic	- Hemorrhagic is the most common sign of shock - Presents pale and cold with weak pulses and collapsed neck veins
Obstructive	- Cardiac Tamponade: Requires emergent pericardiocentesis - Tension Pneumothorax: Requires emergent needle decompression
Cardiogenic	- After trauma, can be caused by myocardial contusion - Cold, clammy, signs of CHF, weak/rapid pulse
Vasomotor	- Spinal cord injury can cause diffuse circulatory collapse from loss of peripheral vascular tone. Will appear pink/well perfused.

TRAUMA (HEAD-TO-TOE)

Trauma Surgery

Shock (in trauma)

Five Major Sources of Bleeding:
1) Chest (hemothorax)
2) Abdomen (liver, splenic injury)
3) Pelvis/Retroperitoneum (pelvic fracture, kidney injury)
4) Long Bones (femur fractures)
5) External (scalp lacerations, other extremity injuries)

Head Trauma

[See: Neuro] for full discussion on head trauma

DDx:
- TBI (concussion or more severe injury)
- Bleeds (epidural/subdural hematoma, diffuse axonal injury)
- Skull fractures (linear, basilar)

Diagnosis: CT scan (all with head trauma deserve head CT)

Penetrating Neck Injury

General: Any injury to the neck that penetrates the platysma. Classically anatomically split into three zones, displayed below:

Zone 1	Clavicles up to cricoid	- Great vessels, carotids/jugular, distal trachea, esophagus, lung apex
Zone 2	Cricoid to angle of mandible	- Carotid/jugular/vertebral vessels, vagus/phrenic/recurrent laryngeal nerve, esophagus, larynx, trachea
Zone 3	Angle of mandible to base of skull	- Proximal carotids, jugular vein, vertebral artery, oropharynx, C-spine

Clinical: Variable depending on organ involved
- "Hard Signs" of vascular injury: Severe hemorrhage, expanding hematoma, hemodynamic instability
- "Hard Signs" of airway/esophageal injury: Hemoptysis, hematemesis, resp failure, air bubbling from wound

Diagnosis: Multidetector helical CTA (MDCT-A) is now preferred test (if stable)
- This replaces previous "zone based" method, which (depending on zone involved) employed some combination of arteriography, esophagrams, esophagoscopy, bronchoscopy to rule out injury

Management:
- Intubation (for anyone with compromised airway)
- Emergent surgical intervention (hemodynamic instability, expanding hematoma, clear "hard sign" of esophageal, tracheal, or vascular injury)
- If no injury demonstrated on CT, conservative monitoring

TRAUMA (HEAD-TO-TOE)

Trauma Surgery

Spinal Trauma

General: Acute spinal cord injuries most commonly occur with MVA, but also after falls, sports accidents, and violence

Injury Type	Clinical Features
Complete Cord	- Complete loss of motor and sensory below the level of the lesion
Incomplete Cord	- Motor/sensory deficits, depending on injury
Spinal Shock	- Like a spinal concussion, with flaccid paralysis, sensory loss, and absent bowel/bladder function below the level of the injury - Recovery is highly variable, from hours to weeks
Anterior Cord	- From ASA infarct or direct injury from bone chip or disc - Loss of motor and pain/temp sensation, but fine touch spared
Central Cord	- Upper extremity motor dysfunction - Bladder dysfunction - Sensory dysfunction below level of injury

Diagnosis: CT spine (in suspected areas of injury)

Management:
- Prehospital: Spinal immobilization (cervical collar, backboard)
- ED: Intubation, continued cervical stabilization/immobilization, neuro exam
- Surgery: If unstable fracture, spinal cord compression, or instability

Blunt Chest Trauma

Injury	Features/Management
Cardiovascular	
Blunt Cardiac Injury	- Variety of conditions, including ventricular wall rupture, valve damage, myocardial infarction, or "contusion" (which presents with myocardial stunning and/or dysrhythmia without hemorrhage or structural damage) - Dx: ECG, ECHO, and cardiac enzymes
Traumatic Aortic Rupture	- Often occurs with high-speed deceleration and can create a rapidly expanding hematoma that results in instant death - A minority of patients can have a contained injury that allows for survival until medical care - Dx: CXR. If suspicious for aortic injury, get CT Chest. - Tx: Surgical or endovascular repair
Cardiac Tamponade	[See: Cards]

TRAUMA (HEAD-TO-TOE)

Trauma Surgery

Blunt Chest Trauma

Injury	Features/Management
Lung	
Pneumothorax [See: Pulm]	- Often due to broken rib - Traumatic pneumothoraces can be under tension, which can cause hemodynamic instability, tracheal deviation away from side of lesion, and contralateral mediastinal shift/ipsilateral diaphragm flattening. Management includes urgent needle decompression (if under tension), followed by chest tube.
Hemothorax	- Bleeding from aortic/myocardial rupture, or from lung parenchyma or intercostal vessels - Presents similarly to PTX, but dull to percussion on exam - Requires chest tube placement (in low, dependent spot in chest). If > 1.5 L of blood is collected, patient needs emergent surgery.
Rib Fracture	- [See: Ortho] - Risk for pneumothorax, or atelectasis/PNA development
Flail Chest	- Multiple rib fx in different locations that allow a segment of the chest wall to "float" (caves in during inspiration and bulges out during expiration) - Generally 3 or more ribs fractured in 2 or more places - Presents with hypoxemia, shallow tachypnea, paradoxical chest movement - Tx: Pain control, supplemental O_2, and positive pressure ventilation (if required)
Pulmonary Contusion	- Occurs within 48 hours of chest trauma (alveolar hemorrhage) - Often associated with flail chest - Presents with hypoxemia, ↓ breath sounds, in setting of trauma - Dx: CXR ("white out" of lungs with patchy infiltrates, which do not follow normal anatomic borders) - Tx: Pain control, supplemental O_2, pulmonary toileting, fluid restriction
Diaphragmatic Rupture	- Presents with respiratory distress/XR showing bowel in chest - Tx: Surgical repair
Rupture of Trachea or Bronchus	- Usually instantly fatal - Presents with respiratory distress, hemoptysis, dysphonia - Possible subcutaneous emphysema or recurrent pneumothorax (with chest tube air leakage) - DX: CT Chest or bronchoscopy - Tx: Surgical repair

TRAUMA (HEAD-TO-TOE) — Trauma Surgery

Blunt Abdominal Trauma

General: Majority of blunt abdominal trauma associated with MVC, car vs pedestrian, or from falls. Risk for bleeding from laceration or rupture of internal organ.

Liver	- Most common cause of abdominal bleeding post trauma - Tx: Usually no intervention required, but unstable patients get surgery, while persistent bleeds get IR embolization - Note: Pringle maneuver used during surgery clamps portal triad to control bleeding. If still bleeding, source is hepatic veins.
Spleen	- Most common significant abdominal bleeding post trauma - Often associated with fractured ribs on lower left - Tx: Splenectomy, laceration repair, or IR arterial embolization
Duodenum	- Hematoma formation from compression against posterior ribs - Often occurs in kids due to thin walls/lack of fat - Hematoma causes bowel obstruction, which presents within 1-2 days of injury
Bowel	- Can rupture acutely, or develop ischemia over hours after damage to mesenteric vessels, presenting as bowel ischemia days later
Kidney	- Rare. Includes kidney contusions, lacerations, or renovascular injury. - Can present with gross hematuria (DDx: Bladder injury)

Clinical: Varies from mild symptoms to severe shock/coma. Signs of severe injury:
- Abdominal distension/guarding/rebound tenderness
- Seat belt sign (ecchymosis on abdomen from seat belt)
    - 30% chance of internal injury

Diagnosis/Management:

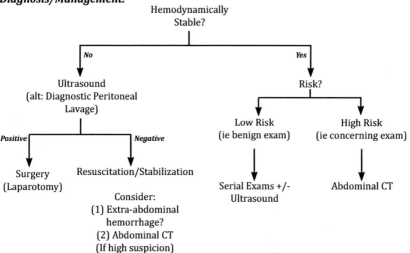

TRAUMA (HEAD-TO-TOE) — Trauma Surgery

Penetrating Abdominal Trauma (Gunshot)

General: Most commonly result in injuries to bowel or liver. The vast majority cause significant intra-abdominal injury that necessitates surgery.

Diagnosis: CT scan w/ contrast (for those without indication for emergent surgery)

Management:
- Emergent Laparotomy: Indicated if hypotension, peritonitis, or evisceration
  - If surgery, patient should be given antibiotics
- Surgical management for anyone that is found to have significant injury on CT imaging (ie bowel injury)
- In rare, select circumstances, nonoperative management is chosen for patients without clear injury on CT scan and are hemodynamically stable

Penetrating Abdominal Trauma (Stab Wounds)

General: Compared to gunshot wounds, stab wounds have a wider range of possible pathology, from simple skin/soft tissue injuries that do not penetrate fascia, to injuries to abdominal organs and vasculature

Management:
- Emergent Laparotomy: Indicated if hypotension, peritonitis, or evisceration
- Local Wound Exploration (for fascial penetration)
  - If negative, provide good wound care, and consider discharge
  - If positive, admit for serial abdominal exam and monitoring
    - Consider CT for further workup
    - Surgery if develops peritonitis, hemodynamic instability, anemia, or leukocytosis

Abdominal Compartment Syndrome

General: Defined as elevated intra-abdominal pressure (called intra-abdominal hypertension), that results in organ dysfunction (including impaired cardiac function, renal impairment, ventilation problems, and gut hypoperfusion)

Risk: Trauma, burns, extensive fluid resuscitation (ie sepsis), abdominal surgery

Clinical: Tensely distended abdomen. Most patients are critically ill and not communicating.

Diagnosis: Measure intra-abdominal pressure (most commonly use bladder pressure)

Management: Surgical decompression (with temporary open abdomen)

TRAUMA (HEAD-TO-TOE) — Trauma Surgery

Pelvic Fracture

General: Significant mechanism, such as MVC or car vs pedestrian, required for pelvic fractures. Includes pelvic ring, sacral, and acetabular fractures. Often results in significant bleed from damage to iliac vessel branches.

Clinical:
- Instability of pelvis with pelvic compression
- Signs of bleeding, hemodynamic instability

Diagnosis: XR (if unstable) and CT (if stable)
- Note: Must perform rectal exam, vaginal exam, bladder imaging to rule out associated injuries

Management:
- Pelvic binder, resuscitation/stabilization
- Consideration for operative stabilization, pelvic packing, or embolization of the bleeding vessel (situation specific)

Genitourinary Trauma

Posterior Urethra	- Almost all occur with men. Often occurs with pelvic fractures. - Presents as blood at meatus, difficulty/inability to void, and high-riding prostate on DRE - Dx: Retrograde Urethrogram (do NOT place foley) - Tx: Suprapubic catheter placement for bladder drainage, +/- delayed surgical repair weeks later
Extraperitoneal Bladder	- Presents as suprapubic tenderness, gross hematuria, difficulty voiding - Dx: Retrograde cystography (including post-void) - Tx: Conservative (urethral catheter drainage, allowing for spontaneous healing)
Intraperitoneal Bladder	- Presents as suprapubic tenderness, gross hematuria, difficulty voiding, peritonitis (from urine leakage into peritoneum) - Dx: Retrograde cystography (including post-void) - Tx: Primary repair
Female Genitalia	- Bruising/lacerations usually occur in setting of sexual abuse
Male Genitalia	- Penile fracture [See: Urology] - Other external injuries include skin/soft tissue injuries, scrotal hematoma (which are often large/impressive) - Should use US to rule out testicular rupture or loss of continuity of the tunica albuginea, and retrograde cystogram to rule out urethral injury

Surg17

TRAUMA (HEAD-TO-TOE)   Trauma Surgery

Extremity/Vascular Injuries

General: Trauma to extremity can include vascular, nervous, bone, and soft tissue damage. If 3/4 of these tissues are involved, the extremity is considered "mangled."

Clinical:
- Fracture: Deformity, point tenderness
- Vascular: Hard signs of injury include active bleed, growing hematoma, absent distal pulses. Classic signs of extremity ischemia ("6 P's"):
    - Pain, pallor, paresthesias, paralysis, pulselessness, poikilothermia
- Nerve: Weakness or paresthesia (in nerve-specific cutaneous distributions)

Diagnosis:
- XR
- Injured Extremity Index (like Ankle-brachial index, but comparing BP between two extremities). < 0.9 is considered abnormal.
    - CT Angiography if the IEI is abnormal

Management:
- Prehospital:
    - If bleeding, direct pressure, or tourniquet if pressure not sufficient
- Surgical
    - Hard signs of vascular injury → Surgical repair
- Compartment Syndrome: Common, especially. with crush injuries
    - Fasciotomy
- Traumatic Amputation (ie of finger)
    - Out of hospital: Patient should clean with saline, wrap in saline-soaked gauze, and place in sealed bag on ice
    - Surgical repair at hospital

Select Vascular Injuries

Artery	Mechanism of Injury
Axillary	- Anterior shoulder dislocation
Subclavian	- Clavicular fracture
Brachial	- Supracondylar humeral fracture, elbow dislocation
Iliac Branches	- Pelvic fractures
Femoral	- Anterior hip dislocation
Superficial Femoral	- Femoral shaft fracture
Popliteal	- Posterior knee dislocation, tibial plateau fracture

BURNS

Trauma Surgery

Burns: Overview

General: Injury to skin and possibly underlying tissue from exposure to one of the following
- Thermal injury
- Electricity
- Chemicals
- Radiation

Degree	Anatomy	Clinical
1st (Superficial)	- Epidermis only	- Blanching, painful, erythematous skin (looks like sunburn)
2nd (Superficial partial thickness)	- Epidermis and portions of dermis	- Weeping, erythematous skin - Still painful - Blisters present
2nd (Deep partial thickness)	- Epidermis and portions of dermis	- Weeping blisters, variable colors (red and white) - Painless
3rd (Full thickness)	- All epidermis/dermis	- Dry, leathery, waxy white and/or dark charred skin - Painless
4th	- Skin, fat, fascia, muscle, all involved	- Severe, disfiguring injury with deep tissue exposure

Diagnosis: Clinical diagnosis. Important to determine extent of injury through use of scoring system, such as Lund-Browder chart or Rule of Nines (seen below).

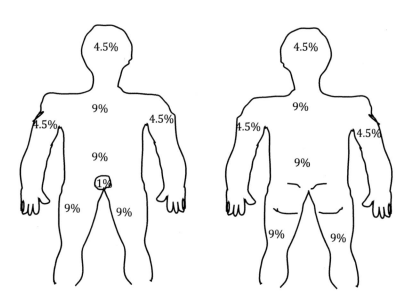

Surg19

BURNS — Trauma Surgery

Burns- Management

Fluids	Parkland Formula (estimated fluid requirement): - mL of LR = Kg x % Body Surface Burned x 4mL - Fluid given first half over 8 hours and second half over 16 hours - Despite the classic formula above, most burn centers provide fluids to maintain urine output (at least 0.5 mL/kg/hr)
Wound Care	- Antimicrobial Agents: Silver Sulfadiazine, Mafenide Acetate, Chlorhexidine, others - Covered by gauze or nonadherent film products
Analgesia	- Opioid analgesics
Other	- PPI prophylaxis (Curling Ulcers) - Ensure proper nutrition (as patients are hypermetabolic). Tube feeds or TPN if necessary.
Surgical	- Escharotomy for circumferential burns (can cause limb ischemia) - Surgical grafting (following conservative therapy, for select severe, but isolated burn wounds)

Special Situations:
- Inhalation Injury
    - Diagnosis: Bronchoscopy
    - Requires intubation if signs of airway edema, blistering, elevated carboxyhemoglobin > 10%, or impending respiratory failure
- Chemical Burn
    - Tap water irrigation
- Electric [See: EM]
    - Watch for arrhythmia, rhabdo, posterior shoulder dislocation

Note: Burn patients are often in an elevated metabolic state, and are hyperthermic, tachycardic, tachypnic.

Burns- Infection

General: Highest risk for mortality with burns. Organisms:
- Early: *Staphylococcus* and *Streptococcus*
- > 5 days: Gram negatives (*Pseudomonas, E. Coli*, etc) and fungi (*Candida*)

Clinical:
- Presents as rapid change in clinical condition of patient (ie increasing pain, change in appearance of burn wound, or systemic signs like hemodynamic changes)
- Note: Traditional sepsis criteria cannot be used due to hypermetabolic state

Diagnosis: Tissue biopsy and culture (> 10^5 colonies per gram tissue)

Management: Surgical debridement, broad spectrum antibiotics, wound care

ANESTHESIA

Anesthesia Surgery

	Mechanism	Indication	Side Effects/Management Concerns
Inhaled			
Desflurane Isoflurane Sevoflurane	Unknown	Unconscious Deep Sedation	- Most commonly used agents currently due to best side effect profile
Halothane			- Hepatotoxicity (still used in third world countries)
Enflurane			- Proconvulsant, ↓ myocardial contractility
Methoxyflurane			- Acute kidney injury
Nitric Oxide		Conscious Sedation	- Rapid onset/offset. Frequent nausea/vomit after.
Neuromuscular Blockade			
Succinylcholine	- Depolarizing agent (ACh agonist)	- Endotracheal Intubation	- Hyperkalemia, myalgias - Risk for malignant hyperthermia (if predisposed)
Rocuronium Vecuronium	- Nondepolarizing agent (ACh antagonist)	- Endotracheal Intubation - Surgery	- Excreted via hepatic and renal clearance (be careful in those with underlying dysfunction) - Reversed with acetylcholinesterase inhibitors (ie Neostigmine) or Sugammadex (directly inactivates paralytic agent)
Atracurium Cisatracurium	- Nondepolarizing agent (ACh antagonist)	- Endotracheal Intubation - Surgery	- Eliminated via Hoffman mxn (spontaneous degradation, not dependent on hepatic or renal clearance)
IV Agents			
Propofol	- GABA potentiation	- Induction, ICU sedation	- ↓ BP/HR/CO,bronchodilation, antiemetic, antiseizure
Etomidate	- GABA potentiation/agonist	- Induction	- ↔ BP/HR/CO. Nausea/vomiting.
Ketamine	- NMDA antagonist	- Induction	- ↑ BP/HR/CO, bronchodilation. Hallucinations.
Midazolam	- GABA agonist	- Adjuvant agent	
Opioids	- Opioid receptor agonist	- Adjuvant agent	

ANESTHESIA
Anesthesia Surgery

General Anesthesia: Basic Principles

General: General anesthesia aims to create a state of amnesia, analgesia, and muscle paralysis during surgery

Steps:

Induction	- Initial step: Put patient to sleep - Usually IV Propofol with an opioid (ie Fentanyl) as adjunct agent - Next, paralytic agent administered and patient intubated
Maintenance	- Inhaled or IV agents (or, most commonly, a combination of both) - Neuromuscular blocking agent
Emergence	- Discontinuation of anesthetic agents - Reversal of residual neuromuscular blockade effects - Extubation

Inhaled Anesthetic Pharmacology
- Blood Solubility → Determines onset/offset time (↓ solubility more rapid)
- Lipid Solubility → Potency (↑ solubility in lipids increases potency)
    - Related to the inverse of MAC (minimal alveolar concentration), which is the amount of agent needed to prevent response to noxious stimulus in 50% of people
- In general, inhaled agents result in:
    - Increased cerebral blood flow, cerebral vasodilatation
    - ↓ SVR and MAP
    - Pulm: ↓ Tidal Volume, ↑ CO_2
    - ↓ GFR

Malignant Hyperthermia

General: A hypermetabolic state that is caused when a susceptible person is exposed to Succinylcholine or inhaled anesthetic (ie Halothane, Sevoflurane, etc). Most commonly due to AD RYR-R mutations (leading to unregulated amounts of calcium channel activation in muscle).

Clinical:
- Hyperthermia, tachycardia, hypercapnia
- Muscle rigidity, rhabdomyolysis
- Mixed metabolic and respiratory acidosis

Management:
- Discontinue anesthetics (and start non-triggered drug if still in surgery)
- 100% O_2
- Dantrolene
- Monitor and treat arrhythmia, hyperkalemia, rhabdo, acidosis, etc

ANESTHESIA

Anesthesia Surgery

Spinal/Epidural Anesthesia

General: Injection of anesthetic medication into the subarachnoid space (for spinal) or epidural space (for epidural). Commonly used for lower abdominal, lower extremity, OB-GYN surgery.

Technique: Performed via needle or catheter inserted between the vertebrae in the lumbar spinal level. Anesthetic usually Bupivacaine or Lidocaine.

Adverse Events:

High Spinal	- Excess anesthetic or improper needle position, resulting in ascending motor/sensory blockade with hypotension, bradycardia, and dyspnea (due to respiratory muscle involvement)
Postdural Puncture Headache	- Headache within 3 days post any dura puncturing procedure - Positional (worse when upright), possible with nausea/vomiting
Transient Neurologic Sx	- Syndrome of painful paresthesias in lower extremity < 24 hours after spinal - Considered benign and transient

Regional Anesthesia

Peripheral Nerve Block:
- Injection or infusion of local anesthetic agent (-caine)
- Utilizes US or electrical nerve stimulator to identify proper nerve
- Variety of different upper and lower extremity nerves can be blocked

Intravenous Regional Anesthesia
- Often used for short procedures in the forearm (ie carpal tunnel release)
- Establish IV, exsanguination of extremity, tourniquet placement, and injection of anesthetic through IV catheter
- Limited duration

Local Anesthesia

Esters (duration)	Amides (duration)
Procaine (0.5-1 hr)	Lidocaine (0.75-1.5 hr)
Cocaine (0.5-1 hr)	Mepivacaine (1-2 hr)
Tetracaine (1-6 hr)	Bupivacaine (2-8 hr)

General: The above local agents act to prevent nerve cell depolarization and signal propagation through inhibition of Na channels

Adverse Events:
- Each drug has a limited amount of drug that can be injected
- If over this amount, risk of systemic toxicity
    - Early symptoms include metallic taste, anxiety, perioral numbness
    - Severe symptoms: Seizures, arrhythmia/cardiac arrest

OPIATES

Anesthesia, Medicine, Surgery

Opiates	Mechanism	Indication	Side Effects/Management Concerns
Oxycodone (PO) Hydromorphone (PO/IV) Methadone (PO) Morphine (PO/IV) Fentanyl (IV/patch)	- Opioid receptor agonists (especially μ-opioid receptors)	- Pain control - Air hunger (especially morphine)	- Addiction [See: Psych], tolerance - Respiratory depression/CNS depression - Urinary retention - Common: Nausea, vomiting, headache, lightheadedness - Constipation - Miosis * Tolerance does not develop to constipation or miosis
Codeine		- Antitussive - Pain control	
Dextromethorphan		- Antitussive	
Loperamide Diphenoxylate		- Diarrhea	
Naloxone Naltrexone	- Opioid receptor antagonist	- Reversal of opiate toxicity	- Few side effects if no opioids in system - Can cause signs of withdrawal
Tramadol	- Weak opioid agonist - Serotonin and muscarinic antagonist	- Analgesia	- Common: Nausea/vomiting, dry mouth, dizziness (similar to opiates, but severe respiratory depression less common) - Serotonin syndrome (if paired with SNRIs or other serotonergic drugs)
Buprenorphine	- Partial opioid agonist	- Opioid misuse disorder (paired with naloxone, so inactive if injected)	- Similar to other opiates

NORMAL PREGNANCY

Obstetrics / OB-GYN

Basic Terminology of Pregnancy

Gravidity: Number of times a woman has been pregnant
Parity:
- T: Number of pregnancies leading to birth > 37 weeks gestational age
- P: Preterm
- A: Abortion
- L: Living children

Developmental age: The number of weeks/days since fertilization
Gestational age: The number of weeks/days since the last menstrual period

Trimesters: (These ranges are defined slightly differently depending on source)
1st: Weeks 1-12 weeks GA   2nd: Weeks 13-26 week GA   3rd: Weeks 27- birth GA

Diagnosis of Pregnancy

β-hCG	- Most common. Either urine or serum (more sensitive). - Generally positive by the time of expected period (ie ~ 2 weeks after ovulation and conception) - β-hCG doubles ~ 48 hours during early pregnancy and peaks around 100,000 mIU/mL by 10 weeks GA, declining slowly after this point, to around 10,000-20,000 mIU/mL at term
Ultrasound	- Most often used to confirm intrauterine pregnancy - Gestational sac visible on transvaginal US at ~5 weeks GA (β-hCG ~ 1,500 mIU/mL) - Yolk sac visible at ~ 5-6 weeks - Fetal heart motion measurable ~ 6 weeks GA (β-hCG ~ 5,000 mIU/mL)

Dating of Pregnancy

Naegele Rule: Estimated date of delivery is three months minus date of last menses, plus 7 days

Ultrasound (if LMP is uncertain):

Test	Timing	Accuracy
Crown-Rump Length	< 13 weeks	+/- 5 Days (early) to +/- 7 Days (later) Most accurate at 7-10 weeks (+/- 3 days)
Biparietal Diameter Head Circumference Femur Length	> 13 weeks	+/- 7 days (during early 2nd trimester) to +/- 3-4 weeks (by end of 3rd trimester)

Notes:
- If assisted reproduction, can simply add 266 days to date of conception
- If discrepancy between LMP and ultrasound: Can redate (ie use US date) if the patients LMP falls outside the above confidence interval for the US test
- Fundal height should be ~ 1 cm/week pregnant
- Fetal heart tones appear ~ 10-12 weeks
- Fetal movements ("quickening") occurs ~ 17-18 weeks

NORMAL PREGNANCY

Obstetrics OB-GYN

Clinical Signs of Pregnancy

Clinical Symptoms	Examination Findings
- Amenorrhea - Nausea +/- vomiting - General fatigue - Breast enlargement - Mild uterine cramping	- Telangiectasias, palmar erythema, linea nigra - Softening of cervix (Goodell sign) - Softening of uterus (Ladin sign) - Blue discoloration of vagina/cervix (Chadwick sign)

Physiologic Changes of Pregnancy

Cardiovascular	- ↑ HR, CO, SV; ↓ BP, Peripheral vascular resistance
Pulmonary	- ↑ TV, Minute/Alveolar Ventilation; ↓ CO_2
Renal	- ↑ GFR
Gastrointestinal	- ↓ Sphincter tone
Heme	- ↑ Plasma volume, ↓ Hematocrit
Endocrine	- ↑ TBG (increases total T3, T4)
Weight Gain (BMI)	< 18.5: 1 lb/wk (28-40 lbs total) 18.5-25: 0.75 lb/wk (25-35 lbs total) 25-30: 0.5 lb/wk (15-25 lbs total) > 30: 0.25 lb/wk (10-20 lbs total)

Common (Benign) Problems During Pregnancy

Back Pain	- Most common in 3rd trimester, as enlarged uterus exaggerates lordosis and changes center of gravity - Tx: Supportive (stretch, heat, massage, Acetaminophen)
Constipation	- Tx: Increased PO fluids, bulking agents, laxatives
Edema	- Lower extremity edema from IVC compression - Tx: Positional change (avoid IVC compression), elevated LE
GER	- Increased relaxation of sphincters - Tx: Antacids
Hemorrhoids	- From venous congestion/IVC compression - Tx: Topical anesthetics/steroids
Round Ligament Pain	- Adnexal pain from stretching of uterus/ligament attachments - Tx: Self-limited
Urinary Frequency	- From increased circulating volume/GFR - Tx: Rule-out UTI

ROUTINE PRENATAL CARE
Obstetrics OB-GYN

First Trimester (Initiate care by 10 weeks gestation)	Lab Tests: - Rh type/RBC screen, H/H, and MCV - Rubella, Varicella antibody screen - RPR/VDRL, chlamydia, offer HIV - HBsAg - Pap Smear (if none within 6 months) - UA and culture, urine protein - PPD If MCV low AND suspicion for possible hemoglobinopathy: - Hemoglobin analysis (via HPLC or IEF) of mom - Test dad if mom carries concerning gene If concern over family history of genetic condition (Cystic Fibrosis, Tay-Sachs): - Genetically test mom - Test dad if mom carries concerning gene Consider Hgb A1C, TSH if risk factors or symptoms
Second Trimester	- Aneuploidy screening (either late first or early second trimester) - Neural tube defect screen (US + AFP) - Fetal anatomic US (18-22 weeks) - Diabetes screen (24-28 weeks): 1 hour glucose challenge
Third Trimester	- RhoGAM for Rh- women (at 28 weeks) - H/H - GBS Culture (35-37 weeks)

Note: Visits q4 week (up to 28 wk), q2 week (28 - 36 wk), q1 week (36 wk - birth)

Other Routine Advice:

Vaccinations	- Give all Tdap and influenza - Give (if not immunized) HepA, HepB, PCV, HFlu, Meningococcus - Contraindicated: HPV, MMR, live flu, Varicella
Nutrition	- Require additional ~300 kCal/day (normal woman is ~2000) - Note: Should avoid undercooked meats, unpasteurized dairy, excessive seafood consumption, deli meats/soft cheeses, limit excessive caffeine intake Supplements: - Iron supplementation - Calcium (1000 mg /day) - Folate (0.4-0.8 mg/day, with 4 mg if risk factor for NT defect)
Exercise	- 20-30 minutes of moderate intensity exercise daily - Avoid high impact sports - Contraindicated if amniotic fluid leak, cervical incompetence, placental abnormalities, severe preeclampsia

PRENATAL TESTING
Obstetrics OB-GYN

Prenatal Aneuploidy Screening

Test	Timing	Features
First-Trimester Combined	9-13 weeks	- Uses PAPP-A, β-hCG, US for nuchal translucency <table><tr><th></th><th>NT</th><th>PAPP-A</th><th>β-hCG</th></tr><tr><td>T21</td><td>↑</td><td>↓</td><td>↑</td></tr><tr><td>T18</td><td>↑</td><td>↓</td><td>↓</td></tr><tr><td>T13</td><td>↑</td><td>↓</td><td>↓</td></tr></table>
Second-Trimester Quad	15-22 weeks	- AFP, β-hCG, estriol, inhibin <table><tr><th></th><th>AFP</th><th>β-hCG</th><th>Estriol</th><th>Inhibin</th></tr><tr><td>T21</td><td>↓</td><td>↑</td><td>↓</td><td>↑</td></tr><tr><td>T18</td><td>↓</td><td>↓</td><td>↓</td><td>Variable</td></tr><tr><td>T13</td><td colspan="4">Variable findings</td></tr></table>
Cell Free DNA	> 10 weeks	- Increasingly being offered as primary screening test, but also used as secondary screening test to avoid invasive procedure after (+) 1st/2nd trimester screen - Has high sensitivity (and high NPV), but is not diagnostic - Must have adequate amount of DNA (must be > 10 weeks, ↑ risk for inadequate sample if obese)

AFP Interpretation

Reduced AFP (< 0.5 MoM)	Increased AFP (> 2.5 MoM)
- Trisomy 21 and 18 - Fetal demise - Incorrect gestational dating	- Open-neural tube defects: Anencephaly, spina bifida - Abdominal wall defects: Gastroschisis, omphalocele - Multiple gestation - Incorrect gestational dating

Invasive Diagnostic Tests

	CVS	Amniocentesis
Age	10-13 weeks	15-20 weeks
Gen	Transcervical or transabdominal aspiration of chorionic tissue	Transabdominal aspiration of amniotic fluid (using US guidance)
Cons	- Risk of fetal loss ~1:100 - Risk for bleed/fetomaternal bleed, infection - Limb defects associated with early CVS	- Risk of fetal loss ~1:300-500 - Rarely causes leakage of amniotic fluid or direct fetal injury - Note: Discolored (brown) samples are a sign of ↑ risk of fetal demise

PRENATAL TESTING

Obstetrics OB-GYN

Antepartum Fetal Surveillance

Test	Features
Nonstress Test	- Continuous FHR monitoring Reactive NST (for ≥ 32 weeks) - Two accelerations > 15 bpm above baseline HR lasting > 15 sec over a 20 minute period Nonreactive NST - Insufficient (< 2) accelerations over a 40 minute period - Need to perform further tests (ie biophysical profile) or go out over longer period of time - Lack of FHR accelerations may occur with fetal sleeping (most commonly), fetal CNS anomalies, maternal sedatives * Can perform vibroacoustic stimulation to try to wake up baby
Contraction Stress Test	- Continuous FHR monitoring with contractions from oxytocin or natural labor (test rarely performed now) - Observe for late or significantly variable decelerations in FHR occurring with contractions (sign of fetal stress)
Biophysical Profile	- Uses 5 parameters to score 2 (normal) or 0 (abnormal) (1) Tone (≥ 1 flexion/extension movement of spine or limb) (2) Breathing (breathing episode for > 30 seconds) (3) Fetal movement (≥ 3 limb movements) (4) Amniotic fluid volume (single deepest vertical pocket ≥ 2cm) (5) Nonstress test (reactive) - Score: 8-10 → Reassuring for fetal well being 6 → Equivocal (repeat test soon) 0-4 → Worrisome for asphyxia. Delivery (usually) indicated.
Modified Bio-physical Profile	- Combination of NST and AF measurement
Amniotic Fluid Index	- Can measure depth of pocket in all 4 quadrants and add them together (> 25 polyhydramnios, < 5 oligohydramnios)
Other Tests (used to monitor certain high risk conditions)	
Umbilical Artery Velocimetry	- Used to assess IUGR/placental insufficiency - Flow can be halted or even reversed during diastole with IUGR
Transcranial Doppler	- US monitoring of cerebral artery flow velocity - Evaluates for fetal anemia (high rates of flow found in anemic fetuses)

TERATOGENESIS (DRUGS)
Obstetrics — OB-GYN, Pediatrics

Select Teratogenic Drugs/Exposures

Drug	Fetal Findings
ACEi	- Renal abnormalities, ↓ fetal GFR, oligohydramnios
Aminoglycoside	- Neurosensory hearing loss
Androgens	- Virilization (females)
Anticonvulsants	Carbamazepine - Neural tube defects, facial dysmorphia, CV defects Phenytoin - "Fetal Hydantoin Syndrome" (facial dysmorphia, cleft palate, VSD, intellectual disability) Valproate - Risk for neural tube defects, facial dysmorphia, cleft palate, CV defects (ASD), polydactyly/other limb abnormalities
Caffeine	- Possible ↑ risk for abortion at > 300 mg/day levels
DES	- Genital issues (ie abnormal uterine shapes, vaginal septa) - Clear cell adenocarcinoma of vagina in adolescents
Folate Antagonist (ie MTX, TMP)	- Risk for neural tube defects - MTX also linked to spontaneous abortion, growth restriction, microcephaly, intellectual disability
Lead	- Increased spontaneous abortion rate (at high levels)
Lithium	- Ebstein's anomaly, other congenital heart defects
Mercury	- Unclear risk, but recommended to limit possible exposure
Methimazole	- Aplasia cutis
Radiation	- Risk for microcephaly, growth or mental retardation
Statins	- Limb abnormalities, congenital heart malformations
Tetracycline	- Bone/teeth staining
Thalidomide	- Bilateral limb malformations (ie phocomelia), microtia, other cardiac/GI malformations
Tobacco	- Placental insufficiency (↑ risk for placental abruption/previa, low birth weight, PPROM, ectopic pregnancy)
Vitamin A/ Retinoids	- CNS, cardioaortic, ear, and clefting defects
Warfarin	- Nasal hypoplasia, stippling of bone epiphysis, IUGR

TERATOGENESIS (DRUGS)
Obstetrics
OB-GYN, Pediatrics

Fetal Alcohol Spectrum Disorder

General: Fetal alcohol exposure can result in a highly variable degree of impact on the developing fetus, with a variety of clinical phenotypes possible

Clinical:
- Facial abnormalities (short palpebral fissures, thin vermillion border, smooth philtrum)
- Growth retardation (↓ height/weight percentiles)
- CNS
    - Structural: Microcephaly, focal neurologic defects, other structural abnormalities
    - Neurobehavioral impairment: Developmental delay, intellectual disability, behavioral abnormalities

Diagnosis:

Fetal Alcohol Syndrome	- Characteristic facial features, growth retardation, CNS involvement, and neurobehavioral impairment
Alcohol-related Neurodevelopmental Disorder	- Neurobehavioral impairment with documented EtOH exposure - Other features may or may not be present
Alcohol-Related Birth Defects	- Specific malformation with documented EtOH exposure

Other Drugs

Marijuana	- Use discouraged during pregnancy (evidence is controversial and lacking, but concern about potential neurodevelopmental impact)
Amphetamines	- Increased risk of fetal demise, IUGR, preeclampsia, and placental abruption
Cocaine	- Risk for placental insufficiency, leading to placental abruptions, spontaneous abortion, premature births

Neonatal Abstinence Syndrome

General: Neonatal withdrawal from maternal heroin (or other opiate abuse) during pregnancy

Clinical:
- Presents within a few days of life with irritability, high-pitched cry, poor sleep, feeding difficulty, poor tone, tremors, GI disturbances, failure to thrive

Management:
- Supportive: Adequate nutrition, decreasing sensory stimulation, swaddling
- If supportive care fails, small doses of methadone or morphine are used

TERATOGENESIS (TORCH INFECTIONS)

Obstetrics
OB-GYN, Pediatrics

	General	Clinical	Management/PPX
Toxoplasma	- Due to protozoan *Toxoplasma gondii* - Usually acquired by fecal-oral transmission of sporozoite on contaminated food/water - Transplacental transmission - Mothers are asymptomatic	- Often subclinical at birth, but can present with fever, maculopapular rash, HSM, seizures, jaundice - Classic Triad: Hydrocephalus, intracranial calcifications, chorioretinitis - If untreated: Intellectual disability, seizures, motor deficits, hearing/vision loss - Dx: Serology (Toxo IgM/IgG)	Tx: Pyrimethamine + Sulfadiazine (plus Leucovorin) for neonatal infection Spiramycin, (or the above combo), for confirmed maternal infection PPX: Avoid undercooked meats, wash fruit/veg, avoid raw shellfish, do not change cat's litter box
Other (see next page)			
Rubella	- Due to rubivirus that causes "German Measles" - Transplacental transmission - Presents in mom as mild, self-limited febrile illness with classic rash	- Associated with fetal demise/abortion and IUGR - Classic signs include cataracts, hearing loss, and congenital heart disease (PDA, pulm artery stenosis) - Other signs include microcephaly, HSM, jaundice, purpuric rash, radiolucent bone disease - Dx: Rubella IgM/IgG or viral culture	Tx: Supportive PPX: MMR vaccine (before preg)
CMV	- Most common TORCH infection - Transplacental transmission - Presents as self-limited febrile illness in mom	- Usually asymptomatic, but can present at birth with small size, microcephaly, jaundice, petechiae, ↑ LFTs, thrombocytopenia, chorioretinitis - Periventricular intracranial calcifications - Can cause long term disability (sensorineural hearing loss, intellectual disability, vision loss) - Dx: PCR or viral culture (NOT serology)	Tx: Ganciclovir or Valganciclovir (for any symptomatic baby) PPX: No medical intervention (just general good hand hygiene and avoidance of close contact with young children)
HSV	- Most commonly acquired at birth from actively infected maternal genital tract - Can rarely be passed in utero if mom has primary HSV infection	- Presents in three different possible ways (normal at birth, but then subsequently developing): (1) Local: Vesicular skin, oral, and eye lesions (2) CNS: Irritability, seizures, lethargy, poor feeding (3) Disseminated: Neonatal sepsis - Dx: HSV culture or serum/CSF PCR	Tx: Acyclovir (for any type of neonatal infection) PPX: Acyclovir at 36 weeks until birth if genital HSV lesion during pregnancy * C-Section: If active lesion or prodrome

OBGYN8

OTHER PERINATAL INFECTIONS

Obstetrics — OB-GYN, Pediatrics

	General	Clinical	Management/PPX
Syphilis	- Transplacental transmission of the spirochete *T. pallidum* - Most commonly occurs in pregnant women with untreated primary and secondary syphilis (not latent)	- Associated with ↑ risk of stillbirth, IUGR, prematurity - Early Features: Fever, HSM, jaundice, LA, failure to thrive, rhinitis ("snuffles"), maculopapular rash, condyloma lata, cytopenias - Later Features (> 2 y/o): Frontal bossing, saddle nose, Hutchinson teeth (pegged shaped incisors), Mulberry molars, gummas, saber shins (anterior bowing), CNS disease (intellectual disability, seizures) - Dx: RPR/VDRL, with confirmation via FTA-ABS	Tx: - Penicillin (maternal infection) Note: If allergy, check skin allergy test, and if positive → Desensitize - Penicillin (neonatal infection)
Parvovirus	- DNA virus, causes mild febrile illness in mom (Erythema infectiosum) - Transplacental transfer	- Associated with first trimester spontaneous abortions - Infection during 2nd-3rd trimester can cause fetal hydrops - Dx: Serology (+ maternal IgM)	Tx: Monitor fetal MCA velocity for signs of severe anemia. If severe, give intrauterine RBC transfusions.
VZV	- Rare, primary varicella infection - Transplacental transmission during late 1st-2nd trimester (Shingles has no impact on baby)	- Intrauterine growth retardation, dermatologic scarring - CNS (microcephaly, intellectual disability), ocular (cataracts, chorioretinitis, etc), and limb hypoplasia - Dx: Clinical	Tx: Acyclovir (for neonatal and maternal infections), VariZIG (for babies exposed at birth) PPX: - VZV vaccine PRIOR to pregnancy if mom seronegative - If mom is seronegative and exposed to Varicella: VariZ Ig
Zika	- Due to mosquito transmitted Zika virus - Transplacental transmission, most dangerous in the 1st trimester	- Causes microcephaly, facial abnormalities, vision/hearing issues, hypertonia, and seizures - CNS findings (calcifications, ventriculomegaly, structural abnormalities) all possible - Dx: Zika serology or rt-PCR	Tx: Supportive PPX: Avoid Zika affected areas (Central America, South America, parts of Asia/Africa)

OTHER PERINATAL INFECTIONS
Obstetrics OB-GYN

Management of Maternal HIV During Pregnancy

General: HIV can be transmitted transplacentally, at the time of delivery, and via breast milk

Prenatal	Initiate all HIV + women on ART therapy:
	- Dual NRTI Backbone
	  (ie Abacavir/Lamivudine or Tenofovir/Emtricitabine)
	  PLUS
	- Protease inhibitor (Atazanavir or Darunavir) OR
	- Integrase inhibitor (Raltegravir)
	
	(Note: The above agents are all considered safe during pregnancy)

Intrapartum	- Continue ART throughout pregnancy/delivery - If viral load > 1000 copies/mL: Schedule C-section at 38 weeks plus IV Zidovudine
Postnatal	- Moms: Continue ART therapy - Infants: Zidovudine (4-6 weeks). Note: If mom was not on ART therapy or had high viral load (ie > 1000 copies/mL), baby gets combined ART therapy.

Other Infectious Disease During Pregnancy

Hepatitis B	- Transplacental transmission occurs with active hepatitis B infection (Note: HBeAg + moms have ~90% transmission rates) - Newborns of HBsAg-positive mothers should receive HBIG and hepatitis B vaccine within 12 hours of delivery - Mothers with active hepatitis B can receive tenofovir
Hepatitis C	- Transplacental transmission in ~5-10% of HCV infected women (exclusively if HCV RNA (+)) - Babies are usually asymptomatic at birth, and should check anti-HCV antibody at ~ 18 months to see if infected
Chlamydia	- Causes conjunctivitis (< 2 weeks) and pneumonia (~4-12 weeks) in newborns - Maternal infection associated with preterm, PPROM, low birth weight - Tx: Erythromycin (for neonate)
Gonorrhea	- Associated with miscarriage, PPROM, prematurity - Causes ophthalmia neonatorum (conjunctivitis) - Rarely can disseminate in newborn - Tx: Ceftriaxone + Azithromycin

ABORTION

Obstetrics
OB-GYN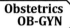

Elective Abortion

General: ~50% of pregnancies are unintended, and ~20% are terminated electively. Legalized nationwide in 1973 as part of Rowe vs Wade. Can be performed up until viability (~24 weeks), unless medical indication to terminate later.

Procedure:

Type	Timing	Features
Medical	< 10 weeks GA	- Mifepristone, followed by Misoprostol in 24-48 hr
Aspiration	< 14 weeks GA	- Mechanical cervical dilatation and aspiration of uterine contents
Surgical	14-24 weeks GA	- Dilation and evacuation (using osmotic or pharm dilators, followed by extraction/curettage)
Induction	14-24 weeks GA	- Misoprostol plus mifepristone (Note: Usually use feticidal injection to ensure no live birth)

Management:
- RhoGAM if Rh (-)
- Antibiotic prophylaxis (usually given, but controversial)

Spontaneous Abortion (Miscarriage)

General: The loss of products of conception prior to the 20th week of pregnancy. Most common in first trimester, and most commonly due to chromosomal abnormalities.

Risk: ↑ Maternal age, smoking, history of spontaneous abortion

Etiology:

Fetal	- Chromosomal abnormalities (ie aneuploidy [Trisomy 16]) - Trauma - Congenital abnormalities (from teratogens, etc)
Maternal	- Maternal uterine structural abnormalities - Systemic maternal disease (infection, endocrinopathy, hypercoagulable state, etc)

Clinical: See next page

Diagnosis: Pelvic exam and US
- US can confirm fetal viability if POC still in utero (ie lack of cardiac activity)

Management:
- See next page for specifics depending on classification of abortion
- RhoGAM if Rh (-)

Complications:
- Hemorrhage: Usually due to retained products. D&C indicated.
- Endometritis/septic abortion

OBGYN11

ABORTION

Obstetrics — OB-GYN

	Symptoms	Findings	Management
Threatened	- Uterine bleeding +/- abdominal pain - No POC expulsion	- Closed Os - Intact Membranes - Live fetus	- Supportive care (until symptoms resolve or progress to complete abortion) - Associated w/ ↑ risk for preterm/PPROM, but can still proceed to viable birth
Inevitable	- Vaginal bleeding + cramping	- Open Os - POC present on US (at level or above os) - Fetus may still have heartbeat	- Can be managed one of three ways, based on preference: (1) Surgery (dilation and curettage) (2) Medically (Mifepristone/Misoprostol) (3) Expectant Management (allow natural passage. Can monitor β-hCG to measure completeness. If spontaneous passage does not occur, can then proceed to surgical or medical intervention)
Incomplete	- Vaginal bleeding + cramping - Passage of large clots/tissue	- Open Os - POC present on US (within/being expelled from cervical canal)	
Missed	- Fetal death without any passage of POC - Variable presentation (asymptomatic to vaginal bleeding) - Often presents as failure of pregnancy to progress	- Closed OS - US shows nonviable conceptus with no fetal cardiac activity	
Complete	- Vaginal bleeding + cramping - Complete passage of POC, followed by resolution of symptoms	- Closed OS - US shows no conceptus	- Supportive
Septic	- Foul-smelling vaginal discharge - Most often occurs after elective abortion, but can occur with spontaneous abortion (especially if retained POC)	- Sepsis (fever, hypotension) - Enlarged, tender uterus/cervix	- IV Antibiotics (same as PID) - Suction D&C

OBGYN12

ABORTION

Obstetrics OB-GYN

Recurrent Spontaneous Abortion

General: Defined as three or more consecutive pregnancy losses

Risk:

Uterine	- Polyps/fibroids/adhesions - Cervical insufficiency
Genetic	- Aneuploidy - Parents with balanced or Robertsonian translocations
Immunologic	- Antiphospholipid syndrome
Endocrine	- Uncontrolled diabetes - Hypothyroidism - PCOS
Hematologic	- Inherited or acquired hypercoagulable states

Diagnosis:
- Uterine hysterosalpingogram (workup for structure)
- Karyotypes of mom/dad, and abortus if available (for genetic)
- Anticardiolipin IgM/IgG, lupus anticoagulant titers
- TSH

Management:
- Treat underlying (surgical correction of structural abnormalities, manage endocrinopathy, etc)

Cervical Insufficiency

General: The inability of the uterine cervix to retain a pregnancy in the 2nd trimester due to painless dilation of the cervix

Etiology:
- Cervical Trauma: Repeated D&C, cervical cone, loop electrocautery excision procedure (LEEP), prior labor/delivery
- Congenital cervical abnormalities

Clinical:
- History of 2nd trimester pregnancy loss
- Cervical dilation and effacement on physical exam
- Can be asymptomatic or present with mild cramping/contractions

Diagnosis: Transvaginal US (< 25 mm long before 24 weeks)

Management:
- Cerclage (suture stabilization of the cervical os)
- Hydroxyprogesterone

ABORTION

Obstetrics OB-GYN

Intrauterine Fetal Demise

General: Absence of fetal cardiac activity > 20 weeks GA

Risk: ↑ Age, obesity, multiple gestation, smoking, underlying medical conditions

Etiology:
- Perinatal infection
- Placental injury (ie abruption)
- Maternal systemic disease
- Uterine abnormalities
- Hydrops/Alloimmune disease
- Fetal cord accident (diagnosis of exclusion)

Clinical:
- Uterus small for GA
- Reported lack of movement

Diagnosis: US (without fetal heart activity, confirmed by 2 MDs)

Management:
- GA 20-24 weeks
    - Dilation and evacuation or induction and delivery
- GA > 24 weeks
    - Prostaglandins and Oxytocin for induction and delivery
- Note: If not delivered within a few weeks, risk for maternal DIC

Workup:
- Autopsy
- Placental analysis
- Fetal karyotype
- Maternal labs (for Antiphospholipid, fetomaternal hemorrhage)

ECTOPIC PREGNANCY

Obstetrics OB-GYN

Ectopic Pregnancy

General: Implantation at a site other than the endometrium. Locations include:
- Tube ampulla (~80%), tube isthmus (~10%), fimbriae (~5%)
- Abdominal, ovarian, cervical, cesarean scar (all rare)

Risk: History of ectopic, PID, IVF, endometriosis, pelvic surgery, smoking
- IUD (lower risk for pregnancy, but elevated risk for ectopic if failure)

Clinical: Abdominal pain and vaginal bleeding

Diagnosis: Serial β-hCG and Transvaginal US (see algorithm below)
- Note: β-hCG should rise by at least 35% in 48 hours (normally it doubles)

Management:

Surgical	Indicated if:
Salpingectomy OR Salpingostomy	- Hemodynamically unstable or tubal rupture - β-hCG > 5,000 OR fetal cardiac activity present on US - Contraindications to MTX (ie coexisting intrauterine pregnancy, immunodeficiency, hematologic/hepatic/renal disease) - Patient not reliable/able to comply with medical follow up
Medical Methotrexate	- 50 mg/m² dose of MTX given day 1 - β-hCG checked on days 4, 7 - If inadequate decline (ie < 15%), second dose of MTX given - Follow β-hCG until undetectable

Complications: Tubal Rupture
- Presents as diffuse abdominal pain (peritonitis), cervical motion tenderness
    - +/- Severe vaginal bleeding
    - Possible hypovolemic shock
- Dx: FAST US
- Tx: Stabilize in ED (ie ABCs, blood transfusions), emergent laparotomy

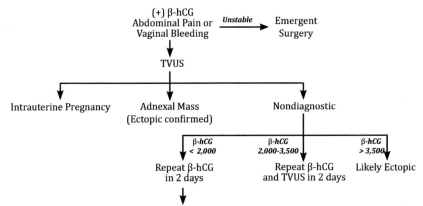

OBGYN15

GESTATIONAL TROPHOBLASTIC DISEASE
Obstetrics OB-GYN

Hydatidiform Mole

	Complete Mole (~90%)	Partial Mole (~10%)
Mxn	- Sperm fertilizes empty ovum	- Normal ovum fertilized by 2 sperm
Karyo	- 46 XX; 46 XY (all paternal) - p57 negative	- 69 XXY; 69 XYY; 69 XXX (extra paternal set) - p57 positive
Histo	- Diffuse villi swelling/hyperplasia - No fetal tissue	- Focal villi swelling/hyperplasia - Fetal tissue present (RBC, body parts)
Clin	- Presents as abnormal vaginal bleed - Uterus enlarged for date - β-hCG high (> 100,000) - Signs of high β-hCG (hyperemesis, preeclampsia, hyperthyroid, theca lutein cyst)	- Presents as missed abortion - Uterus expected size for date - β-hCG mildly elevated
US	- "Snow-storm" pattern, grape-like clusters	- Variable
Prog	- Up to 25% chance of malignancy - 4% chance of metastatic disease	- Up to 4% chance of malignancy - 0% chance of metastatic disease

General: Moles are considered benign trophoblastic disease (while invasive moles, placental site trophoblastic tumors, and choriocarcinoma are considered gestational trophoblastic neoplasia)

Risk: History of gestational trophoblastic disease, age > 35 or < 20

Clinical: See above

Diagnosis: Based on US features, symptoms, and β-hCG. Confirmed with histology.

Management: Dilation and Suction Curettage (D&C)
- Follow β-hCG until normalized (+ 6 month period after normalized)
- Usually 14 weeks for complete, 8 weeks partial
- Ensure good contraception during this period of time

GESTATIONAL TROPHOBLASTIC DISEASE

Obstetrics
OB-GYN

Gestational Trophoblastic Neoplasia (Overview)

General: Refers to group of malignant trophoblastic neoplasms associated with either a hydatidiform mole or normal pregnancy. Types include:
- Invasive mole
- Placental site trophoblastic tumor
- Choriocarcinoma

Risk: History of molar pregnancy, ↑ maternal age (ie > 40), Asian ancestry

Clinical:
- Variable depending on subtype of disease
- Can include symptoms from ↑ β-hCG (hyperthyroidism, theca lutein cysts, pelvic pain, abnormal uterine bleeding)

Diagnosis: Clinical (Tissue not required for diagnosis. Based on ↑ β-hCG, uterine enlargement, metastatic disease, etc)
- Workup (if suspicious) should include CXR (common metastatic site)

Management:
- Low Risk: Single Agent Chemo (Methotrexate or Actinomycin D)
    - Generally defined as local disease without significant mets
- High Risk: Multi-Agent Chemo
    - Generally defined as highly metastatic disease
- Always trend β-hCG and provide good contraception
- Placental site trophoblastic tumor should be treated with hysterectomy

Gestational Trophoblastic Neoplasia (Subtypes)

Invasive Mole	- Hydropic villi invading into myometrium - Rarely metastasize, and can spontaneously regress - Presents as ↑ β-hCG after treatment of molar pregnancy. Can also present with persistent vaginal bleeding. - Tx: Single Agent Chemo (Methotrexate or Actinomycin D). Trend β-hCG, reliable contraception. Note: Hysterectomy is alternative treatment for those without desire for fertility.
Placental Site Trophoblastic Tumor	- Proliferation of intermediate trophoblasts (ie no villi) - Presents as irregular vaginal bleeding and enlarged uterus - Note: β-hCG not significantly elevated (because no syncytiotrophoblast, but hPL is ↑) - Tx: Hysterectomy (poor chemotherapy sensitivity)

Choriocarcinoma	- Can occur with molar pregnancy (50%), abortion, or normal pregnancy
	- Proliferation of cytotrophoblast and syncytiotrophoblast with chorionic villi
	- Common metastasis to vagina and lungs
	- Tx: Chemotherapy
	    - Single-agent used if local (Methotrexate or Actinomycin D)
	    - Multi-agent used for high risk, metastatic disease
	    - Follow β-hCG, provide reliable contraception

PLACENTAL PATHOLOGY

Obstetrics OB-GYN

	General/Risk	Clinical/Diagnosis	Management
Placenta Previa	- Abnormal placental implantation Subtypes: - Complete: Placenta covers the cervical os - Partial: Partially covers cervical os - Marginal: Extends to the margin of the os - Low lying: In close proximity to the os - Risk: History of placenta previa or cesarean delivery, history of D&C or myomectomy, multiple gestation	- Painless vaginal bleeding - Rarely causes uterine contractions/cramps - Associated with placenta accreta, preterm labor, PROM, vasa previa - Dx: Ultrasound (before digital exam due to risk for hemorrhage) Note: Once placenta is > 2 cm from cervical os, vaginal delivery is considered safe	- If asymptomatic: Follow with US (most previa resolve on own) - Counsel patients to reduce bleeding risk by avoiding sexual activity, strenuous exercise, or prolonged standing - Supportive care/blood transfusions for acute episodes of bleeding - Delivery (at 36-37 weeks) by C-section - C-section also indicated if patient goes into labor, has life-threatening bleed, or severe fetal distress
Vasa Previa	- Presence of fetal blood vessels in membranes covering the cervical os - Commonly associated with velamentous umbilical cord or succenturiate lobe - Risk: Velamentous cord insertion, low-lying placenta/previa, IVF, multiple gestation	- Presents as painless bleeding at time of rupture of membranes - Fetal HR may show signs of distress (bradycardia, decelerations, sinusoidal pattern, etc) - Apt test can be used to confirm fetal blood (mix NaOH with blood → Turns pink if fetal) - Dx: Transvaginal US (w/ doppler)	- Emergent C-section (indicated if acute bleeding, labor, or PROM) - Antepartum: Weekly nonstress testing, betamethasone at 28-32 weeks, schedule C-section at 34-35 weeks - Planned C-section/Hysterectomy at 34-35 weeks
Placenta Accreta	- Accreta: Anchoring of placental villi to the myometrium - Increta: Chorionic villi invade the myometrium - Percreta: Anchoring of placental villi through the myometrium and into serosa/abdominal organs Risk: Hx of myomectomy/C-section/D&C	- Generally asymptomatic prior to delivery (but may be identified via US) - At delivery: Lack of placenta delivery - Retained parts, possible cord avulsion, and severe hemorrhage Dx: US (shows irregularity or absence of placental myometrial interface). MRI if diagnosis uncertain.	- If diagnosed due to hemorrhage at the time of vaginal delivery, emergent hysterectomy is indicated

PLACENTAL PATHOLOGY
Obstetrics OB-GYN

Placental Abruption

General: Separation of the placenta prior to delivery of fetus. Usually due to:
- Underlying chronic placental disease (see risk factors below)
- Acute traumatic event (blunt trauma, deceleration injury)
- Rapid uterine decompression (ie delivery of twin, relief of polyhydramnios)

Risk: History of placental abruption, hypertension/eclampsia, tobacco/cocaine use, chorioamnionitis

Clinical:
- Severe vaginal bleeding
- Abdominal pain/contractions
- Uterine rigidity/tenderness
- Fetal distress
- High risk for DIC, hemorrhagic shock

Diagnosis: US (retroplacental clot)
- Note: US findings not consistent, so diagnosis may be based on clinical findings

Management:
- Initial: FHR monitoring, IV access, other supportive care
- Delivery (choice depends on stability of mom/baby)
    - If both are stable (and > 36 weeks): Vaginal delivery
    - If either is unstable: C-section (unless vaginal delivery imminent)

Uterine Rupture

General: Complete disruption of all uterine layers

Etiology:
- Prior C-section (especially history of rupture, vertical hysterotomy)
- Uterine myomectomy with cavity entry
    - Rarely seen in those without history of scarred uterus
- Increased risk with prolonged labor, excess uterotonic drugs, multiple gestation, ↑ maternal age

Clinical:
- Sudden worsening of abdominal pain
- Possible vaginal bleeding, fetal distress
- Classic signs: Loss of fetal station, or palpation of fetal parts outside uterus
- Can be complicated by urinary tract injury, hemorrhagic shock
- Symptoms brought on or exacerbated by oxytocin

Diagnosis: Clinical + US confirmation (of disruption of all uterine layers)

Management:
- Crash C-section
- Hysterectomy. Occasionally uterine repair may be possible.

MULTIPLE GESTATION
Obstetrics / OB-GYN

Overview of Multiple Gestation

General: ~3% rate of multiple gestation pregnancies in US

Risk: ↑ Maternal Age, IVF

Clinical:
- Moms can experience rapid weight gain, excessive uterus size for age
- ↑ β-hCG, AFP, hPL for expected age

Diagnosis: Most commonly picked up on US
- Can see two amniotic sacs or "twin-peaks" sign (fused membranes)

Management:
- Twin Delivery:
    - Cephalic/Cephalic: Vaginal Delivery
    - Cephalic/Non-cephalic: C-section or trial of vaginal delivery
    - Non-cephalic/Non-cephalic: C-section
- Triplets: Almost always require C-section

Maternal Complications:
- Moms are more likely to require hospitalization, have placental abnormalities (ie previa), and require C-section

Fetal Complications:
- Prematurity and low birth weight (common, risk ↑ with fetal number)
- Fetal Growth Restriction (from crowding or uteroplacental insufficiency)
- Increased risk of congenital malformations
- Twin-twin Transfusion
    - Unbalanced vascular flow to two monochorionic twins
    - "Donor twin" (hypovolemic, growth restriction, oligohydramnios)
    - "Recipient twin" (hypervolemia, organomegaly, polyhydramnios)
    - Rarely, there can be a significant intertwin hemoglobin difference
        - Called twin anemia polycythemia sequence
    - Management:
        - Fetal laser coagulation (tries to correct flow difference)
        - Amnioreduction (helps prevent preterm contractions)

MULTIPLE GESTATION

Obstetrics OB-GYN

Multiple Gestation (Subtypes)

Class	Features
Dizygotic	
Dichorionic Diamniotic	- Implantation of two separate fertilized ovum ("fraternal twins") - Can be different sexes - Separate placenta/amniotic sacs
Monozygotic	
Dichorionic Diamniotic	- One fertilized ovum, which splits (~days 1-3) and implant separately - Separate placenta/amniotic sacs
Monochorionic Diamniotic	- One fertilized ovum, which splits after blastocyst forms (~days 4-8), and implant separately - Share placenta, separate amniotic sac
Monochorionic Monoamniotic	- One fertilized ovum, which implants, and then later splits (~days 8-13) - Same placenta, same amniotic sac - Highest risk for fetal mortality
Conjoined	- Same as monochorionic-monoamniotic above, except split occurs at ~14 days after embryonic disk has formed

NORMAL LABOR AND DELIVERY
Obstetrics OB-GYN

Overview and Definition of Labor

General: Labor is defined as painful contractions PLUS cervical change

Stage	Definition	Nulliparous	Multiparous
First (Latent)	Onset of labor until 4-6 cm dilation	< 20 hours (average 10-12)	< 14 hours (average 6-8)
First (Active)	4-6 cm until complete 10 cm cervical dilation	4-6 hr (> 1-1.2 cm/hr)	2-3 hr (> 1.2-1.5 cm/hr)
Second	Complete cervical dilation to delivery of infant	< 2 hours (3 hr if epidural)	< 1 hour (2 hr if epidural)
Third	From delivery of infant to delivery of placenta	< 30 minutes	< 30 minutes

Evaluation of Labor

- Leopold Maneuvers: Used to determine fetal lie (ie longitudinal or transverse, etc)
- Cervical Examination
    - Dilation (measured at internal os)
        - Dilation can cause "bloody show" (small cervical bleed)
    - Effacement (thinning of cervix from normal length of 3-5 cm)
    - Station: Based on position relative to imaginary line between ischial spines
        - Negative is inside of uterus, positive is outside of uterus
    - Cervical position and consistency
- Speculum Examination (look for ROM)
    - Pooling of fluid (after asking patient to bear down), nitrazine paper (amniotic fluid is alkaline), ferning (microscopically)
    - Other tests: Indigo-carmine dye injection, amnisure immunoassay
- Ultrasound: Can evaluate for effacement or new oligohydramnios (suggests ROM)

Bishop Score

Cervical Status	0	1	2	3
Dilatation	Closed	1-2 cm	3-4 cm	> 5 cm
Effacement	< 30%	30-50%	50-80%	> 80%
Station	-3	-2	-1 or 0	≥ +1
Consistency	Firm	Intermediate	Soft	
Position	Posterior	Intermediate	Anterior	

Cardinal Movements and Occiput Presentation

Cardinal Movements:
Engagement, descent & internal rotation, complete rotation, complete extension, external rotation, anterior shoulder delivery, posterior shoulder delivery

Occiput Presentation:
Vertex presentation with anterior occiput is ideal. Occiput posterior and transverse can lead to longer delivery time.

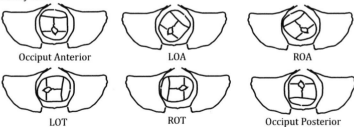

Occiput Anterior   LOA   ROA

LOT   ROT   Occiput Posterior

NORMAL LABOR AND DELIVERY

Obstetrics
OB-GYN

Fetal Heart Rate Monitoring

General: Fetal heart rate can be monitored via external doppler monitor or via fetal scalp electrode. Often combined with tocometry, which measures intrauterine pressure to help establish timing, length, and strength of contractions.

Component	Features
Rate	< 110 (bradycardia): Congenital heart defects, severe hypoxemia (uterine hyperstimulation, cord prolapse, rapid fetal descent) > 160 (tachycardia): Hypoxia, maternal fever, fetal anemia, drugs
Variability	- Absent: Indicates severe fetal distress - Minimal: < 6 bpm (indicates fetal hypoxia, drugs, or sleep) - Can attempt fetal scalp stimulation to induce variability - Normal: 6-25 bpm - Marked: > 25 bpm - Sinusoidal: Fetal anemia
Accelerations	- 15 bpm above baseline for 15 seconds (at least 2 in 20 minutes) Note: At < 32 weeks it is 10 bpm/10sec, at least 2 in 20 min

Decelerations

Type	Description	Cause	Tracing
Early	- Gradual (onset to nadir > 30 sec) ↓ in FHR that mirrors uterine contraction	- Head Compression (vagal tone)	
Late	- Gradual (onset to nadir > 30 sec) ↓ in FHR with onset after peak of contraction and recovery of FHR after contraction is over	- Uteroplacental Insufficiency - Fetal hypoxemia	
Variable	- Abrupt (onset to nadir < 30 sec) ↓ in FHR lasting no more than 2 minutes - Not correlated with contractions	- Umbilical Cord Compression	

VEAL-CHOP
- Variable → Cord compression
- Early → Head compression
- Acceleration → Okay
- Late → Placental insufficiency

NORMAL LABOR AND DELIVERY
Obstetrics / OB-GYN

Induction and Augmentation of Labor

Induction:
- Indicated if:
  - Postterm
  - Preeclampsia, DM
  - IUGR
  - Signs of fetal distress on antenatal testing
- Techniques:
  - May begin spontaneously after cervical ripening
  - Oxytocin
  - Amniotomy (ie artificial ROM)

Cervical Ripening
- Indicated in those with poor Bishop's score (< 6) prior to induction
- Methods include:
  - Misoprostol (PGE1)
  - PGE2 gel or vaginal inserts (Prepidil/Cervidil)
  - Mechanical bulb dilator

Augmentation:
- Indications: Inadequate contractions or prolonged phase of labor
- Oxytocin: Stimulates uterus for stronger and more frequent contractions
  - Side Effects: Tachysystole, ADH like effect (hyponatremia), hypotension, fetal distress

Analgesia and Pain Management

General: Visceral pain from uterine and cervical distension/cramping (Stage 1) and somatic pain from Stage 2 of labor as vagina and perineal structures are stretched
- Block must reach T10 for visceral first stage pain, S2-S4 for second stage

Indications: Maternal request (sufficient to provide, assuming no contraindications)

Lamaze	- Coping/relaxation techniques taught in classes during pregnancy
Opiates	- Generally inferior to neuraxial block and avoided - If used, rapid acting agents used (ie Fentanyl) - Can cause fetal bradycardia and neonatal respiratory depression
Neuraxial	- Options include epidural, combined spinal-epidural, or spinal - Generally given continuously via catheter (can be via "single-shot") - Continuous allows easy transition to operative delivery - Drug Choice: Local anesthetic (Bupivacaine) plus opiate (Fentanyl) - [See: Surgery] for discussion of complications
Nerve Block	- Pudendal nerve block: Used as adjunct if patient suffering from somatic vaginal/perineal pain
General Anesthesia	- Reserved for cases of emergent C-section when there is no time for neuraxial block

OPERATIVE LABOR AND DELIVERY

Obstetrics — OB-GYN

Cesarean Delivery

Indications:

Maternal	Fetal
Failure to Progress, including: - Cephalopelvic disproportion - Failed labor induction Structural: - Obstructive tumors, fibroids - Placental abruption, previa - Vasa previa or cord prolapse Medical Conditions - HIV infection (untreated) - Active HSV - Cervical cancer - Obstructive tumors, fibroids	- Fetal distress (ie on FHR monitoring) - Fetal malpresentation - Multiple gestation (ie triplets or malpresenting first twin) Fetal Anomalies - Macrosomia (ie > 5000 g)

Surgical Technique:
- Neuraxial anesthesia is preferred (general anesthesia for emergencies)
- Transverse Incision (Pfannenstiel)
    - Better cosmetics, less postoperative pain
    - Occasionally vertical incisions are used in severe emergencies
- Low transverse hysterotomy
- Delivery of fetus and placenta
- Ensure no retained parts/bleeding (uterine massage/oxytocin)
- Abdominal wall closure

Postoperative Issues:
- Pain, urinary retention, infection, bleeding

Long-Term Complications:
- Scarring (↑ risk for uterine rupture, placenta previa/accreta)

Trial of Labor After Cesarean (TOLAC)

General: Although primary C-section is often followed by C-section during future pregnancies, some women elect for trial of labor. Called TOLAC for labor trial, and VBAC for vaginal birth after cesarean.

Risk in these patients for uterine rupture at site of C-section scar

Lower Risk	- Only 1 prior C-section, prior vaginal birth or VBAC
Higher Risk	- > 1 prior cesarean delivery, "classical" cesarean delivery - Prior C-section for cephalopelvic disproportion - Last cesarean within 18 months

Management:
- In general, TOLAC can be considered if 1 prior C-section with transverse incision. Otherwise, repeat deliveries should be via C-section.

OBGYN25

OPERATIVE LABOR AND DELIVERY

Obstetrics OB-GYN

Operative Vaginal Delivery

General: Refers to the use of forceps or vacuum to assist in the extraction of fetus from vagina

Indications:
- Generally indicated when normal labor needs to be terminated
- In general, cesarean delivery is performed rather than forceps/vacuum, but there are some situations where they are indicated:
    - Prolonged 2nd stage of labor (ie from maternal exhaustion)
    - Fetal compromise
    - Maternal disorder that contraindicates valsalva
- Note: In all the above cases, operative delivery must be safe/possible. This means baby has head engaged (with station > 0), full dilation/cervical effacement, membranes ruptured, and adequate anesthesia.

Type	Features	Adverse Events
Forceps	- Forceps used to grasp the anterior occiput	- ↑ Risk of maternal genital trauma (ie vaginal lacerations, bladder injury, etc) - ↑ Risk of fetal CN VII injury
Vacuum	- Suction cup applied to fetal scalp	- ↑ Risk of cephalohematoma, retinal hemorrhage compared to forceps

* All operative vaginal deliveries have rare risk of fetal CNS hemorrhage
* Above adverse events can happen with either forceps or vacuum, but are classified with the operative technique that they are more highly associated with

Episiotomy/Lacerations

Episiotomy:
- Surgical enlargement of the vagina via incision into the perineum, in order to widen the birth canal and facilitate delivery
- No specific indications for episiotomy (occasionally used by some OB physicians when rapid vaginal delivery is needed or shoulder dystocia)
- Approach
    - Mediolateral (↓ risk of sphincter injury, but harder to repair)
    - Medial (Easiest to repair, but painful and ↑ risk of sphincter injury)
- Complications: Sphincter injury, bleeding, infection, rectovaginal fistula

Lacerations:
- Vaginal lacerations are commonplace with vaginal delivery
- Types:
    - Grade 1: Vaginal only
    - Grade 2: Perineal body
    - Grade 3: Into anal sphincter
    - Grade 4: Through anal mucosa
- Complications: Wound abscess, sphincter injury, rectovaginal fistula

COMPLICATIONS OF LABOR & DELIVERY

Obstetrics — OB-GYN

	General/Clinical	Management
Spontaneous Rupture of Membranes (ROM)	- Occurs after the onset of labor - Required for fetal head engagement - Can be confirmed via history of gush of fluid & speculum examination confirming leakage of amniotic fluid (presentation is similar for all the ROM conditions)	- Normal Delivery Management Note: Can confirm ROM with nitrazine paper test, fern testing, US (for oligohydramnios), indigo carmine dye injection
Premature ROM (PROM)	- Rupture of the membranes prior to regular contractions - Women at full term (vs PPROM) - ↑ Risk of maternal and fetal infections	- Induction of labor (Oxytocin)
Preterm Premature ROM (PPROM)	- Rupture of membranes prior to contractions at < 37 weeks GA - Risk for complications, including intrauterine infection/neonatal sepsis, oligohydramnios, umbilical cord prolapse or compression, fetal malpresentation	See Algorithms Below - Urgent delivery is indicated for any PPROM associated with intrauterine infection, placental abruption, fetal distress, or concern about cord prolapse

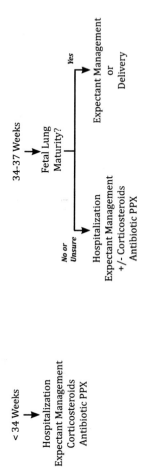

COMPLICATIONS OF LABOR & DELIVERY
Obstetrics — OB-GYN

Premature Labor

General: Birth prior to 37 weeks gestational age

Risk: History of premature labor, multiple gestation, smoking, history of cervical surgery (ie those with cervical insufficiency)

Etiology: Premature labor can be induced by infection, PROM, polyhydramnios, placental abruption

Clinical: Presents similarly to normal term labor (cramping, contractions, vaginal discharge of clear fluid/mucus/blood tinged fluid)

Diagnosis: Painful Contractions (> 4 in 20 min or > 8 in 60 min) AND cervical change (ie dilation > 3 cm or effacement)
- Fetal Fibronectin (used between weeks 22-34)
    - High negative predictive value
    - Positive levels support likely true preterm labor

Management: All should receive full H&P, speculum exam (r/o PROM), and US

≥ 34 Weeks	- Admit and deliver *Note: If no progression (and fetal well being is confirmed) then patient can be discharged home

32-33 Weeks	- Betamethasone
	- Tocolytic Drugs (48 hours for steroid effects). Drugs include:
	  - β2-mimetics (Ritodrine or Terbutaline)
	  - $MgSO_4$
	  - Ca-Channel Blockers (Nifedipine)
	  - PG Inhibitors (Indomethacin)
	- GBS Antibiotic PPX (Penicillin G, Ampicillin, or Clindamycin)

< 32 Weeks	- Same as 32-33 weeks, but add $MgSO_4$ (proven neuroprotection)

Complications:
- Fetal: Intraventricular hemorrhage, NRDS, PDA, necrotizing enterocolitis, retinopathy of prematurity, bronchopulmonary dysplasia

Prophylaxis:
- If history of spontaneous premature birth: Progesterone supplementation
- If Short Cervix (on TVUS 16-24 weeks):
    - No history of prematurity: Give progesterone
    - Plus history of prematurity: Progesterone plus cerclage

COMPLICATIONS OF LABOR & DELIVERY
Obstetrics / OB-GYN

Postterm Pregnancy

General: Consider postterm at ≥ 42 weeks GA

Risk: History of postterm, obesity, fetal endocrinopathy, male fetus, nulliparity

Management:
- Induce labor if:
    - Non-reassuring fetal testing or oligohydramnios
    - ≥ 42 weeks
    - Consider at 41 weeks GA (especially if favorable cervix)
- If expectant management: Monitor with biophysical profile

Complications:
- Fetal: Macrosomia, oligohydramnios, meconium aspiration
    - Dysmaturity syndrome (dry peeling nails, flaking skin, lots of hair)
- Maternal: Birth trauma, increction, hemorrhage

GBS Infection

General: Organism that routinely colonizes GU tract in women. Can cause UTI (both cystitis and pyelonephritis), chorioamnionitis, endomyometritis, neonatal sepsis.

Diagnosis:
- Screened for at 35-37 weeks in all pregnant women (vaginal/rectal swab)

Management:
- Antibiotic PPX: Penicillin G or Ampicillin (alt: Cefazolin, Clindamycin)
- Started at the onset of labor (but not C-section without labor)
    - Indications include:
        - (+) Routine GBS screening
        - History of infant with early-onset GBS infection
        - GBS bacteriuria during current pregnancy
        - Unknown status, plus:
            - Preterm labor, intrapartum fever, or prolonged ROM (> 18 hours)

Chorioamnionitis

General: Infection of the amniotic fluid, membranes, placenta, and/or decidua. Usually polymicrobial (from vaginal flora in women with rupture membranes), but can be due to iatrogenically introduced bacteria from procedures.

Clinical: Clinical diagnosis made with fever > 100.4°F PLUS ≥ 1 of the following:
- FHR > 160
- Maternal WBC count > 15,000
- Purulent vaginal/cervical discharge

Diagnosis: Confirmed with positive gram stain/culture of amniotic fluid

Management: Ampicillin + Gentamicin +/- Clindamycin or Metronidazole (if C-section).
- Prompt delivery is indicated (normal vaginal delivery is okay unless patient has some usual indication for C-section)

COMPLICATIONS OF LABOR & DELIVERY

Obstetrics — OB-GYN

Failure to Progress	General	Management
First Stage (Latent)	- Normal: < 20 hrs (prima), < 14 hrs (multip) - Risk: Unfavorable cervix	- Therapeutic rest (ie Morphine and rest) - Oxytocin augmentation - Amniotomy - Most will eventually pass into active labor or will stop having contractions
First Stage (Passive)	- Normal: > 6 cm, 1-2 cm/hr progression - Protracted: Dilating < 1 cm/hr - Arrest: No cervical change in 4 hours despite adequate contractions Causes include: - Lack of Power: Normal power is > 200 Montevideo units (MVUs) (defined as sum of the peak uterine pressure - baseline uterine pressure for each contraction) - Passenger/Pelvis Issue: Cephalopelvic disproportion	- Initial: Oxytocin and amniotomy - If ineffective → C-section
Second Stage	- Normal: < 3 hours (null), < 2 hours (prima), plus longer for those with epidural anesthesia - Cause: Most often passenger/pelvis issue (including mal-presentation, macrosomia, cephalopelvic disproportion)	- Trial of Oxytocin (if infrequent contractions > 3 mins) - Consideration for operative delivery OR C-section - Decision of operative vs C-section is highly based on experience and clinical judgement
Third Stage (Placental Delivery)	- Normal: < 30 minutes - Risk: Prior C-section, D&C, or fibroids	- Oxytocin, uterine massage [See: Postpartum Hemorrhage] - Retained Placenta: Manual extraction or D&C

COMPLICATIONS OF LABOR & DELIVERY
Obstetrics / OB-GYN

Shoulder Dystocia

General: Failure of the shoulders to spontaneously deliver after the fetal head

Risk: Maternal obesity, diabetes mellitus, macrosomia, post-date, history of shoulder dystocia. Note: > 50% of cases are idiopathic and have none of the above risk factors.

Clinical:
- Recoil of fetal head into the perineum ("turtle sign")

Management:

B	- Breathe
E	- Elevate legs (McRoberts Position: Sharp flexion of the hips)
C	- Call for help
A	- Apply suprapubic pressure (downward to release anterior shoulder)
L	- enLarge vaginal opening with episiotomy
M	- Maneuvers

Complications of Shoulder Dystocia

Erb Palsy	- C5-C6 injury - Presents with decreased reflexes on affected side, as well as "Waiter's tip" (extended elbow, pronated forearm, flexed wrist) - Tx: 80% are self-limited and improve over following months. Massage and physical therapy.
Klumpke	- C8-T1 injury - Presents with "claw hand" (extended wrist, extended MCPs, and flexed IPs) - Possible Horner syndrome
Clavicle Fx	- Presents with clavicular bony crepitus, deformity, and/or decreased Moro reflex on the affected side
Humeral Fx	- Presents with upper-arm bony crepitus, deformity, and/or decreased Moro reflex on the affected side
Asphyxia	- Can result in hypoxic-ischemic encephalopathy or death if severe

COMPLICATIONS OF LABOR & DELIVERY

Obstetrics OB-GYN

Breech Presentation

Frank Breech (50-75%)	- Presents rear first, with flexed hips and extended knees
Footling Breech (20%)	- Presents with one or both legs presented first
Complete Breech (5-10%)	- Presents rear first, with flexed hips and flexed knees

Diagnosis: Leopold maneuvers or ultrasound

Management:
- 75% spontaneously change to vertex by week 38
- External cephalic version: Performed after week 37
    - Apply directed pressure to abdomen to turn infant to vertex
    - Risks: Placental abruption and cord compression
      (must be prepared for emergency C-section, give RhoGAM)
    - Contraindications: Ruptured membranes/oligohydramnios, extended head, non-reassuring tracing, fetal/uterine abnormalities, multiple gestation
    - Active labor is relative contraindication
- Trial of breech vaginal delivery:
    - Attempt only if delivery is imminent with favorable situation (flexed head, low-to-normal fetal weight, favorable pelvis)
    - Complications: Cord prolapse or head entrapment
- Elective C-section: Recommended to be scheduled at 39-40 weeks and preferred to vaginal delivery given lower risk of fetal morbidity
- Internal Podalic Version
    - Performed to flip around second twin in vaginal delivery of cephalic/non-cephalic twins

Other Fetal Malpresentation

Face	- Fetal face (from forehead to chin) is leading in birth canal - Higher chance for arrested labor and may require C-section
Brow	- Fetal forehead (from anterior fontanelle to the brow) leading
Transverse	- Fetal longitudinal axis is perpendicular to long axis of uterus - Usually converts to cephalic or breech presentation prior to labor - If persists, perform external cephalic version at 37 weeks (like breech) - If converts to vertex, deliver vaginally like normal. If does not convert after 2x attempt at external cephalic version (at 37, 38 weeks), then C-section is indicated. - If in active labor and transverse: C-section indicated

COMPLICATIONS OF LABOR & DELIVERY

Obstetrics OB-GYN

Fetal Distress

Decelerations	- Late decelerations are always concerning and indicate need for rapid delivery In case of variable decelerations, attempt the following: - Face mask O_2 - Turn on left side to decrease IVC compression - Bolus IVF - Discontinue oxytocin - If prolonged contraction (hypertonus) or tachysystole (too many contractions): Can give one dose of Terbutaline - Amnioinfusion (relieves cord compression)
Bradycardia	- Heart rate < 110 for at least 10 minutes Causes: - Pre-placental (due to maternal hypoxia, from seizure, AFE, PE, MI, resp failure, over-sedation) - Uteroplacental (abruption, infarction, hemorrhage) - Post-placental (cord prolapse, compression, or vasa previa) - Tx: See variable deceleration above (similar maneuvers)
Tachycardia	- Causes include: Anemia, drugs, infection, arrhythmia - Tx: Underlying cause

Cord Emergencies

Nuchal Cord	- Umbilical cord wrapped around fetal neck - Tx: Manually reduce. If unable, but delivery is imminent, clamp in two places and cut.
Cord Prolapse	- Cord protrusion past the presenting part of the fetus and into the cervical canal or vagina - Presents most often with fetal bradycardia/decelerations - Tx: Urgent C-section

FETAL COMPLICATIONS

Obstetrics OB-GYN

Fetal Growth Restriction

General: Defined as < 10th percentile or 2500 g. Note:
- Small for Gestational Age: Includes < 10th percentile (including those that are simply constitutionally small due to parental factors)
- Fetal Growth Restriction (or intrauterine growth restriction) refers to those with failure to reach expected in utero growth potential due to genetic or environmental factors

Symmetric FGR	Asymmetric FGR
- Reductions in size of all organs with the body, head, and height proportionally affected	- Disproportionate growth restriction with normal head size, but decreased length, and severely decreased weight
- Usually present before 20 weeks	- Usually presents after 20 weeks
- Chromosomal defects - Genetic disorders - Infection	- Uteroplacental insufficiency - Malnutrition

Management:
- Prenatal: Serial ultrasound, monitoring:
    - Fetal growth
    - Biophysical profile
    - Umbilical artery doppler (IUGR can result from decreased, absent, or even reversed flow)
- Delivery: Try to maximize growth by delaying delivery
    - Deliver at term if no issues with BPP or umbilical doppler
    - Deliver if decreased flow and BPP becomes abnormal
    - Deliver if reverse flow (> 32 weeks) or absent flow (> 34 weeks)

Complications: Increased risk for
- Prematurity, perinatal asphyxia
- Hypothermia, hypoglycemia, polycythemia

Large for Gestational Age

General: > 90 percentile or 4000 g

Risk: Maternal diabetes mellitus (both gestational and preexisting), excessive weight gain, fetal sex (male), ↑ gestational age, genetic disease (ie Beckwith-Wiedemann)

Management: Planned cesarean delivery, if:
- EFW > 4500 g in women with diabetes
- EFW > 5000 g in women without diabetes

Complications:
- Hypothermia, hypoglycemia, hypocalcemia, polycythemia
- Birth injuries common (clavicle fracture, brachial plexus injury, facial nerve palsy, shoulder dystocia)

FETAL COMPLICATIONS
Obstetrics OB-GYN

Amniotic Fluid Disorders

	Oligohydramnios	Polyhydramnios
Gen	- AFI < 5 on US	- AFI > 25 on US
Etio	- Fetal urinary tract abnormalities: GU obstruction, renal agenesis - Chromosomal abnormalities - Uteroplacental insufficiency - Rupture of membranes - Often idiopathic	- Maternal DM - Multiple gestation - Twin-twin transfusion syndrome - Fetal anemia, isoimmunization - Pulmonary abnormalities - Fetal anomalies (Duodenal atresia, TE fistula, anencephaly)
Dx	- AFI: The sum of the deepest amniotic fluid pocket in all four quadrants - Single deepest pocket: Alternative, arguably better test (< 2 cm oligohydramnios, > 8 cm polyhydramnios)	
Tx	- Amnioinfusion (limited to use when increased volume is temporarily needed, such as fetal anatomic US) - Delivery (at 37-38 weeks)	- Consider workup for underlying condition (US for fetal anemia, karyotype) - If severe, amnioreduction +/- Indomethacin (at < 32 weeks)
Comp	- High risk of fetal mortality (esp. if occurring earlier in pregnancy) - Cord compression - Potter sequence	- Prematurity/PROM - Fetal malpresentation - Cord prolapse

OBGYN35

FETAL COMPLICATIONS
Obstetrics — OB-GYN

Rh(D) Alloimmunization

General: RhD (-) moms exposed to fetal Rh(+) blood in prior pregnancy can lead to maternal anti-Rh IgG that can cross the placenta and result in fetal hemolytic anemia. During first pregnancy, IgM builds (which does not pass placenta), but subsequent pregnancies can have IgG that crosses placenta.

Risk: Transplacental fetomaternal bleeding history (more likely if history of pregnancy without prenatal care or in third world country)

Clinical: Generally asymptomatic. If severe:
- Kernicterus/jaundice
- Hydrops fetalis
    - Hyperdynamic state with heart failure, diffuse edema, ascites, pericardial effusion

Diagnosis: anti-Rh(D) antibody in maternal serum (screen at first visit)

Management:
- Check father's Rh status (if Rh [-] in mom/dad then baby must Rh [-])
    - If father not available, confirm fetal Rh typing with cell free DNA
- If fetus is Rh (+)
    - Serial IgG Rh titers (Anything ≥ 1:16 has high risk for fetal anemia)
    - If high titers, transcranial MCA doppler (high flow → Anemia)
    - If ↑ MCA doppler, check fetal H/H via umbilical cord sampling
- If severe fetal anemia:
    - Deliver if ≥ 35 weeks
    - Fetal transfusion < 35 weeks

Prevention: Applies to RhD (-) women plus possibility fetus can be RhD (+)
- RhoGAM at 28 Weeks
- Within 72 hours of Rh (+) birth (but can be given later if its forgotten)
- Also give RhoGAM in any situation of possible fetomaternal hemorrhage:
    - Abortion
    - Ectopic pregnancy, molar pregnancy
    - CVS/amniocentesis
    - Vaginal bleeding 2nd/3rd trimester
    - Placenta previa/abruption
    - External cephalic version
    - Abdominal trauma

Note: If major bleeding suspected, Rosette test can confirm large bleed, with Kleihauer Betke test (measures fetal RBCs in maternal serum) to determine dose of RhoGAM

Other RBC Antigens

ABO Incompatibility	- O-type mothers have IgG against AB antigen - Causes mild hyperbilirubinemia within 24 hours of birth
Lewis	- Mild hemolysis
Duffy	- Moderate hemolysis
Kell	- Severe hemolysis
Rh (C)	- Similar to Rh (D)

MATERNAL PREGNANCY COMPLICATIONS

Hyperemesis Gravidarum

General: Disorder of persistent vomiting during pregnancy

Risk: Nulliparity, multiple gestation, molar pregnancy, history of nausea with estrogen exposure

Clinical:
- Nausea and vomiting, beyond the degree expected from typical morning sickness
- No clear definition, but the following suggest hyperemesis:
    - Persistence of symptoms into second trimester
    - Ketonuria
    - Starvation and weight loss (> 5% from prepregnancy weight)

Diagnosis: Clinical

Management:
- Pharm
    - Pyridoxine-Doxylamine
    - Diphenhydramine
    - Promethazine, Metoclopramide, Ondansetron (if severe)
- If present with hypovolemia:
    - IV fluids, IV antiemetics
    - Give thiamine (high risk for thiamine deficiency)

MATERNAL PREGNANCY COMPLICATIONS

Obstetrics OB-GYN

Fetal and Obstetric Complications with Diabetes

Fetal Complications:

Exposure	Potential Risks to Fetus
First Trimester	- Congenital heart defects - Neural tube defects - Risk for abortion - Small left colon syndrome - Caudal regression syndrome
Second / Third Trimester	- Macrosomia/Organomegaly - Neonatal hypoglycemia - Increased risk for birth trauma (brachial plexus injury, shoulder dystocia, clavicle fracture, etc)

Obstetric Complications:
- Polyhydramnios
- Preeclampsia
- Miscarriage
- Infection
- Postpartum hemorrhage
- ↑ Risk for C-section

Pregestational Diabetes

General: Pregnancy can worsen hyperglycemia in patients with pre-existing diabetes mellitus. Insulin requirements can go up significantly.

Management:

Mother	- Strict glucose control with insulin (if necessary) - Basal-bolus insulin dosing preferred (oral agents discontinued) - Ensure weight gain is consistent with expected (careful diet control) - Try to maintain A1C < 6%
Fetus	- Anatomic US at 18-20 weeks (for congenital abnormalities) - Weekly non-stress tests (starting at 32 weeks) - Twice weekly non-stress tests (starting at 36 weeks) - Deliver at 39-40 weeks (or earlier if another indication)

MATERNAL PREGNANCY COMPLICATIONS

Obstetrics OB-GYN

Gestational Diabetes

General: Glucose intolerance that newly develops during pregnancy, due to increased insulin resistance. Typically diagnosed in later 2nd to 3rd trimester.

Class A1	Gestational diabetes (diet controlled)
Class A2	Gestational diabetes (insulin controlled)
Class B-D	Pregestational diabetes (exact class dependent on onset age and duration)

Risk: ↑ BMI, previous history of gestational DM, prediabetes, Hispanic/Pacific Islander

Clinical: Typically asymptomatic, but can present due to diabetic complication (ie large for GA infant, polyhydramnios, etc)

Diagnosis:
- Screening: 1 hr 50g GTT. Performed at 24-28 weeks.
    - Glucose > 140 at 1 hr considered abnormal
- Diagnostic: 3 hr 100g GTT. Normal cutoffs below.

Fasting	95 mg/dL
One Hour	180 mg/dL
Two Hour	155 mg/dL
Three Hour	140 mg/dL

Management:
- Nonpharmacologic: Exercise, careful diet, and strict glucose monitoring
    - ~ 2200 Calories, with 40% carbs, 40% fats, 20% protein
    - Glucose Targets:
        - Fasting < 95
        - 1 hr Postprandial < 140
        - 2 hr Postprandial < 120
- If poor control despite nonpharmacologic therapy, give insulin
- Delivery:
    - A1 (Diet Controlled): No special requirements
    - A2 (Insulin-Controlled): Deliver at 37-38 weeks
        - Offer C-section if > 4500 g
        - Nonstress tests weekly started at 32 weeks

Note: Mom at increased risk for type II DM after pregnancy, as well as gestational diabetes at future pregnancies. Should have 2-hour 75 gram oral glucose tolerance test between 6-12 weeks postpartum.

MATERNAL PREGNANCY COMPLICATIONS
Obstetrics OB-GYN

Chronic and Gestational Hypertension

Chronic	- Essential hypertension (> 140/90) present prior to pregnancy
Gestational	- Idiopathic hypertension (> 140/90) after 20 weeks without proteinuria or organ dysfunction

Patients are at risk for prematurity, FGR, placental abruption, or to progress to preeclampsia

Management:
- Monitor Blood Pressure
    - BP not treated with pharm unless in severe range (> 160/110)
    - If severe, drug choices include Methyldopa, Labetalol, Nifedipine
        - Acute blood pressure control with Labetalol/Hydralazine
        - Avoid ACEi/ARB in pregnancy
- Careful screening for progression to eclampsia (ie urine protein, renal function, LFTs, etc)
- Monitor with weekly biophysical profiles starting at 32 weeks
- Delivery
    - Early delivery (37-39 weeks) if uncomplicated hypertension
    - Delivery at 34-36 weeks if poorly controlled severe hypertension

Eclampsia and Preeclampsia

General: Clinical syndrome of hypertension, edema, and proteinuria. Believed to be due to abnormal development of the uteroplacental circulation, but is overall not fully understood. The resulting ischemic placenta leads to systemic vasoconstriction and ischemia of organs, resulting in the symptoms seen.

Risk:
- History of preeclampsia in prior pregnancy
- Extreme ages (< 20, > 40), nulliparity
- Black race
- Chronic hypertension, renal disease, diabetes, or collagen vascular disease
- Multiple gestation

Clinical:
- Syndrome of hypertension and proteinuria (see next page for criteria)
- Occurs after 20 weeks gestation
- Maternal Complications
    - Seizures
    - Intracerebral hemorrhage
    - Pulmonary edema
    - DIC
    - End organ failure (ie renal, hepatic)
- Obstetric Complications
    - Uteroplacental insufficiency
    - Fetal growth restriction
    - Oligohydramnios

MATERNAL PREGNANCY COMPLICATIONS — Obstetrics OB-GYN

	Clinical Criteria	Management
Preeclampsia	- Systolic BP ≥ 140 mmHg or diastolic BP ≥ 90 mmHg PLUS - Proteinuria (ie ≥ +1 on dipstick or > 300 mg/24 hr)	- Deliver if at term (≥ 37 weeks) - Conservative management if preterm, then deliver at 37 weeks - IV Magnesium Sulfate (seizure ppx at time of delivery)

Preeclampsia with Severe Features	- Systolic BP ≥ 160 mmHg or diastolic BP ≥ 110 mmHg
	OR
	- Systolic BP ≥ 140 mmHg or diastolic BP ≥ 90 mmHg PLUS end organ damage, such as:
	  - Neuro: Blurred vision, new persistent headaches, or scotomata
	  - Renal: Acute, progressive renal insufficiency
	  - GI: Severe RUQ pain, elevations of AST/ALT
	  - Pulmonary Edema
	  - Thrombocytopenia (< 100k)
		- Deliver if ≥ 34 weeks
		- Controversial prior to 34 weeks (may necessitate delivery, versus conservative management)
		- Magnesium Sulfate (seizure ppx at time of delivery)
		- Antihypertensives (for control < 160/110 mmHg)
		- Glucocorticoids (if < 34 weeks)

Eclampsia	- Seizures (generalized tonic-clonic) in women with preeclampsia - Often have prodromal symptoms (headache, visual changes, RUQ pain, etc) - Can be complicated by abruption, DIC, or cardiac arrest	- ABC's, supplemental O_2, place women in lateral position - Antihypertensives (for control < 160/110 mmHg) - IV Mag Sulfate (Diazepam/Phenytoin if refractory) - Delivery (either trial of labor if baby is stable after seizure, versus emergent C-section if fetal distress)

Mg Level	Clinical
4-7 mEq/L	Therapeutic range for seizure prophylaxis
7-10 mEq/L	Loss of DTRs
10-15 mEq/L	Respiratory paralysis, altered cardiac conduction
> 25 mEq/L	Cardiac Arrest

Note: In general, a trial of labor is indicated (rather than C-section), unless there is fetal distress that would necessitate surgical delivery

MATERNAL PREGNANCY COMPLICATIONS

Obstetrics OB-GYN

	Clinical Criteria	Management
HELLP Syndrome	- Rare complication of pregnancy, associated with preeclampsia - Microangiopathic hemolytic anemia (schistocytes, LDH, ↑ bilirubin, thrombocytopenia) - Elevated liver enzymes (with RUQ abdominal pain due to stretched Glisson capsule)	- ≥ 34 weeks: Deliver - < 34 weeks: Corticosteroids, deliver if fetal or maternal distress - Antihypertensives, IV $MgSO_4$ (similar to preeclampsia)

Acute Fatty Liver of Pregnancy	- Liver dysfunction and fatty infiltration of hepatocytes
	- Associated with abnormal long-chain fatty acid metabolism
	- Presents as diffuse hepatic failure (jaundice, encephalopathy, coagulopathy)
	  - Elevated LFTs (AST/ALT, bilirubin, PT/INR)
	  - Increased creatinine
	  - Hypoglycemia
		- Delivery (regardless of age)
		- Supportive care
		- May require liver transplantation in severe cases

Intrahepatic Cholestasis of Pregnancy	- Presents with diffuse pruritus (palms, soles, worst at night) - Elevated total serum bile acid levels - Mildly elevated bilirubin, AlkPhos, AST/ALT	- Delivery at term (≥ 37 weeks) - Ursodeoxycholic acid
Appendicitis	- Presents with nausea, vomiting, and RLQ abdominal pain - Fever and leukocytosis may be present - Can present with RUQ pain later in pregnancy (due to shifting of GI tract) - Dx: US	- Appendectomy (generally via laparotomy)

MATERNAL PREGNANCY COMPLICATIONS
Obstetrics OB-GYN

UTI/Pyelonephritis During Pregnancy

General: Women are at an increased risk for urinary tract infections during pregnancy, due to relaxation of smooth muscle in the urinary tract. *E. Coli* most common (others include *Staphylococcus saprophyticus*, GBS, *Enterococcus*).

Risk: Increased risk with multiple gestation, gestational diabetes

Clinical:
- Asymptomatic Bacteriuria (generally picked up on routine screening)
- Acute Cystitis (urgency, increased frequency, dysuria, suprapubic pain)
- Acute Pyelonephritis (fever, flank pain, CVA tenderness)

Diagnosis:
- > 10^5 Colony Forming Units on culture, plus the above clinical symptoms

Management:

Asymptomatic Bacteriuria/UTI	- Antibiotics (Nitrofurantoin, Amoxicillin, Fosfomycin) - 7 day course - Follow up cultures to confirm eradication - If repeat UTI, prophylactic antibiotics likely needed
Pyelonephritis	- Admission for fluids, parenteral antibiotics - Abx choice includes Ceftriaxone, Cefepime, Ampicillin + Gentamicin, etc. - Suppressive antibiotics for the remainder of pregnancy

Thyroid Abnormalities During Pregnancy

Hypothyroidism
- Estrogen causes ↑ in TBG, while hCG causes increase in T4 due to TSH receptor stimulation
- If hypothyroid, may not have adequate increase in T4, and will become hypothyroid during pregnancy
- Typically women will require increase doses (~25%) of Levothyroxine

Hyperthyroidism
- Similar symptoms and criteria as hyperthyroidism outside of pregnancy
- Usually due to Graves or β-HCG induced
- Treatment:
    - Beta-blocker
    - Propylthiouracil (PTU) in 1st trimester, Methimazole in 2nd/3rd
    - Radioiodine therapy contraindicated in pregnancy

POSTPARTUM COMPLICATIONS

Obstetrics OB-GYN

	Risk	Clinical/Diagnosis	Management
Postpartum Hemorrhage	- Defined as loss of > 500 mL of blood during vaginal delivery, or 1000 mL during C-section - Generally managed with two large bore IVs, fluids, RBC transfusions - If severe, may require uterine artery embolization or ligation, or hysterectomy - Can be complicated by hypovolemic shock and Sheehan syndrome		
Uterine Atony	- Exhausted myometrium - Rapid or prolonged labor - Operative deliveries - ↑↑↑ Oxytocin stimulation - Tocolytics - Conditions interfering with contractions (anesthesia, myomas, MgSO$_4$) - Macrosomic fetus - Multiparity	- Soft, enlarged, "boggy" uterus - Most common cause of postpartum bleed	- Uterine massage - Oxytocin - Methylergonovine (CxI if ↑ BP) - Carboprost (CxI if asthma) - Bakri Balloon - Uterine artery embolization - Hysterectomy
GU Tract Trauma	- Precipitous labor - Operative vaginal delivery - Macrosomia	- Normal uterus - Visualize bleeding laceration	- Hold pressure over defect - Surgically repair defect
Retained Placenta	- Placenta accreta - Placenta previa - Uterine fibroids - History of C-section, other uterine surgery	- Firm uterus	- Manual removal of retained tissue - Curettage - Hysterectomy

OBGYN44

POSTPARTUM COMPLICATIONS — Obstetrics OB-GYN

Uterine Inversion

General: Uterus "births" itself through the cervix. Occurs with too much power, traction (ie pulling on placenta), or extensive fundal pressure.

Risk: Macrosomia, rapid L&D, placenta accreta

Clinical:
- Absent uterus upon palpation of abdomen
- Smooth, round mass protruding from vagina
- Severe hemorrhage, hemodynamic instability, lower abdominal pain

Diagnosis: Clinical

Management:
- Manual replacement
- Tocolytics or Nitroglycerin (may be required before replacement)
- Uterine Atony (occurs after successful replacement): Oxytocin

Amniotic Fluid Embolus

General: Amniotic fluid enters maternal circulation due to breakdown in the barrier of the uterine vessels, resulting in acute right ventricular failure, respiratory failure, and systemic inflammation

Clinical:
- Acute onset of hypotension due to cardiogenic shock
- Hypoxemic respiratory failure
- Disseminated intravascular coagulation

Diagnosis: Clinical

Management: ABCs, supportive care

Sheehan's Syndrome

General: Ischemic infarction of the pituitary after hypovolemic shock from postpartum hemorrhage

Clinical: Anterior pituitary insufficiency, including failure to lactate, hypotension, amenorrhea, weight loss, loss of sexual hair

Diagnosis:
- Hormone testing (TSH, cortisol, estradiol)
- MRI of pituitary/hypothalamus to rule out other pathology

Management: Hormone replacement

POSTPARTUM COMPLICATIONS — Obstetrics OB-GYN

Postpartum Fever

Note: Low grade fever is normal for first 24 hours post delivery. Postpartum fever is temperature > 100.4°F 2-10 days post delivery.

Wound Infection	- Surgical site infection (ie laceration, episiotomy) - Usually presents with swelling, erythema, exudate - Requires opening wound, debridement
UTI/Cystitis Pyelonephritis	- Similar presentation and treatment to normal upper or lower UTI
Mastitis/Breast Engorgement	- Diffuse swelling versus acute cellulitis of breast tissue
Endometritis	- Infection of the uterine lining, usually polymicrobial - Risk: C-section, prolonged labor - Presents with T > 100.4°F, leukocytosis, tachycardia, abdominal pain, uterine tenderness - Rarely can present with toxic shock syndrome - Dx: Clinical - Tx: Gentamicin + Clindamycin
Septic Pelvic Thrombophlebitis	- Rare complication of delivery, where endothelial injury results in ovarian or deep venous thrombosis and polymicrobial infection - Presents with fever +/- severe abdominal pain, refractory to antibiotic therapy (usually started empirically for endometritis) - Dx: CT or MRI to evaluate for thrombi (Note: Usually picks up ovarian venous thrombus, but can be falsely negative) - Tx: Antibiotics + anticoagulation

POSTPARTUM MANAGEMENT
Obstetrics OB-GYN

Routine Postpartum Care

Pain
- NSAIDs, Acetaminophen, low dose opioids as necessary

Perineal Care
- Ice packs, monitor for intact repair

Usual Findings
- Transient fevers (for 24 hours), chills
- Breast engorgement
- Lochia
    - Rubra (red for 1-2 days postpartum)
    - Serosa (brown around day 3-4 postpartum)
    - Alba (yellow for weeks postpartum)
- Mild hair loss

Common Postpartum Complications

Urinary Retention
- Common ~ 6 hours post delivery
- Presents with inability to void, dribbling, suprapubic pain
- Bladder scan to confirm
- Tx: Analgesics, ambulation, urinary catheterization as necessary

Pubic Symphysis Diastasis
- Injury from separation of pubic diaphysis
- Usually due to traumatic delivery usually of big baby
- Presents with midline abdominal pain with radiation down both legs
    - Pain worse with ambulation
    - Tenderness of symphysis pubis
- Tx: Supportive care, NSAIDs, PT

Postpartum Depression

Blues	- Presents with 2-3 days of delivery, usually resolving in 2 weeks - Mild depression, irritability, tearfulness - Tx: Reassurance
Depression	- Presents within 4 weeks of delivery - Presents with SIGECAPS symptoms [See: Psych] - Often has ambivalence to the baby - Tx: Antidepressants + psychotherapy
Psychosis	- Can present at anytime after delivery, usually in someone with history of depression or bipolar disorder - Presents with delusions, hallucinations, disorganized thoughts - Tx: Antipsychotics, mood stabilizers - Often requires hospitalization given risk of infanticide

OBGYN47

POSTPARTUM MANAGEMENT

Obstetrics — OB-GYN

Breastfeeding

General: After pregnancy, the estrogen and progesterone levels drop, prolactin rises, and milk production/lactation is stimulated

Colostrum
- Early breast milk
- Protein, fat, secretory IgA, and minerals

Mature Milk
- Transitioned within 1 week postpartum
- Contains protein, fat, lactose, water

	Benefits	Contraindications
Infant	- Improved immunity (decreased risk of acute illnesses, such as sepsis, respiratory disease, gastroenteritis, UTI) - Improvement of GI function/maturity	- Galactosemia
Maternal	- ↓ rates of breast and ovarian cancer - Maternal-infant bonding - Accelerated recovery from childbirth - Quicker return to prepartum weight - Improved child spacing - Reduced expense	- Active herpetic breast lesions - HIV or HTLV infection - Current chemotherapy or radiation therapy - Abuse of street drugs or alcohol

Complication	Findings
Engorgement	- Common. Warm, firm, tender, swollen breast. Low-grade fever. - Tx: Continue breastfeeding. Ice packs, analgesia as needed.
Mastitis	- Cellulitis of periglandular tissue caused by nipple trauma - Most commonly MSSA/MRSA - Presents with unilateral breast swelling, tenderness, erythema, purulence, and possibly fever/leukocytosis - Tx: Continue breastfeeding. Antibiotics: Dicloxacillin or Cephalexin, with TMP-SMX or Clindamycin reserved for suspected MRSA.
Abscess	- Focal area of erythema and fluctuance, often associated with mastitis - Dx: Clinical +/- US - Tx: Antibiotics and needle drainage. I&D if refractory.

Lactation Suppression
- Utilized for those not trying to breastfeed
- Engorgement will have negative feedback and stop prolactin production
- Tx: Use supportive bra, minimize nipple stimulation, cold packs, NSAIDs
    - Bromocriptine is not indicated

MENSTRUAL CYCLE

Gynecology OB-GYN

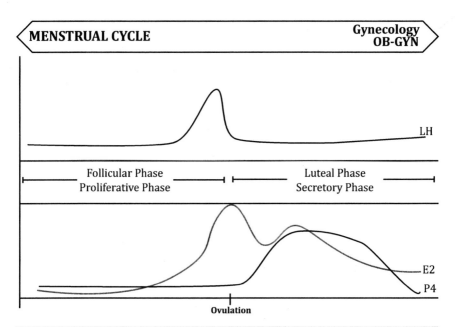

Menstrual Phases

Follicular (Proliferative)	- Starts with menstruation, ends at LH surge/ovulation - Variable in length, but averages 13 days - Development of straight glands and thin secretions - At end of follicular phase, a dominant follicle is selected
Ovulation	- Estradiol reaches a peak, causing positive feedback to the pituitary, resulting in LH surge - Follicle releases ovum, and then transitions to corpus luteum - "Mittelschmerz" = Ovulation pain resulting from ovulation and leakage of blood that irritates peritoneum
Luteal	- Corpus luteum produces progesterone, stimulating endometrial proliferation and secretions - Corpus luteum eventually breaks down without LH or β-hCG, with resulting drop in progesterone, and eventual sloughing of endometrial lining - Ends when menses begins

OBGYN49

MENSTRUAL CYCLE

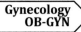
Gynecology
OB-GYN

Premenstrual Syndrome (PMS)/Dysphoric Disorder (PMDD)

General: A group of symptoms that can occur within 3-5 days preceding menses
- PMS: Presence of one or more of the below symptoms
- PMDD: Below symptoms, PLUS significant socioeconomic impairment

Clinical:
- Affective lability, irritability, depressed mood, anxiety
- Anhedonia, problems concentrating, anergia, appetite changes
- Hypersomnia/insomnia, physical symptoms (bloating, breast tenderness)

Diagnosis:
- Prospective symptom diary for at least two months
- Rule out other medical disorders (ie hypothyroidism)

Management:
- PMS: Regular exercise, stretching, stress relief techniques
- PMDD: SSRI (alt: OCPs)

Primary Ovarian Insufficiency

General: Impaired ovarian function in women < 40 years old

Etiology:
- Autoimmune
- Prior chemotherapy or radiation therapy
- Genetic (ie Fragile X [FMR gene mutation])
- Other genetic disorders (often have family history)

Clinical:
- Progressive oligomenorrhea
- Hot flashes, vaginal dryness, fatigue, etc

Diagnosis:
- ↑ FSH (in menopausal range)

Management:
- Emotional support
- Hormone replacement (combined estrogen/progesterone)

MENSTRUAL CYCLE

Gynecology
OB-GYN

Menopause

General: Physiologic cessation of menstruation in a woman > 45 y/o.
- Average age ~51

Clinical:
- Irregular menses for years leading up to final menstrual period
- Hot flashes
- Vaginal dryness, sexual dysfunction
- Fatigue, sleep disturbance
- Irritability, mood changes

- ↑ FSH, FSH:LH ratio > 1
- Osteoporosis/progressive bone loss (loss of estrogen)
- ↑ Risk of cardiovascular events and atherosclerosis

Diagnosis: Cessation of menses for 12 months (no further workup required)

Management:

Vaginal Atrophy	- Topical vaginal estrogen
Hot Flashes	- Hormone Replacement Therapy (Combo E2/P4) - SSRI, SNRI, gabapentin are options if HRT contraindicated

Hormone Replacement:
- Indicated if moderate-to-severe vasomotor symptoms (< 60 y/o and menopause within last 10 years)
- Transdermal HRT preferred, with combination estrogen/progestin
- Risk: ↑ risk of CV event, stroke, VTE, breast cancer
- Contraindications:
    - Thromboembolic history
    - Endometrial or breast cancer

CONTRACEPTION

Gynecology OB-GYN

Method	Mechanism	Positives/Indications	Side Effects
Surgical			
Vasectomy	- Bilateral vas deferens ligation	- Permanent efficacy	- Must use contraception for 6-8 weeks - Ensure azoospermia with semen analysis
Tubal Ligation	- Variety of surgical methods to ligate tubes	- Permanent, safe	- Generally irreversible, but reversal procedures may be able to restore fertility - Increased risk for ectopic pregnancy
Hysteroscopic ("Essure")	- Hysteroscopic placement of metal coil device in tubes, inducing fibrosis **OFF MARKET STARTING 2019**	- Minimally invasive	- Needs backup contraception for 12 weeks - Confirm placement with hysterosalpingogram
IUD			
Levonorgestrel (Mirena, Skyla)	- Local hormonal release, increasing cervical mucus viscosity and inducing endometrial atrophy	- Effective for 3-5 years depending on model - Immediate fertility when removed - Safe with breastfeeding - Highly efficacious	- Irregular bleeding/spotting (usually worse in initial 3-6 months, then improves) - Increased ectopic pregnancy rate
Copper (Paragard)	- Induces inflammation that creates hostile environment for implantation	- Effective for 10 years - Immediate fertility when removed - Safe with breastfeeding - Highly efficacious	- Cramping, heavier bleeding during periods - Increased ectopic pregnancy rate
	IUD Contraindications: - Pregnancy, undiagnosed abnormal uterine bleeding, active gynecologic infection - Relative contraindications include structural uterine abnormality, recent STI, prior ectopic		

CONTRACEPTION

Gynecology OB-GYN

Method	Mechanism	Positives/Indications	Side Effects
Hormonal			
Implant (Nexplanon)	- Progestin (Etonogestrel) implant in arm - Inhibits ovulation - Increases cervical mucus viscosity	- 3 year lifespan - Immediate fertility when removed - Safe with breastfeeding	- Irregular, lighter periods
Injections (Depo Provera)	- Depo progestin (Medroxyprogesterone) - Inhibits ovulation - Increases cervical mucus viscosity	- Given every 3 months	- Irregular, possibly heavy bleeding (during initial months) - Amenorrhea (usually develops after a year) - Decreased bone mineral density (reversible, encourage exercise and Ca/Vit D)
Mini-pill	- Progestin only pill - Affects cervical mucus and endometrium - Ovulation not consistently suppressed	- Pill taken daily	- Must be taken at same time every day - Irregular bleeding possible
OCPs	- Combined estrogen-progestin - Inhibits gonadotropin surge/ovulation	- Pill taken daily (with 1 week hormone free period) - Decrease ovarian and endometrial ca risk - Decreases benign breast conditions - Predictable, lighter less painful menses - Improves acne - Immediate fertility on cessation	- Bloating, nausea, breast tenderness common - Breakthrough bleeding - Increased risk of venous thromboembolism - ↑ Stroke risk (especially in those that smoke, older age, or history of migraine w/ aura) - ↑ Risk of MI (very small risk now with low dose pills) - ↑ Blood pressure (mild effect) Estrogen Contraindications: - > 35 y/o and daily smoker - Severe, uncontrolled hypertension - History of VTE, stroke, or CAD - Breast cancer - Cirrhosis or hepatocellular adenoma
Ring		- Placed in vagina for 3 weeks, then removed (with 1 week ring free)	
Patch		- Weekly patch application (wear for 3 weeks, then 1 week off)	

OBGYN53

CONTRACEPTION

Gynecology OB-GYN

Other Contraceptive Methods

Option	Benefits
Male/Female Condoms	- Provide STI/HIV protection
Fertility Awareness	- Timing ovulation via use of a calendar and possibly basal body temperature - Effective way of trying to get pregnant, not preventing it
Spermicide (Nonoxynol-9 Octoxynol-9)	- Not a primary method of birth control, but can be added to others - Can increase risk of UTI
Lactational Amenorrhea	- Must breastfeed every 3 hours and remain amenorrheic - Not 100% reliable, and should use another form of contraception - Options postpartum for those breastfeeding include IUDs and progestin-only pills or depots

Emergency Contraception Options

Method	Timing	Efficacy	Mechanism
Copper IUD	Up to 5 days	99%	- Inflammatory reaction that is toxic to sperm and ova, preventing implant
Ulipristal ("Ella")	Up to 5 days	98%	- Antiprogestin - Delays ovulation
Levonorgestrel ("Plan B")	Up to 3 days	60-90%	- Delays ovulation
OCPs (Yuzpe regimen)	Up to 5 days	50-75%	- Delays ovulation

OBGYN54

INFERTILITY

Gynecology OB-GYN

Overview of Infertility

General: Inability to conceive within 12 months of active attempts (> 80% of those trying for this period of time will conceive)
- Infertility workup should begin at 12 months, but it is reasonable to start earlier (ie 6 months) in those > 35 years old

Etiology	Select Examples	Clinical Findings
Male Factors - Should always start with semen analysis, which should be repeated if abnormal - If sperm counts are decreased, LH/FSH/Testosterone should be checked - If normal semen analysis, either this is a female problem, or idiopathic male infertility		
Testicular Defect	- Testicular insults (toxins, torsion, infection, varicoceles)	- Oligo or azoospermia - Normal endocrine testing
Hypogonadism	Primary Hypogonadism (↓ T, ↑ FSH/LH) - Klinefelter, other genetic disorder Secondary Hypogonadism (↓T/FSH/LH) - Prolactinoma, hypothyroidism	- Oligo or azoospermia
Sperm Abnormalities		- Abnormal sperm morphology or motility
Sperm Transport	- Ejaculatory duct obstruction - Congenital absence of vas deferens	- Oligo or azoospermia - Normal endocrine testing - GU ultrasound may reveal structural cause

Female Factors
- Assessment of ovulatory status (ie history of regular menstrual cycles, can check midluteal progesterone level)
- Hysterosalpingogram (to evaluate tubal patency/uterine cavity abnormalities)
- Ovarian reserve analysis:
   - Day 3 FSH (abnormally elevated with ↓ follicles), estradiol (↑ with low follicle reserve)
   - Anti-Müllerian hormone level (declines over time with decreasing follicle pool)		

Ovarian Factors	- Hypogonadotropism - PCOS - Decreased ovarian reserve	- Abnormal menstrual history, endocrine analysis - Abnormal reserve analysis
Tubal Factors	- Pelvic inflammatory disease - Endometriosis - Any other cause of pelvic adhesions	- Hysterosalpingogram abnormalities
Cervical Factors	- History of cervical surgery	
Uterine Factors	- Fibroids, polyps, or adhesions	- Hysterosalpingogram or TVUS abnormalities

INFERTILITY

Gynecology OB-GYN

Management of Infertility

Method	Features
Ovulation Induction	- Used for ovulatory disorders - Clomiphene is most common drug used (selective SERM at pituitary/hypothalamus, induces ovulation ~ 1 weeks after use) - Alternative agents: Aromatase inhibitors (Letrozole), GnRH agonists (Leuprolide) - Often associated with hot flashes and ovarian hyperstimulation (syndrome of ovarian enlargement, pain, ascites, etc)
Intrauterine Insemination	- Used for cervical dysfunction or severe sexual dysfunction - Concentrated sperm injected into uterus at proper time of cycle OR after stimulation (ie with Clomiphene)
In-Vitro Fertilization	- Used in those with severe structural abnormalities (blocked tubes, severe endometriosis), severe male factor infertility, poor response to pharm induction agents, diminished ovarian reserve - Ovaries are stimulated, oocytes aspirated, fertilized in laboratory, then transferred into the uterine cavity

Disorder Specific Therapy:

Endometriosis	- Surgical resection and lysis of adhesions - Assisted reproductive technologies if this fails
Uterine Abnormalities	- Consider surgical correction (not great data for this either way)
Cervical Factor Infertility	- Intrauterine insemination

AMENORRHEA

Gynecology
OB-GYN, Pediatrics

Primary Amenorrhea

General: Defined as
- Absence of menses by 15 years old OR
- Absence of menses and secondary sexual characteristics by age 13

Etiology	Axis	Anatomy	Features	Diagnosis
Central Hypogonadism	-	+	Etiologies vary, including: - Stress/exercise/low BMI - Hyperprolactinemia - Sellar mass - Kallmann syndrome (low GnRH production, anosmia) - Constitutional pubertal delay	↓ FSH/LH MRI
Ovarian Insufficiency	-	+	Etiologies vary, including: - Turner's syndrome - Prior chemotherapy, radiation	↑ FSH/LH Karyotype
Outflow Tract Disorders				
Müllerian Agenesis	+	-	- Congenital absence of upper vagina, cervix, and uterus	Ultrasound
Lower GYN	+	+	- Transverse vaginal septum - Imperforate hymen	Clinical exam
Enzyme/Hormonal Issues				
Androgen Insensitivity	+	-	- XR disorder in 46XY patients in which there is a defect in androgen receptor - Normal external genitalia, but no upper vagina, uterus, tubes - Testes often undescended or in labia majora - Sparse sexual hair, but breast development present - ↑ Testosterone - Dx: Clinical, plus XY karyotype, and genetic testing for AR gene - Tx: Gonadectomy (after pubertal development), hormone replacement, vaginal dilation	
5α reductase Deficiency	+	-	- AR disorder of lack of male virilization from abnormal conversion of T to DHT - Normal internal male urogenital tract, but external genitalia is typically female or indeterminate - Individual otherwise appears male, and will develop further male sex characteristics during puberty - Dx: Increased T:DHT ratio - Tx: Assign male gender OR gonadectomy/estrogen	

Diagnosis: See next page for steps in workup of primary amenorrhea

Management:
- Treat/manage underlying condition
- Estrogen replacement (if necessary)
- Surgical management of structural disorders

AMENORRHEA

Gynecology — OB-GYN, Pediatrics

Primary Amenorrhea -- Workup

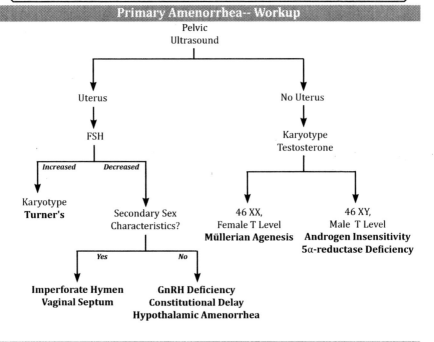

Secondary Amenorrhea

General: Absence of menses for 6 consecutive months (if normally irregular) or 3 consecutive months (if previously regular cycles)

Etiology	Features
Pregnancy	- Most common cause
Ovarian	- Primary ovarian insufficiency - PCOS
Hypothalamic	- Functional hypothalamic (low weight, excess exercise, stress) - Systemic illness
Pituitary	- Prolactinoma - Sheehan syndrome - Other sellar masses
Uterine	- Asherman syndrome (adhesions from prior uterine surgery or infection) - Cervical stenosis
Other	- Hypothyroidism - Medications: Atypical antipsychotics, dopamine antagonists

Diagnosis: See workup algorithm on next page
- Always start with urine β-hCG pregnancy test
- FSH, E2, TSH, prolactin

AMENORRHEA

Gynecology OB-GYN

Secondary Amenorrhea-- Workup

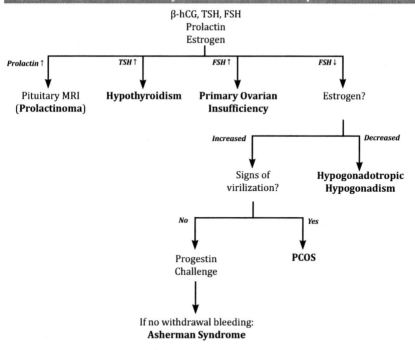

Secondary Amenorrhea-- Management

Etiology	Management
Hypothalamic	- Lifestyle changes (increased caloric intake, decreased exercise) - CBT (especially if under stress)
Hyperprolactinemia	- [See: Endocrine] - Bromocriptine or Cabergoline
Primary Ovarian Insufficiency	- Estrogen therapy (prevent bone loss)
Asherman	- Hysteroscopic lysis of adhesions
PCOS	- Weight loss, OCPs

HYPERANDROGENISM

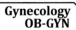
Gynecology
OB-GYN

Overview of Hirsutism and Virilization

General: Excess androgen production from ovary or adrenal glands
- Testosterone (ovary)
- DHEAS (adrenal gland)

Clinical:

Hirsutism	- Excess hair growth (dark, coarse hairs) in androgen-dependent areas (upper lip, chin, torso, buttocks) - Although hirsutism refers to hair growth, it is often associated with acne and male-pattern hair loss
Virilization	Hirsutism as above, PLUS the following: - Clitoral enlargement - Increased muscle mass - Deepening of voice - Male-pattern hair loss

Diagnosis:
- DHEAS and T levels
- Depending on concern for source: Ovarian US or Adrenal CT/MRI

Differential of Hyperandrogenism

Etiology	T	DHEAS	Features	Management
Ovarian Causes				
PCOS	↑	↔	- Hirsutism, insulin resistance, oligomenorrhea	- Weight loss, OCPs
Sertoli-Leydig	↑↑	↔	- Severe virilization, rapid onset - Androgen production from ovarian tumor	- Surgical excision +/- chemotherapy
Hyperthecosis	↑↑	↔	- Excess active luteinized stromal cells in the ovaries - US demonstrates increased size of ovaries (bilateral), increased stroma	- Bilateral oophorectomy
Adrenal Causes				
Adrenal Tumor	↔	↑↑	- Excess androgen production from adrenal adenoma or carcinoma - Dx: CT or MRI (unilateral mass)	- Surgical resection
CAH (non-classical)	↔	↑	- 21-hydroxylase deficiency - Presents similarly to PCOS (ie hirsutism without virilization) - Dx: ↑ 17-hydroxyprogesterone	- Steroids
Other Causes				
Cushing Disease				
Idiopathic Hirsutism (normal menstrual cycles, labs)				

HYPERANDROGENISM

Gynecology
OB-GYN

Polycystic Ovarian Syndrome

General: Syndrome caused by elevated androgens. Multifactorial and complex, the disorder occurs in those with genetic susceptibility and insulin resistance, resulting in excessive LH release, abnormal ovarian follicular development, and excessive production of androgens.

Risk: Often comorbid with metabolic syndrome, OSA

Clinical:
- Androgen excess (acne, male pattern hair loss, hirsutism)
- Menstrual irregularities (from decreased ovulation or anovulation)
- Obesity, insulin resistance
- ↑ Risk for endometrial hyperplasia/adenocarcinoma
- Lab findings:
    - ↑ LH/FSH ratio
    - ↑ Testosterone levels
    - ↑ Estrogen levels

Diagnosis: Rotterdam criteria (≥ 2/3 of the following)
- Oligomenorrhea
- Hyperandrogenism (acne, balding, hirsutism, ↑ serum T)
- Polycystic ovaries on TVUS

Management:
- Weight loss
- Combined estrogen-progestin contraceptives (for menstrual irregularity, symptoms of excess androgens)
- Ovulation induction: Either Letrozole or Clomiphene

DYSMENORRHEA

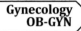
Gynecology
OB-GYN

Primary Dysmenorrhea

General: Recurrent, crampy, midline lower abdominal pain that occurs during menses in the absence of pathology that could cause the pain. Caused by uterine ischemia from vasoconstriction associated with prostaglandin release.

Clinical:
- Presents with low, midline, spasmodic pelvic pain
- Occurs in first 1-3 days of menstruation
    - Versus endometriosis, which is pain days to weeks before cycle
- Associated with nausea, diarrhea, flushing, headache

Diagnosis: Clinical diagnosis of exclusion

Management:
- NSAIDs (Ibuprofen, Mefenamic acid)
- Combined OCPs
- Others: Heat, exercise, massage

Secondary Dysmenorrhea

General: Menstrual pain associated with pathologic process

Etiology:
- Adenomyosis
- Endometriosis
- Cervical Stenosis
- Pelvic inflammatory disease
- Others: Adhesions, fibroids

Diagnosis/Management:
- Differs based on etiology

Adenomyosis

General: Invasion of endometrial glands/stroma into the uterine musculature
- Myometrium becomes hypertrophic and hyperplastic in response

Risk: Endometriosis, fibroids

Clinical:
- Dysmenorrhea
- Menorrhagia
- Enlarged, boggy, uterus

Diagnosis: TVUS or MRI
- Definitive diagnosis is histologic (but typically imaging is utilized)

Management:
- Progestins (IUDs, pills): Can control menorrhagia short term
- Definitive therapy: Hysterectomy or uterine artery embolization

DYSMENORRHEA

Gynecology
OB-GYN

Endometriosis

General: Functional endometrial glands and stroma outside uterus. Pathophysiology unknown, but current theories include:
- Retrograde menstruation
- Lymphatic or vascular spread
- Metaplastic transformation of tissue

Risk: ↑ risk with nulliparity, early menarche, heavy menstrual bleeding, family history

Clinical:
- Cyclic pelvic and/or rectal pain (classically 1-2 weeks before menses)
- Abnormal uterine bleeding
- Dyspareunia
- Dyschezia (painful defecation)
- Ovarian mass (endometrioma, "chocolate brown")
- Infertility
- Physical exam can reveal: Posterior vaginal fornix tenderness or nodules, fixation of the cervix or uterus from adhesions, or adnexal mass

Diagnosis:
- Laparoscopy (biopsy for histologic confirmation, plus staging of disease)
- Patients are often treated empirically without surgical/histologic diagnosis, and the response to therapy dictates whether laparoscopy is necessary

Management:

Pain	- First line: NSAIDs plus combined oral contraceptives (hormones used continuously) - Second line: GnRH agonist (ie Leuprolide) plus add back estrogen/progestin - Refractory: Aromatase inhibitors (Anastrozole, Letrozole) - If refractory to the pharmacologic measures above, laparoscopy is often required, both diagnostically and therapeutically
Infertility	- Laparoscopy and lysis of adhesions - Assisted reproduction technologies
Endometrioma	- Laparoscopic cystectomy

OBGYN63

MENORRHAGIA

Gynecology OB-GYN

Menorrhagia Definitions

Normal	- Menses every 28 days (can range from 21-35 day cycles) - 3-5 days of bleeding, ~ 30 mL
Menorrhagia	- Heavy bleeding (> 80 mL) and/or prolonged (> 7 days)
Metrorrhagia	- Bleeding occurring between normal menses
Menometrorrhagia	- Heavy bleeding occurring between normal menses
Oligomenorrhea	- Irregular cycles > 35 days apart

Differential Diagnosis of Abnormal Uterine Bleeding

General: Bleeding outside the typical 2-7 days period of a normal 28 day cycle

Etiology: "PALMCOIN"
- Polyp
- Adenomyosis
- Leiomyoma
- Malignancy
- Coagulopathy
- Ovulatory dysfunction
- Endometrial
- Iatrogenic (IUDs)
- Not yet classified (ie pregnancy, the most common cause)

Diagnosis:
- Broad workup, including β-hCG, CBC, coags, TSH, prolactin, pap smear
- Any postmenopausal women with uterine bleeding deserves endometrial biopsy

Management of Abnormal Uterine Bleeding

Pharm	- Combined contraceptives or progestin IUD/injectable - NSAIDs or Tranexamic acid for those with contraindication
Surgical	Definitive: - Endometrial ablation - Uterine artery embolization - Hysterectomy
Acute Bleeding	- Supportive care (2x large bore IV, crystalloids, RBC transfusions) - Uterine tamponade with balloon or gauze - Hemodynamically stable: IV estrogens - Hemodynamically unstable: Uterine curettage

VAGINITIS

Gynecology / OB-GYN

	Bacterial Vaginosis	Trichomoniasis	Vulvovaginal Candidiasis
Microbiology	- Shift in vaginal flora away from lactobacilli, to diverse bacteria including anaerobes - *Gardnerella vaginalis* predominant	- Protozoan *Trichomonas vaginalis* infection	- Overgrowth of *Candida albicans* (part of normal vaginal flora) - Other *Candida* also possible (ie glabrata)
Risk	- Sexual activity - Frequent douching	- Unprotected sex (passed person-to-person via sexual contact)	- Diabetes mellitus, antibiotic use, immunocompromised states
Clinical	- Odor, increased discharge	- Increased discharge, odor, pruritus, dysuria	- Vulvar pruritus, with possible burning, irritation
Exam	- Homogenous thin gray-white discharge	- Erythema of the vulva and vaginal mucosa - Punctate hemorrhages of upper vagina/cervix ("Strawberry cervix") - Profuse, malodorous yellow-green discharge	- Erythematous, excoriated vagina - Thick, white, discharge with curdy texture without odor
pH	> 4.5	5.0-6.0	4.0-4.5
Whiff test	Positive	Occasionally positive	Negative
Wet Mount	Clue cells (epithelial cells with bacteria)	Motile trichomonads (bigger than WBC, smaller than epi cells)	Pseudohyphae
KOH Prep	Negative	Negative	Positive (pseudohyphae)
Management	PO Metronidazole (500 mg PO BID 5-7 days) Topical Metronidazole (5 days) (Vaginal or oral Clindamycin can also be used)	PO Metronidazole or Tinidazole (single dose) * Partners should also be evaluated and treated	PO Fluconazole (1 time) or topical azoles * Cases of recurrent disease may require longer PO or topical regimens * Glabrata treated with intravaginal boric acid
Other	Amsel Criteria (≥ 3/4): Classic vaginal discharge, elevated pH, clue cells, fishy odor		

OBGYN65

UPPER GYN INFECTIONS

Gynecology
OB-GYN

Pelvic Inflammatory Disease

General: Acute bacterial infection of the upper genital tract, including uterus, fallopian tubes (salpingitis), ovaries, peritonitis. Typically due to ascending infection from lower genital tract.

Etiology:
- Gonorrhea and Chlamydia
- Other assorted bacteria also implicated less commonly (*Mycoplasma genitalium*, group A/B *Strep*, *E. Coli*, *Klebsiella*, etc)

Risk: Sexually active (esp. multiple partners), lack of barrier protection, history of PID or STI
- Pregnant women usually not at risk given mucus plug

Clinical:
- Acute onset lower abdominal or pelvic pain
- Uterine, cervical ("Chandelier sign"), and/or adnexal tenderness
- Purulent cervical discharge, possible bleeding/spotting
- Systemic symptoms: Fevers, chills, leukocytosis

Diagnosis: Clinical diagnosis
- Lower abdominal/pelvic pain + uterine, cervical, or adnexal tenderness
   - Generally the above is enough to warrant empiric therapy
- Pelvic imaging (ie TVUS, CT) supportive, but unnecessary for diagnosis

Management:

Hospitalized	- "Foxy Doxy": Cefoxitin IV + Doxycycline PO - Clindamycin + Gentamicin (alternative regimen) - Should admit: Pregnant women, poor compliance (ie teenagers), TOA, perihepatitis, failed outpatient therapy, women unable to tolerate PO, severe presentations
Outpatient	- Ceftriaxone 1x IM + Doxycycline (14 days)

Complications:
- Infertility, ↑ ectopic pregnancy risk
- Pelvic adhesions
- Perihepatitis (Fitz-Hugh-Curtis)
    - Inflammation of the liver capsule/peritoneum
    - RUQ abdominal pain (often pleuritic), possible abnormal LFT's
    - Laparoscopy: Purulent/fibrinous exudates surrounding the liver
- Tubo-Ovarian Abscess (TOA)
    - 10% of patients with PID develop TOA, an inflammatory mass of the tubes and/or ovaries
    - Typically polymicrobial
    - Presents like PID, but may be extra sick or not responding to abx
    - Rupture TOA can present with acute abdomen and sepsis
    - Dx: Imaging (TVUS)
    - Tx: Antibiotics for uncomplicated cases, but surgical drainage or salpingo-oophorectomy if unresponsive or severe infections

CONGENITAL GYN ABNORMALITIES

Gynecology
OB-GYN, Pediatrics

	General/Clinical	Management
Vaginal Abnormalities		
Imperforate Hymen	- Hymenal epithelium normally degenerates, but can abnormally persist - Obstruction can cause hydrocolpos, mucocolpos, or hematocolpos - Rarely can cause primary amenorrhea	- Surgery
Transverse Vaginal Septum	- Failure of canalization between the lower 2/3 and upper 1/2 of the vagina (Müllerian ducts do not fuse to the urogenital sinus) - Presents with short vagina with blind pouch - Can also present with primary amenorrhea, cyclic pelvic pain	- Surgery
Vaginal Agenesis	- Complete absence of vagina - Frequently associated with Mayer-Rokitansky-Küstner-Hauser, with associated absence of uterus and cervix	- Vaginal dilators or surgical vaginoplasty
Uterine Abnormalities		
Congenital Uterine Anomalies	- Congenital uterine abnormalities due to abnormal Müllerian duct fusions during embryonic development - Generally idiopathic, but can be associated with DES exposure - Increased risk for associated renal abnormalities or inguinal hernia - Rarely symptomatic - Dx: TVUS, MRI, or hysterosalpingogram	- Generally no intervention required - Surgical correction if recurrent pregnancy loss

Normal   Septate   Bicornuate   Didelphus   Unicornate

OBGYN67

MISC VAGINAL LESIONS
Gynecology / OB-GYN

		General/Clinical	Management
Skin Lesions	**Lichen Sclerosus**	- Presents with thin, white, wrinkled skin localized on the labia ("paper thin") - Shrinkage and agglutination of labia minora - Often causes severe pruritus, dyspareunia - Increased risk of SCC in this area	Dx: Biopsy Tx: High potency topical steroids
	Lichen Simplex Chronicus	- Localized thickening of the vulvar skin from excess scratching and pruritus	Tx: Topical steroids (to break itch-scratch cycle)
	Vulvar Lichen Planus	- Presents with vulvar pain, pruritus, discharge - Brightly erythematous erosions with "lacy" white striae - Lesions also can be intravaginal or involve other mucosal areas	Dx: Biopsy Tx: High potency topical steroids
	Vulvar Psoriasis	- Classic scaling red plaques, typically also located elsewhere on body - Typically asymptomatic or only mild pruritus	Dx: Clinical or biopsy Tx: Topical steroids, UV light
Cysts	**Bartholin's Cyst**	- Obstruction of Bartholin's duct and dilation of the gland - Can occur idiopathically or from trauma - Presents with cysts lateral to the vaginal orifice	- If asymptomatic: Observation If infected or symptomatic: - I&D PLUS word catheter placement - Marsupialization (second line) - Antibiotics if recurrent, high risk, or appearing septic
	Skene's Gland Cyst	- Paraurethral gland cysts, located in the anterior vagina near the opening of the urethra	
	Gartner's Cyst	- Remnants of mesonephric ducts, typically located on the lateral vaginal wall - Generally asymptomatic	

OBGYN68

MISC CERVICAL LESIONS

Gynecology / OB-GYN

	General/Clinical	Management
Cervical Cysts	- Nabothian cysts most common, caused when glandular columnar cells become covered by squamous epithelial, but still produce mucus - Generally asymptomatic	- Self-limited
Cervical Polyps	- Polyps often originate from the endocervical canal, appear as broad based or pedunculated lesions - Often asymptomatic, but can cause intermenstrual or postcital bleed	- Polypectomy if symptomatic
Cervical Stenosis	- Narrowed endocervical canal, which can cause buildup of menstrual flow - Risk: Cervical surgery, cancer - Presents with severe dysmenorrhea, relieved with increased flow - Diagnosis: Clinical exam (try to pass dilator)	- Cervical dilation (laminaria, stent, or surgical dilation)

PELVIC ORGAN PROLAPSE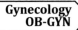

General: Herniation of the pelvic organs past the vaginal walls. Commonly seen after menopause due to decreased estrogens, vaginal atrophy, and effects of gravity.

Subtype	Definition
Cystocele	- Bladder bulge into the anterior vagina
Rectocele	- Rectum bulge into the posterior vagina
Enterocele	- Protrusion of the small intestines and peritoneum into vagina
Urethrocele	- Prolapse of urethra into the vagina - Often occurs concurrently with cystocele
Uterine Prolapse	- Prolapse of the uterus into the vagina

Risk: ↑ Age, high parity or history of traumatic delivery, history of pelvic surgery, obesity, chronic constipation

Clinical:
- Pelvic pressure, heaviness or sensation of bulging
- Protrusion of tissue from the vagina
- Can be associated with urinary, bowel, or sexual issues (ie dyspareunia)
    - Urinary incontinence, a sense of incomplete bladder emptying
    - Defecatory issues (may need to "splint," ie apply pressure to the posterior vagina to allow for defecation)

Diagnosis: Clinical exam. POP-Q score can be utilized to characterize and risk stratify.

Management:

Conservative	- Pelvic floor exercises
	- Vaginal Pessaries
	   - Silicone devices that support the pelvic organs
	   - Regularly remove and clean to avoid infection

Surgical	- Indicated for symptomatic prolapse or failure of conservative tx Types Include: - Hysterectomy with colpopexy (vaginal vault suspension) - Colporrhaphy (fix the hernia) - Colpocleisis: Close the vaginal opening (done in those at high risk of surgery and don't need vagina)

Vesicovaginal Fistula

General: Fistula between vagina and bladder. Associated with recent pelvic surgery, radiation, malignancy, history of traumatic labor.

Clinical: Painless continuous leakage of urine into vagina

Diagnosis: Dye tests, cystoscopy

Management: Surgical correction

CERVICAL NEOPLASIA

Gynecology OB-GYN

Cervical Cancer

General: Cancer of the cervix, either squamous cell (~70%) or adenocarcinoma (~25%). Highly associated with HPV (16, 18, 31, 45). Usually originates at the transformation zone (junction between squamous epithelium of ectocervix and glandular epithelium of the endocervix).

Risk:
- Early onset of sexual activity
- Multiple or high risk sex partners
- History of other STI's
- Immunocompromised (such as HIV)
- Smoking

Clinical:
- Often asymptomatic
- Metrorrhagia, postcoital spotting, cervical ulceration all possible

Diagnosis: Biopsy for definitive diagnosis
- Often picked up on Pap smear screening, which should be followed by colposcopy and directed biopsy
    - Colpo performed by staining cervix with acetic acid
        - Findings include acetowhite epithelium, mosaicism, punctuations, atypical vessels

Dysplasia	Location	Bethesda	CIN
Mild	- Bottom 1/3 of cervical epithelium	LSIL	I
Moderate	- Bottom and middle 1/3 of cervical epithelium	HSIL	II
Severe or Carcinoma in situ	- > 2/3 of cervical epithelium	HSIL	III

Stage	Description

I	- Confined to cervix:
	  - IA: Microscopically diagnosed
	  - IB1: Clinically visible, < 4 cm in greatest dimension
	  - IB2: Clinically visible, > 4 cm in greatest dimension

II	- Spread beyond cervix (ie upper vagina or parametrium)
III	- Spread to lower vagina or pelvic side wall
IV	- Invades bladder, rectum, or distant metastasis

CERVICAL NEOPLASIA

Gynecology OB-GYN

Management of Cervical Malignancy

Lesion	Intervention
CIN 1	- Monitor Pap +/- HPV q12 months. Repeat colposcopy if abnormal. - If CIN 1 persists for 2 years: Conization/LEEP
CIN 2/3	- Conization/LEEP - If plans to become pregnant: Can consider q6 month cytology + colposcopy for one year if CIN 2
Cancer	- Early Disease (Stage IA-IB): Surgical conization or hysterectomy - Advanced Disease (Stage IB2 or higher): Chemo + radiation therapy

If Pregnant:
- LSIL or HSIL paps should be investigated with colposcopy
- CIN I: Defer further management to 6 weeks postpartum
- CIN II-III: Follow routine colposcopy during pregnancy
- Invasive Cervical Cancer: Depends on patient's wishes, but can consider abortion with treatment, localized excision procedure, or defer treatment until after delivery

Types of Procedures:
- Cold knife conization
- LEEP (loop electrical excision procedure)
- Side Effects:
    - Cervical stenosis
    - Cervical insufficiency (↑ preterm risk or second trimester loss)

Prophylaxis: HPV 9-valent vaccine (okay to use ages 9-45 y/o)

Cervical Cancer Screening

Normal Risk Individuals	
21-29 y/o	- Pap test q3 years
30-65 y/o	- Pap test q3 years OR - Pap + HPV cotest q5 years
> 65 y/o	- If normal risk, and patient has 3 negative paps or 2 negative cotests in the last 10 years, screening can stop
Special Situations	
Smokers	- Reasonable to extend screening to 75-80 y/o
Immuno-suppressed	- Start screening at time of first sexual activity - Screen q1 year
Hysterectomy	- If total hysterectomy (ie cervix removed), no screening needed UNLESS history of CIN grade II or higher lesion (in which case vaginal cytology is reasonable)
Post-ablative for CIN	- After surgery for CIN, pap + HPV q1 years for 2 years - If normal, return to normal screening schedule for at least 20 years

CERVICAL NEOPLASIA
Gynecology OB-GYN

Interpretation of Screening

AGC (Atypical Glandular Cells)	- Colposcopy, endocervical sampling - Endometrial biopsy if > 35 y/o OR < 35 but at risk for endometrial dysplasia (obesity, PCOS, etc)
ASC-US (≥ 25 y/o)	- Check HPV if available (otherwise, repeat cytology in one year) - ASC-US + HPV (+): Colposcopy - ASC-US + HPV (-): Cotest in 3 years
LSIL (≥ 25 y/o)	- LSIL + HPV (-): Repeat co-test in 1 year - LSIL + HPV (+ or unknown): Colposcopy
ASC-US or LSIL (21-24 y/o)	- Repeat cytology in 12 months - If cytology remains abnormal → Colposcopy
HSIL or ASC-H	- Colposcopy - If negative, follow with q6M colposcopy for 2 years
NILM but HPV(+)	- Either repeat cotest in 1 year OR DNA type HPV - If HPV 16 or 18 positive → Colposcopy

OBGYN73

ENDOMETRIAL NEOPLASIA

Gynecology
OB-GYN

Endometrial Polyps

General: Hyperplastic overgrowth of endometrial glands/stroma. Generally benign, but are possibly malignant (especially in those that are postmenopausal).

Risk: High estrogen levels (obesity, Tamoxifen, hormone replacement therapy)

Clinical: Often asymptomatic, but can cause abnormal uterine bleeding

Diagnosis: TVUS or hysteroscopy is suggestive, but definitive diagnosis on histology

Management:

Premenopausal	- Polypectomy if symptomatic or if at high risk for endometrial hyperplasia/cancer
Postmenopausal	- Polypectomy for all

Uterine Leiomyoma (Fibroids)

General: Benign smooth muscle tumors arising from the myometrium. Sensitive to estrogen and progesterone. Malignant transformation to leiomyosarcoma is very rare.
Subtypes:

Intramural	- Located within uterine wall
Submucosal	- Located beneath endometrium, extending into and distorting uterine cavity - Highest risk for bleeding
Subserosal	- Extend from myometrium to the serosal surface of the uterus
Cervical	- Located within cervix

Risk:
- African-Americans
- Increased estrogen exposure (low parity, early menarche)
- Alcohol ↑ risk, smoking possibly protective

Clinical:
- Abnormal uterine bleeding
- Bulk Symptoms: Bloating, constipation, ↑ urinary frequency or retention
- Pelvic pain: Dysmenorrhea, dyspareunia
- Exam demonstrates firm, nontender, irregularly shaped uterus

Diagnosis: TVUS (first line)
- Saline sonography or hysteroscopy (can characterize uterine cavity)

Management:

Expectant	- Reasonable to monitor patient if asymptomatic or postmenopausal - Growing fibroid in postmenopausal patient concerning for malignancy
Pharmacologic	- OCPs, progestin IUDs, GnRH agonists can be trialed for symptomatic patients, but evidence for efficacy lacking
Surgical	- Indicated if symptomatic (abnormal uterine bleeding, infertility) - Myomectomy (if patient wishes to maintain fertility) - Hysterectomy or uterine arterial embolization (if done childbearing)

OBGYN74

ENDOMETRIAL NEOPLASIA
Gynecology — OB-GYN

Endometrial Hyperplasia

General: Hyperplastic proliferation of endometrial glands, typically associated with continuous estrogen exposure. Categorized into the following groups:

Subtype	Findings	Cancer Risk
Simple Hyperplasia w/o Atypia	- Mildly crowded glands	< 5%
Complex Hyperplasia w/o Atypia	- Crowded glands, elevated gland-to-stroma ratio	< 5%
Simple Atypical Hyperplasia	- Mildly crowded glands - Nuclear atypia (enlargement, prominent nucleoli)	> 10%
Complex Atypical Hyperplasia	- Crowded glands, elevated gland-to-stroma ratio - Nuclear atypia (enlargement, prominent nucleoli)	> 20%

Risk: Obesity, PCOS, anovulation, isolated estrogen therapy, estrogen producing tumor

Clinical: Abnormal uterine bleeding, most commonly postmenopausal
- US may show thickened endometrial stripe (> 4 mm)

Diagnosis: Endometrial Biopsy. Indicated if:
- ≥ 45 with abnormal uterine bleeding or postmenopausal bleeding
- < 45 with abnormal uterine bleeding + unopposed estrogen, lynch syndrome, or failed medical management
- > 35 with atypical glandular cells on Pap test

Management:
- No atypia: Progestin IUD
- Atypia: Hysterectomy. Progestin IUD if wish to preserve fertility.

Endometrial Carcinoma

General: Most common gynecologic malignancy in US. Subtypes:

Type I	Endometrioid	- Derives from atypical endometrial hyperplasia - Favorable prognosis (compared to type II)
Type II	Serous, Clear cell, Carcinosarcoma	- Unrelated to estrogen exposure, associated with p53 mutation - See in older aged individuals - Poor prognosis

Risk: Same as hyperplasia: Obesity, PCOS, anovulation, isolated estrogen therapy. Plus:
- Hypertension, diabetes
- Lynch syndrome (should receive regular screening)

Clinical: Asymptomatic or abnormal uterine bleeding

Diagnosis: Biopsy

Management: TAH, bilateral salpingo-oophorectomy, lymphadenectomy
- Surgery is used to stage patients, establish type of disease (for all patients)
- Adjuvant therapy dictated by stage/risk
    - Radiation therapy for locally invasive tumor (myometrium, cervix)
    - High risk disease (ie Stage ≥ III, or type II histology) receives chemotherapy +/- radiation

OVARIAN NEOPLASIA
Gynecology OB-GYN

Differential Diagnosis of Adnexal Mass

Etiology	Features	Management
Benign Cysts		
Follicular	- Most common, occurs when follicle fails to rupture after follicular maturation	- Self-limited
Corpus Luteal	- Corpus luteum failure to involute, continues enlargement after ovulation - Normal in early pregnancy	- Self-limited
Theca-Lutein	- Luteinized follicle cysts from overstimulation due to β-hCG	- Self-limited
Benign Mass		
Teratoma	- Dermoid cyst - Characteristic US finding: Hyperechoic contents, hyperechoic lines or dots, fluid, and areas of acoustic shadowing	- Cystectomy
Cystadenoma	- Serous or mucinous cystadenomas are most common benign ovarian tumors - Thin walls with multiple locules possible, > 5 cm in size	- Cystectomy (especially if symptomatic) - Observation (also reasonable)
Pathologic Masses		
Endometrioma	- Endometriosis of the ovary - Presents with mass, pelvic pain, dysmenorrhea - "Chocolate Cyst," which appears complex on US (homogeneous internal echoes)	- Laparoscopy
Tubo-Ovarian Abscess	- Inflammatory mass associated with PID	- Antibiotics, surgery [See: PID]
Malignant Masses		
Epithelial Carcinoma	- See discussion for full details	
Pregnancy Associated		
Luteal Cyst or Luteoma	- Cystic or solid corpus luteum	Self-limited
Ectopic	- Pain, vaginal bleeding, etc	[See: Ectopic Preg]

Workup of Adnexal Mass

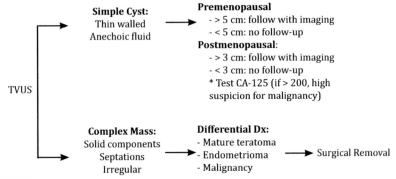

TVUS

Simple Cyst: Thin walled, Anechoic fluid

Premenopausal
- > 5 cm: follow with imaging
- < 5 cm: no follow-up

Postmenopausal:
- > 3 cm: follow with imaging
- < 3 cm: no follow-up
* Test CA-125 (if > 200, high suspicion for malignancy)

Complex Mass: Solid components, Septations, Irregular

Differential Dx:
- Mature teratoma
- Endometrioma
- Malignancy

→ Surgical Removal

OVARIAN NEOPLASIA

Gynecology OB-GYN

Adnexal Mass Complications

Etiology	Features	Management
Hemorrhagic Cyst	- Most commonly physiologic cyst that develops internal bleeding - Often presents with mild to severe abdominal pain - US demonstrates cystic mass with internal echoes	- Usually self-limited (supportive care) - Hospitalization, blood products may be required in more severe cases
Ruptured Cyst	- Rupture of a benign or pathologic cyst, with resulting fluid/blood leakage into peritoneum - Presents with severe, unilateral lower abdominal pain - US shows ovarian cyst + serous fluid in pelvis	- Surgery if bleeding continues or unstable
Ovarian Torsion	- Complete or partial rotation of ovary around suspensory ligaments, resulting in ischemia - Risks: Cystic mass (esp > 5 cm) or ovulation induction - Presents as acute onset pelvic pain, adnexal mass, nausea/vomiting - US shows mass, doppler may show limited blood flow	- Ovarian detorsion - Cystectomy - Oophorectomy if fully necrotic

Epithelial Ovarian Neoplasia

General: Majority of primary ovarian neoplasms are epithelial histology. Subtypes include serous (most common), mucinous, clear cell, endometrioid.

Risk:
- ↑ Age, low parity, infertility
- Positive family history (first degree relative), BRCA, Lynch II
- Decreased risk: OCPs, multiparity, breast feeding, chronic anovulation

Clinical:
- Pelvic/abdominal pain, bloating, early satiety adnexal mass
- US: Complex, cystic mass with solid components, thick septations

Diagnosis: Histology after surgical removal

Management:
- Total hysterectomy and salpingo-oophorectomy + lymph node dissection
- Adjuvant chemotherapy in most
- CA-125 surveillance

OVARIAN NEOPLASIA

Gynecology OB-GYN

		General	Clinical	Management
Germ Cell	Dysgerminoma	- Primarily arise in young women (10-30 y/o) - Associated with β-hCG, AFP, LDH production - Tumor of undifferentiated germ cells - LDH, placental AlkPhos production	- Present with abdominal mass or pain - Bleeding, precocious puberty (β-hCG)	- Oophorectomy or cystectomy - Oophorectomy or cystectomy
	Mature Teratoma	- "Dermoid Cyst." Benign, mature tissues of ectodermal, mesodermal, endodermal origin.	- Generally asymptomatic (torsion possible) - TVUS: Characteristic appearance	
	Immature Teratoma	- Immature, trilineage malignancy		
	Yolk Sac Tumor	- AFP elevation		
	Choriocarcinoma	- Nongestational choriocarcinoma is very rare - β-hCG producing	- Precocious puberty (kids) - Postmenopausal bleeding (adults)	
	Embryonal	- Undifferentiated, often part of mixed tumor		
Stromal	Granulosa	- Produce estrogen or Inhibin A or B	- Precocious puberty - Postmenopausal bleeding	- Unilateral oophorectomy (if wish to preserve fertility) - TAH-BSO (adults who complete child bearing)
	Sertoli-Leydig	- Produces androgens	- Virilization	
	Fibroma	- Benign solid stromal neoplasms	- Meigs: Fibroma + ascites + pleural effusion	- Unilateral oophorectomy
Fallopian Tube		- Typically adenocarcinoma derived from tubes	- Latzko's triad: Profuse watery discharge, pelvic pain, mass	- Similar to epithelial ovarian cancer

VULVAR/VAGINAL NEOPLASIA

Gynecology OB-GYN

Vulvar Neoplasia

General: Most commonly squamous cell carcinoma of the vulva

Risk:
- HPV/cervical cancer
- Vulvar lichen sclerosus
- Immunodeficiency
- Smoking

Clinical:
- Mass that can cause pruritus, pain, bleeding
- Varied appearance: Plaque, ulcers, nodular mass all possible

Diagnosis: Biopsy

Management:
- Surgical Excision (partial vulvectomy) +/- lymph node dissection
- Chemotherapy or radiation for advanced disease

Other Histologic Subtypes

Melanoma	- Presents as a black itchy mass, with biopsy revealing proliferation of melanocytes - Treated similarly to vulvar SCC with vulvectomy and LN dissection
Paget's	- Rare, intraepithelial adenocarcinoma of the vulva - Presents with pruritus, erythematous "eczematous" appearing lesion - 20% have coexisting adenocarcinoma elsewhere (ie breast) - Diagnosis and management with biopsy and excision as above

Vaginal Neoplasia

General: Most commonly squamous cell carcinoma of the vagina, with similar risk factors as cervical cancer. Rarely adenocarcinoma or clear cell carcinoma.

Risk:
- HPV, immunosuppression, chronic inflammation
- DES (adenocarcinoma or clear cell carcinoma)

Clinical:
- Presents with vaginal bleeding, discharge, or postcoital bleeding
- Most likely upper 1/3 of vagina

Diagnosis: Biopsy. Colposcopy used if difficulty identifying lesion.

Management:

VAIN (Squamous atypia without invasion)	- Excision, laser ablation, or topical therapy
Stage I (Limited to vaginal wall)	- Local excision
Stage II-IV	- Chemotherapy and/or radiation therapy

BREAST

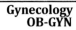
Gynecology OB-GYN

Evaluation of Nipple Discharge

General: Nipple discharge can range from normal lactation, galactorrhea, or pathologic discharge

Etiology	Presentation	Differential Diagnosis
Lactation	- Milk production - Occasionally bloody during pregnancy (benign)	- Pregnancy - Post-partum (up to 6 months after cessation of breastfeeding)
Galactorrhea	- Bilateral milky discharge - Typically white, clear, or straw colored - Caused by hyperprolactinemia	- Chronic breast stimulation (ie from clothing) - Medications (dopamine inhibitory meds) - Prolactinoma - Hypothyroidism
Pathologic	- Usually unilateral production of fluid from single duct - Can be serous or blood tinged	- Intraductal papilloma - Malignancy - Duct ectasia - Mastitis or abscess

Diagnosis:
- Ultrasound +/- mammography (used if > 30 y/o)
- If multi-ductal: Pregnancy test, prolactin, TSH
- Biopsy if mass found

Management:
- Physiologic: Treat underlying, remove meds, etc
- Pathologic: Surgical (duct excision)

Intraductal Papilloma	- Benign proliferation of ductal epithelium - Present with bloody nipple discharge - Dx: Imaging (mammo), following by core needle biopsy - Tx: Excision
Duct Ectasia	- Inflammation and fibrosis of the ductal system - Often presents with green, sticky nipple discharge

Evaluation of New Breast Mass

General: New breast masses can represent benign or malignant processes. Often found on patient self-breast exam.

Etiology: See next page for full DDx

Diagnosis:
- < 30 y/o: Ultrasound +/- mammogram (if highly suspicious)
- > 30 y/o: Mammogram (even if recent normal)
- MRI diagnostically difficult cases

Management:
- Core needle biopsy (generally preferred method for tissue diagnosis)
- FNA: Reasonable alternative if US highly suggestive of simple cyst

BREAST

Gynecology OB-GYN

	General	Clinical	Management
Benign Breast Masses			
Cyst	- Simple Cyst: Simple fluid filled lesion, always benign - Complex Cyst: Also typically benign, but should confirm with FNA, follow with imaging	- Solitary mass, possibly painful Ultrasound: - Simple: Ovoid, homogenous, anechoic - Complex: Thick walled, septated, solid components	- Can observe simple, asymptomatic cysts - FNA (symptomatic or complex) - Surgically remove if recurrent
Fibroadenoma	- Most common benign breast tumor - Slow growing proliferation of epithelial and stromal components	- Well defined, mobile, rubbery mass - US: Well-defined, solid mass - Dx: Core needle biopsy (can also repeat imaging in 3-6 months)	- Reassurance or Surgical Excision
Fibrocystic Changes	- Not a specific condition, but rather a term to describe nonspecific nonproliferative breast lesions (cysts, hyperplasia, etc)	- Bilateral breast swelling, pain, tenderness, lumpiness - Symptoms are often cyclic, worst before menses occurs, improving after menses	- Reassurance - For pain: Supportive bra, NSAIDs - Tamoxifen if severe
Galactocele	- Cystic collections of fluid, usually caused by an obstructed milk duct - Common with breastfeeding	- Soft cystic mass on exam - US shows complex cystic mass - Dx: FNA (resulting in milky substance)	- Reassurance
Fat Necrosis	- Benign lesion that occurs after chest trauma or breast surgery/radiation	- Presents with irregular breast mass - Can appear similar to malignancy on US - Dx: Biopsy (fat, foamy macrophages)	- Reassurance
Malignant Breast Masses			
Phyllodes	- Rare, breast tumors of fibroblast and stromal proliferation	- Large, smooth, irregular, painless mass - Appears smooth, with multiple lobules on mammography - Dx: Core biopsy	- Wide Local Excision

BREAST

Gynecology OB-GYN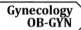

Breast Cancer

General: Most common cancer in women and second most common cause of death. Most commonly derived from epithelial tissues.

Premalignant	
Atypical Ductal Hyperplasia	- Proliferation of atypical ductal cells similar to DCIS but less extensive - Surgical excision is indicated
DCIS	- Premalignant lesion, with atypical ductal cells restricted above the ductal basement membrane
LCIS	- Often found incidentally on breast biopsy performed for some other reason - Premalignant expansion of epithelial cells contained within breast lobules - Most commonly multicentric and bilateral
Malignant	
Invasive Ductal	- Most common type of breast cancer - Cords and nests of cells with possible gland formation
Invasive Lobular	- Single-file cellular infiltrate the mammary stroma and adipose tissue (associated with loss of E-cadherin) - Elevated risk for bilateral disease
Inflammatory	- Extremely aggressive, rapid subtype with dermal lymphatic invasion - Clinically presents with edema, erythema, peau d'orange (dimpling, pitting)
Paget's	- Epidermal spread of malignant ductal cells, resulting in eczematous changes to the nipple - Often concomitant with invasive carcinoma

Risk:

↑ Risk	- Age > 70 (very high relative risk) - BRCA1/2 - Mother or sister with breast cancer - Excess estrogen exposure (Age < 12 at menarche, age > 30 at first birth, age > 55 at menopause, hx of OCP or HRT use) - > 2 EtOH drinks/day
↓ Risk	- Breastfeeding, increased parity, normal BMI, regular exercise

Clinical:
- Early Findings: Single, nontender, firm mass with ill defined margins OR mammographic abnormalities on routine screening
- Late Findings:
    - Regional lymphadenopathy or other metastatic disease
    - Peau D'Orange skin (invasion of dermal lymphatics)
    - Dimpling (tethering of Cooper ligament)

Diagnosis:
- Core needle biopsy (often image guided)
    - Preferred to FNA given higher diagnostic yield, ability to test receptor status (ER/PR/HER2)

BREAST — Gynecology OB-GYN

Management of Breast Cancer

DCIS	- Mastectomy OR - Breast conserving therapy (BCT) (Lumpectomy + Radiation) - Adjuvant hormonal therapy if ER positive (Tamoxifen or Anastrozole)
LCIS	- Observation - Surgically remove those high risk histologic features (ie necrosis)
Early Stage (Stage I, IIA, IIB)	Defined as disease limited to breast with only limited spread to axillary nodes Primary Surgery - Mastectomy OR breast conserving therapy - Sentinel lymph node biopsy (for all), with dissection if positive Note: Large or multifocal disease should undergo mastectomy Adjuvant Therapy - Hormone therapy if ER/PR+ (Tamoxifen) or HER2 + (Trastuzumab) - Chemotherapy (if high risk, ie large tumors or triple negative disease)
Locally Advanced (Stage III, also subset of IIB)	Defined as extension to chest wall/skin, > 5 cm in size, or extensive regional lymphadenopathy - Neoadjuvant Chemotherapy - Surgery (mastectomy or breast conserving therapy)
Metastatic (Stage IV)	- Hormone therapy and/or systemic chemotherapy

BREAST — Gynecology OB-GYN

Screening for Breast Cancer

Age	Screening Recommendation
< 40	- Not indicated for average risk women
40-50	- Guidelines vary by expert group - Overall, an individualized "shared decision making" model is encouraged
50-75	- Screening recommended for all (q2 years) - Note: Frequency is debated and varies between expert groups (q1-2 years)
>75	- Not indicated, unless life expectancy >10 years

High Risk:
- Defined as BRCA mutation +, personal history of ovarian/breast cancer, radiation therapy earlier in life, or strong family history (as determined by risk calculator with > 20% risk)
- Should start screening early with alternating q6 month mammogram/MRI

Modality:
- Mammography (primary modality used for all, including dense breasts)
- Ultrasound (used to follow up certain lesions on mammography)
- MRI (used as adjunct is certain high risk patients)

- Screening clinical or self breast exam: Not indicated

Mammography:

BI-RADS Category	Management	Cancer Risk
0: Incomplete	- Additional imaging	N/A
1: Negative	- Continue routine screening	0%
2: Benign	- Continue routine screening	Near 0%
3: Probably Benign	- 6 month follow up	< 2%
4: Suspicious	- Core needle biopsy	2-95%
5: Highly Suggestive	- Core needle biopsy	> 95%
6: Known Malignancy		N/A

Benign Findings:
- Skin or vascular calcifications
- Eggshell or rim calcifications

Pathologic Findings:
- Clustered, granular microcalcifications
- Fine pleomorphic, linear, or linear-branching calcifications

BREAST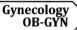

BRCA

General: BRCA1 and 2 genes code for tumor suppressor proteins involved in DNA damage detection and repair (double strand breaks). Autosomal dominant inheritance. Mutations in these genes place patients at risk for malignancy, specifically breast and ovarian, as below.

BRCA 1	- Breast cancer (50-70% risk) - Ovarian cancer (~40% risk)
BRCA 2	- Breast cancer (50-70% risk) - Ovarian cancer (~15% risk) - Male breast and pancreatic cancer

Management:

Screening for Mutation	Indicated if: - Personal history of breast cancer PLUS age < 50, strong family history, or multiple breast cancers in same patient - Family history of BRCA gene variant - > 3 cancers on same side of family (breast, ovarian) - Strong family history (cancer diagnosis at age < 45, > 2 primary breast cancers in an individual or on the same side of family with one < 50)
Screening in BRCA Patient	- Breast Ca: Annual MRI and mammogram, starting at age 25-30 - Ovarian Ca: q6 month ultrasound + CA125, starting at age 30 Note: The above screening is assuming the patient has not undergone risk reducing surgery like mastectomy or BSO
Prophylaxis in BRCA +	Surgical - Bilateral mastectomy (any age per patient preference) - Bilateral salpingo-oophorectomy (age 35-45 after childbearing) Pharm - If no mastectomy, can consider Tamoxifen

OB-GYN PHARM

Gynecology OB-GYN

	Mechanism	Indication	Side Effects/Management
Reproductive Hormones			
Estrogen Ethinyl estradiol	- Estrogen receptor agonists	- Hormone replacement therapy - Contraception	- Increased risk of venous thromboembolism - Increased risk of endometrial cancer
Progestins Levonorgestrel Medroxyprogesterone Etonogestrel Norethindrone	- Progesterone receptor agonists	- Hormone replacement therapy - Contraception	
GnRH Agonists Leuprolide	- GNRH agonist - If used continuously, acts as an antagonist	- Fibroids, endometriosis - Precocious puberty - Infertility (pulsatile) - Prostate cancer	- Menopausal symptoms when used continuously
SERMs			
Clomiphene	- Antagonist at estrogen receptors in hypothalamus	- Infertility	- Hot flashes - Vision changes (blurring, double vision, scotomata) → Warrants discontinuation of therapy
Tamoxifen Raloxifene	- Antagonist of estrogen at breast, but agonist at bone	- ER/PR + breast cancer - Osteoporosis	- Hot flashes - Increased risk of venous thromboembolism
Other Hormone Antagonists			
Mifepristone Ulipristal	- Progesterone receptor antagonist	- Emergency contraception or abortifacients	- Abdominal pain, uterine cramping, and vaginal bleeding
Anastrozole Letrozole	- Aromatase inhibitors	- ER/PR + breast cancer (if postmenopausal)	- Osteoporosis

OBGYN86